The Role of Pregnancy Nutrition
in Maternal and Offspring Health

The Role of Pregnancy Nutrition in Maternal and Offspring Health

Special Issue Editor

Ekaterina Maslova

MDPI • Basel • Beijing • Wuhan • Barcelona • Belgrade

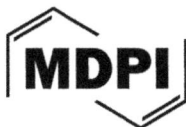

MDPI

Special Issue Editor
Ekaterina Maslova
ICON plc
UK

Editorial Office
MDPI
St. Alban-Anlage 66
4052 Basel, Switzerland

This is a reprint of articles from the Special Issue published online in the open access journal *Nutrients* (ISSN 2072-6643) in 2019 (available at: https://www.mdpi.com/journal/nutrients/special_issues/role_pregnant_health).

For citation purposes, cite each article independently as indicated on the article page online and as indicated below:

LastName, A.A.; LastName, B.B.; LastName, C.C. Article Title. *Journal Name* **Year**, *Article Number, Page Range.*

ISBN 978-3-03921-996-4 (Pbk)
ISBN 978-3-03921-997-1 (PDF)

Contents

About the Special Issue Editor

Ekaterina Maslova is Senior Epidemiologist at ICON plc and holds an Honorary position at the School of Public Health, Imperial College London. Dr. Maslova is a trained nutritional epidemiologist with a track record of publishing on maternal nutrition and offspring chronic disease outcomes using large population-based cohorts and randomized clinical trials. Following the completion of her doctoral degree from the Harvard School of Public Health in 2012, Dr. Maslova went on to do a postdoctoral fellowship at Statens Serum Institut in Copenhagen, Denmark, where she developed her own research agenda examining dietary mitigation of offspring outcomes in high-risk obstetric populations. Dr. Maslova has taught both undergraduate and graduate students at US, Danish, and UK institutions, and continues to supervise master's and PhD students in her field of research.

Preface to "The Role of Pregnancy Nutrition in Maternal and Offspring Health"

In pregnancy, maternal nutrition sustains and nourishes the developing fetus. Imbalances in either the direction of nutritional excess or deficiency can have detrimental consequences for offspring health. Furthermore, a cumulation of research now points to the importance of good pregnancy nutrition beyond immediate fetal outcomes. This includes modifying the risk of offspring outcomes as they enter childhood and adulthood through influences on placental development, hormonal pathways, and organ structure and function. Suboptimal nutrition during the gestational period may also compromise maternal outcomes during pregnancy, some of which have long-term consequences for women's health. There is a clear need to understand the biological and social mechanisms that underpin the development of these outcomes to better target clinical and public health interventions. It is also important to gather insight into population subgroups that may be especially vulnerable to nutritional insults during pregnancy for further personalization of any future interventions. This Special Issue on "The Role of Pregnancy Nutrition in Maternal and Offspring Health" includes etiological and mechanistic studies of pregnancy nutrition with short- and long-term maternal and child health outcomes, including original research, narrative reviews, and systematic reviews and meta-analyses. Together this body of work provide important insights into the influence of dietary patterns, food groups, and nutrients on pregnancy outcomes, and long-term offspring neurodevelopmental, respiratory, and metabolic health. It also highlights the nutritional consequences for specific groups of women, including those with pregnancy complications and eating disorders.

Ekaterina Maslova
Special Issue Editor

nutrients

MDPI

Review

The Effects of Vegetarian and Vegan Diet during Pregnancy on the Health of Mothers and Offspring

Giorgia Sebastiani [1,*], Ana Herranz Barbero [1], Cristina Borrás-Novell [1],
Miguel Alsina Casanova [1], Victoria Aldecoa-Bilbao [1], Vicente Andreu-Fernández [2],
Mireia Pascual Tutusaus [1], Silvia Ferrero Martínez [3], María Dolores Gómez Roig [3] and
Oscar García-Algar [1]

1   Neonatology Unit, Hospital Clinic-Maternitat, ICGON, BCNatal, 08028 Barcelona, Spain;
    HERRANZ@clinic.cat (A.H.B.); CBORRASN@clinic.cat (C.B.-N.); MMALSINA@clinic.cat (M.A.C.);
    VALDECOA@clinic.cat (V.A.-B.); mireiapascualt@gmail.com (M.P.T.); OGARCIAA@clinic.cat (O.G.-A.)
2   Grup de Recerca Infancia i Entorn (GRIE), Institut d'investigacions Biomèdiques August Pi i
    Sunyer (IDIBAPS), 08028 Barcelona, Spain; VIANDREU@clinic.cat
3   BCNatal | Barcelona Center for Maternal Fetal and Neonatal Medicine Hospital Sant Joan de Déu,
    08028 Barcelona, Spain; sferrero@sjdhospitalbarcelona.org (S.F.M.);
    lgomezroig@sjdhospitalbarcelona.org (M.D.G.R.)
*   Correspondence: GSEBASTI@clinic.cat; Tel.: +34-610602714

Received: 30 January 2019; Accepted: 1 March 2019; Published: 6 March 2019

Abstract: Vegetarian and vegan diets have increased worldwide in the last decades, according to the knowledge that they might prevent coronary heart disease, cancer, and type 2 diabetes. Althought plant-based diets are at risk of nutritional deficiencies such as proteins, iron, vitamin D, calcium, iodine, omega-3, and vitamin B12, the available evidence shows that well planned vegetarian and vegan diets may be considered safe during pregnancy and lactation, but they require a strong awareness for a balanced intake of key nutrients. A review of the scientific literature in this field was performed, focusing specifically on observational studies in humans, in order to investigate protective effects elicited by maternal diets enriched in plant-derived foods and possible unfavorable outcomes related to micronutrients deficiencies and their impact on fetal development. A design of pregestational nutrition intervention is required in order to avoid maternal undernutrition and consequent impaired fetal growth.

Keywords: vegetarian diets; vegan diets; plant-based diets; nutrition; pregnancy; breastfeeding; human milk; micronutrients; fetal development

1. Introduction

Balanced maternal nutrition during pregnancy is imperative for the mother's health status and, consequently, for offspring, and is crucial to maintain an adequate environment for optimal fetal development. According to the theory of "early life programming" environmental factors and lifestyle during pregnancy determine the risk of developing chronic diseases later in life and also influence lifelong health in offspring [1]. Pregnancy requires an increased intake of macro and micronutrients and balanced diet. For that, it offers a critical window of opportunity to acquire dietetic habits that are beneficial for fetal healthy [2].

Pre-pregnancy and pregnancy adherence to food-safety recommendations, according to the updated Dietary Guidelines for American and Mediterranean Diet, should avoid inadequate levels of key nutrients and micronutrients (proteins, iron, folic acid, vitamin D, calcium, iodine, omega-3, and vitamin B12) that may predispose the offspring to chronic condition later in life such as obesity, diabetes, cardiovascular disease, and neurodevelopmental delays [3].

The percentage of vegetarians and vegans in the general population has increased over the last years partly due to evidence that vegetarianism is linked to improved health. Thus, cohort data have shown that low-fat diets enriched with fruit, vegetables, and fiber can lead to a reduction of risk factors for coronary heart diseases, a better lipid profile [4], lower body mass index (BMI) [5], and lower blood pressure [6]. In addition vegetarian diets appear to prevent cancer and type 2 diabetes [7,8]. Nevertheless, some data suggest that vegetarians and vegans may be at greater risk of increased plasma homocysteine levels, an arising risk factor for cardiovascular disease [9,10], and of low bone mineral density, which predisposes to osteoporosis [11]. Plant-based diets are reported to contain less saturated fatty acids, animal protein and cholesterol, and more folate, fibre, antioxidants, phytochemicals, and carotenoids. However, plant-based diets have a low content of essential micronutrients such as iron, zinc, vitamin B 12, vitamin D, omega-3 (*n*-3) fatty acids, calcium, and iodine. Consequently, the risk of adverse effects due to micronutrient deficiencies that lead to the risk of malnutrition should not be underestimated [12].

The reasons for choosing a vegetarian or vegan lifestyle are variable and range from evidence-based health consciousness to environmental concerns, socioeconomic considerations, ethical grounds, or spiritual/religious beliefs. Medical reasons also exist in some occasions; for instance, women of childbearing age affected by chronic kidney disease (CKD) may be conditioned to the choice of low-protein vegetarian diet [13]. According to the American Dietetic Association, well planned vegetarian diets are safe for all age groups and in all physiological conditions, including childhood, adolescence, pregnancy, and lactation [12,14]. On the contrary, the German Nutrition Society does not recommend vegetarian or vegan diets during pregnancy, lactation, and childhood, due to the inadequate supply of essential nutrients [15].

Vegetarian diets typically comprise of plant foods such as grains, legumes, nuts, seeds, vegetables, and fruit, and exclude all kinds of animal food including meat (pork, beef, mutton, lamb, poultry, game, and fowl), meat products (sausages, salami, and pâté), fish, mollusks, and crustaceans. Vegetarian diets usually include dairy products like eggs and honey. Accordingly, there are two main directions:

(1) Lacto-ovo-vegetarianism (LOV). This excludes meat but includes dairy products, eggs, and honey, together with a wide variety of plant foods. Subcategories are lacto-vegetarianism (LV), which excludes eggs, and ovo-vegetarianism (OV), which excludes dairy products.
(2) Veganism (VEG), which excludes meat, dairy products, eggs, and honey, but includes a wide variety of plant foods [16].

However, some people adhere to other plant-based diets that limit the foods consumed:

- Raw food diet: consisting exclusively of vegetables, including sprouted cereals and pulses, fresh and dried fruits, and seeds, as well as milk and eggs, all of which are mainly eaten raw.
- Fruit diet: consisting exclusively of fresh and dried fruits, seeds, and some vegetables.
- Macrobiotic diet: the strictly vegetarian version of this diet consists of cereals, pulses, vegetables, seaweed, and soy products; while dairy products, eggs, and some vegetables are avoided. Fish is consumed by people who adhere to a macrobiotic diet.

Despite the concrete definition of such categories there is a wide variety of dietary pattern. Vegetarians can be divided into other subgroups: semivegetarians, who are defined as consuming red meat and poultry once per month or more and all meats—including fish—once per month or more, but no more than once per week; pesco-vegetarians, who consume fish once per month or more but all other meats less than once per month; lacto-vegetarians, who consume eggs and dairy once per month or more, but fish and other meats less tan once per month; and lastly, vegans or strict vegetarians are defined as those who do not consume eggs, dairy, or fish [16].

In Europe and North America vegetarians are LOV [17], while Asian Indian vegetarians are mostly lacto-vegetarians [18]. Moreover, it has been described that Chinese vegetarians consume considerably smaller amount of dairy products than Western vegetarians [19].

In 2006, approximately 2.3% of the US adult population (4.9 million people) strictly followed a vegetarian diet, asserting that they never ate meat, fish, or poultry. In 2012 the percentage increased to 5%. Approximately 1.4–2% of the US adult population is vegan [20]. The percentage of young people who are vegetarian is still higher (6–11%), with similar levels of vegetarian teenagers reported in both the United Kingdom and Australia [21]. On the basis of dietary recall data from the 1999–2004 National Health and Nutrition Examination Survey (NHANES), 7.5% of American women were reported adhering to a vegetarian diet [22]. The distribution of women of childbearing age who follow a vegetarian diet is different between developed and developing countries. In developing countries, the prevalence of vegetarian diet may increase due to poverty and economic reasons. In India, 20–30% of the total population is considered to be vegetarian for religious reasons, but normally they do not eat meat because of economic causes. In developed countries, vegetarians comprehend more women than men, and tend to be of higher educational or socioeconomic status, with low probabilities to plan children, and generally they are under 40 years of age. There are also variations between ethnic groups. In the United Kingdom, people of non-White ethnic origin are more likely to indicate themselves as vegetarian than white (15% vs. 6% of white respondents) [23].

Despite the assessment of the importance of a healthy diet in pregnancy, data have demonstrated that women don't change diet during pregnancy, so optimal preconception dietary pattern is determinant for a healthy pregnancy [24]. In addition, the period of lactation is extremely important for growing patterns of infants and the effectiveness of breastfeeding depends on maternal nutritional status. The lack of macro- and micronutrient intake during lactation may lead to the reduction of micronutrients and energy content in breast milk that could lead to severe illness in breastfed infant [25].

The aim of this narrative review was to analyze the existing studies in humans focused on the effects of vegetarian (LOV) and vegan (VEG) diets during pregnancy on maternal outcomes and nutritional status and on fetal healthiness and complications, valuing the risks and benefits of such nutritional choice. Moreover our aim was to study the period of lactation and breast milk composition of vegetarian and vegan mothers and if the breastfeeding is safe for optimal child growth, because there are no specific clinical guidelines about lactation for vegetarian mothers. The publications reviewed in this paper mainly concern plant-based diets as LOV and VEG. Consequently, the results mainly pertain to these diets, which are generally defined as "vegetarian". We did not assess studies about raw food, fruit, and macrobiotic diets. A research for English written articles was performed using MEDLINE/PubMed/Cochrane databases (since 2000 up to 31 December 2018). The research was based on the combination of the following keywords: vegetarian diet, vegan diet, plant-based nutrition, pregnancy outcomes, fetal development, vegetarian/vegan, and breastfeeding/human milk, combined with words related to nutritional status and to the nutrients of interest (protein, vitamin B12, folate, calcium, iron, zinc, iodine, and *n*-3 fatty acids). Studies were identified and examined for methodology and key results. Researches about preconception period were also analyzed. Review team members screened titles and abstracts and selected articles that seemed pertinent to the topics, excluding those not in English or not concerned with humans. The full papers were read to select potentially eligible articles and to assess the scientific merit and relevance of each paper valued. The manuscripts were also analyzed according with the type of study (case–control, review, longitudinal cohort, and cross-sectional), type of diets, number of cases, and possible bias. We performed a narrative review because we expected high heterogeneity of results and lack of randomised trials in pregnant vegetarians in the literature. We included American Dietetic Association Guidelines in pregnancy and International Guidelines for vegetarian and vegan diets; moreover, we also included scientific papers about the nutritional status of mothers, reflecting fetal nutrition and possible detrimental effects on fetal development. We included few data before 2000, only those with crucial results.

Especially, our main goal was to highlight if vegetarian or vegan diets could be considered safe for the mother's health and for offspring during pregnancy and lactation. We also focused on the effect of these dietary patterns on the lack of micronutrients in order to find a target therapy that could avoid fetal complication.

2. Review

2.1. International Guidelines for a Healthy Nutrition in Pregnancy: Omnivores and Vegetarians (see Table S1)

Pregnancy is a critical period during which the mother requires different amount of nutrients for healthy gestation, in order to promote optimal fetal development and to avoid the "reprogramming" of fetal tissue, predisposing the infant to lifelong chronic conditions [26]. Preconception body mass index (BMI) is determinant to avoid adverse outcomes during pregnancy. Overweight and caloric excess are related to maternal and fetal health risk including diabetes, preeclampsia and cardiovascular disease, so gestational weight gain during pregnancy must be kept into the normal range recommended [27]. On the contrary, low BMI and malnourished mothers could impair fetal development and nutrients supply, leading to adverse birth outcomes, physical and cognitive delays in childhood, and metabolic disorders in adulthood [28].

In the course of normal gestation plasma volume expands, producing a decrease of vitamins and minerals concentrations; however, plasma lipids and cholesterol arise. During early gestation the fat stores of mothers increase, whereas the last gestation is characterized by increased insulin resistance: these are metabolic changes essential to support fetal growth [29].

According to the 2015–2020 Dietary Guidelines for Americans (DGA), pregnant women have to consume a variety of foods to maintain energy and nutrient requirements and to gain recommended amounts of weight. According to the Dietary Reference Intakes (DRIs) and Institute of Medicine (IOM), caloric necessities are no higher than the estimated energy requirement for nonpregnant women until the second trimester. The extra energy requirement per day is 340 kcal in the second trimester and 452 kcal in the third trimester (IOM), or 260 kcal and 500 kcal, respectively (according to European Food Safety Authority—EFSA) [30,31]. The Guidelines recommend practicing moderate intensity physical activity during pregnancy for benefits to both the mother and fetus [32].

All pregnant women need appropriate nutritional supplementation. Iron supplementation is essential for iron deficiency anemia during gestation [33]. Folic acid consumption of 600 mcg/day from fortified foods and dietary supplements is needed to avoid neural tube defects (NTD) [34]. In addition adequate levels of vitamin D (600 UI/day), choline (450 mg/day), and iodine (220 mcg/day) are needed for normal fetal growth and brain development [35–37]. During a normal pregnancy the efficiency of calcium absorption increases, so the intake of calcium is equal to a nonpregnant woman of the same age. During pregnancy and lactation, adequate calcium intake is considered to be 1000 mg/day. Women with calcium intakes less than 500 mg/day need additional amounts to achieve maternal and fetal bone requirements [38]. Supplementary Materials Table S1 shows the daily nutrients requirements of the principal macro- and micronutrients during pregnancy and lactation, as well as a comparison between the American Guidelines, IOM, EFSA, and International Federation of Gynecology and Obstetrics (FIGO) [39,40].

The Physicians Committee for Responsible Medicine suggests that vegetarian pregnant women have to follow the recommendations for protein intake and should increase up to 25 g of protein each day to reach 1.1 g/kg/day as in pregnancy the demand of protein increases [40,41]. The recommendations are to consume daily portions of dark green vegetables (1–2 servings), other vegetables and fruits (4–5 servings), bean and soy products (3–4 servings), whole grains (six or more servings), and nuts, seeds, and wheat germ (1–2 servings). Vegetarians should include sources of protein, iron, and vitamin B-12 intake, as well as calcium and vitamin D if avoiding milk products. Charts listed in these guidelines are useful for substituting beans, tofu, nuts, eggs, and seeds for meats, and include alternative food sources for calcium if milk and dairy products are rejected [3,41].

2.2. International Guidelines for Vegetarian and Vegan Diets

According to the Academy of Nutrition and Dietetics a well planned plant-based eating pattern could be appropriate for all stages of life if adequate and healthy recommendations are followed. For example, in the vegetarian population, if the diet includes a variety of plant products, it would provide the same protein quality as a diet that included meat. Venti et al. provided a modified food guide pyramid for vegetarian and vegan diets [42]. According to these recommendations, the normal intake of protein is 0.8 g/kg/day for an adult woman who follows diets containing high quality protein such as egg, meat, milk, or fish. If dairy products, whole grains, beans, nuts, and seeds are the primary protein sources in the diet, the protein digestibility falls, so the recommendation for dietary protein should increase 20% for vegetarian adult woman until 1 g/kg/day. The protein quality of foods is assessed by their Protein Digestibility Corrected Amino Acid Score (PDCAAS), which measures the score for amino acid digestibility. Values close to 1 correspond to animal products supplying all nine essential amino acids, while values below 0.7 are typical of plant foodstuffs. Even if the score is lower, the combination of more vegetable foods with different amino acid composition could enhance the overall quality of their protein component [31].

According to Messina's guide for North American vegetarians, this population have to consume more legumes, nuts, tofu, beans, seeds, fortified breakfast cereals, milk, cheese or yogurt, and fortified soymilk, which are good sources of vitamin B12, vitamin D, iron, and calcium (the recommendation is the intake of 1200 to 1500 mg/day of calcium, 20% more than omnivores). People who adhere to vegan diets would have to intake daily supplements of vitamin D, vitamin B12, and calcium because the average of these nutrients is insufficient [43].

Although the vegetarian and vegan population tries to compensate the adequate intake of micronutrients, these types of diets limit their amounts. Alfa-linolenic acid (omega-3 or ALA) derives from foods such as flax seeds, chia seeds, mungo beans, walnuts, and canola and soybean oils, so vegetarians consume an abundance of ALA. One teaspoonful of walnuts, soybeans, and mungo beans or one teaspoonful of flaxseed oil or ground flaxseed will supply the daily requirement of ALA. High temperature damages this oil, so it should not be fried. Linoleic acid (n-6 or LA) is derived from nuts, seeds, leafy vegetables, grains, and vegetable oils (corn, safflower, sesame, and sunflower). Unsaturated fatty acids are crucial for cell membrane function and the production of eicosanoids (thromboxanes, leukotrienes, prostaglandins, and prostacyclins). LA (*n*-6) is converted to arachidonic acid (AA) and ALA (*n*-3) is converted to eicosapentaenoic acid (EPA) and docosahexaenoic acid (DHA). High intake of LA (*n*-6) inhibits the synthesis of DHA from ALA (*n*-3). Consequently, a balanced ratio intake of *n*-6 and *n*-3 as 1:2 or 1:3 would be most advantageous for vegetarians. To improve the conversion of ALA to more physiologically active fatty acids like EPA and DHA is essential for the development of brain and nervous system. Vegetarians should guarantee that their diet contains sufficient proteins, pyridoxine, biotin, calcium, copper, magnesium, and zinc. In addition, they should reduce intake of n-6 fatty acids and trans fatty acids that inhibit such conversion, by limiting consumption of processed and deep-fried foods, and alcohol [44]. However, people who adhere to vegetarian or vegan diets steadily show low plasma EPA or DHA, especially vegans compared to nonvegetarians [45].

Moreover vegetarian diets have been associated with iron deficiency but not to iron deficiency anemia so the recommendation for vegetarians is to enrich the diet with iron-fortified breads and cereals, beans and lentils, raisins, and blackstrap molasses, as well as sources of vitamin C, like tomatoes and citrus fruits for optimal iron absorption, cooked in cast iron pans [46]. The iron from vegetarian diets is less available for absorption because these diets contain nonheme iron from plants that is worst absorbed than heme iron contained in animal food like meat. In contrast the absorption of nonheme iron in vegetarian people is high to compensate low body iron stores compared to nonvegetarians. The mean iron absorption from a vegetarian diet is estimated 10% compared to 18% of a diet containing meat. Moreover, nonheme iron absorption is inhibited by whole grains, legumes, and nuts because they contain phytic acid so a balanced diet is needed [47]. Zinc deficiency is also common in people who adhere to vegetarian diets due to the inhibition of zinc absorption from plant food with phytic acid, an inhibitor of zinc bioavailability, so the recommendation is a 50% greater intake of zinc [48]. Calcium intake is high in LOV but vegans show low intake of calcium than recommended. Calcium can be found in low-oxalate (high bioavailability) foods such as bokchoi, broccoli, Chinese cabbage, collards, kale, okra, turnip greens, and soy products. Other foods with slightly less calcium bioavailability are fortified soymilk, sesame seeds, almonds, and red and white beans. Calcium bioavailability from plant foods can be affected by oxalates and phytates, which are inhibitors of calcium absorption; for example spinach and rhubarb have a low calcium bioavailability, whereas kale, broccoli, and bokchoi have high calcium bioavailability. Another important calcium source is water, in particular, hard water that has high calcium and magnesium levels derived from groundwater, particularly from limestone and dolomite [31]. If dietary intake of calcium is low, calcium supplemention should be recommended in divided doses [49–51].

Low vitamin D is the most common deficiency among LOV and vegan people so they may need sun exposure, food fortified with vitamin D, and daily supplements to maintain adequate serum levels. Good sources of vitamin D are found in fish liver oils, fatty fish, and egg yolks, but vitamin content in these foods varies. However, reaching adequate levels of vitamin D from fortified foods is a challenge for vegans because few plant foods are fortified with this vitamin. In such cases, especially in vegan population, vitamin D supplements seem to be the most adequate way to ensure correct vitamin D status [52].

Vegetarian diets are at serious risk of vitamin B12 depletion and/or deficiency, an essential micronutrient that plays a specific role in the synthesis of DNA and red blood cell division and in one carbon metabolism. Vitamin B12 is an essential nutrient that transfers the methyl group in a methionine synthase-requiring reaction, converting homocysteine to methionine. It is essential for the synthesis of energy in mitochondria and for erythropoiesis in the bone marrow. In addition, it is also necessary for the synthesis of myelin and the maintenance of neural axons. Vitamin B12, also called cobalamin, is found in adequate ranges only in animal and dairy foods. If the consumption of animal foods is absent as seen in vegetarian diets it results in low intake and cobalamin deficiency due to its scarce presence in plant foods, although vegetarians consume some fortified foods as cereals and soy products. This deficiency generates hematological alterations, impairment of erythropoiesis, and neurologically-poor outcomes as it plays a key role in neuronal myelinization [53]. The DRI for Vitamin B12 is 2.4 µg/day for adults [54]. The European Food Safety Authority (EFSA) Panel on Dietetic Products, Nutrition and Allergies established an Adequate Intake (AI) of cobalamin nearly 4 µg/day for adults [55]. A high intake of plant-based foods may result in high folate levels, which may cause vitamin B-12 depletion by rectifying the hematologic alterations that are present with vitamin B12 insufficiency. A high prevalence of deficiency, assessed by methylmalonic acid and/or holotranscobalamin II levels, is frequent among vegetarians, and a high prevalence of increased concentration of homocysteine. Vegan subjects reported the most compromised status of vitamin B12 because they do not consume eggs, yoghurt, cheese, and milk, which are natural sources of cobalamin. Chronic low intake of vitamin B12 can lead to a depletion status, and this progressive deficiency may become clinically evident after years, resulting in permanent neurologic damage [56–58].

2.3. The Effects of Vegetarian and Vegan Diets during Pregnancy on Maternal Nutritional Profile (see Table S2)

Vegetarian and vegan diets have been considered a nutritional challenge during pregnancy, and they require strong awareness to achieve complete intake of essential nutrients, as such, these diets are at risk of nutritional deficiencies. As described, several studies have demonstrated the insufficient supply of essential nutrients such as vitamin B12, vitamin D, calcium, zinc, iron, proteins, essential fatty acids, and iodine in vegetarian and vegan diets [46]. Here we discuss the published evidence of the effect of plant food diets on maternal nutritional profile. The choice of vegetarian or vegan diet is always in preconception, period so well adjusted preconception nutrition is essential for healthy pregnancy. The nutritional pattern depends on the socioeconomic status of the mother, ethnicity, and the reason for choosing vegetarian diets. If the choice is not cultural but is due to ethical beliefs and good socioeconomic status, the probability of a balanced diet increases [59]. In a case–control poblational study called the KOALA Birth Cohort Study (a prospective cohort of 2834 mother–infant pairs in the Netherlands), vegetarian pregnant women who chose organic foods, had higher education and calculated good intake of macro- and micronutrients for a balanced diet [60]. In the same cohort, vegetarian pregnant women had lower BMI if compared to women following a conventional dietary pattern, and lower prevalence of overweight and obesity 4–5 years after delivery [61]. Generally it is difficult to verify the effect of such diets and to separate them from other determinant factors such as ethnicity, lifestyles, or smoking.

2.3.1. Vitamin B12

A recent review shows that there is a high prevalence of vitamin B12 depletion or deficiency among vegetarians [62]. During pregnancy the intestinal absorption of vitamin B12 increases; absorption is better in small amounts and frequent intervals as fetal needs are not high. Vitamin B12 derived from maternal tissue stores does not cross the placenta, but the absorbed vitamin B12 is transferred across the placenta. Low maternal serum concentration of vitamin B12 during the first trimester is a risk factor for NTD and poor maternal outcomes such as preeclampsia, macrocytic anemia, and neurological impairment [63]. The estimated average requirement (EAR) of vitamin B12 is 2.2 μg/day for pregnancy and 2.4 μg/day for lactation [39]. Many people with vitamin B12 deficiency present signs of clinical anemia or mild anemia. The macrocytosis may be masked by a concomitant disorder, such as iron deficiency, thalassemias, or typical high folate levels in vegetarian women [63]. Dietary deficiency of vitamin B12 is frequent in some developing countries or population with marginal status like India, the Middle East, Africa, China, and Central America [64].

In the prospective PREFORM study in Toronto (*n* = 368), the prevalence of suboptimal B12 status (serum total B12 <210 pmol/L) was 35% at 12–16 gestational weeks and 43% at delivery; the prevalence of B12 deficiency (serum total B12 <148 pmol/L) was 17% and 38%, respectively. Maternal dietary vitamin B12 intake during pregnancy was weakly associated with maternal vitamin B12 levels [65]. Another prospective longitudinal study conducted during pregnancy showed that the prevalence of B12 deficiency increased between the second and third trimester from 8% to 35% in healthy pregnant women with B12 intake >RDA (2.6 μg/day). This decrement of plasma total B12 during pregnancy could be the consequence of increased metabolic rate, active B12 transport across the placenta, and hemodilution [66], so it is important to distinguish if very low serum vitamin B12 in pregnancy represents a true deficiency or an exaggerated physiological fall.

Koebnick et al., in a longitudinal cohort study, compared serum vitamin B12 and homocysteine concentrations in pregnant women consuming a LOV diet, low meat diet (LMD = <300 g/wk), or a diet with larger amounts of meat (>300 g/wk). Dietary vitamin B12 intake, serum levels of vitamin B12, and plasma total homocysteine concentrations were measured once in each trimester. This data included 27 pregnant LOV, 43 pregnant low meat consumers and 39 pregnant controls who consumed more meat as a 'Western diet' (WD). The following criteria were used to consider "low serum concentration of vitamin B12"; <130 pmol/L in the first trimester, <120 pmol/L in the second trimester, and <100 pmol/L in the third trimester. The prevalence of B12 deficiency, based on these cutoffs in at least one trimester, was found to be 39% of LOV, 9% of low-meat eaters, and 3% of the control group. Also, the odds ratio of having a low serum B12 during at least one trimester was 3.9 (95% confidence interval, 1.9–6.1) times higher among LOV and 1.8 (1.0–3.9) times higher among low meat consumers compared with the odds among women of control group. The deficiency rate for women was 33% in the first trimester, 17% in the second, and 39% in the third trimesters. The limitations of this study are that the sample did not include vegan participants, the inclusion of a small population, and that some comparisons were more cross-sectional than longitudinal due to the study design. Moreover high folate intake and folate supplementation during pregnancy may cover the real effects of low vitamin B12 intake on plasma. The higher deficiency in vegetarian pregnant women in the third trimester pointed out a depletion of vitamin B12 stores instead of expanded blood volume.

The authors recommend a higher intake of vitamin B-12 of more than 3.0 mcg/daily for pregnant women consuming a LOV diet [67].

Gibson et al. conducted a cross-sectional study in 99 pregnant women from Ethiopia and included participants whose diet was based on either maize (*Zea mays* L.) and fermented enset (*Enset ventricosum*) products that are the major staple foods consumed. As in the Sidama Zone of Southern Ethiopia, animal products often provide <1% of total energy, this low intake of animal products is coincident with infections and bacterial overgrowth, meaning that pregnant women in Sidama are at high risk of vitamin B-12 deficiency and possibly of folate deficiency. They described that 23% of pregnant women had low plasma vitamin B12 (<150 pmol/L), but 62% had elevated plasma methylmalonic acid (MMA) (>271 nmol/L). None had elevated plasma cystathionine or total homocysteine. Even though they were diagnosed with vitamin B-12 deficiency, there were no signs of macrocytic anemia. This data was limited by the small sample and it was conducted in a specific population [68]. In a cross-sectional study conducted in 284 Canadian pregnant women in Vancouver, the authors found that pregnant South Asian women had suboptimal B12 status (11.5%) or B12 deficiency (61.5%) and showed more MMA plasma concentrations. Plasma total B12 concentration was positively associated with age, education, and B12 supplements. Pre-pregnancy BMI was the strongest independent predictor of plasma total B12 concentration. One limitation of this data was the absence of a dietary assessment to quantify B12 intake, as this specific population promoted vegetarianism [69]. A study conducted in small sample of pregnant Indian women showed that hyperhomocystinemia leads to global DNA hypermethylation in vegetarian population due to low dietary intake of vitamin B-12 during pregnancy and that this could predispose to cardiovascular risk and obesity [70]. All these studies provide evidence that vegetarian and vegan pregnant women are at high risk of vitamin B12 depletion.

On the contrary, a longitudinal case–control study recruited 109 participants and showed that high folate intake in LOV pregnant women and low risk of folate deficiency [71].

2.3.2. Vitamin D and Calcium

Plasma levels of vitamin D during pregnancy depend on sunlight exposure and intake of foods high in vitamin D, fortified foods, or supplements. During pregnancy there is not an increment of vitamin D requirements. Vitamin D deficiencies exist among the general population, especially those with dark skin and vegetarians. Data from the third NHANES indicate that ~42% of African American women and 4% of white women show vitamin D insufficiency [72]. Vegan diets have shown lower average intakes of vitamin D than lacto-vegetarians and omnivores [73]. Sachan et al. performed a cross-sectional data describing the levels of serum vitamin D, calcium, and parathormone (PTH) in 207 urban and rural pregnant women (84.3% of urban and 83.6% of rural women). They found vitamin D values below the cutoff (<22.5 ng/mL) and low calcium intake in the population who does not consume meat. In this study, 14% of the mothers had biochemical osteomalacia [74]. Another data found similar results in Iranian pregnant women at the delivery [75]. Dasgupta et al. recruited a total of 50 pregnant female aged 20–40 years of the Northern Eastern Part of India and assessed vitamin D during the first trimester. Nearly 42% of the cases had vitamin D deficiency and 14% had vitamin D insufficiency in the first trimester; 63.63% who had 25(OH)D levels <20 ng/mL were vegetarians. They did not find any association between vitamin D levels and multivitamin supplements or dietary calcium intake [76]. These studies were limited by the recruitment of a specific population.

During pregnancy and lactation, adequate calcium intake is considered to be 1000 mg/day. Vegetarians and vegans should consume 1200 to 1500 mg/day of calcium, 20% more than omnivores. Pregnant and lactating women should consume a minimum of eight servings of calcium-rich foods [12].

Despite recommendations about a good intake during pregnancy, vegetarian pregnant women are at high risk of vitamin D deficiency and may suffer bone impairment, osteoporosis, and hypocalcemia [77]. In a population-based cross-sectional survey conducted in Shaanxi Province in Northwest China, pregnant women who followed a vegetarian pattern had low calcium intake [78].

2.3.3. Iron

During pregnancy, mild anemia is physiologic as a consequence of the normal hemodilution status. During the second and third trimesters of pregnancy there is a rise in maternal blood volume and iron transportation to the placenta and fetus, showing an increased necessity for iron. Iron absorption from plant (nonheme) and animal (heme) supply is improved during pregnancy and increases with each trimester. Inhibitors of iron absorption include calcium, coffee, and fiber. Vitamin C can help to enhance absorption by reducing the inhibitory effects of phytate. [79,80]. The average of dietary iron needed in pregnancy is dependent on maternal preconception stores and estimated requirements are shown in Table S1.

A systematic review and meta-analysis showed that vegetarian population exhibits lower stores of iron compared to nonvegetarian [81]. In pregnant vegetarian women the results are controversial. A British study, conducted in a cohort of 1274 pregnant women aged 18–45 years, showed that vegetarians had adequate iron intakes from diet and they followed the recommended iron supplementation during the first and second trimesters of pregnancy more than nonvegetarians [82]. Sharma et al. described a high prevalence of anemia in Indian pregnant women because of very low frequency of meat eating. However, this study was cross-sectional and limited to a specific population [83].

2.3.4. Essential Fatty Acids

LA (*n*-6) and ALA (*n*-3) are polyunsaturated fatty acids which are obtained from food sources. LA (*n*-6) is converted to arachidonic acid (AA), and ALA is converted to EPA and DHA. DHA is an important component of neural and retinal membranes. It accumulates in the brain and retina during the end of gestation and early postnatal life. Polyunsaturated fatty acids are transferred via the placenta to the developing fetus from the mother's plasma. Adequate provision of DHA is thought to be essential for optimal visual and neurologic development during early life [84]. A significant percentage of women of childbearing age in Europe are vegetarian and the majority of the population in countries such as India. This group is particularly at risk as the exclusion of meat or fish from the diet may determine very low intakes of DHA. According to a more comprehensive database and improved questionnaire, vegetarian women can achieve higher intakes of DHA (30 mg/day) [85]. For example, women consuming diets with marine products or eating marine oil supplements can reach very high intakes of DHA (>1000 mg/day). The adequate ingestion of DHA is especially important in the last stage of pregnancy as placenta is able to channel the uptake of DHA to the fetus [86].

The literature regarding DHA levels in pregnancy is limited. Pregnant and lactating women increase the necessity of a source of preformed DHA. Lower proportions of DHA have been found in the fetal plasma of vegetarian mothers if compared with mothers who are omnivores [87].

2.3.5. Zinc

Zinc is less bioavailable and it is likely to be present in lower ranges when obtained from plant-derived compared to animal food sources [47]. Vegetarians usually have lower zinc consumption compared with omnivores and their serum zinc levels are lower but in the normal range [88].

During pregnancy the need of Zinc increases so women are encouraged to enhance the intake of zinc and adopting food preparation methods which improve its absorption (soaking, germination fermentation, and sourdough leavening of bread) and reduce phytate levels in zinc rich foods [89].

Although high zinc intake is essential during pregnancy, the consequences of zinc deficiency are not described, so it has been postulated that the body adapts the absorption according to the average intake [90]. The current recommendation of dietary intake for zinc in pregnant women aged 19–50 years is 11 mg/day [48]. A meta-analysis compared the dietary zinc intake of pregnant vegetarian and nonvegetarian (NV) groups: the zinc intake of vegetarians was found to be lower than that of NV (-1.38 ± 0.35 mg/day; $p < 0.001$); the exclusion of low meat eaters from the analysis revealed a greater difference (-1.53 ± 0.44 mg/day; $p = 0.001$). Neither vegetarian nor NV groups met the recommended dietary allowance (RDA) for zinc. In contrast, the evidence evaluated in this systematic review suggests that there is no difference between groups in biomarkers of zinc status (concentrations of zinc in serum/plasma, urine, and hair) or in functional outcomes associated with pregnancy (period of gestation and birth weight) [91].

2.3.6. Iodine, Magnesium

Vegetarian or vegan diets may result in low iodine intake because the main dietary sources of iodine are meat, fish, and dairy products, but iodine in the salt could avoid the risk of deficiency [92].

An adequate magnesium status during pregnancy is essential for fetal development. Serum magnesium levels physiologically decrease during pregnancy due to high demand, higher renal excretion, and haemodilution. In a longitudinal study conducted in 108 healthy pregnant women, significant higher dietary magnesium intakes were observed in pregnant women consuming a plant-based diet (508,714 mg/day for LOV and 504,711 mg/day for low-meat eaters) than in pregnant women consuming a control diet (41,279 mg/day). Urinary magnesium excretion was higher in LOV, followed by low-meat eaters, when compared to the control group [93]. So vegetarian or vegan diets result in high magnesium levels.

2.3.7. Proteins

Proteins demand during pregnancy and lactation increases up to 71 g/day (1.1–1.2 g/kg/day) compared to 46 g/day (0.8 g/kg/day) for nonpregnant women. Protein deposition in maternal and fetal tissues increases throughout pregnancy, much more during the third trimester. Enhanced protein synthesis occurs, combined with decreased amino acid catabolism and urea synthesis. The increment of circulating plasma amino acids is a conservation mechanism for retention of protein during a period of increased demand. Additional protein is needed in pregnancy to reach the estimated 21 g/day deposited in fetal, placental, and maternal tissues during the second and third trimesters. Proteins derived from plants are sufficient to reach these needs. Legumes, nuts, tofu, and eggs are good sources of proteins. Soy protein can reach adequate protein needs as animal protein. Cereals content is low in lysine, so this essential amino acid can be acquired by the intake of more beans and soy products. An increase in all sources of protein can compensate a low lysine average [63]. Pregnant women who adhere to vegan diet are at higher risk of protein deficiency so additional protein is indicated for the vegan diet in the second and third trimesters: 25 g of protein may be added by including 1.5 cups of lentils or 2.5 cups of soy milk per day [94].

2.4. The Effects of Vegetarian and Vegan Diets during Pregnancy on Mother's Health (see Table S3)

2.4.1. Preeclampsia (PE)

Studies about the effects of vegetarian and vegan diet on maternal outcome have yielded incongruent results. The most ancient retrospective data conducted by Carter et al. [95], in 775 vegan mothers in "the Farm"—a vegan community in Summertown, Tennessee—reported only one case of preeclampsia (0.13%).

PE may be caused by a relative prostacyclin deficiency secondary to an excessive production of thromboxane A2. A vegan diet (low in AA) might provide protection against this condition, especially if the conversion of LA to AA is inhibited by decreased activity of the enzyme delta-6-desaturase. Another observational prospective study enrolled 1.538 pregnant Washington state residents and used food frequency questionnaire (FFQ) to assess maternal dietary intake three months before and during pregnancy [96]. They reported that dietary fiber might reduce dyslipidaemia, a condition related to PE. In the group of fiber intake the relative risk (RR) of PE for women in the highest ($\geq$21.2 g/day) vs. the lowest quartile (<11.9 g/day) was 0.28 (95% CI = 0.11–0.75). The same was for water-soluble fiber and insoluble fiber.

Vegetarian diet combined with physical activity seems to reduce the risk of PE. A longitudinal study conducted in 238 black pregnant women from Congo showed that the incidence of arterial hypertension was 4.6% overall (2.9% of whom had PE and 1.7% of whom showed transient hypertension). Women who did not usually consume daily servings of vegetables during pregnancy (33.3%) showed higher frequency of PE compared to women who consumed more than three servings of vegetables per day (3.7%) [97]. In a case–control study, conducted in 172 preeclamptic pregnant women and 339 normotensive controls, the authors described that foods that were beneficial in decreasing the risk of preeclampsia were fruits, vegetables, cereals, dark bread, and low-fat dairy products for their high content of fiber, calcium, and potassium [98]. Despite the evidence support the protective effect of plant based diets on PE, these results might be read with caution because PE is a multifactorial condition.

2.4.2. Gestational Diabetes

Vegetarian diets and high intake of fiber could avoid the development of Gestational Diabetes (GD). In a prospective cohort study of 13,110 pregravid women of Nurses' Health Study II (USA) the authors conducted a self-reported FFQ. They described 758 cases of GD in an 8-year period. Dietary total fiber and cereal and fruit fiber were negatively associated with GD risk after adjustment. Each 10 g/day increment in total fiber intake was associated with 26% (95% CI 9–49) reduction in GD risk. Each 5 g/day increment in cereals was linked to a 23% (9–36) risk reduction and fruit fiber with a 26% (5–42) risk reduction. The combination of high-glycemic load and low-cereal fiber diet was linked to a 2.15-fold (1.04–4.29) increased risk of GD [99]. Another randomized controlled clinical trial included 52 women with GD who were randomly assigned to receive control ($n = 26$) vs. DASH (Dietary Approaches to Stop Hypertension) diet ($n = 26$) only for four weeks. The control diet was composed of 45–55% carbohydrates, 15–20% protein, and 25–30% fat. The DASH diet was rich in fruits, vegetables, whole grains, low-fat dairy products, lower saturated fats, cholesterol, and refined grains with a total of 2400 mg/day of sodium. In addition, the DASH diet is low energy-dense and contains high amounts of dietary fiber, phytoestrogens, potassium, calcium, magnesium, and folic acid. Women who consumed the control diet had more incidence of cesarean section—46.2% vs. 80.8% of control group—as well as less need for insulin after intervention: 23% vs. 73% for control group [100]. Assaf et al. [101] conducted a case–control study of 697 normoglycemic women who were randomized (at 8–12 weeks of gestation) in control group (337), of which fat consumption was limited to 30% of total caloric intake, or the intervention group (360), where a MedDiet was offered, enhanced with Extra Virgin Olive Oil (EVOO) and pistachios (40–42% fats of total caloric intake). The composite outcome was defined as having one event of emergency C-section, perineal trauma, pregnancy-induced hypertension and preeclampsia, prematurity, large for gestational age (LGA), and small for gestational age (SGA). The authors found a significant reduction in the risk of composite outcome in the group who received the MedDiet enhanced with EVOO and nuts. The data involved an Indian population and found that Indian vegetarians display a high prevalence of GD; however this concern is of a specific population with high susceptibility to diabetes [102]. Moreover a cross-sectional study in India enrolled 995 white British pregnant women, described that low circulating levels of vitamin B12 were correlated to high maternal BMI and high insulin resistance (assessed by HOMA method) [103].

Nevertheless, a recent Cochrane review showed that dietary interventions in pregnancy for preventing gestational diabetes mellitus need more high-quality evidence to determine their potential effects in pregnancy [104]. In addition, according to a systematic review of observational studies on gestational weight gain (GWG), the intake of carbohydrates and vegetarian diets was associated with lower GWG, contrary to diets with higher intakes of proteins, animal fats, and energy-dense foods, suggesting that plant-based dietary patterns could be beneficial in preventing GWG and consequently GD [105].

2.4.3. Preterm Delivery

Data correlating preterm delivery and vegetarian diets are controversial. A retrospective study conducted in Australia analyzed maternal dietary patterns in the 12 months before conception on fetal growth and preterm delivery [106]. They studied three patterns: (1) high-protein/fruit (characterized by fish, meat, chicken, fruit, and some whole grains); (2) high-fat/sugar/takeaway (takeaway foods, potato chips, and refined grains); and (3) vegetarian-type (vegetables, legumes, and whole grains). A 1-SD (standard deviation) increase in the scores on the high-protein/fruit pattern was associated with decreased likelihood of preterm birth, whereas the reverse direction was apparent for the high-fat/sugar/takeaway pattern. A 1-SD increase in the scores on the high fat/sugar/takeaway pattern was also associated with shorter gestation and low birth length. A longitudinal prospective study conducted on Danish National Birth Cohort enrolled 35,530 nonsmoking women, investigated the association of maternal intake of a Mediterranean-type diet (MD) assessed by FFQ and preterm birth [107]. MD was defined as fish twice a week or more, use of olive or rape seed oil, consumption of five fruits and vegetables a day, ate meat (other than poultry and fish) at most twice a week, and drank at most two cups of coffee a day. For early preterm birth Odds ratio was 0.61 (95% CI: 0.35–1.05) in women fulfilling all criteria for MD and 0.28 (0.11–0.76) in women with none, adjusted for possible confounders (parity, BMI, maternal height, socioeconomic status and cohabitant status). So MD during pregnancy may reduce the risk of early delivery in Danish women. Data including the Norwegian Mother and Child Cohort Study (MoBa) enrolled 26,115 pregnant women using FFQ and divided them in three groups: 569 of full criteria of MD, 25,397 1–4 criteria of MD, and 159 none criteria. No differences were found in preterm birth (OR: 0.73; 95% CI: 0.32, 1.68). A significantly lower rate of preterm birth was found in women with fish intake twice or more a week (OR: 0.84; 95% CI: 0.74, 0.95) [108]. A randomized clinical trial conducted in Norway on 290 pregnant White women (BMI 19–32), analyzed the effect of a cholesterol-lowering diet on maternal, cord, and neonatal plasma lipids and pregnancy outcomes [109]. Maternal total and low-density lipoprotein (LDL) cholesterol levels were lowered in the intervention compared with the control group, but lipid levels in cord blood and in neonates born to mothers in the intervention versus the control groups did not differ. Preterm birth (< 37 weeks) was lower in the intervention group (RR 0.10; 95% CI 0.01–0.77). In addition a prospective data performed in Denmark found the relationship of low consumption of seafood with a strong risk of preterm delivery and low birth weight, OR = 3.6 (95% confidence interval 1.2 to 11.2) showing that low plasma concentration of EPA and DHA during pregnancy is a strong risk factor for subsequent early preterm birth in Danish women [110,111].

2.4.4. Consequences of Unbalanced Nutrition on Mother's Mental Health

Recently, maternal depression has been linked to inadequate nutrition during pregnancy. Pregnant women are particularly vulnerable to the adverse effects of poor nutrition on mood because pregnancy and lactation increase nutrient requirements. Plausible links between nutrition and mood have been reported for folate, vitamin B12, calcium, vitamin D, iron, selenium, zinc, and PUFAs, which are required for the biosynthesis of several neurotransmitters such as serotonin, dopamine, and norepinephrine [112]. Numerous studies have found a positive association between low *n*-3 levels and a higher incidence of maternal depression. The two *n*-3 fatty acids most correlated to brain development and function are EPA and DHA, of which, the latter is the most prominent in the brain. Nevertheless the current evidence from randomised controlled trials is inconclusive [113]. A recent study assessed that self-reported postpartum depression was more prevalent among vegetarians than omnivorous subjects, probably due to inadequate micronutrients intake [114].

2.5. The Effects of Vegetarian and Vegan Diets during Pregnancy on Fetal Outcomes (see Table S4)

Fetal outcomes depend on a balanced interchange between maternal nutrients, placental transport and fetal growth factors. Maternal undernutrition may lead impairment of fetal development due to nutrient limitations and decreased nutrient source for fetal growth, changes in placental functions, and epigenetic modifications in the fetal genome. Macro- and micronutrients may directly regulate DNA stability and phenotypic adaptation by influencing the availability of methyl donors thereby modulating epigenetics mechanisms. In animal models, the metabolism of amino acids (glycine, histidine, methionine, and serine) and vitamins (B6, B12, and folate) provide methyl donors for DNA and protein methylation, emphasizing the critical role of balanced nutrient supply through placenta [115].

Dietary patterns may involve very different foods that contain a multitude of nutrients with interactive functions. Many of them are also correlated, so it is difficult to separate their effects. Thus, the cumulative effects of nutrients may be easier to identify than those of a single nutrient.

The increase of women adopting vegetarian or vegan diets has raised concerns about these risks during pregnancy. Nevertheless, the effect of vegetarian or vegan diets on fetal anthropometrics differs considerably between studies. Many studies have found positive correlation between birth weight (BW) and maternal intake of certain food items such as milk, fruits, and green leafy vegetables [116,117]. A recent review included papers that assessed diet by FFQ and studied the association among different dietary patterns and BW. Authors found that the patterns positively associated with BW were labeled "nutrient dense", "protein-rich", "health conscious", and "Mediterranean". Those negatively associated with BW were labeled "Western", "processed", "vegetarian", "transitional", and "wheat products". The dietary patterns "Western" and "wheat products" were also associated with higher risk of SGA babies, whereas a "traditional" pattern in New Zealand was inversely associated with having a SGA baby [118]. Wen et al. [119] found an association between vegetarian diet and lower fetal growth during the second trimester. In a prospective data reported by Reddy et al. [120], birth weight and head circumference and length were lower in the infants born from South Asian vegetarians, even after adjusting for maternal height, duration of gestation, parity, gender of infants, and smoking habits. A systematic review of the literature performed by Murphy et al. [121], studied the associations of consumption of fruits and vegetables during pregnancy with infant birth weight or SGA births. This data identified limited evidence of a positive association between fruit and vegetable consumption during pregnancy and birth weight.

On the contrary, there are data demonstrating a protective effect of plant-based dietey patterns on anthropometric fetal development explained by the high content of vitamins in such diets. A case–control study enrolled 787 pregant women and assessed fruit and vegetable consumption during pregnancy using FFQ (in-person interview). The authors reported that women with lower intake of vegetables during the first trimester had higher incidence of SGA and no association was found between fruit consumption and birth outcomes [122]. Four multiethnic birth cohorts in Canada (the NutriGen Alliance) involving 3997 pairs of full-term neonates and mothers assessed dietary patterns by FFQ. Among White Europeans, a plant-based dietary pattern was inversely associated with birth weight and increased risk of SGA. Not adjusted for cooking methods (among South Asians) maternal consumption of a plant-based diet was associated with a higher birth weight [123]. The heterogeneus results may be due to the different dietary context between developed or developing Countries and most of the included studies concerning low BW provided no maternal information on body mass index or gestational weight gain for vegetarians or controls. Other prospective studies showed that average birthweights of infants born from vegetarian mothers do not differ significantly from omnivorous mothers. Clinical relevance of these data is at least doubtful and the heterogeneity of the results suggests the presence of confounding factors. As fetal growth is directly affected by maternal protein intake, pregnant women need to consume an optimal variety of food plants in vegetarian or vegan diets to achieve the same biodisponibility of proteins of omnivorous population as several studies have demonstrated [124–126].

Micronutrients such as vitamin B12 and zinc are deficient in vegetarian and vegan diets, as the main source are animal products [127]. It has been suggested that the supposed lower BW observed among infants born from mothers who adhere to vegetarian diets may be related to poor nutritional status with regard to iron or vitamin B12. As is highlighted in Fikawati et al.'s longitudinal study, infants may be born as well with low vitamin B12 stores if the maternal intake during pregnancy is inadequate [124]. Maternal B12 status is a key determinant of infant B12 status and is an independent factor for NTD [128]. A recent review demonstrated an association between vitamin B12 status, low BW and preterm delivery [129]. The effects of vegetarian diet on the development of NTD are contradictory [130,131]. Although the direct effect on fetal development has not been well described, vegetarian women may include extra sources of vitamin B12 in their diet to avoid fetal depletion.

Iron deficiency during pregnancy has been associated with low BW and neonatal anemia [132]. Iron derived from meat has better bioavailability than iron provided by plants, therefore vegetarian and vegan women should take a higher content of iron to avoid depletion of internal stores [94]. In fact, a British study found that iron deficiency during pregnancy was not higher in vegetarians and that iron intake was higher in vegetarian women during the first trimester [82], probably due to an awareness of risks and a consequent well planned diet. A recent review showed that vitamin D deficiency is also linked to fetal poor growth and vegetarians are at risk of vitamin D deficiency [133].

An increased risk of hypospadias has been associated to vegetarian or vegan diet during pregnancy, based in the increased intake of phytoestrogens. It was first reported in one prospective study, which obtained an adjusted OR of 4.99 (2.10–11.88) in vegetarian women compared to their omnivorous counterparts. However, this work failed to demonstrate a relationship between the incidence of hypospadias and the intake of soya products, which were supposed to be the first source of phytoestrogens in this lifestyle [134]. Another Scandinavian prospective case–control study reported an increased risk of hypospadias in women with diets excluding meat and fish diet. The study was based in the hypothesis that the lack of some essential amino acids may produce a deficiency during organogenesis [135]. However, these large and well-designed studies had the limitation that their conclusions were based on indirect correlations derived from retrospectively self-administered questionnaires. On the contrary, more recent works, which have focused on the relationship of nutrients to estrogen metabolism and the quantity of phytoestrogens in the diet to hypospadias, have not found positive correlation [136,137]. Furthermore, one Italian study found a positive correlation between hypospadias and a frequent consumption of fish during pregnancy [138]. This contradictory data, together with other studies, suggest that the imbalance of some nutrients or the intake of food contaminants may play roles in the genesis of hypospadias; however, at this point in time, there is not enough information to conclude that vegetarian or vegan diets increase the risk of disruption during the genital organogenesis [139,140].

Plant-based and vegetarian diets, characterized by a high consumption of fruits and vegetables and low or no intakes of cured meat and smoked fish, which represent the principal exogenous dietary sources of nitrate, nitrite, and N-nitroso compounds, associated with a higher risk of developing NTD, would be protective to the risk of congenital malformations [92]. However, it has been described that pickled vegetables are also a source of nitrite and NOCs. A study showed the association between maternal periconceptional consumption of pickled vegetables and NTD in four Chinese countries [141]. They found that >6 pickled vegetable meals/wk increased the risk of NTD, compared with less frequent (i.e., <1 meal/week) consumption. In addition, the authors showed that maternal intake (>1 meal/week) of meat, eggs, or milk had protective effect against the risk of NTD, so the literature is controversial.

2.6. The Effects of Vegetarian and Vegan Diet on the Composition of Human Milk

Vegetarian diets differ between individuals: without good information and well planned diets, vegetarians may be at risk for some deficiencies during pregnancy and consequently during breastfeeding period. In the Table S1 we recollected the daily nutrient requirements during pregnancy and lactation. Although vegetarian diets are usually rich in carbohydrates, the need to develop energy reserves during lactation increases demand for more calories. Both vegetarian and nonvegetarian mothers need caloric reserves to reach sufficient energy average for breastfeeding during the postpartum period [142]. The composition of human milk changes dynamically and can vary according to many maternal factors, such as diet and nutritional status. A recent study analyzed the association of maternal nutrition and body composition with human milk composition. They did not find a significant statistical relationship between human milk composition and nutrients in women's diet during the first six months of lactation. For women in the third month postpartum, they observed moderate to strong correlations between total protein content in milk and the body composition measures such as percentage of fat mass, fat-free mass, and muscle mass. The variance in milk fat content was related to body mass index (BMI), with a significant positive correlation in the first month postpartum. These findings suggest that maternal body composition may be associated with the nutritional value of human milk, with independence of type of diet [143]. Nutritional supplements do not change milk composition in observational studies maybe due to compensatory physiological mechanisms that conserve stable milk macronutrient composition related to the nutritional modifications of maternal diet [144]. Also protein concentration in human milk does not vary in relation to maternal intake of vegetal or animal proteins [145]. Nevertheless, Agostoni et al. [146] reported that animal proteins, compared to plant proteins, are associated with positive psychomotor development indices for infants and young children.

Vegetarian mothers might have low pre-pregnancy nutritional status that can lead to low maternal fat stores for lactation. Fikawati et al. [147] conducted a longitudinal data on mother–infant breastfeeding pairs in Indonesia. They followed 42 pairs of vegetarian and 43 pairs of nonvegetarian. Sociodemographic characteristics did not differ between the two dietary groups except in maternal parity. Vegetarian mothers had lower pre-pregnancy BMI but higher pregnancy weight gain compared to nonvegetarian. This study showed that vegetarian mothers had significantly lower BMI during lactation than nonvegetarian and the breastfeeding had no effect on infant weight and length but had significant effect on mothers' BMI and weight loss. The mothers in the nonvegetarian group in this study had a significantly greater energy intake compared with the vegetarians. Without adequate intake of energy during lactation the postpartum nutritional profile of vegetarian mothers decreased, so the maternal nutritional stores are sacrificed to support infant normal growth.

Low maternal vitamin B-12 intake during lactation can lead to low vitamin B12 content in breast milk which can cause permanent neurological disabilities in infants with low vitamin B12 levels. Maternal vitamin B12 status is the major factor affecting the severity of cobalamin deficiency in breast-fed infants and vegetarian and vegan population are at increasing risk [148]. In regions where animal source food consumption is low and prenatal supplementation is not common, infants are at risk of vitamin B12 deficiency, as shown in prospective data which found that maternal and infant serum/plasma and breast milk total vitamin B12 concentrations were significantly higher among Canadian mothers compared to Cambodian mothers [149]. Breastfed infants of mother who adhere to vegan diets are at increased risk of vitamin B12 deficiency [150]. Pawlak et al. [151], conducted a cross-sectional study in which 74 vegan, vegetarian, and nonvegetarian women were recruited. The prevalences of low vitamin B-12 (<310 pmol/L) were 19.2% for vegans, 18.2% for vegetarians, and 15.4% for nonvegetarians, which was independent of diet. Approximately 85% of participants categorized as having low vitamin B-12 were taking vitamin B12 supplements at doses in excess of the Recommended Dietary Allowance but this study had limitation of small sample.

Specific fatty acids that form the total lipid fraction are influenced by maternal nutrition. Fatty acids intake derives from the maternal plasma, or they synthesized endogenously by the mammary glands. Both of these sources are influenced by maternal diet composition [143].

The breast milk of vegetarians and particularly vegans in the United Kingdom showed lower DHA levels if compared to omnivores, but in the United States, vegetarians do not have lower levels of DHA in breast milk lipids, probably due to higher ingestion of ALA from soybean oil or preformed DHA [63]. Compared to nonvegetarians, the breast milk of vegetarians was found to have more than twice the amount of LA and ALA, but less than half the amount of DHA [84]. The levels of DHA in human milk augment with DHA supplementation. Supplementation with DHA during lactation is more useful to raise DHA content in breast milk than supplementing only during pregnancy [152]. A recent review analyzed 13 low- and middle-income countries and showed that the content of DHA in breast milk was very low in populations living mainly on plant-based diets but higher in fish-eating countries [153].

A cross-sectional observational study of 74 lactating women following a vegan (*n* = 26), vegetarian (*n* = 22), or omnivore (*n* = 26) diet pattern was conducted in the United States [154]. They found that breast milk from vegans had significantly higher unsaturated fat and total omega-3 fats, and lower saturated fats, trans fats, and omega-6 to omega-3 ratios than vegetarian and omnivore. DHA concentrations in breast milk were low regardless of maternal diet pattern, and were reflective of low seafood intake and supplement use. Supplement use was relatated to high DHA levels. The study was limited to small sample. The vegan diet contains essentially no ARA and DHA, as plants thought to have fatty acids (such as hempseed, rapeseed, flaxseeds, soy beans, and walnuts) are poorly converted into DHA by the body [155].

In addition, in the developed world, vitamin D deficiency is most frequently diagnosed exclusively in breastfed infants of vegetarian or vegan mothers [156].

More data are needed to evaluate the milk composition of mother following vegetarian or vegan diets.

2.7. Vegetarian and Vegan Diet during Pregnancy and Lactation: Target Therapy and Health Intervention

Specific dietary interventions before, during, and after gestation that are aimed in improving diet quality and setting appropriate intakes of macro- and micronutrients are important to avoid maternal health impairment with consequent physical and neurological fetal abnormalities.

The Mediterranean diet pattern, characterized by low total fat (<30% of energy), low saturated fat (<10% of energy), high complex carbohydrates (but relatively low total carbohydrate), and high dietary fiber intake, is generally considered healthy for all people, and has been recommended as a good preconception and pregnancy diet. The intake of pulses, green leafy vegetables, cereals, and fruit that is associated with best adherence to the Mediterranean diet provides a relatively high intake of folate, which is particularly important in the preconception period. Following a Mediterranean diet also increases the likelihood of achieving adequate intakes of zinc, B vitamins, vitamin A, vitamin E, magnesium, and vitamin C [40].

A strict plant-based diet is suitable during pregnancy but it must be well planned in order to provide all the energy requirements and meet critical nutrients, such as protein, fiber, omega-3, fatty acids, zinc, iodine, calcium, vitamin D, and vitamin B12. The vegetarian-type pattern is not associated to any outcome as preterm birth, BW or SGA if requirements are met [106,127]. Educational resources and food recommendations help vegetarians to consume adequate and complete diets. Some tools could be used for educating vegetarian patients as recording dietary intake by food diaries, providing charts that list of different sources of nutrients or sample menus [63]. Providers should regularly assess a woman's diet and her energy intake [121]. Guidelines on what to eat during pregnancy and lactation are essentially the same for vegetarians as for meateaters, but women who choose restricted diets may need to consume supplements or fortified food in order to reach the recommended requirements [9].

2.7.1. Proteins

Protein needs are particularly high during pregnancy and lactation. Although protein requirements are easily met in a vegan diet, it is recommended an increase by 10% of protein intake during pregnancy [157]. Adding 1.5 cups of lentils or 2.5 cups of soy milk per day could cover additional protein need [94]. Essential amino acids can be full obtained from both grains and legumes. An increase in all sources of protein can compensate for low lysine intake [63]. Lysine is an amino acid that can be more readily obtained from beans and soy and less readily obtained from cereals.

Some plant foods, such as soy, lupines, spinach, pseudocereals (buckwheat, quinoa, and amaranth), and hemp seeds, have all the essential amino acids in similar proportions to animal foods. But some other foods, such as antinutritional factors or fiber, interfere in the absorption of plant proteins. Plant proteins have low digestibility (on average 85%) [157]. If protein consumption in a vegan diet is well planned, no differences in infant birth weight in vegan mothers in comparison with omnivorous mothers have been observed [16]. Balanced energy and protein supplementation reduce the risk of stillbirth and SGA, but high-protein supplementation is not recommended [158]. Plasma quantization of amino acids could be performed in a laboratory to detect deficiencies [159].

2.7.2. Fibers

Fiber intake is recommended in pregnancy because it improves the richness of microbiota and avoids constipation but an excessive consume can difficult the meeting of appropriate nutrient and energy absorption. Therefore, during second and third trimester, alternative foods are preferred (fruits and vegetables, refined grains, peeled beans, and high-protein, high-energy, fiber-free foods such as soy milk, tofu, and soy yoghurt) [157].

2.7.3. Fatty acids/Omega-3

Due to the limited vegetable sources of DHA, pregnant vegetarian women are encouraged to consume an algae-based supplement. ALA is the only *n*-3 fatty acid present in plant foods (flaxseeds, hempseeds, chia seeds, walnuts, and their oils), but ALA elongation to EPA and DHA is limited, and influenced by diet. High dietary LA intake, excessive intakes of trans fatty acids, inadequate intakes of energy, protein, pyridoxine, biotin, calcium, copper, magnesium, or zinc can impair EPA and DHA synthesis [16]. A balanced intake of *n*-3 and *n*-6 fatty acids is important in order to produce sufficient amounts of DHA and EPA. Vegans and vegetarians can be at a disadvantage in balancing this ratio, because they may limit sources of ALA (n-3) or DHA in their diet, and they typically consume an abundance of LA [63]. Good plant sources of omega-3 fatty acids include ground flaxseeds and flaxseed oil, ground chia seeds, and walnuts. Seed oils rich in omega-6, trans fats (margarine), and tropical oils (coconut, palm, and palm kernel oils), which are rich in saturated fats, should be avoided in order to maintain an optimal omega-6/omega-3 ratio and favor the conversion of ALA into polyunsaturated fatty acids (PUFAs). Olive oil has a low influence in this ratio and, in addition to flaxseed oil, and should be the only additional oil to use as omga-3 source. In a recent Cochrane review, the authors studied supplement of omega-3 fatty acids in pregnant women. They found increased prolonged gestation > 42 weeks from 1.6% to 2.6% in women who received omega-3 LCPUFA compared with no omega-3 (moderate-quality evidence); reduced risk of perinatal death (moderate-quality evidence); fewer neonatal care admissions (moderate-quality evidence); reduced risk of low BW babies (15.6% versus 14% (high-quality evidence)); and a small increase in LGA babies (moderate-quality evidence). PE might possibly be reduced with omega-3 LCPUFA but with low-quality evidence. No differences were found for SGA or intrauterine growth restriction. It seems reasonable to recommend a daily supplementation of DHA for all pregnant women [160]. Even at the pregestational level, an intake of adequate amounts of n–3 PUFAs and DHA plays a major role; indeed, small variations in the habitual maternal dietary composition before pregnancy are likely to be more effective in improving the delivery of long-chain PUFAs to the fetus than large dietary changes in the late stages of pregnancy [92]. In these stages, a daily intake of 100 to 200 mg microalgae-derived DHA supplement is suggested [157].

2.7.4. Zinc

Vegetarians should be encouraged to consume more dietary zinc than the Population Reference Intake (PRI) suggested for omnivores, especially when the dietary phytate/zinc ratio is high [16]. Legumes, soy, nuts, seeds, and grains are all rich in zinc [157]. Zinc absorption can be improved by adopting food preparation methods (soaking, germination fermentation, sourdough leavening of bread) that reduce phytate levels in zinc rich foods. Zinc-fortified foods (e.g., breakfast cereals) can also be used. Zinc-rich foods should be eaten together with foods that contain organic acids such as fruit, and vegetables of Brassicaceae family [16] in order to improve zinc absorption.

2.7.5. Iodine

Vegan diets could provide low intake of iodine, although iodine deficiencies are quite uncommon in Western countries. Iodized salt is the safest way to reach iodine requirements in vegan pregnant and lactating women. Iodized salt varies among countries. The estimated average requirement for iodine in pregnant women is 200 µg/day [157]. Higher salt intake during pregnancy in vegans is considered harmless because of the low incidence of hypertension in this population, and can facilitate to meet the iodine requirements. Another option can be an algae-derived supplement.

2.7.6. Iron

Iron supplementation is only recommended if iron status has been shown to be low by appropriate blood tests [16]. A well planned vegan diet can meet iron needs. Iron content in vegan diets is in nonheme form, with lower bioavailability than heme-forms from animal sources (1–34% and 15–35%, respectively). During pregnancy it is recommended a daily consumption of iron rich foods as soy, beans, seeds, nuts, and green leafy vegetables as well as vitamin-C in combination. Some cooking considerations and food preparations should also improve iron absorption [157].

2.7.7. Calcium

A vegan diet can protect calcium stocks by increasing absorption [94]. Therefore, supplementation is rarely needed. Vegetarians and vegans should consume 1200 to 1500 mg/day of calcium, which is ~20% more calcium than that recommended for omnivores [63]. Ideally, low-oxalate foods (high bioavailability), such as broccoli or bokchoi, must be preferred. Other foods with slightly less calcium bioavailability are fortified soymilk, sesame seeds, almonds, and red and white beans. Another important source of calcium is hard water. Most of the varied diets above 2400 kcal should completely cover calcium needs [157]. Villar et al. [161] conducted a randomized clinical trial in 8325 pregnant women with dietary calcium intake <600 mg/day. In the intervention group the intake was 1.5 g/day calcium. They did not find differences in PE. They found a reduction of severe preeclamptic complications index. Preterm delivery was reduced only in women <20 years. Neonatal mortality rate was lower in the calcium group. Another data from Cochrane database evaluated calcium supplementation ($\geq$1 g/day) during pregnancy in 13 studies. This supplement was associated with a significant reduction in the risk of preeclampsia, particularly for women with low calcium diets but the significant reduction in the risk of PE associated with calcium supplementation might be overestimated (small effect, high heterogeneity and publication bias) [162]. The World Health Organization recommends 1.5 g to 2 g of calcium daily for pregnant women with low dietary calcium intake [40].

2.7.8. Vitamin D

Vegans must rely strongly on ultraviolet B rays—the band of ultraviolet that causes synthesis of vitamin D-3—from direct sunlight, to obtain sufficient vitamin D. Extending sunlight exposure and consuming vitamin D fortified foods may be appropriate strategies to avoid possible vitamin D deficiencies [92]. Adequate levels of this molecule and the maintenance of proper metabolism during pregnancy need to be emphasized because some beneficial effects have been reported. For example vitamin D enhances insulin responsiveness for glucose transport, through the modulation of insulin receptor expression. Vitamin D induces insulin secretion and decreases insulin resistance preventing gestational diabetes. In addition, it plays a critical role in the regulation of blood pressure and electrolyte and plasma volume homeostasis; therefore, normal serum vitamin D levels help to prevent hypertension and PE through suppression of the renin–angiotensin system [163]. Nevertheless, excess vitamin D may also have detrimental effects because it might decrease progesterone concentrations causing a preterm labor or impair fertility outcomes, so supplementation should be selective [164].

Vitamin D supplements are the usual remedy for meeting the recommended requirements (15 µg/day). Good sources of vitamin D are found in fish, liver oils, fatty fish, and egg yolks, but vitamin content in these foods varies by the time of year [63]. Plant sources of vitamin D are beans, broccoli, and leafy greens, but its content of this molecule without fortification is low, except for some wild mushrooms that contain a relevant concentration of this vitamin; therefore, vegetarian and vegan women are at risk of vitamin D deficiency. These source of vitamin D can be further fortified with calcium supplements, including cow's milk, some soymilk products, and some breakfast cereals. Serum levels of vitamin D are easily measured if there is concern regarding intake of this essential nutrient [94]. Optimal serum 25-OH vitamin levels for pregnant women are above 75 nmol/L (30 ng/mL). Most of prenatal vitamins contain insufficient vitamin D in order to prevent infant vitamin D deficiency, so to get the recommended doses of 1000 to 2000 IU per day, are considered safe in pregnancy [157]. A recent Cochrane review underlines that supplementing pregnant women with vitamin D in a single or continued dose increases serum 25-hydroxyvitamin-D, and may reduce the risk of preeclampsia, low BW, and preterm delivery. However, when vitamin D and calcium are combined, the risk of preterm birth is increased. Further studies are needed to evaluate vitamin D supplementation and the correct dose during pregnancy [165].

2.7.9. Vitamin B12

Vitamin B12 is not found in plant sources, and therefore must be obtained through animal consumption or via supplements [94]. Since vitamin B12 deficiency may appear in pregnant vegetarian women, in particular vegans, an adequate B12 status should be improved, so the use of B12 supplements is necessary. Pregnant and lactating vegans should be advised to supplement their diets with 4 µg/d of vitamin B12 [150]. Foods fortified with vitamin B12 include meat substitute products, breakfast cereals, soymilks, tofu, cereals, and nutritional yeast. Seaweed and tempeh are generally not reliable sources of vitamin B12. Four servings daily of vitamin B12-fortified foods are recommended in pregnancy and lactation [63]. Even if common pre- and postnatal multivitamins contain 100% of the RDA for vitamin B12, they are not positively associated with B12 concentration in breastmilk of vegetarian women because only a fraction of the B12 they provide is absorbed. Pregnant and lactating vegetarian and vegan mothers should be encouraged to take an individual B12, supplement and dissolve it under the tongue or chew it slowly in order to increase absorption [157]. In the case of vitamin B12 deficiency, the majority of clinical studies suggest starting with high parenteral doses of B12, after which oral treatment is continued. Considering the importance of adequate intake of vitamin B12 during pregnancy and considering that supplementation is not toxic, an ingestion of higher dose of B12 supplement (50 µg/day) would ensure correct vitamin status [92]. Vitamin B12 status (serum B12, along with homocysteine and folic acid) should be regularly checked throughout pregnancy also in women with optimal B12 levels in the first trimester, and it is necessary to adjust supplementation schemes according to the laboratory results [157].

3. Limitations

The present study corresponds to a descriptive review in which the majority of papers evaluated maternal dietary intake through a food frequency questionnaire. The main limitations of these questionnaires are the different food list and the possible mistakes of reporting.

Most studies analyzed in this review concluded that vegetarian and/or vegan diets exert diverse effects on pregnant outcome and nutritional profile. However, some of them describe specific populations in India or Africa with lower economic status and particular idiosyncrasy. For that, ethnicity and poverty have to be taken into account as a cause of an unbalanced diet, micronutrient deficiency, and poor pregnancy outcome. Furthermore, epidemiological and biochemical studies need to be done in Western countries to corroborate the conclusions obtained in African and/or Asian regions.

Mother undernutrition could be multifactorial, so it is important to mention the difficulties to determine the molecular mechanisms promoted by each micronutrient which may affect specifically the maternal nutritional profile.

4. Conclusions

Diet is one of the most significant lifestyle-related factors in determining health state and predisposing the offspring to develop several diseases. Vegetarian and vegan diets are emerging worldwide due to the evidence that plant-based dietary patterns reduce the risk of coronary heart disease, high blood pressure, type 2 diabetes, and cancer. Pregnancy is a critical window of opportunity to provide dietetic habits that are beneficial for fetal healthy. It is also an exclusive condition in which the requirements of energy and micronutrients intake increase to maintain the supply of essential nutrients for fetal development. Each stage of fetal growth is dependent on appropriate maternal nutrient transfer, so a balanced diet is essential to avoid fetal complications. The choice of vegetarian or vegan diet is always in the preconception period due to ethical reasons or poor social condition, so a well-adjusted preconception nutrition is essential for healthy pregnancy. Available data demonstrated that micronutrients insufficiency and caloric restriction are more common in developing countries, where vegetarian diets are chosen because of socioeconomic reasons. On the contrary in developed countries, the consciousness and the concern of a balanced diet is taken more into account. Generally it is difficult to verify the effects of such diets on pregnancy outcomes and to separate them from other confounding factors such as ethnicity, lifestyles or smoking.

Although more high quality evidence is needed, balanced plant-based diets rich in fibers and low in fat are considered to be protective against poor pregnancy outcomes such as PE, DG, and preterm delivery. However, these protective effects disappear if micronutrients deficiencies emerge. Moreover unbalanced dietary patterns with lack of macro- and micronutrients such as proteins, vitamin B12, vitamin D, calcium, DHA, and iron are at more risk of fetal impairment (low BW, neurological disabilities, and fetal malformations). Maternal undernutrition may potentially alter fetal growth trajectory by modifying placental weight and nutrient transfer capacity; depending on the severity of the nutritional deprivation and on the timing of depletion. Thus, plant-based diets during pregnancy and lactation require a strong awareness for a complete intake of essential key nutrients and vitamin supplements, according to international guidelines.

In addition, during breastfeeding both vegetarian and nonvegetarian mothers need caloric reserves to reach sufficient energy average. The composition of human milk changes dynamically and may vary according to many maternal factors, such as nutritional status. Nutritional supplements do not change milk composition in observational studies, also proteins concentration in human milk does not vary in relation to maternal intake of vegetal or animal proteins, but maternal body composition may be associated with the nutritional value of human milk. So maternal undernutrition, producing lack of vitamin B12, vitamin D, calcium, and DHA during lactation may lead to low vitamin content in breast milk, which can cause permanent neurological disabilities in infants or low bone mineralization.

Finally, the current manuscript supports the evidence that maternal nutritional status is the key condition for health benefits of plant-based diets. Vegetarians and vegans are at risk of nutritional deficiencies, but if the adequate intake of nutrients is upheld, pregnancy outcomes are similar to those reported in the omnivorous population. So updated evidence highlights that well-balanced vegetarian and vegan diets should be considered safe for the mother's health and for offspring during pregnancy and lactation. In this regard, specific dietary interventions before, during, and after gestation that are aimed at improving diet quality and adjusting appropriate intakes of macro- and micronutrients might avoid maternal health impairment, mental diseases during pregnancy, and consequent physical and neurological fetal disabilities. The vegetarian-type pattern should be considered safe and it is not associated with preterm birth, BW, or SGA if the requirements are met. Therefore, healthcare professionals might have knowledge about plant-based diets characteristics in order to implement balanced dietary patterns, enhancing supplement intake, and paying attention to critical nutrients to avoid dangerous health outcomes. Further large-scale observational studies would help to define correlations between plant-based diets, gestation, and health, and might be suitable to design pregestational nutrition intervention strategies.

Supplementary Materials: The following are available online at http://www.mdpi.com/2072-6643/11/3/557/s1, Table S1: Selected daily nutrient requirements during pre-pregnancy, pregnancy, and lactation; Table S2: Studies about the effects of vegetarian and vegan diet on maternal nutritional profile; Table S3. Studies about the effects of Vegetarian and vegan diet on maternal outcomes; Table S4: Studies about the effects of vegetarian and vegan diets on fetal outcomes.

Author Contributions: All authors contributed to the work reported. G.S. carried out the reference search of bibliographic source, selecting papers, and Writing—Original Draft Preparation; she made the tables and the review of manuscript. A.H.B., C.B.-N., M.A.C., V.A.-B., M.P.T., and S.F.M. contributed to the bibliographic source and elaboration of the initial manuscript and tables. V.A.-F. supervised the methodology and reviewed the manuscript. M.D.G.R. and O.G.-A. performed the final check of the manuscript from a gynaecologist's and neonatologist's point of view, respectively.

Funding: This research received no external funding.

Acknowledgments: This work was supported by grant from Red de Salud Materno-Infantil y del Desarrollo (SAMID) (RD16/0022/0002) from Instituto de Salud Carlos III, Madrid (Spain).

Conflicts of Interest: The authors declare no conflicts of interest.

References

1. Fall, C.H. Fetal programming and the risk of noncommunicable disease. *Indian. J. Pediatr.* **2013**, *80* (Suppl. 1), S13–S20. [CrossRef] [PubMed]
2. Barker, D.J.P.; Bergmnann, R.L.; Ogra, P.L. (Eds.) *The Window of Opportunity: Pre-Pregnancy to 24 Months of Age*; Karger, Nestle Nutrition Institute: Basel, Switzerland, 2008; pp. 1–266.
3. Procter, S.B.; Campbell, C.G. Position of the Academy of Nutrition and Dietetics: Nutrition and Lifestyle for a Healthy Pregnancy Outcome. *J. Acad. Nutr. Diet.* **2014**, *114*, 1099–1103. [CrossRef] [PubMed]
4. Wang, F.; Zheng, J.; Yang, B.; Jiang, J.; Fu, Y.; Li, D. Effects of Vegetarian Diets on Blood Lipids: A Systematic Review and Meta-Analysis of Randomized Controlled Trials. *J. Am. Heart. Assoc.* **2015**, *27*, e002408. [CrossRef] [PubMed]
5. Rosell, M.; Appleby, P.; Spencer, E.; Key, T. Weight gain over 5 years in 21,966 meat-eating, fish-eating, vegetarian, and vegan men and women in EPIC-Oxford. *Int. J. Obes.* **2006**, *30*, 1389–1396. [CrossRef] [PubMed]
6. Berkow, S.E.; Barnard, N.D. Blood pressure regulation and vegetarian diets. *Nutr. Rev.* **2005**, *63*, 1–8. [CrossRef] [PubMed]
7. Khan, N.; Afaq, F.; Mukhtar, H. Cancer chemoprevention through dietary antioxidants: Progress and promise. *Antioxid. Redox. Signal.* **2008**, *10*, 475–510. [CrossRef] [PubMed]
8. Jenkins, D.J.; Kendall, C.W.; Marchie, A.; Jenkins, A.L.; Augustin, L.S.; Ludwig, D.S.; Barnard, N.D.; Anderson, J.W. Type 2 diabetes and the vegetarian diet. *Am. J. Clin. Nutr.* **2003**, *78*, 610S–616S. [CrossRef] [PubMed]
9. Phillips, F. Vegetarian nutrition. *British Nutrition Foundation. Nutr. Bull.* **2005**, *30*, 132–167. [CrossRef]
10. Chang-Claude, J.; Hermann, S.; Eilber, U.; Steindorf, K. Lifestyle determinants and mortality in German vegetarians and health-conscious persons: Results of a 21-year follow-up. *Cancer Epidemiol. Biomark. Prev.* **2005**, *14*, 963–968. [CrossRef] [PubMed]
11. Ho-Pham, L.T.; Nguyen, N.D.; Nguyen, T.V. Effect of vegetarian diets on bone mineral density: A Bayesian meta-analysis. *Am. J. Clin. Nutr.* **2009**, *90*, 943–950. [CrossRef] [PubMed]
12. Position of the American Dietetic Association: Vegetarian diets. *J. Amer. Diet. Assoc.* **2009**, *109*, 1266–1282. [CrossRef]
13. Piccoli, G.B.; Attini, R.; Vasario, E.; Gaglioti, P.; Piccoli, E.; Consiglio, V.; De Agostini, C.; Oberto, M.; Trodos, T. Vegetarian supplemented low-protein diets. A safe option for pregnant CKD patients: Report of 12 pregnancies in 11 patients. *Nephrol. Dial. Transplant.* **2011**, *26*, 196–205. [CrossRef] [PubMed]
14. U.S. Department of Agriculture; U.S. Department of Health and Human Services. *Dietary Guidelines for Americans 2010*, 7th ed.; U.S. Government Printing Office: Washington, DC, USA, 2010.

15. Richter, M.; Boeing, H.; Grünewald-Funk, D.; Heseker, H.; Kroke, A.; Leschik-Bonnet, E.; Oberritter, H.; Strohm, D.; Watzl, B.; The German Nutrition Society (DGE). Vegan Diet Position of the German Nutrition Society (DGE). *Ernaehrungs. Umschau. Int.* **2016**, *4*, 92–102.

16. Agnoli, C.; Baroni, L.; Bertini, I.; Ciappellano, S.; Fabbri, A.; Papa, M.; Pellegrini, N.; Sbarbati, R.; Scarino, M.L.; Siani, V.; et al. Nutrition, Metabolism & Cardiovascular Diseases Position paper on vegetarian diets from the working group of the Italian Society of Human Nutrition. *Nutr. Metab. Cardiovasc. Dis.* **2017**, *27*, 1037–1052. [PubMed]

17. Davey, G.K.; Spencer, E.A.; Appleby, P.N.; Allen, N.E.; Knox, K.H.; Key, T.J. Epic-oxford: Lifestyle characteristics and nutrient intakes in a cohort of 33 883 meat-eaters and 31 546 non meat-eaters in the UK. *Public Health Nutr.* **2003**, *6*, 259–269. [CrossRef] [PubMed]

18. Jayanthi, V. Vegetarianism in India. *Perit. Dial. Int.* **2001**, *21*, S322–S325. [PubMed]

19. Lee, H.Y.; Woo, J.; Chen, Z.Y.; Leung, S.F.; Peng, X.H. Serum fatty acid, lipid profile and dietary intake of Hong Kong Chinese omnivores and vegetarians. *Eur. J. Clin. Nutr.* **2000**, *54*, 768–773. [CrossRef] [PubMed]

20. Stahler, C. How Often Do Americans Eat Vegetarian Meals? And How Many Adults in the U.S. Are Vegetarian? Available online: http://www.vrg.org/journal/vj2011issue4/vj2011issue4poll.php (accessed on 10 October 2017).

21. Vegetarian Resource Group. How Many Youth Are Vegetarians? How Many Kids Don't Eat Meat? *Veg. J.* **2005**, *4*, 26–27.

22. Farmer, B.; Larson, B.T.; Fulgoni, V.L., III; Rainville, A.J.; Liepa, G.U. A vegetarian dietary pattern as a nutrient-dense approach to weight management: An analysis of the national health and nutrition examination survey 1999–2004. *J. Am. Diet. Assoc.* **2011**, *111*, 819–827. [CrossRef] [PubMed]

23. Sabate, J.; Ratzin-Turner, R.A.; Brown, J.E. Vegetarian Diets: Descriptions and Trends. In *Vegetarian. Nutrition*; CRC Series in Modern Nutrition; CRC: Boca Raton, FL, USA, 2001; pp. 3–18.

24. Crozier, S.R.; Robinson, S.M.; Godfrey, K.M.; Cooper, C.; Inskip, H.M. Women's dietary patterns change little from before to during pregnancy. *J. Nutr.* **2009**, *139*, 1956–1963. [CrossRef] [PubMed]

25. Allen, L.H. Multiple micronutrients in pregnancy and lactation: An overview. *Am. J. Clin. Nutr.* **2005**, *81*, 1206S–1212S. [CrossRef] [PubMed]

26. Shapira, N. Prenatal nutrition: A critical window of opportunity for mother and child. *Womens Health* **2008**, *4*, 639–656. [CrossRef] [PubMed]

27. Rasmussen, K.M.; Yaktine, A.L. (Eds.) *Weight Gain During Pregnancy: Reexamining the Guidelines*; National. Academies. Press: Washington, DC, USA, 2009.

28. Black, R.E.; Victora, C.G.; Walker, S.P.; Bhutta, Z.A.; Christian, P.; de Onis, M.; Ezzati, M.; Grantham-McGregor, S.; Katz, J.; Martorell, R.; et al. Maternal and child undernutrition and overweight in low-income and middle-income countries. *Lancet* **2013**, *382*, 427–451. [CrossRef]

29. Academy of Nutrition and Dietetics. Practice Paper of the Academy of Nutrition and Dietetics: Nutrition and Lifestyle for a Healthy Pregnancy Outcome. Available online: http://www.eatright.org/members/practicepapers/ (accessed on 22 May 2014).

30. US Department of Agriculture. Dietary Guidelines for Americans, 2015–2020. Available online: http://www.cnpp.usda.gov/dgas2010-policydocument.htm (accessed on 3 March 2019).

31. EFSA (European Food Safety Authority). *Dietary Reference Values for Nutrients: Summary Report*; EFSA Supporting Publication: London, UK, 2017.

32. US Department of Health and Human Services. Physical activity for women during pregnancy and the postpartum period. In *2008 Physical Activity Guidelines for Americans*; Office of Disease Prevention & Health Promotion: Washington, DC, USA, 2008; pp. 41–42.

33. Gautam, C.S.; Saha, L.; Sekhri, K.; Saha, P.K. Iron deficiency in pregnancy and the rationality of iron supplements prescribed during pregnancy. *Medsc. J. Med.* **2008**, *10*, 283–288.

34. Centers for Disease Control and Prevention. Folic Acid: Recommendations. Available online: http://www.cdc.gov/ncbddd/folicacid/recommendations.html (accessed on 24 September 2012).

35. Thorne-Lyman, A.; Fawzi, W.W. Vitamin D during pregnancy and maternal, neonatal and infant health outcomes: A systematic review and meta-analysis. *Paediatr. Perinat. Epidemiol.* **2012**, *26* (Suppl. 1), 75–90. [CrossRef] [PubMed]

36. Caudill, M.A. Pre- and postnatal health: Evidence of increased choline needs. *J. Am. Diet. Assoc.* **2010**, *110*, 1198–1206. [CrossRef] [PubMed]

37. Obican, S.G.; Jahnke, G.D.; Soldin, O.P.; Scialli, A.R. Teratology public affairs committee position paper: Iodine deficiency in pregnancy. *Birth Defects Res.* **2012**, *94 Pt A*, 677–682. [CrossRef]
38. Hacker, A.N.; Fung, E.B.; King, J.C. Role of calcium during pregnancy: Maternal and fetal needs. *Nutr. Rev.* **2012**, *70*, 397–409. [CrossRef] [PubMed]
39. Kominiarek, M.A.; Rajan, P. Nutrition Recommendations in Pregnancy and Lactation. *Med. Clin. North. Am.* **2016**, *100*, 1199–1215. [CrossRef] [PubMed]
40. Hanson, M.A.; Bardsley, A.; De-Regil, L.M.; Moore, S.E.; Oken, E.; Poston, L.; Ma, R.C.; McAuliffe, F.M.; Maleta, K.; Purandare, C.N.; et al. The International Federation of Gynecology and Obstetrics (FIGO) recommendations on adolescent, preconception, and maternal nutrition: "Think Nutrition First". *Int. J. Gynaecol. Obstet.* **2015**, *131*, S213–S253. [CrossRef]
41. Physicians Committee for Responsible Medicine Website. Vegetarian Diets for Pregnancy. Available online: www.pcrm.org/health/veginfo/pregnancy.html (accessed on 28 March 2007).
42. Venti, C.A.; Johnston, C.S. Modified Food Guide Pyramid for Lactovegetarians and Vegans. *J. Nutr.* **2002**, *132*, 1050–1054. [CrossRef] [PubMed]
43. Messina, V.; Melina, V.; Mangels, A.R. A new guide for North American Vegetarians. *J. Am. Diet. Assoc.* **2003**, *103*, 771–775. [CrossRef] [PubMed]
44. Davis, B.C.; Kris-Etherton, P.M. Achieving optimal essential fatty acid status in vegetarians: Current knowledge and practical implications. *Am. J. Clin. Nutr.* **2003**, *78*, 640S–646S. [CrossRef] [PubMed]
45. Welch, A.; Shakya-Shrestha, S.; Lentjes, M.; Wareham, N.; Khaw, K. Dietary intake and status of n-3 polyunsaturated fatty acids in a population of fish-eating and non fish-eating meat-eaters, vegetarians, and vegans and the precursor-product ratio of a-linolenic acid to long-chain n-3 polyunsaturated fatty acids: Results from the EPIC-Norfolk cohort. *Am. J. Clin. Nutr.* **2010**, *92*, 1040–1051. [PubMed]
46. Position of the Academic of Nutrition and Dietetics: Vegetarian diets. *J. Acad. Nutr. Diet.* **2015**, *115*, 801–810. [CrossRef] [PubMed]
47. Hunt, J.R. Bioavailability of iron, zinc, and other trace minerals from vegetarian diets 1-4. *Am. J. Clin. Nutr.* **2003**, *78*, 633–642. [CrossRef] [PubMed]
48. Foster, M.; Chu, A.; Petocz.; Samman, S. Effect of vegetarian diets on zinc status: A systematic review and meta-analysis of studies in humans. *J. Sci. Food. Agric.* **2013**, *93*, 2362–2371. [CrossRef] [PubMed]
49. Institute of Medicine. Dietary Reference Intakes for Calcium and Vitamin D. Available online: http://www.iom.edu/Reports/2010/Dietary-Reference-Intakes-for-calcium-and-vitamin-D.aspx (accessed on 17 October 2013).
50. Larsson, C.L.; Johansson, G.K. Dietary intake and nutritional status of young vegans and omnivores in Sweden. *Am. J. Clin. Nutr.* **2002**, *76*, 100–106. [CrossRef] [PubMed]
51. Weaver, C.M.; Proulx, W.R.; Heaney, R. Choices for achieving adequate dietary calcium with a vegetarian diet. *Am. J. Clin. Nutr.* **1999**, *70*, 543S–548S. [CrossRef] [PubMed]
52. Crowe, F.L.; Steur, M.; Allen, N.E.; Appleby, P.N.; Travis, R.C.; Key, T.J. Plasma concentrations of 25-hydroxyvitamin D in meat eaters, fish eaters, vegetarians and vegans: Results from the EPIC-Oxford study. *Public Health Nutr.* **2011**, *14*, 340–346. [CrossRef] [PubMed]
53. Rizzo, G.; Laganà, A.S.; Rapisarda, A.M.C.; La Ferrera, G.M.G.; Buscema, M.; Rossetti, P.; Nigro, A.; Muscia, V.; Valenti, G.; Sapia, F.; et al. Vitamin B12 among vegetarians: Status, assessment and supplementation. *Nutrients* **2016**, *8*, 767. [CrossRef] [PubMed]
54. Otten, J.J.; Hellwig, J.P.; Meyers, L.D. *Dietary Reference Intakes: The Essential Guide to Nutrient Requirements*; Institute of Medicine of the National Academies: Washington, DC, USA, 2006.
55. Panel on Dietetic Products, Nutrition, and Allergies. Scientific opinion on dietary reference values for cobalamin (Vitamin B12). *EFSA J.* **2015**, *13*, 4150.
56. Pawlak, R.; Lester, S.E.; Babatunde, T. The prevalence of cobalamin deficiency among vegetarians assessed by serum vitamin B12: A review of literature. *Eur. J. Clin. Nutr.* **2014**, *68*, 541–548. [CrossRef] [PubMed]
57. Obersby, D.; Chappell, D.C.; Dunnett, A.; Tsiami, A.A. Plasma total homocysteine status of vegetarians compared with omnivores: A systematic review and metaanalysis. *Br. J. Nutr.* **2013**, *109*, 785–794. [CrossRef] [PubMed]
58. Herrmann, W.; Schorr, H.; Obeid, R.; Geisel, J. Vitamin B-12 status, particularly holotranscobalamin II and methylmalonic acid concentrations, and hyperhomocysteinemia in vegetarians. *Am. J. Clin. Nutr.* **2003**, *78*, 131–136. [CrossRef] [PubMed]

59. Northstone, K.; Emmett, P.; Rogers, I. Dietary patterns in pregnancy and associations with socio-demographic and lifestyle factors. *Eur. J. Clin. Nutr.* **2008**, *62*, 471–479. [CrossRef] [PubMed]
60. Simões-Wüst, A.P.; Moltó-Puigmartí, C.; Van, Dongen; Martien, C.J.M.; Dagnelie, P.C.; Thijs, C. Organic food consumption during pregnancy is associated with different consumer profiles, food patterns and intake: The KOALA Birth Cohort Study. *Public Health Nutr.* **2017**, *20*, 2134–2144.
61. Simões-Wüst, A.P.; Kummeling, I.; Mommers, M.; Huber, M.A.; Rist, L.; van de Vijver, L.P.; Dagnelie, P.C.; Thijs, C. Influence of alternative lifestyles on self-reported body weight and health characteristics in women. *Eur. J. Public Health* **2013**, *24*, 321–327. [CrossRef] [PubMed]
62. Pawlak, R.; James, P.S.; Raj, S.; Cullum-Dugan, D.; Lucus, D. How prevalent is vitamin B12 deficiency among vegetarians? *Nutr. Rev.* **2013**, *71*, 110–117. [CrossRef] [PubMed]
63. Penney, D.S.; Miller, K.G. Nutritional Counseling for Vegetarians During Pregnancy and Lactation. *J. Midwifery Women's Health* **2008**, *53*, 37–44. [CrossRef] [PubMed]
64. Stabler, S.P.; Allen, R.H. Vitamin B12 deficiency as a worldwide problem. *Annu. Rev. Nutr.* **2004**, *24*, 299–326. [CrossRef] [PubMed]
65. Visentin, C.E.; Masih, S.P.; Plumptre, L.; Schroder, T.H.; Sohn, K.J.; Ly, A.; Lausman, A.Y.; Berger, H.; Croxford, R.; Lamers, Y.; et al. Low serum vitamin B-12 concentrations are prevalent in a cohort of pregnant Canadian women. *J. Nutr.* **2016**, *146*, 1035–1042. [CrossRef] [PubMed]
66. Koebnick, C.; Heins, U.A.; Dagnelie, P.C.; Wickramasinghe, S.N.; Ratnayaka, I.D.; Hothorn, T.; Pfahlberg, A.B.; Hoffmann, I.; Lindemans, J.; Leitzmann, C. Longitudinal concentrations of vitamin B(12) and vitamin B(12)-binding proteins during uncomplicated pregnancy. *Clin. Chem.* **2002**, *48*, 928–933. [PubMed]
67. Koebnick, C.; Hoffmann, I.; Dagnelie, P.C.; Heins, U.A.; Wickramasinghe, S.N.; Ratnayaka, I.D.; Gruendel, S.; Lindemans, J.; Leitzmann, C. Long-Term Ovo-Lacto Vegetarian Diet Impairs Vitamin B-12 Status in Pregnant Women. *J. Nutr.* **2004**, *134*, 3319–3326. [CrossRef] [PubMed]
68. Gibson, R.S.; Abebe, Y.; Stabler, S.; Allen, R.H.; Westcott, J.E.; Stoecker, B.J.; Krebs, N.F.; Hambidge, K.M. Zinc, gravida, infection, and iron, but not vitamin B-12 or folate status, predict hemoglobin during pregnancy in Southern Ethiopia. *J. Nutr.* **2008**, *138*, 581–586. [CrossRef] [PubMed]
69. Jeruszka-Bielak, M.; Isman, C.; Schroder, T.H.; Li, W.; Green, T.J.; Lamers, Y. South Asian Ethnicity is related to the highest risk of vitamin B12 deficiency in pregnant canadian women. *Nutrients* **2017**, *23*, 317. [CrossRef] [PubMed]
70. Gadgil, M.S.; Joshi, K.S.; Naik, S.S.; Pandit, A.N.; Otiv, S.R.; Bhushan, K.; Patwardhan, B.K. Association of homocysteine with global DNA methylation in vegetarian Indian pregnant women and neonatal birth anthropometrics. *J. Matern. Fetal Neonatal Med.* **2014**, *27*, 1749–1753. [CrossRef] [PubMed]
71. Koebnick, C.; Heins, U.A.; Hoffmann, I.; Dagnelie, P.C.; Leitzmann, C. Folate status during pregnancy in women is improved by long-term high vegetable intake compared with the average western diet. *J. Nutr.* **2001**, *131*, 733–739. [CrossRef] [PubMed]
72. Nesby-O'Dell, S.; Scanlon, K.S.; Cogswell, M.E.; Gillespie, C.; Hollis, B.W.; Looker, A.C.; Allen, C.; Doughertly, C.; Gunter, E.W.; Bowman, B.A. Hypovitaminosis D prevalence and determinants among African American and white women of reproductive age: Third Health and Nutrition Examination Survey, 1988–1944. *Am. J. Clin. Nutr.* **2002**, *76*, 187–192. [CrossRef] [PubMed]
73. Smith, A.M. Veganism and osteoporosis: A review of the current literature. *Int. J. Nurs. Pract.* **2006**, *12*, 302–306. [CrossRef] [PubMed]
74. Sachan, A.; Gupta, R.; Das, V.; Agarwal, A.; Awasthi, P.K.; Bhatia, V. High prevalence of vitamin D deficiency among pregnant women and their newborns in northern India. *Am. J. Clin. Nutr.* **2005**, *81*, 1060–1064. [CrossRef] [PubMed]
75. Kazemi, A.; Sharifi, F.; Jafari, N.; Mousavinasab, N. High prevalence of vitamin D deficiency among pregnant women and their newborns in an Iranian population. *J. Womens Health* **2009**, *18*, 835–839. [CrossRef] [PubMed]
76. Dasgupta, A.; Saikia, U.; Sarma, D. Status of 25(OH)D levels in pregnancy: A study from the North Eastern part of India. *Indian J. Endocrinol. Metab.* **2012**, *16* (Suppl. 2), S405–S407. [PubMed]
77. Elsori, D.H.; Hammoud, M.S. Vitamin D deficiency in mothers, neonates and children. *J. Steroid. Biochem. Mol. Biol.* **2018**, *175*, 195–199. [CrossRef] [PubMed]
78. Yang, J.; Dang, S.; Cheng, Y.; Qui, H.; Mi, B.; Jiang, Y.; Yan, H. Dietary intakes and dietary patterns among pregnant women in Northwest China. *Public Health Nutr.* **2017**, *20*, 282–293. [CrossRef] [PubMed]

79. Graves, B.S.; Barger, M.K. A "conservative" approach to iron supplementation during pregnancy. *J. Midwifery Women's Health* **2001**, *46*, 159–166. [CrossRef]

80. Williamson, C. Nutrition in pregnancy. *Nutr. Bull.* **2006**, *31*, 28–59. [CrossRef]

81. Haider, L.M.; Schwingshackl, L.; Hoffmann, G.; Ekmekcioglu, C. The effect of vegetarian diets on iron status in adults: A systematic review and meta-analysis. *Crit. Rev. Food. Sci. Nutr.* **2018**, *58*, 1359–1374. [CrossRef] [PubMed]

82. Alwan, N.A.; Greenwood, D.C.; Simpson, N.A.; McArdle, H.J.; Godfrey, K.M.; Cade, J.E. Dietary iron intake during early pregnancy and birth outcomes in a cohort of British women. *Hum. Reprod.* **2011**, *26*, 911–919. [CrossRef] [PubMed]

83. Sharma, J.B.; Soni, D.; Murthy, N.S.; Malhotra, M. Effect of dietary habits on prevalence of anemia in pregnant women of Delhi. *J. Obs. Gynaecol. Res.* **2003**, *29*, 73–78. [CrossRef]

84. Jensen, C.L. Effects of n-3 fatty acids during pregnancy and lactation. *Am. J. Clin. Nutr.* **2006**, *83*, S1452–S1457. [CrossRef] [PubMed]

85. Masson, L.F.; McNeill, G.; Tomany, J.O.; Simpson, J.A.; Peace, H.S.; Wei, L.; Grubb, D.A.; Bolton-Smith, C. Statistical approaches for assessing the relative validity of a food-frequency questionnaire: Use of correlation coefficients and the kappa statistic. *Public Health Nutr.* **2003**, *6*, 313–321. [CrossRef] [PubMed]

86. Haggarty, P. Effect of placental function on fatty acid requirements during pregnancy. *Eur. J. Clin. Nutr.* **2004**, *58*, 1559–1570. [CrossRef] [PubMed]

87. Sanders, T.A.B. Essential fatty acid requirements of vegetarians in pregnancy, lactation and infancy. *Am. J. Clin. Nutr.* **1999**, *70*, 555S–559S. [CrossRef] [PubMed]

88. Foster, M.; Samman, S. Vegetarian diets across the lifecycle: Impact on zinc intake and status. *Adv. Food. Nutr. Res.* **2015**, *74*, 93–131. [PubMed]

89. Baroni, L.; Goggi, S.; Battino, M. VegPlate: A Mediterranean-Based Food Guide for Italian Adult, Pregnant, and Lactating Vegetarians. *J. Acad. Nutr. Diet.* **2018**, *118*, 2235–2243. [CrossRef] [PubMed]

90. King, J.C. Determinants of maternal zinc status during pregnancy. *Am. J. Clin. Nutr.* **2000**, *71*, 1334S–1343S. [CrossRef] [PubMed]

91. Foster, M.; Herulah, U.; Prasad, A.; Petocz, P.; Samman, S. Zinc Status of Vegetarians during Pregnancy: A Systematic Review of Observational Studies and Meta-Analysis of Zinc Intake. *Nutrients* **2015**, *7*, 4512–4525. [CrossRef] [PubMed]

92. Pistollato, F.; Sumalla Cano, S.; Elio, I.; Masias Vergara, M.; Giampieri, F.; Battino, M. Plant-Based and Plant-Rich Diet Patterns during Gestation: Beneficial Effects and Possible Shortcomings. *Adv. Nutr. An. Int. Rev. J.* **2015**, *6*, 581–591. [CrossRef] [PubMed]

93. Koebnick, C.; Leitzmann, R.; García, A.L.; Heins, U.A.; Heuer, T.; Golf, S.; Katz, N.; Hoffmann, I.; Leitzmann, C. Long-term effect of a plant-based diet on magnesium status during pregnancy. *Eur. J. Clin. Nutr.* **2005**, *59*, 219–225. [CrossRef] [PubMed]

94. Tyree, S.; Baker, B.R.; Weatherspoon, D. On veganism and pregnancy. *Int. J Child. Educ.* **2012**, *27*, 43–49.

95. Carter, J.P.; Furman, T.; Robert Hutcheson, H. Preeclampsia and reproductive performance in a community of vegans. *South. Med. J.* **1987**, *80*, 692–697. [CrossRef] [PubMed]

96. Qiu, C.; Coughlin, K.B.; Frederick, I.O.; Sorensen, T.K.; Williams, M.A. Dietary fiber intake in early pregnancy and risk of subsequent preeclampsia. *Am. J. Hypertens.* **2008**, *21*, 903–909. [CrossRef] [PubMed]

97. Longo-Mbenza, B.; Kadima-Tshimanga, B.; Buassa-bu-Tsumbu, B.; M'Buyamba, K., Jr. Diets rich in vegetables and physical activity are associated with a decreased risk of pregnancy induced hypertension among rural women from Kimpese, DR Congo. *Niger. J. Med.* **2008**, *17*, 45–49. [PubMed]

98. Frederick, I.O.; Williams, M.A.; Dashow, E.; Kestin, M.; Zhang, C.; Leisenring, W.M. Dietary fiber, potassium, magnesium and calcium in relation to the risk of preeclampsia. *J. Reprod. Med.* **2005**, *50*, 332–344. [PubMed]

99. Zhang, C.; Liu, S.; Solomon, C.G.; Hu, F.B. Dietary fiber intake, dietary glycemic load, and the risk for gestational diabetes mellitus. *Diabetes Care* **2006**, *29*, 2223–2230. [CrossRef] [PubMed]

100. Asemi, Z.; Samimi, M.; Tabassi, Z.; Esmaillzadeh, A. The effect of DASH diet on pregnancy outcomes in gestational diabetes: A randomized controlled clinical trial. *Eur. J. Clin. Nutr.* **2014**, *68*, 490–495. [CrossRef] [PubMed]

101. Assaf-Balut, C.; García de la Torre, N.; Duran, A.; Fuentes, M.; Bordiú, E.; del Valle, L.; Familiar, C.; Valerio, J.; Jiménez, I.; Herraiz, M.A.; et al. A Mediterranean Diet with an Enhanced Consumption of Extra Virgin Olive Oil and Pistachios Improves Pregnancy Outcomes in Women Without Gestational Diabetes Mellitus:

A Sub-Analysis of the St. Carlos Gestational Diabetes Mellitus Prevention Study. *Ann. Nutr. Metab.* **2019**, *74*, 69–79. [CrossRef] [PubMed]

102. Arora, G.P.; Thaman, R.G.; Prasad, R.B.; Almgren, P.; Brons, C.; Groop, L.C.; Vaag, A.A. Prevalence and risk factors of gestational diabetes in Punjab, North India: Results from a population screening program. *Eur. J. Endocrinol.* **2015**, *173*, 257–267. [CrossRef] [PubMed]

103. Knight, B.A.; Shields, B.M.; Brook, A.; Hill, A.; Bhat, D.S.; Hattersley, A.T.; Tajnik, C.S. Lower Circulating B12 Is Associated with Higher Obesity and Insulin Resistance during Pregnancy in a Non-Diabetic White British Population. *PLoS ONE.* **2015**, *10*, 8. [CrossRef] [PubMed]

104. Muktabhant, B.; Lawrie, T.A.; Lumbiganon, P.; Laopaiboon, M.; Ta, L.; Lumbiganon, P.; Laopaiboon, M.; Tieu, J.; Shepherd, E.; Middleton, P. Dietary advice interventions in pregnancy for preventing gestational diabetes mellitus (Review). *Cochrane Database Syst. Rev.* **2017**, *1*, CD007145.

105. Streuling, I.; Beyerlein, A.; Rosenfeld, E.; Schukat, B.; von Kries, R. Weight gain and dietary intake during pregnancy in industrialized countries—A systematic review of observational studies. *J. Perinat. Med.* **2011**, *39*, 123–129. [CrossRef] [PubMed]

106. Grieger, J.A.; Grzeskowiak, L.E.; Clifton, V.L. Preconception Dietary Patterns in Human Pregnancies Are Associated with Preterm Delivery. *J. Nutr.* **2014**, *144*, 1075–1080. [CrossRef] [PubMed]

107. Mikkelsen TB Association between a Mediterranean diet and risk of preterm birth among Danish women: A prospective cohort study. *Acta Obs. Gynecol. Scand.* **2008**, *87*, 325–330. [CrossRef] [PubMed]

108. Haugen, M.; Meltzer, H.M.; Brantsaeter, A.L.; Mikkelsen, T.; Østerdal, M.L.; Alexander, J.; Olsen, S.F.; Bakketeig, L. Mediterranean-type diet and risk of preterm birth among women in the Norwegian Mother and Child Cohort Study (MoBa): A prospective cohort study. *Acta Obs. Gynecol. Scand.* **2008**, *87*, 319–324. [CrossRef] [PubMed]

109. Khoury, J.; Henriksen, T.; Christophersen, B.; Tonstad, S. Effect of a cholesterol-lowering diet on maternal, cord, and neonatal lipids, and pregnancy outcome: A randomized clinical trial. *Am. J. Obs. Gynecol.* **2005**, *193*, 1292–1301. [CrossRef] [PubMed]

110. Olsen, S.F.; Secher, N. Low consumption of seafood in early pregnancy as a risk factor for preterm delivery: Prospective cohort study. *BMJ* **2002**, *324*, 447. [CrossRef] [PubMed]

111. Olsen, S.F.; Halldorsson, T.I.; Thorne-Lyman, A.L.; Strøm, M.; Gørtz, S.; Granstrøm, C.; Nielsen, P.H.; Wohlfahrt, J.; Lykke, J.A.; Langhoff-Roos, J.; et al. Plasma Concentrations of Long Chain N-3 Fatty Acids in Early and Mid-Pregnancy and Risk of Early Preterm Birth. *Ebiomedicine* **2018**, *35*, 325–333. [CrossRef] [PubMed]

112. Leung, B.M.; Kaplan, B.J. Perinatal depression: Prevalence, risks, and the nutrition link—A review of the literature. *J. Am. Diet. Assoc.* **2009**, *109*, 1566–1575. [CrossRef] [PubMed]

113. Gould, J.F.; Best, K.; Makrides, M. Perinatal nutrition interventions and post-partum depressive symptoms. *J. Affect. Disord.* **2017**, *15*, 2–9. [CrossRef] [PubMed]

114. Hogg-Kollars, S.; Mortimore, D.; Snow, S. Nutrition health issues in self-reported postpartum depression. *Gastroenterol. Hepatol. Bed Bench* **2011**, *4*, 120–136. [PubMed]

115. Cetin, I.; Mando, C.; Calabrese, S. Maternal predictors of intrauterine growth restriction. *Curr. Opin. Clin. Nutr. Metab. Care* **2013**, *16*, 310–319. [CrossRef] [PubMed]

116. Olsen, S.F.; Halldorsson, T.I.; Willett, W.C.; Knudsen, V.K.; Gillman, M.W.; Mikkelsen, T.B.; Olsen, J.; NUTRIX Consortium. Milk consumption during pregnancy is associated with increased infant size at birth: Prospective cohort study. *Am. J. Clin. Nutr.* **2007**, *86*, 1104–1110. [CrossRef] [PubMed]

117. Rao, S.; Yajnik, C.S.; Kanade, A.; Fall, C.H.; Margetts, B.M.; Jackson, A.A.; Shier, R.; Joshi, S.; Rege, S.; Lubree, H.; et al. Intake of micronutrient-rich foods in rural Indian mothers is associated with the size of their babies at birth: Pune maternal nutrition study. *J. Nutr.* **2001**, *131*, 1217–1224. [CrossRef] [PubMed]

118. Kjøllesdal, M.K.R.; Holmboe-Ottesen, G. Dietary Patterns and Birth Weight—A Review. *AIMS Public Health* **2014**, *1*, 211–225. [CrossRef] [PubMed]

119. Wen, X.; Justicia-Linde, F.; Kong, K.; Zhang, C.; Chen, W.; Epstein, L. Associations of diet and physical activity with the three components of gestational weight gain. *Am. J. Epidemiol.* **2013**, *11*, S11–S81.

120. Reddy, S.; Sanders, T.A.B.; Obeid, O. The influence of maternal vegetarian diet on essential fatty acid status of the newborn. *Eur. J. Clin. Nutr.* **1994**, *48*, 358–368. [PubMed]

121. Murphy, M.M.; Stettler, N.; Smith, K.M.; Reiss, R. Associations of consumption of fruits and vegetables during pregnancy with infant birth weight or small for gestational age births: A systematic review of the literature. *Int. J. Womens. Health* **2014**, *6*, 899–912. [CrossRef] [PubMed]

122. Ramón, R.; Ballester, F.; Iñiguez, C.; Rebagliato, M.; Murcia, M.; Esplugues, A.; Marco, A.; García de la Hera, M.; Vioque, J. Vegetable but not fruit intake during pregnancy is associated with newborn anthropometric measures. *J. Nutr.* **2009**, *139*, 561–567. [CrossRef] [PubMed]

123. Zulyniak, M.A.; De Souza, R.J.; Shaikh, M.; Desai, D.; Lefebvre, D.L.; Gupta, M.; Wilson, J.; Wahi, G.; Subbarao, P.; Becker, A.B.; et al. Does the impact of a plant-based diet during pregnancy on birth weight differ by ethnicity? A dietary pattern analysis from a prospective Canadian birth cohort alliance. *BMJ* **2017**, *7*, e017753. [CrossRef] [PubMed]

124. Fikawati, S.; Syafiq, A.; Wahyuni, D. Nutrient intake and pregnancy outcomes among vegetarian mothers in Jakarta, Indonesia. *Veg. Nutr. J.* **2013**, *20*, 15–25.

125. Robic, T.; Benedik, E.; Bratanic, B.; Fidler Mis, N.; Rogelj, I.; Golja, P. Body composition in (NON) vegetarian pregnant women and their neonates. *Clin. Nutr. Suppl.* **2012**, *7*, 108. [CrossRef]

126. Gomez Roig, M.D.; Mazarico, E.; Ferrero, S.; Montejo, R.; Ibanez, L.; Grima, F.; Vela, A. Differences in dietary and lifestyle habits between pregnant women with small fetuses and appropriate-for- gestational-age fetuses. *J. Obs. Gynaec. Res.* **2017**, *43*, 1145–1151. [CrossRef] [PubMed]

127. Piccoli, G.; Clari, R.; Vigotti, F.; Leone, F.; Attini, R.; Cabiddu, G.; Mauro, G.; Castelluccia, N.; Colombi, N.; Capizzi, I.; et al. Vegan-vegetarian diets in pregnancy: Danger or panacea? A systematic narrative review. *BJOG* **2015**, *122*, 623–633. [CrossRef] [PubMed]

128. Molloy, A.M. Should vitamin B_{12} status be considered in assessing risk of neural tube defects? *Ann. N. Y. Acad. Sci.* **2018**, *1414*, 109–125. [CrossRef] [PubMed]

129. Molloy, A.M.; Kirke, P.N.; Brody, L.C.; Scott, J.M.; Mills, J.L. Effects of folate and vitamin B12 deficiencies during pregnancy on fetal, infant, and child development. *Food. Nutr. Bull.* **2008**, *29* (Suppl. 2), S101–S111. [CrossRef] [PubMed]

130. Larsen, P.S.; Nybo Andersen, A.M.; Uldall, P.; Bech, B.H.; Olsen, J.; Hansen, A.V.; Strandberg-Larsen, K. Maternal vegetarianism and neurodevelopment of children enrolled in The Danish National Birth Cohort. *Acta Paediatr.* **2014**, *103*, e507–e509. [CrossRef] [PubMed]

131. Deb, R.; Arora, J.; Meitei, S.Y.; Gupta, S.; Verma, V.; Saraswathy, K.N.; Saran, S.; Kalla, A.K. Folate supplementation, MTHFR gene polymorphism and neural tube defects: A community based case control study in North India. *Metab. Brain Dis.* **2011**, *26*, 241–246. [CrossRef] [PubMed]

132. Haider, B.A.; Olofin, I.; Wang, M.; Spiegelman, D.; Ezzati, M.; Fawzi, W.W. Anaemia, prenatal iron use, and risk of adverse pregnancy outcomes: Systematic review and meta-analysis. *BMJ* **2013**, *346*, 3443. [CrossRef] [PubMed]

133. Hu, Z.; Tang, L.; Xu, H.L. Maternal Vitamin D Deficiency and the Risk of Small for Gestational Age: A Meta-analysis. *Iran. J. Public. Health* **2018**, *47*, 1785–1795. [PubMed]

134. North, K.; Golding, J. A maternal vegetarian diet in pregnancy is associated with hypospadias. The ALSPAC Study Team. Avon Longitudinal Study of Pregnancy and Childhood. *BJU* **2000**, *85*, 107–113. [CrossRef]

135. Akre, O.; Boyd, H.A.; Ahlgren, M.; Wilbrand, K.; Westergaard, T.; Hjalgrim, H.; Nordenskjöld, A.; Ekbom, A.; Melbye, M. Maternal and gestational risk factors for hypospadias. *Environ. Health Perspect.* **2008**, *116*, 1071–1076. [CrossRef] [PubMed]

136. Carmichael, S.L.; Cogswell, M.E.; Ma, C.; Gonzalez-Feliciano, A.; Olney, R.S.; Correa, A.; Shaw, G.M.; National Birth Defects Prevention Study. Hypospadias and maternal intake of phytoestrogens. *Am. J. Epidemiol.* **2013**, *178*, 434–440. [CrossRef] [PubMed]

137. Carmichael, S.L.; Ma, C.; Feldkamp, M.L.; Munger, R.G.; Olney, R.S.; Botto, L.D.; Shaw, G.M.; Correa, A. Nutritional factors and hypospadias risks. *Paediatr. Perinat. Epidemiol.* **2012**, *26*, 353–360. [CrossRef] [PubMed]

138. Giordano, F.; Carbone, P.; Nori, F.; Mantovani, A.; Taruscio, D.; Figa Talamanca, I. Maternal diet and the risk of hypospadias and cryptorchidism in the offspring. *Paediatr. Perinat. Epidemiol.* **2008**, *22*, 249–260. [CrossRef] [PubMed]

139. Christensen, J.S.; Asklund, C.; Skakkebæk, N.E.; Jørgensen, N.E.; Andersen, H.R.; Jørgensen, T.M.; Olsen, L.H.; Høyer, A.P.; Moesgaard, J.; Thorup, J.; et al. Association between organic dietary choice during pregnancy and hypospadias in offspring: A study of mothers of 306 boys operated on for hypospadias. *J. Urol.* **2013**, *189*, 1077–1082. [CrossRef] [PubMed]

140. De Kort, C.A.; Nieuwenhuijsen, M.J.; Mendez, M.A. Relationship between maternal dietary patterns and hypospadias. *Paediatr. Perinat. Epidemiol.* **2011**, *25*, 255–264. [CrossRef] [PubMed]

141. Li, Z.W.; Zhang, L.; Ye, R.W.; Liu, J.M.; Pei, L.J.; Zheng, X.Y.; Ren, A.G. Maternal periconceptional consumption of pickled vegetables and risk of neural tube defects in offspring. *Chin. Med. J.* **2011**, *124*, 1629–1633. [PubMed]

142. Wilson, P.R.; Pugh, L.C. Promoting nutrition in breastfeeding women. *J. Obs. Gynecol. Neonatal Nurs.* **2005**, *34*, 120–124. [CrossRef] [PubMed]

143. Bzikowska-Jura, A.; Czerwonogrodzka-Senczyna, A.; Olędzka, G.; Szostak-Węgierek, D.; Weker, H.; Wesołowska, A. Maternal Nutrition and Body Composition During Breastfeeding: Association with Human Milk Composition. *Nutrients* **2018**, *27*, 10. [CrossRef] [PubMed]

144. Keikha, M.; Bahreynian, M.; Saleki, M.; Kelishadi, R. Macro- and micronutrients of human milk composition: Are they related to maternal diet? A comprehensive systematic review. *Breastfeed. Med.* **2017**, *12*, 517–527. [CrossRef] [PubMed]

145. Boniglia, C.; Carratu, B.; Chiarotti, F.; Giammarioli, S.; Sanzini, E. Influence of maternal protein intake on nitrogen fractions of human milk. *Int. J. Vitam. Nutr. Res.* **2003**, *73*, 447–452. [CrossRef] [PubMed]

146. Agostoni, C.; Decsi, T.; Fewtrell, M.; Goulet, O.; Kolacek, S.; Koletzko, B.; Michaelsen, K.F.; van Goudoever, J. Complementary feeding: A commentary by the ESPGHAN committee on nutrition. *J. Pediatr. Gastroenterol. Nutr.* **2008**, *46*, 99–110. [CrossRef] [PubMed]

147. Fikawati, S.; Syafiq, A.; Irawati, A.; Karima, K. Comparison of Lactational Performance of Vegetarian and Non-Vegetarian Mothers in Indonesia. *Malays. J. Nutr.* **2014**, *20*, 15–25.

148. Honzik, T.; Adamovicova, M.; Smolka, V.; Magner, M.; Hruba, E.; Zeman, J. Clinical presentation and metabolic consequences in 40 breastfed infants with nutritional vitamin B12 deficiency—What have we learned? *Eur. J. Paediatr. Neurol.* **2010**, *14*, 488–495. [CrossRef] [PubMed]

149. Chebaya, P.; Karakochuk, C.D.; March, K.M.; Chen, N.N.; Stamm, R.A.; Kroeun, H.; Sophonneary, P.; Borath, M.; Shahab-Ferdows, S.; Hampel, D.; Barr, S.I.; et al. Correlations between Maternal, Breast Milk, and Infant VitaminB12 Concentrations among Mother-Infant Dyads in Vancouver, Canada and Prey Veng, Cambodia: An Exploratory Analysis. *Nutrients* **2017**, *9*, 270. [CrossRef] [PubMed]

150. Pawlak, R. To vegan or not to vegan when pregnant, lactating or feeding young children. *Eur. J. Clin. Nutr.* **2017**, *71*, 1259–1262. [CrossRef] [PubMed]

151. Pawlak, R.; Vos, P.; Shahab-Ferdows, S.; Hampel, D.; Allen, L.H.; Perrin, M.T. Vitamin B-12 content in breast milk of vegan, vegetarian, and nonvegetarian lactating women in the United States. *Am. J. Clin. Nutr.* **2018**, *108*, 525–531. [CrossRef] [PubMed]

152. Boris, J.; Jensen, B.; Salvig, J.D.; Secher, N.J.; Olsen, S.F. A randomized controlled trial of the effect of fish oil supplementation in late pregnancy and early lactation on the n-3 fatty acid content in human breast milk. *Lipids* **2004**, *39*, 1191–1196. [CrossRef] [PubMed]

153. Michaelsen, K.F.; Dewey, K.G.; Perez-Exposito, A.B.; Nurhasan, M.; Lauritzen, L.; Roos, N. Food sources and intake of n-6 and n-3 fatty acids in lowincome countries with emphasis on infants, young children (6–24 months), and pregnant and lactating women. *Matern. Child. Nutr.* **2011**, *7* (Suppl. 2), 124–140. [CrossRef] [PubMed]

154. Perrin, M.T.; Pawlak, R.; Dean, L.L.; Christis, A.; Friend, L. A cross-sectional study of fatty acids and brain-derived neurotrophic factor (BDNF) in human milk from lactating women following vegan, vegetarian, and omnivore diets. *Eur. J. Nutr.* **2018**. [CrossRef] [PubMed]

155. Blanchard, D.S. Omega 3: Fatty acid supplementation in perinatal settings. *Am. J. Matern. Child Nurs.* **2006**, *31*, 250–256. [CrossRef]

156. Baatenburg de Jong, R.; Bekhof, J.; Roorda, R.; Zwart, P. Severe nutritional vitamin deficiency in a breast-fed infant of a vegan mother. *Eur. J. Pediatr.* **2005**, *164*, 259–260. [CrossRef] [PubMed]

157. Baroni, L.; Goggi, S.; Battaglino, R.; Berveglieri, M.; Fasan, I.; Filippin, D.; Griffith, P.; Rizzo, G.; Tomasini, C.; Tosatti, M.A.; et al. Vegan Nutrition for Mothers and Children: Practical Tools for Healthcare Providers. *Nutrients* **2018**, *20*, 5. [CrossRef] [PubMed]

158. Ota, E.; Hori, H.; Mori, R.; Farrar, D. Antenatal dietary education and supplementation to increase energy and protein intake. *Cochrane Database Syst. Rev.* **2015**. [CrossRef] [PubMed]

159. Manta-vogli, P.D.; Schulpis, K.H.; Dotsikas, Y.; Yannis, L. The significant role of amino acids during pregnancy: Nutritional support. *J. Matern. Fetal Neonatal Med.* **2018**, *30*, 1–7. [CrossRef] [PubMed]

160. Middleton, P.; Shepherd, E.; Makrides, M. Omega-3 fatty acid addition during pregnancy. *Cochrane Database Syst. Rev.* **2018**, *15*, CD003402. [CrossRef] [PubMed]

161. Villar, J.; Abdel-Aleem, H.; Merialdi, M.; Mathai, M.; Ali, M.M.; Zavaleta, N.; Purwar, M.; Hofmeyr, J.; Thi Nhu Ngoc, N.; Campódonico, L.; et al. World Health Organization randomized trial of calcium supplementation among low calcium intake pregnant women. *Am. J. Obs. Gynecol.* **2006**, *194*, 639–649. [CrossRef] [PubMed]

162. Hofmeyr, G.J.; Lawrie, T.A.; Atallah, A.N.; Duley, L.; Torloni, M.R. Calcium supplementation during pregnancy for preventing hypertensive disorders and related problems. [Review][Update of Cochrane Database Syst. Rev. 2010;(8):CD001059; PMID: 20687064]. *Cochrane Database Syst. Rev.* **2014**, *6*, CD001059.

163. Colonese, F.; Laganà, A.S.; Colonese, E.; Sofo, V.; Salmeri, F.M.; Granese, R.; Triolo, O. The pleiotropic effects of vitamin D in gynaecological and obstetric diseases: An overview on a hot topic. *Biomed. Res. Int.* **2015**, *2015*, 986281. [CrossRef] [PubMed]

164. Laganà, A.S.; Vitale, S.G.; Ban Frangež, H.; Vrtačnik-Bokal, E.; D'Anna, R. Vitamin D in human reproduction: The more, the better? An evidence-based critical appraisal. *Eur. Rev. Med. Pharm. Sci.* **2017**, *21*, 4243–4251.

165. De-Regil, L.M.; Palacios, C.; Lombardo, L.K.; Peña-Rosas, J.P. Vitamin D supplementation for women during pregnancy. *Cochrane Database Syst. Rev.* **2016**. [CrossRef] [PubMed]

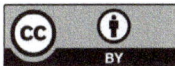

Communication

Supplementation of Plants with Immunomodulatory Properties during Pregnancy and Lactation—Maternal and Offspring Health Effects

Aneta Lewicka [1], Łukasz Szymański [2], Kamila Rusiecka [3], Anna Kucza [3], Anna Jakubczyk [4], Robert Zdanowski [3] and Sławomir Lewicki [3,*]

1 Laboratory of Epidemiology, Military Institute of Hygiene and Epidemiology, Kozielska 4, 01-163 Warsaw, Poland

2 Department of Microwave Safety, Military Institute of Hygiene and Epidemiology, Kozielska 4, 01-163 Warsaw, Poland

3 Department of Regenerative Medicine and Cell Biology, Military Institute of Hygiene and Epidemiology, Kozielska 4, 01-163 Warsaw, Poland

4 Department of Biochemistry and Food Chemistry, University of Life Sciences, Skromna 8, 20-704 Lublin, Poland

* Correspondence: slawomir.lewicki@wihe.pl; Tel.: +48-261816108

Received: 29 June 2019; Accepted: 16 August 2019; Published: 20 August 2019

Abstract: A pregnant woman's diet consists of many products, such as fruits, vegetables, cocoa, tea, chocolate, coffee, herbal and fruit teas, and various commercially available dietary supplements, which contain a high number of biological active plant-derived compounds. Generally, these compounds play beneficial roles in women's health and the development of fetus health. There are, however, some authors who report that consuming excessive amounts of plants that contain high concentrations of polyphenols may negatively affect the development of the fetus and the offspring's health. Important and problematic issues during pregnancy and lactation are bacterial infections treatment. In the treatment are proposals to use plant immunomodulators, which are generally considered safe for women and their offspring. Additional consumption of biologically active compounds from plants, however, may increase the risk of occurrences to irreversible changes in the offspring's health. Therefore, it is necessary to carry out safety tests for immunomodulators before introducing them into a maternal diet. Here, we present data from animal experiments for the four most-studied plants immunomodulators genus: *Rhodiola*, *Echinacea*, *Panax*, and *Camellia*, which were used in maternal nutrition.

Keywords: immunomodulators; maternal nutrition; pregnancy; *Rhodiola*; *Echinacea*; *Panax*; *Camellia*

1. Introduction

The antibiotic treatments of bacterial infections during pregnancy and lactation are very problematic because of their negative effects on embryo and newborn development. The food and drug administration agency divided all known antibiotics into five groups (A, B, C, D, X) depending on the potential risk of harmful effects on the offspring. In general, only group A antibiotics are considered to be safe when used during pregnancy and lactation [1]. Prenatal exposure to the antibiotics from the remaining groups may modify the immunological system of the offspring. The offspring of mothers treated during pregnancy with the group B antibiotics, such as penicillin and cephalosporin, showed, after pathogen stimulation, a decrease of the specific immune response and increase of the nonspecific immune response [2]. Also, prenatal treatment with antibiotics increased the risk of childhood asthma and obesity [3]. The alternative therapy, which could potentially support or even replace antibiotic treatment, would be the use of plant-derived immunomodulators. Nowadays, there are more than 300 plants which exhibit beneficial properties for humans. Plant-derived compounds which affect the immune system belong to chemical groups of compounds such as: alkaloids (i.e., leonurine [4], piperine [5], and sophocarpine [6]), terpenoids (i.e., ginsan [7] or oleanolic acid [8]), polysaccharides (from licorice *Glycyrrhiza uralensis Fisch* [9], or from *Lentinus edodes* [10]), lactones (from *Datura quercifolia* [11] or sesquiterpene lactones from *Loranthus parasiticus*), and essential oils (Z-ligustilide [12] or Tetramethylpyra-zine [13]). However, the most well-known and numerous group of immune-affecting compounds belongs to flavonoids, which are divided into flavones, flavanones, flavanols, flavonols, catechins, isoflavones, and anthocyanins [14]. Some of the flavonoids, such as genistein or quercetin, are commonly-used supplements in human nutrition [15,16]. Plant-derived immunomodulators affect the immune system in various ways: [1] directly by affecting the immune cell functions in both adaptive and innate immunity [17] and by direct anti-microbial, anti-viral, or anti-fungal properties [18] or [2] indirectly by modulation of non-immune cell function [19], reduction of inflammation [20], the influence of cytokines secretion [21], or modulation of angiogenesis [22]. Most importantly, plant-derived immunomodulators are generally considered as safe for humans and therefore are a good alternative for the use of most synthetic immunomodulators, which cause various side effects. This statement is mostly true for people in a normal state of life, however, for pregnant women and their offspring, this can become dangerous. Several researchers had shown that theobromine and cocoa catechins administered to pregnant mice affected embryonic angiogenesis and morphology and function of some of their progeny organs, among them the lymphoid system and kidneys [23–27]. Therefore, before the recommendation of supplementation of plant-derived immunomodulators in the maternal diet, experiments on animals should be performed. Here, we presented data from animal experiments for the four most-studied plants' immunomodulators genus, *Rhodiola*, *Echinacea*, *Panax*, and *Camellia*, which were used in maternal nutrition. The summarized effects of Rhodiola, *Echinacea*, Ginseng, and Camellia, or its extracts supplemented in pregnancy and/or lactation on mothers and offspring health, are presented in Table 1.

Table 1. Summarized effects of *Rhodiola*, *Echinacea*, *Ginseng*, and *Camellia*, or its extracts, supplemented in pregnancy and/or lactation on mothers and offspring health.

Herb or Extract	Key Substances	Pharmacological Action	
		Mother	Offspring
Rhodiola	phenylethanoid salidroside and tyrosol, phenolic acids (i.e., chlorogenic, ferulic, ellagic and p-coumaric), and flavonoids (i.e., fisetin, naringenin, kaempferol, epicatechin, luteolin, quercetin, epigallocatechin and (+)-catechin)	reduces the percentage of cells with a respiratory burst in granulocytes (supplementation with RKW) [28] increases in the percentage of granulocytes and monocytes in the blood with the respiratory burst (supplementation with RKW-A) [28] contributes to changes in spleen morphology and structure [29] increases the concentration of VEGF and bFGF [30] reduces the number of CD4+ and CD19 + cells and the total number of NK cells [31]	increases hemoglobin concentration (about 0.6 mg/dL) [32] decreases in the mean percentage of lymphocytes in peripheral blood, and an increase in the mean percentage of granulocytes [32] decreases in the percentage of CD3+ cells and CD4+ [32] increases the concentration of IL-10 in the serum [33] stimulate the phagocytosis process [32] significant difference in tissue localization and the number of CD8+ cells [34] contributes to a higher number of CD8+ cells in the central part of the spleen [34] influence cell proliferation in response to mitogen supplementation (LPS, PHA and ConA) [29] decreases the number of apoptotic cells [35] decreases the concentration of VEGF in the sera [30]
Echinacea	alkamides, ketoalkenes, caffeic acid derivatives, polysaccharides, glycoproteins, and caftaric acid	does not affect hematological and reproductive parameters [36] no influences on the enzyme results [37] decreases the level of crude protein in colostrum [37] decreases the level of antibodies in the plasma [37] decreases the number of spleen lymphocytes and nucleated erythroid cells [38] contributes to more frequent miscarriages in the early stages of pregnancy [38]	decreases the number of embryos in litter and significantly diminished VEGF and bFGF content of embryos tissue [39] increases phagocytic activity in blood [40] increases bacterial diversity [40] non-teratogenic, does not increase the risk of malformations [41–43]
Ginseng	polysaccharides, flavonoids, fatty acids, peptides, and saponins (mainly ginsenosides)	increases the total IgG concentration in milk and serum of sows, which was associated with elevated levels of cytokines: IL-2, IL-6, TNF- α, and IFN-γ [44] stimulates the effect of isolated lymphocytes after pokeweed mitogen stimulation [45] stimulates the innate immunity in cows with *Staphylococcus aureus* infection [46] increases phagocytosis, oxidative burst activity of blood neutrophils and number of monocytes [46]	increases IL-2 and TNF-α concentration in the piglets' serum [44] reduces the incidence of schizophrenia in the offspring [47] alleviates the toxic effects of phthalates and bisphenol A [48] reverses the negative effect of dexamethasone on the synthesis of testosterone in Leydig cells [49] teratogenic effect [50]

Table 1. *Cont.*

Herb or Extract	Key Substances	Pharmacological Action	
		Mother	Offspring
Camellia	epigallocatechin, epicatechin, epicatechin gallate	increases the ratio of IL-10/TNF-α and IL-1β in mesenteric adipose tissue and causes a decrease in catalase in the liver [51]	increases the risk of premature birth [58]
		inhibits the penetration of macrophages and increases the expression of AMPK (during lactation) [52]	risk factor for low birth weight of offspring [59]
		contributes to alterations in urinary calcium, creatinine, and urea during the prenatal period, nephrotoxicity [53]	protect against dyslipidemia, glucose intolerance, and fat accumulation [60]
		increases levels of proinflammatory cytokines and decreases anti-inflammatory cytokines levels in serum [53]	pro-inflammatory effect on the adipose tissue (not on a high-fat diet) [60]
		decreases of hemoglobin concentration and loss of the biconcave structure of erythrocytes [54]	decreases the retroperitoneal adipose tissue relative weight and SOD activity but increases adiponectin, LPS, IL-10 and IL-6 content and IL-10/TNF-α ratio in retroperitoneal, IL-10 and TNF-α content in gonadal, and IL-6 content in mesenteric adipose tissues [51]
		increases of WBC level in the mother's blood and induced significant changes in the histology of liver and serum enzymes [54]	improves the results of treatment of maternal gestational diabetes [61]
		increases the efficacy of oral nifedipine treatment in severe pregnancy-induced preeclampsia [56]	reduces neonatal complications [61]
		may be associated with an increased risk of pre-eclampsia [57]	can decreases the number of malformations in fetuses after exposure to cyclophosphamide, but too high dose increases the toxicity of cyclophosphamide [62]
		decreases the level of folic acid [55]	

2. Rhodiola

2.1. Characteristic and Immunomodulatory Properties

Genus *Rhodiola* (family *Crassulaceae*) consists of 200 species, out of which over 20 species have medicinal properties. *Rhodiola* extracts contain phenylethanoid salidroside and tyrosol, phenolic acids (i.e., chlorogenic, ferulic, ellagic, and p-coumaric), and flavonoids (i.e., fisetin, naringenin, kaempferol, epicatechin, luteolin, quercetin, epigallocatechin, and (+)-catechin) [63–65]. They have been used in traditional Asian and European medicine such as tonics, adaptogens, antidepressants, and anti-inflammatory compounds [66]. The extracts from these plants also have anticancer, antibacterial, and immunomodulatory properties [67–70]. *Rhodiola* extracts, given for seven days to mice infected with *Pseudomonas aeruginosa*, decrease the infection. These mice have a higher number and higher metabolic activity of blood leukocytes [71]. *Rhodiola* extracts also have a direct antiviral and antibacterial effect against hepatitis C virus (HCV) and *Mycobacterium tuberculosis* [72,73]. At present, there are several clinical therapies available, which use *Rhodiola* plants to stimulate the immune system [74]. One of the well-characterized plant species from the *Rhodiola* genus which was supplemented in pregnancy and lactation is *Rhodiola kirilowii*, which was supplemented as lyophilized water extract (RKW) or 50% hydro-alcoholic extract (RKW-A) in the pregnancy and lactation period in mice (about 42 days of supplementation).

2.2. Effects on Mothers

Supplementation of mice during pregnancy and lactation with water extract (RKW) or 50% hydro-alcoholic extract (RKW-A) of *Rhodiola kirilowii* (concentration 20 mg extract/kg body weight) had no effect on the average body weight as compared to the control group (receiving sterile water). There were no differences in the mean weight and mass index of selected organs: liver, kidneys, spleen, brain, and eyeballs, between the study groups. Macroscopic assessment of organs also did not reveal any changes in their structure. The morphological elements of blood: WBC (number of white blood cells/mm^3), RBC (number of red blood cells/mm^3), HGB (hemoglobin, g/dL), HCT (hematocrit, %), MCH (mean corpuscular hemoglobin, pg), MCHC (mean hemoglobin concentration, g/dL), RDW (red blood cell distribution width, %), PLT (platelet count /mm^3), and MPV (mean platelet volume, fL), did not differ between the control group and the groups receiving extracts from *Rhodiola kirilowii*. There were no differences in the population of cells belonging to the adaptive immunity system, T cells (CD3+, CD4+, CD8+) and B cells (CD19+), in the blood. However, some small changes in the composition and functioning of innate immunity cells were noticed. Mice fed with RKW extracts showed a lower percentage of cells with a respiratory burst in granulocytes (PhagoBurst test) [28]. In contrast, supplementation with RKW-A extract caused an increase in the percentage of granulocytes and monocytes in the blood with the respiratory burst. Other components of non-specific immunity have not changed (including the number and percentage of NK (natural killer) cells and the percentage of phagocytic cells). There were no changes in the concentration of selected cytokines in the serum: Th1 (IL-2, TNF-α, INF-γ), Th2 (IL-4, IL-6, IL-10), and Th17 (IL-17a) [30].

Despite the lack of differences in the weight and mass index of the spleen in mothers fed with *Rhodiola kirilowii* extracts, significant changes in spleen morphology and structure were observed. Spleens from mothers fed during pregnancy and the lactation water or hydroalcoholic extracts from *Rhodiola kirilowii* contained a significantly lower number of cells per gram of organ [29]. In the cytometric study, a significant reduction in the percentage of lymphocytes was associated with an increase in the percentage of monocytes and granulocytes in the spleen only in the group receiving a 50% hydro-alcoholic extract of *Rhodiola kirilowii*. However, no significant changes in the percentage of the innate (CD335+) and adaptive (CD3+, CD4+, CD8+, CD19+) cell populations between the study groups were observed. Analysis of the total number of cell populations per gram of organ showed no difference in the number of CD3+ and CD8+ cells between groups. However, we found that both extracts reduced the number of CD4+ and CD19+ cells. In addition, water extract significantly reduced the total number of NK cells (CD335+) [31]. The observed changes in the number of cells in the spleen suggest that treatment caused a certain degree of impairment of the adaptive immune response. Therefore, we decided to examine the spleen cells' (mainly T and B cells) proliferation response to mitogens stimulations (ex vivo studies). We found that there were no significant differences in the proliferative activity of splenocytes stimulated with lipopolysaccharide (LPS), phytohemagglutinin (PHA), or concanavalin A (ConA). This means that the functionality of these cells, despite the lower number in the spleen, has been preserved. However, the observed, unfavorable reduction in the number of splenocytes is a disturbing sign, which should be taken into account in the long-term administration of extracts from *Rhodiola kirilowii* to pregnant women [29,30].

The RKW-A group had a higher concentration of VEGF (vascular endothelial growth factor) and bFGF (basic fibroblast growth factor) than the control group. These trends were associated with decreased proliferation of endothelial cells (HECa10) after the supplementation of medium with the serum isolated from mothers fed during pregnancy and lactation with (RKW-A). However, the RKW group showed increased migration of HECa10 cells [30]. The obtained results led to the conclusion that supplementation of hydro-alcoholic extracts of *Rhodiola kirilowii* may cause modulation of angiogenesis processes in developing fetuses. A similar effect was observed in previous studies in which RKW-A extract inhibited tumor angiogenesis and the RKW had no effect [63].

In conclusion, slight changes in adaptive immunity (blood) and in the number of splenocytes with a lack of side effects on the range of morphological blood parameters of mother mice should be considered as a positive effect of supplementation, with such a long period of use. Usually, plant-derived immunomodulatory drugs are used for no more than 2–3 weeks. This is due to the fact that prolonged administration of immunostimulants may cause lack of stimulation, and in extreme situations, deregulations of the immune system, as with what was seen in aquaculture [75]. Authors suggested that for successful use of immunostimulators, not only appropriate timing of administration, but also dosage and period of administration are necessary.

2.3. Effects on Offspring

The animal mass analysis did not show a significant difference between the offspring from the control group and the group supplemented with water extract of *Rhodiola kirilowii*. The mean weight of offspring whose mothers were fed with 50% hydro-alcoholic extract was about 7% lower than in the control group ($p < 0.01$). There were no significant differences in peripheral blood morphometric parameters (WBC, RBC, HCT, MCH, MCHC, RDW, RDW-a, PLT, and MPV) between the control group and the groups receiving *Rhodiola kirilowii* extracts. There was a slight, but significant, increase in hemoglobin concentration (about 0.6 mg/dL) in the group supplemented with *Rhodiola kirilowii* water extract [32].

The analysis of selected components of the adaptive and innate immune system in the blood and spleens of offspring, whose mothers were fed during pregnancy and lactation extracts from *Rhodiola kirilowii*, showed significant differences. A significant decrease in the mean percentage of lymphocytes (approximately 6%, $p < 0.05$) in peripheral blood and an increase in the mean percentage of granulocytes (approximately 20%, $p < 0.05$) were observed in the RKW group (a similar trend was observed in the RKW-A group, however, it was not statistically significant). The analysis of the lymphocyte population showed a significant decrease in the percentage of CD3+ cells (RKW-14%, $p = 0.0434$, RKW-A-10%, $p = 0.0337$) and CD4+ (15%, $p = 0.0184$ and 13%, $p = 0.0116$, respectively). In addition, a lower percentage of CD8+ cells and a higher percentage of NK cells (CD335+) were observed in the RKW group. There were no changes in the percentage of B cells (CD19+) and the percentage of regulatory T cells (CD4+, CD25+, FoxP3+) and CD4+, CD25+ cells between the examined groups [32].

A significant decrease in the percentage of CD4+ in the peripheral blood may indicate a certain impairment of adaptive immunity, which may lead to the disorders in the stimulation of CD19+ cells and the production of specific antibodies. In part, these results were confirmed in the SRBC (sheep red blood cells) test (immunization of mice with sheep red blood cells), in which much lower levels of anti-SRBC antibodies were observed in the serum of mice whose mothers were fed during pregnancy and lactation with RKW-A [33]. The explanation of the lower immune response after RKW-A supplementation may also be associated with an increased concentration of IL-10 in the serum. This cytokine has anti-inflammatory activity and inhibits the synthesis of other pro-inflammatory cytokines that are necessary to activate the immune system in response to antigens. No such changes were observed for water extract (RKW) [33].

Both extracts of *Rhodiola kirilowii* consumed during pregnancy and lactation by mothers stimulated the phagocytosis process in their offspring. There was an increase in the phagocytosis of opsonized *E. coli* bacteria and the intensity of the oxygen burst after stimulation with *E. coli* and zymosan [32]. Interestingly, in the RKW group, there was a significant reduction in serum IL-17a concentration [33]. IL-17a is a cytokine responsible inter alia for supporting phagocytosis of extracellular bacteria. It seems that the observed situation may be related to the activation of granulocytes by polyphenolic compounds present in the extracts, which in turn leads to a reduction of IL-17a secretion (immune system is not "over-activated"). The lack of additional stimulation by IL-17a could also lead to a decrease in the population of phagocytic monocytes and oxygen burst after zymosan stimulation in the RKW group [33].

Spleens of mice fed with *Rhodiola kirilowii* extracts did not differ in mass and mass index (spleen weight/mouse weight) and cellularity compared to the spleens obtained from the control group. There were no significant differences in the morphology of the spleens. In the cytometric study of spleen cells, no significant differences in the percentage of CD3+, CD4+, CD8+, CD19+, and CD335+ cells were noticed [32]. Histological analysis showed no significant difference in the number and location of CD4+ cells, but a significant difference in tissue localization and the number of CD8+ cells. These cells were found not only in usual locations within the spleen but also in the perivascular lymphatic sheath (PALS), the follicular zone of B cells, and in the red pulp. In addition, there was a much higher number of CD8+ cells in the central part of the spleen [34]. This may indicate increased mobility of these cells and thus increased ability to respond to antiviral responses. Supplementation of mothers with extracts from *Rhodiola kirilowii* during pregnancy and lactation also influenced cell proliferation in response to mitogen supplementation: lipopolysaccharide (LPS), phytohaemagglutinin (PHA), and concanavalin A (ConA). A decrease in cell proliferation rate was observed in the RKW-A group after the supplementation of LPS and PHA when compared to the control group. There was a reduction of proliferation rate in the RKW-A group after stimulation with ConA when compared to the RKW group [32]. The presented data indicated attenuation of the ability of adaptive immunity in the hydro-alcoholic *Rhodiola kirilowii* group.

Changes in the percentage of blood cells associated with adaptive immune response (mainly CD3+) suggested a possible negative effect on the maturation of these cells in the thymus in the offspring. The mean thymus weight and the thymic index did not differ between the groups. There were no significant differences in the morphology of the thymus between groups. There were also no abnormalities in the structure of lobules, medulla, cortex ratio, and epithelial cell content. No thymic hypertrophy or atrophy was detected. The offspring of mice whose mothers were fed during pregnancy and lactation RKW and RKW-A extracts had a significantly lower number of apoptotic cells (marker M30) than the control group. However, there was no significant difference in the number of cells synthesizing IL-7 [35]. The obtained data led to the conclusion that extracts from *Rhodiola kirilowii* prolonged the function of thymus cells in the offspring, which may be important for overcoming the infection.

Moreover, Lewicki et al. (2017) [76] found that there were no significant differences in the mass index and macroscopic structure of the kidneys between the examined groups. A higher percentage of individuals with serum creatinine above 0.65 mg % was found in the RKW and RKW-A groups. In addition, the offspring of mothers from RKW-A group had slightly increased urea concentration and decreased cystatin C concentration. These data suggested some abnormalities in the kidneys.

In the RKW-A group, a higher number of tufts per mm^2 was observed and their smaller diameter may indicate their atrophy. These changes may have been caused directly by the active substances in the extracts from *Rhodiola kirilowii* present in the maternal sera, and/or indirectly by affecting the secretion of proangiogenic factors. The differences were observed in the concentration of polyphenols in mice-mothers supplemented with RKW or RKW-A (mainly catechin and salidroside), a lower concentration of VEGF in the sera of the offspring from the RKW-A group [30]. These data indicate that hydro-alcoholic extract should not be long-term supplemented to pregnant women.

3. Echinacea

3.1. Characteristic and Immunomodulatory Properties

Echinacea is a plant belonging to the species from the *Asteraceae* family [77]. There are three species of *Echinacea* with medicinal properties, including *Echinacea purpurea*, *Echinacea pallida*, and *Echinacea angustifolia* [78]. *Echinacea* extracts contained alkamides, ketoalkenes, caffeic acid derivatives, polysaccharides, glycoproteins, and caftaric acid, which are responsible for the medical activity of the plant.

Echinacea-based drugs contribute to a shortening of the various types of infections and colds [79,80]. This is due to the active ingredients such as polysaccharides, alkaloids, coffee acid derivatives [81], and proteoglycans that have immunomodulatory, antiviral, antioxidant, and anti-inflammatory properties [78]. Polysaccharides, especially arabinogalactans, activate macrophages and have a cytotoxic effect against cancer cells [82,83]. During this process, various biological products are formed [84], including nitric oxide, which has a defensive function in the immune system [85]. Bacterial infections contribute to the formation of the inflammatory mediators, which in turn leads to the increase of the nitric oxide levels [86]. This compound is very harmful to healthy cells [87,88]. Studies have shown that the alcohol extracts of the *Echinacea purpurea*, *Echinacea pallida*, and *Echinacea angustifolia* significantly reduce the production of nitric oxide [86]. The extract also increased the number of non-activated macrophage cells that are the first to defend the body against infections [86]. The active ingredients present in *Echinacea* also show antioxidant activity [89–92]. Such components include the alkamids that have an antioxidant effect on the coffee acid derivatives [92].

3.2. Effects on Mothers

Dabboul et al. (2016) conducted a study to check the reproductive and immune parameters of pregnant rabbits during *Echinacea pallida* diet supplementation [36]. The studies were performed on 100 pregnant rabbits at the age of 21 weeks and supplemented with 3 g/day of *Echinacea pallida* for 4 weeks. The tests were carried out on days 0, 14, and 28 of the experiment. The effect of this plant on blood morphology parameters of mothers: red blood cells (n/mm^3), hemoglobin (g/dL), hematocrit (%), mean corpuscular volume (fL), mean corpuscular hemoglobin (pg), mean hemoglobin concentration (g/dL), red blood cell distribution width (%), platelet count (n/mm^3), mean thrombocyte volume (PCT,%), mean platelet volume (fL), platelet distribution width (%), number of white blood cells (n/mm3), lymphocytes (%), monocytes (%), neutrophils (%), eosinophils (%), and basophils (%) has not been observed.

The concentration of total protein (g/dL), glutamic oxoloacetic transaminase (UI/L), blood urea nitrogen (mg/dL), albumin (g/dL), urea (mg/dL), and cholesterol (mg/dL) were also analyzed. The serum protein was determined using semi-automatic agarose gel electrophoresis. Blood and immune parameters were determined in three periods (day 0, day 14, and day 28) and were subjected to statistical analysis using the GLM thematic model. In the case of reproductive parameters, the analysis was carried out for the specific *Echinacea* test and the control sample using the Student's *t*-test. The results of the study showed that *Echinacea* supplementation does not affect hematological and reproductive parameters. Also, in the case of immune parameters, there were no significant differences between the test and control groups.

In another study carried out by Maass et al. (2005), dried *Echinacea purpurea* was introduced in the diet of sows and its effect on the results of plasma enzymes, blood, lymphocyte proliferation, antibodies, and immunoglobulin content in colostrum were checked [37]. The experiments were carried out with the use of various concentrations of *Echinacea* in the diet during different periods of pregnancy and lactation. The period of *Echinacea* supplementation from days 85–110 of pregnancy and in the 4th, 6th, and 9th week of lactation was considered. The study was carried out on 36 sows from the 85th day of pregnancy to the 28th day of lactation. Animals were divided into three experimental groups by weight. The diet during pregnancy and lactation was supplemented by 0%, 1.2%, or 3.6% and 0%, 0.5%, or 1.5% *Echinacea*. Due to the lack of data for pigs, the dose of *Echinacea* was given based on human recommendations (16.5 mg of freshly squeezed juice/kg). Blood analysis was performed on day 85 of pregnancy as well as on day 1 and 28 of lactation. The colostrum was collected manually from 1 to 6 hours after delivery.

Body mass, body temperature, health status, crude protein (6.37 *Kjeldahl-N), immunoglobulins, hematological, and clinic–chemical parameters (alkaline phosphatase, alanine, and aspartate, and gamma-glutamyltransferase aminotransferase) were analyzed using acquired samples. No influence of *Echinacea* on the enzyme results (alkaline phosphatase (U/L), alanine aminotransferase (U/L), aspartate aminotransferase (U/L), gamma-glutamyl transferase (U/L)) was observed. The level of crude protein in colostrum was lower in the *Echinacea* supplemented group. There was no statistical difference in the levels of leukocytes (10^9/L), erythrocytes (10^{12}/L), lymphocytes (%), granulocytes, neutrophils (%), eosinophils (%), basophils (%), or monocytes (%) between the study (*Echinacea* supplemented) and control group. Also, similar results were obtained in a group of breeding pigs. The experiment included two phases of *Echinacea* supplementation (1–3 weeks and 7–9 weeks) and an intermediate phase without supplementation (4–6 weeks). The experiment aimed to investigate the immune effect and the production of antibodies during vaccination of pigs. A differential vaccine was given, which was administered at week 1 and week 5 of the experiment. IgG1 immunoglobulin in colostrum was determined using ELISA technique. From the obtained data, such as the hematological analysis and the varied number of blood cells, supplementation had no effect. The level of antibodies in the plasma showed a significant effect of *Echinacea* in relation to all antibodies, which caused a significantly higher immune response in the control group. The health of the animals was also good.

Chow et al. (2006) focused on studying the effects of *Echinacea* on immunity and spontaneous miscarriages. The study was conducted in mice in which *Echinacea* was fed from the beginning to the 10th, 11th, 12th, 13th, and 14th days of pregnancy [38]. The mother's spleen and bone marrow were collected for examination. The effect of *Echinacea* on hematopoietic cells in the spleen and bone marrow was determined using the Student's *t*-test. The significant differences were found in the results obtained from the immune system analysis in the third trimester in the spleen of pregnant mice. The parameters and number of spleen lymphocytes and nucleated erythroid cells were decreased in *Echinacea*-fed mice. The bone marrow parameters were not influenced by the *Echinacea* supplementation. The results also indicated that miscarriages are more likely to happen in the early stages of pregnancy (10–11 days) in the *Echinacea*-fed mice. Based on these results, it was decided not to suggest the consumption of *Echinacea* in the early stages of pregnancy in women. On the other hand, the results of clinical trials conducted by Heitman et al. (2016) did not show adverse effects of *Echinacea* supplementation of mothers during pregnancy [41].

3.3. Effects on Offspring

Despite the large number of papers which confirmed the immunomodulatory effect of *Echinacea* spp. and a lot of products on the market containing *Echinacea*, there is still a little evidence of offspring safety after uses of the herb in pregnancy and lactation. In 2007, Barcz et al. investigated the effect of alcoholic extracts of *Echinacea* purpurea given to pregnant mice on angiogenic activity and tissue VEGF and bFGF production of their fetuses. Eight pregnant females, from the 1st to the 18th day of pregnancy, were given a 0.06 g solution of *Echinacea* purpurea from different formulations (three mothers were given Esberitox, another three were Echinapur, while two mothers were fed Immunalforte). On day 18, the females were sacrificed, and the fetuses were used for the angiogenesis test. It was found that two *Echinacea* drugs lowered the number of embryos in litter and significantly diminished the vascular endothelial growth factor (VEGF) and the basic fibroblast growth factor (bFGF) content of embryos tissue [39]. The effect of mothers' supplementation in pregnancy and lactation of *Echinacea pallida* on the health of their offspring was also studied by Kovitvadhi et al. (2016) [40]. The authors supplemented sows with *Echinacea* from days 85–110 of pregnancy and in the 4th, 6th, and 9th week of lactation. Offspring from those mothers exhibited an increased phagocytic in blood activity and a higher bacterial diversity compared to other groups. There was no statistically significant difference in animal growth, blood parameters, and humoral immune response against vaccination or against the rabbit hemorrhagic disease virus.

The data from the human studies revealed no effect of *Echinacea* treatment in pregnancy and lactation in mothers on the health of their offspring. The Gallo et al. (2000) study also showed no effect of consuming *Echinacea* during pregnancy on the increased risk of malformations [42]. Also, Perri et al. (2006), in a prospective cohort study, concluded that *Echinacea* is non-teratogenic when used during pregnancy and lactation. The conclusions were based on a lack of evidence that maternal *Echinacea* consumption varied affected major or minor birth defects, differences in pregnancy outcome, delivery method, maternal weight gain, gestational age, infant birth weight, or fetal distress. It should be noted that daily dosage was varied, however, *Echinacea* supplementation was usually used by mothers for up to 7 days [43]. In a cohort study, Heitmann et al. (2016) evaluated the impact of prenatal exposure to *Echinacea* and the consequences of its use on malformations and adverse pregnancy outcomes. Based on the analysis of questionnaires completed by pregnant women at 17 and 30 weeks of pregnancy, 6 months after birth, and information on pregnancy results from the Norwegian birth register, there was no increased risk of malformations or adverse delivery results, such as premature delivery [41].

4. Ginseng

4.1. Characteristic and Immunomodulatory Properties

Ginseng belongs to angiosperms, the *Araliaceae* family, *Panax L.* genus. There are thirteen ginseng species, the most popular of which are *Panax ginseng* C.A. Meyer, *Panax quinquefolium* L., *Panax japonicus* C.A. Meyer. For thousands of years, it has been used in East Asia as a medicinal plant due to the active substances found in the root. These are polysaccharides, flavonoids, fatty acids, peptides, and saponins [93].

The main active substances in the ginseng root are ginsenosides. These are chemical compounds that belong to saponins. Due to the structure, there are three main groups: the protopanaxadiol group, the oleanane group, and the protopanaxatriol group [94]. Ginsenosides have been shown to have anti-inflammatory properties, mainly by inhibiting the production of TNF-α in a mouse macrophage cell line RAW264.7, that was exposed to lipopolysaccharide stimulation [95]. Lee et al. (2005) showed that 20-O-beta-D-glucopyranosyl-20 (S)-protopanaxadiol inhibits TPA-induced expression of COX-2, which in turn may contribute to antitumor activity [96]. Also, Ginsenoside-Re can inhibit the interaction between LPS and TLR4 (toll-like receptor 4) [97]. Other important active substances of ginseng root are polyphenols and polysaccharides [98]. Byeon et al. (2012) have shown that ginseng derived polysaccharides can be used as an immunostimulant via TLR2 (toll-like receptor 2), which mediates the activation of macrophages [99]. Also, TLR2 mediated functional activation of macrophages can be boosted by wortmannin-targeted enzymes. Ginseng polysaccharides also have immunomodulatory, anticancer, and antidiabetic effects [100].

4.2. General Effect of Ginseng

For thousands of years, ginseng root has been used as an immuno-stimulating plant. With the development of science, further properties and mechanisms of ginseng's actions have been discovered.

The administration of the ginseng extract has a positive effect on the spinal cord injury and thus has a neuroprotective effect [101]. However, it has been proven that the use of ginseng extract during pregnancy may have a teratogenic effect. According to research by Khalid et al. (2008), a high dose of the extract may also lead to the development of bone defects [102].

The literature describes many mechanisms of action of ginseng on the immune system. Kim et al. (2009) found that ginsan, ginseng-derived polysaccharide, has immunomodulatory effects on dendritic cells. They showed that ginsan stimulates dendritic cells by inducing their maturation. Ginsan stimulates secretion of cytokines from dendritic cells, increases the proliferation of allogeneic CD4 + lymphocytes, and enhances the expression of CD86 on the surface of dendritic cells [103]. Shin et al. (2002) have shown that ginseng acidic polysaccharides enhance the phagocytic activity of macrophages, stimulates cytokine secretion, and leads to the increased CD14 expression [104]. It has also been proven that ginseng increases the activity of NK cells [105]. Ginseng has been shown to protect mice against sepsis caused by *Staphylococcus aureus* by decreasing the secretion of inflammatory cytokines TNF-α, IL-1β, IL-6, IFN-γ, IL-12, and IL-18 [106]. Chan et al. (2011) focused on bird flu H9N2. They showed that ginsenosides (protopanaxatriol and ginsenoside Re) have protective properties against the H9N2 virus. Protopanaxatriol reduced the expression of IP10 (interferon gamma-induced protein 10), while the second ginsenoside reduces the DNA damage caused by the virus (H9N2-induced inflammation and apoptosis) [107].

4.3. Effects on Mothers

The effects of substances derived from ginseng on pregnant women are not yet fully understood. Xi et al. (2017) investigated the effect of supplementation of polysaccharides derived from ginseng root in a pregnant sow. The extract was given to sows from the 90th day of pregnancy to the 28th day after the birth of the progeny. There was no effect of ginseng supplementation on the total number of piglets, live piglets, weak piglets, and birth weight of piglets, which means that the herb had not affected the reproduction process. Moreover, ginseng treatment in pregnancy and lactation caused a significant increase in the total immunoglobulin G concentration in milk and serum of sows, which was associated with elevated levels of cytokines: IL-2, IL-6, TNF-α, and IFN-γ [44]. Taken together, the results present evidence that ginseng supplemented in pregnancy and lactation modulates the adaptive immunity of mothers.

Also, the positive effect of ginseng supplementation on the function immune system was reported by Concha et al. (1996). Authors investigated ginseng immunomodulatory effects isolated from peripheral blood or milk lymphocyte in an in vitro study. They showed that ginseng has a stimulating effect on both groups of isolated lymphocytes after pokeweed mitogen stimulation [45]. The same scholars have shown, a few years later, that subcutaneous injections of extract from the root of panax ginseng CA Meyer at a dose of 8 mg/kg body weight per day for 6 days can stimulate the innate immunity in cows with staphylococcus aureus infection. In ginseng-treated groups, the numbers of S. aureus-infected quarters and milk somatic cell counts tended to decrease. Moreover, the phagocytosis and oxidative burst activity of blood neutrophils isolated from cows treated with ginseng were significantly increased one week after injection, as well as the number of monocytes in blood [46]. These findings suggested that not only adaptive, but also innate immunity, may be affected after ginseng treatment in pregnant and lactating mothers.

4.4. Effects on Offspring

The supplementation of ginseng extract in the sow's diet may have a beneficial effect on the development of immunity in newborns [44]. This is not only associated with passive immunity delivered to infants by milk (the higher ability of the mother's immune system for the elimination of pathogens) but also with modulation in an immune response in newborns. Maternal supplementation of ginseng significantly increased IL-2 (an important part of organism response to microbial infection) and TNF-α (phagocytosis stimulant) concentration in the piglets' serum.

Ginseng supplementation in pregnancy or the lactation period also plays a protective role against some negative factors. Administration of ginseng extract during pregnancy exposed to prenatal stress reduces the incidence of schizophrenia in the offspring [47]. According to the studies of Saadeldin et al. (2018), administration of an aqueous ginseng extract to pregnant females during exposure to phthalates and bisphenol A alleviates the toxic effects of these compounds in offspring [48]. Wanderly et al. (2013) studied if giving pregnant rats a ginseng extract could reverse the increase in testosterone production induced by dexamethasone. The extract was administered to females from 10 to 20 days of pregnancy by gavage, while dexamethasone was administered by injections from the 14th day to the 21st day of pregnancy. Adult male offspring were sacrificed, and blood, testis, and prostate were removed for further ex vivo examinations and morphological analysis. Plasma was obtained from the blood and the testosterone concentration was tested. The study showed that the ginseng extract is able to reverse the negative effect of dexamethasone on the synthesis of testosterone in Leydig cells [49].

The use of ginseng in pregnancy, however, has some limitations. The study by Belanger et al. (2016) showed that ginseng extracts have a negative effect on pregnancy in mice. Also, in vitro direct exposure to the ginseng extract reduced development in a concentration responsive manner [50].

5. Camellia

5.1. Characteristic and Immunomodulatory Properties

Camellia sinensis (black tea) [108] and *Camellia sinensis, Theaceae* (green tea) [109] are two of the most popular botanical plants. They are cultivated in over 30 countries, especially in tropical areas [53]. Infusions from tea are consumed in different countries, but its consumption is most popular in East Asia [110]. The main active ingredients of tea are polyphenols, more specifically catechins: epigallocatechin, epicatechin, and epicatechin gallate [111–113], which are characterized by antioxidant properties [112,114]. The most biologically active catechins are epigalocatechingallate [108].

Green tea can modulate macrophages and dendritic cells [115,116], as well as immunomodulatory properties of the immune system [117]. Tea can stimulate immunity by stimulating the secretion of antibodies [118,119]. It also acts as an antioxidant and has anticancer activity [120]. Black tea has a positive effect on the cardiovascular system [121]. Due to the limited data regarding the impact of tea consumption on pregnancy, caution is recommended [122]. High concentrations of black tea extract may be toxic during pregnancy [123].

5.2. Effects on Mothers

Losinskas-Hachul et al. (2018) [51] investigated the effect of green tea intake (400 mg/kg of body weight/day) by rat-mothers from the first day of pregnancy until the end of lactation on maternal and offspring metabolism. They showed that the intake of the extract by the mother increases the ratio of IL-10/TNF-α and IL-1β in mesenteric adipose tissue and causes a decrease in catalase activity in the liver. It has been proven that the intake of green tea extract during the lactation period inhibits the penetration of macrophages and increases the expression of AMPK (5′AMP-activated protein kinase), which affects the secretion of insulin [52]. A high dose of black tea extract (100 mg/kg of body weight/day) may contribute to changes in blood and kidneys of pregnant rats. The study by Dey et al. (2017) showed significant alterations in urinary calcium, creatinine, and urea during the prenatal period, while exhibited proteinuria, ketonuria, and histology showed nephrotoxicity during the postnatal period. The herb also affected concentrations of proinflammatory cytokines and decreased anti-inflammatory cytokines compared to the control group [53]. Moreover, the supplementation of black tea extract causes a decrease of hemoglobin concentration and loss of the biconcave structure of erythrocytes. It was also shown that the extract from black tea increases WBC levels in the mother's blood and induced significant changes in the histology of liver and serum enzymes [54].

Kayiran et al. (2013) examined whether black tea consumed during pregnancy affects the oxidative/antioxidant status of breast milk. The mother's milk was analyzed for lipid peroxidation based on malondialdehyde (MDA) levels and reduced glutathione levels (GSH). The study did not show a correlation between the amount of tea consumed and the level of MDA and GSH, which suggests that breast milk is insensitive to the antioxidants present in tea [124].

Deficiency of folic acid increases the risk of neural tube defects in the prenatal period. It has been shown that the levels of folic acid in serum is much lower in pregnant women who consumed more caffeine and tannins (in the form of coffee and oolong tea). According to Otake et al. (2018), pregnant women should minimize the consumption of drinks containing caffeine [55].

Epigallocatechin gallate (EGCG), a natural compound of green tea, has been shown to increase the efficacy of oral nifedipine treatment in severe pregnancy-induced preeclampsia [56]. On the other hand, excessive drinking tea during pregnancy may be associated with an increased risk of pre-eclampsia. Tea components affect this risk through a number of likely mechanisms, for example, as pathways associated with the modulation of angiogenic factors or with oxidative stress [57].

In the Jochum et al. (2017) study, pregnant women were given 300 ml of black tea and the content of flavonoids in milk was evaluated. It was shown that flavonoids (catechin, epicatechin) cannot be detected in milk samples, and the consumption of tea alone did not affect the total antioxidant capacity of breast milk [125].

5.3. Effects on Offspring

It has been shown that the consumption of green tea extract in pregnancy affects offspring's health. The consumption of Japanese and Chinese tea during pregnancy is also associated with an increased risk of premature birth [58]. Yang et al. (2018) showed that drinking tea during pregnancy is a risk factor for low birth weight of offspring [59]. Camelia supplementation of mothers in the pregnancy or lactation period exhibits also health benefits. According to the research by Hachul et al. (2018), the mother's intake of green tea extract exerts a protective action on the progeny that is on a high-fat diet. The extract protects against dyslipidemia, glucose intolerance, and fat accumulation. However, the mother's intake of this extract has a pro-inflammatory effect on the adipose tissue of progeny that is not on a high-fat diet [60]. Also, Losinskas-Hachul et al. (2018) [51] observed this relationship in their rat study. The pump that fed rats the green tea extract was shown to decrease the retroperitoneal adipose tissue relative weight and SOD activity, but increased adiponectin, LPS, IL-10, IL-6 contentl and IL-10/TNF-α ratio in retroperitoneal, IL-10, and TNF-α content in gonadal, and IL-6 content in mesenteric adipose tissues. These changes indicated that the consumption of green tea extracts altered the inflammatory status of 28 day old offspring. Moreover, epigallocatechin 3-gallate supplementation improved the results of treatment of maternal and maternal gestational diabetes. It affects the reduction of neonatal complications, i.e., low birth weight and hypoglycemia, and alleviates the mother's diabetic symptoms [61].

Tea extract showed also a protective role after exposure of compounds which have a negative influence on health. It has been showed that a moderate dose of green tea extract can decrease the number of malformations in fetuses after exposure to a teratogen, such as cyclophosphamide. However, too high a dose increases the toxicity of cyclophosphamide [62].

Due to the limited amount of research on the consumption of tea by pregnant and lactating women and the popularity of tea, further research is necessary.

6. Limitations in Medicinal Herbs Usage

There is no denying the fact that the use of medicinal herbs has its limitations and risks. Plant extracts may contain hundreds of compounds that have specific pharmacologic effects that may be synergistic or antagonistic [126]. Ginseng extract showed contradictory effects in animals, such as histamine and antihistamine-like actions, hypertensive and hypotensive effects, and stimulatory or depressant activity on the central nervous system [127,128]. The synergistic effects of the plant compounds have been shown in Cinchona, which has almost 30 alkaloids [129]. Four of those, cinchonine, l-isomer cinchonidine, quinine, and d-isomer quinidine, have antiplasmodial activity [130].

However, Druilhe et al. (1988) showed that the mixture of alkaloids is two to ten times more effective in vitro than any of the alkaloids used separately [131]. Differences in the bioactivity of extracts of the same plant may result from differences in the composition and concentration of active compounds. However, studies investigating substance that differentiates the extracts often do not lead to the discovery of the active substance responsible for the biological effect, such as in the case of Rhodiola and epigallocatechin [132]. Therefore, it is possible that the positive effects of medicinal herbs are based on the complex relationship between pharmacologic effects of the herb's compounds, and usage of the single compound would not have any significant therapeutic effects.

Also, it is unpractical to isolate and assess every active ingredient from the herbal extract, since the resources required would be huge [133]. Isolation and investigation of every active compound in a plant extract would be laborious and might not render any meaningful results due to synergistic effects between plant compounds.

As another limitation of medicinal herbs usage, one has to consider geographical differences and potential contamination of the extract resulting from the culture, collection, and storage of the herbs [134]. Variation in the secondary metabolites content between plants may be caused by the region of origin, season, cultivar, and nitrogen availability [135,136]. For example, Marrassini et al. (2018) showed that total polyphenols, flavonoids, and tannins content in Urera aurantiaca obtained from two different regions of the same country is significantly different [137].

Therefore, since a simple medication must be a single substance with a proven therapeutic effect, it may never be possible to register any medical herb as a drug, and another unified approach must be implemented for the registration and pharmacovigilance of medicinal herbs.

7. Conclusions

The results presented here suggest that some of the immunomodulators, supplemented in pregnancy and lactation, may affect offspring health. Therefore, before the recommendation to use plant supplementation in the maternal diet to enhance immune system function, the safety of its use should be determined in tests performed on in vivo models. Ideally, if the mechanism of action of these compounds was determined, or the isolation of the substance responsible for the positive biological effect of the plant was achieved. Unfortunately, there is still insufficient knowledge in this topic, which can explain the lack of studies on the effects of medicinal herbs supplementation on the health of pregnant women and their offspring in the database of the national institutes of health (www.clinicaltrials.gov).

Author Contributions: Conceptualization: A.L., S.L. Investigation: A.L., K.R., A.K., Ł.S., A.J., R.Z.; Original draft preparation: A.L., K.R., A.K., Ł.S., R.Z.; Developed search terms and eligibility criteria: A.L., A.J.; Supervision: R.Z. and S.L.; critical evaluation: S.L.; Review and editing—all authors.

Funding: This research received no external funding.

Conflicts of Interest: The authors certify that there is no conflict of interests with any financial organization regarding the material discussed in the paper.

References

1. Hecht, A. Drug safety labeling for doctors. *FDA Consum.* **1979**, *13*, 12–13. [PubMed]
2. Skopińska-Różewska, E.; Mościcka-Wesołowska, M.; Wasiutyński, A.; Małdyk, J.; Malejczyk, M.; Pazdur, J. Lymphatic system of mice born from mothers treated with ampicillin or cloxacillin during gestation. *Arch. Immunol. Ther. Exp.* **1986**, *34*, 203–208.
3. Jedrychowski, W.; Gałaś, A.; Whyatt, R.; Perera, F. The prenatal use of antibiotics and the development of allergic disease in one year old infants. A preliminary study. *Int. J. Occup. Med. Environ. Health* **2006**, *19*, 70–76. [CrossRef] [PubMed]
4. Jin, M.; Li, Q.; Gu, Y.; Wan, B.; Huang, J.; Xu, X.; Huang, R.; Zhang, Y. Leonurine suppresses neuroinflammation through promoting oligodendrocyte maturation. *J. Cell Mol. Med.* **2019**, *23*, 1470–1485. [CrossRef]

5. Soutar, D.A.; Doucette, C.D.; Liwski, R.S.; Hoskin, D.W. Piperine, a Pungent Alkaloid from Black Pepper, Inhibits B Lymphocyte Activation and Effector Functions. *Phytother. Res.* **2017**, *31*, 466–474. [CrossRef]

6. Sang, X.-X.; Wang, R.-L.; Zhang, C.-E.; Liu, S.-J.; Shen, H.-H.; Guo, Y.-M.; Zhang, Y.-M.; Niu, M.; Wang, J.-B.; Bai, Z.-F.; et al. Sophocarpine Protects Mice from ConA-Induced Hepatitis via Inhibition of the IFN-Gamma/STAT1 Pathway. *Front. Pharmacol.* **2017**, *8*, 140. [CrossRef]

7. Song, J.-Y.; Han, S.-K.; Son, E.-H.; Pyo, S.-N.; Yun, Y.-S.; Yi, S.-Y. Induction of secretory and tumoricidal activities in peritoneal macrophages by ginsan. *Int. Immunopharmacol.* **2002**, *2*, 857–865. [CrossRef]

8. Jiménez-Arellanes, A.; Luna-Herrera, J.; Cornejo-Garrido, J.; López-García, S.; Castro-Mussot, M.E.; Meckes-Fischer, M.; Mata-Espinosa, D.; Marquina, B.; Torres, J.; Hernández-Pando, R. Ursolic and oleanolic acids as antimicrobial and immunomodulatory compounds for tuberculosis treatment. *BMC Complement. Altern. Med.* **2013**, *13*, 258. [CrossRef] [PubMed]

9. Ayeka, P.A.; Bian, Y.; Githaiga, P.M.; Zhao, Y. The immunomodulatory activities of licorice polysaccharides (Glycyrrhiza uralensis Fisch.) in CT 26 tumor-bearing mice. *BMC Complement. Altern. Med.* **2017**, *17*, 536. [CrossRef] [PubMed]

10. Zheng, R.; Jie, S.; Hanchuan, D.; Moucheng, W. Characterization and immunomodulating activities of polysaccharide from Lentinus edodes. *Int. Immunopharmacol.* **2005**, *5*, 811–820. [CrossRef] [PubMed]

11. Bhat, B.A.; Dhar, K.L.; Puri, S.C.; Qurishi, M.A.; Khajuria, A.; Gupta, A.; Qazi, G.N. Isolation, characterization and biological evaluation of datura lactones as potential immunomodulators. *Bioorg. Med. Chem.* **2005**, *13*, 6672–6677. [CrossRef]

12. Chung, J.W.; Choi, R.J.; Seo, E.-K.; Nam, J.-W.; Dong, M.-S.; Shin, E.M.; Guo, L.Y.; Kim, Y.S. Anti-inflammatory effects of (Z)-ligustilide through suppression of mitogen-activated protein kinases and nuclear factor-κB activation pathways. *Arch. Pharm. Res.* **2012**, *35*, 723–732. [CrossRef] [PubMed]

13. Hu, J.-Z.; Huang, J.-H.; Xiao, Z.-M.; Li, J.-H.; Li, X.-M.; Lu, H.-B. Tetramethylpyrazine accelerates the function recovery of traumatic spinal cord in rat model by attenuating inflammation. *J. Neurol. Sci.* **2013**, *324*, 94–99. [CrossRef]

14. Jantan, I.; Ahmad, W.; Bukhari, S.N.A. Corrigendum: Plant-derived immunomodulators: An insight on their preclinical evaluation and clinical trials. *Front. Plant Sci.* **2018**, *9*, 1178. [CrossRef]

15. Riva, A.; Ronchi, M.; Petrangolini, G.; Bosisio, S.; Allegrini, P. Improved Oral Absorption of Quercetin from Quercetin Phytosome®, a New Delivery System Based on Food Grade Lecithin. *Eur. J. Drug Metab. Pharmacokinet.* **2019**, *44*, 169–177. [CrossRef]

16. Tyagi, N.; Song, Y.H.; De, R. Recent progress on biocompatible nanocarrier-based genistein delivery systems in cancer therapy. *J. Drug Target* **2019**, *27*, 394–407. [CrossRef] [PubMed]

17. Zhai, Z.; Liu, Y.; Wu, L.; Senchina, D.S.; Wurtele, E.S.; Murphy, P.A.; Kohut, M.L.; Cunnick, J.E. Enhancement of innate and adaptive immune functions by multiple *Echinacea* species. *J. Med. Food* **2007**, *10*, 423–434. [CrossRef] [PubMed]

18. Orhan, D.D.; Ozçelik, B.; Ozgen, S.; Ergun, F. Antibacterial, antifungal, and antiviral activities of some flavonoids. *Microbiol. Res.* **2010**, *165*, 496–504. [CrossRef] [PubMed]

19. Pérez-Cano, F.J.; Massot-Cladera, M.; Rodríguez-Lagunas, M.J.; Castell, M. Flavonoids Affect Host-Microbiota Crosstalk through TLR Modulation. *Antioxid* **2014**, *3*, 649–670. [CrossRef]

20. Serafini, M.; Peluso, I.; Raguzzini, A. Flavonoids as anti-inflammatory agents. *Proc. Nutr. Soc.* **2010**, *69*, 273–278. [CrossRef]

21. Leyva-López, N.; Gutierrez-Grijalva, E.P.; Ambriz-Perez, D.L.; Heredia, J.B. Flavonoids as Cytokine Modulators: A Possible Therapy for Inflammation-Related Diseases. *Int. J. Mol. Sci.* **2016**, *17*, 921. [CrossRef]

22. Mirossay, L.; Varinská, L.; Mojžiš, J. Antiangiogenic Effect of Flavonoids and Chalcones: An Update. *Int. J. Mol. Sci.* **2017**, *19*, 27. [CrossRef]

23. Skopiński, P.; Skopińska-Różewska, E.; Sommer, E.; Chorostowska-Wynimko, J.; Rogala, E.; Cendrowska, I.; Chrystowska, D.; Filewska, M.; Białas-Chromiec, B.; Bany, J. Chocolate feeding of pregnant mice influences length of limbs of their progeny. *Pol. J. Vet. Sci.* **2003**, *6*, 57–59. [PubMed]

24. Skopiński, P.; Szaflik, J.; Duda-Król, B.; Nartowska, J.; Sommer, E.; Chorostowska-Wynimko, J.; Demkow, U.; Skopinska-Rózewska, E. Suppression of angiogenic activity of sera from diabetic patients with non-proliferative retinopathy by compounds of herbal origin and sulindac sulfone. *Int. J. Mol. Med.* **2004**, *14*, 707–711. [CrossRef] [PubMed]

25. Skopińska-Różewska, E.; Balan, B.J.; Sommer, E.; Chorostowska-Wynimko, J.; Bany, J.; Wasiutynski, A.; Siwicki, A.K. The influence of chocolate feeding of pregnant mice on the immunological response of their progeny. *Pol. J. Food Nutr. Sci.* **2004**, *54*, 67–70.

26. Chorostowska-Wynimko, J.; Skopińska-Różewska, E.; Sommer, E.; Rogala, E.; Skopiński, P.; Wojtasik, E. Multiple effects of theobromine on fetus development and postnatal status of the immune system. *Int. J. Tissue React.* **2004**, *26*, 53–60. [PubMed]

27. Patera, J.; Chorostowska-Wynimko, J.; Słodkowska, J.; Borowska, A.; Skopiński, P.; Sommer, E.; Wasiutyński, A.; Skopińska-Różewska, E. Morphometric and functional abnormalities of kidneys in the progeny of mice fed chocolate during pregnancy and lactation. *Folia Histochem. Cytobiol.* **2006**, *44*, 207–211.

28. Lewicki, S.; Skopińska-Różewska, E.; Lewicka, A.; Zdanowski, R. Long-term supplementation of Rhodiola kirilowii extracts during pregnancy and lactation does not affect mother health status. *J. Matern. Fetal Neonatal. Med.* **2019**, *32*, 838–844. [CrossRef]

29. Lewicki, S.; Stankiewicz, W.; Skopińska-Różewska, E.; Wilczak, J.; Leśniak, M.; Suska, M.; Siwicki, A.K.; Skopiński, P.; Zdanowski, R. Spleen content of selected polyphenols, splenocytes morphology and function in mice fed Rhodiola kirilowii extracts during pregnancy and lactation. *Pol. J. Vet. Sci.* **2015**, *18*, 847–855. [CrossRef]

30. Zdanowski, R.; Skopińska-Różewska, E.; Wilczak, J.; Borecka, A.; Lewicka, A.; Lewicki, S. Different effects of feeding pregnant and lactating mice Rhodiola kirilowii aqueous and hydro-alcoholic extracts on their serum angiogenic activity and content of selected polyphenols. *Cent. Eur. J. Immunol.* **2017**, *42*, 17–23. [CrossRef] [PubMed]

31. Lewicki, S.; Skopińska-Różewska, E.; Zdanowski, R. The decrease in number of splenic lymphocytes in mice fed Rhodiola kirilowii during pregnancy and lactation concerns mainly CD19+ and CD4+ cells. *Cent. Eur. J. Immunol.* **2017**, *42*, 331–335. [CrossRef] [PubMed]

32. Lewicki, S.; Skopińska-Różewska, E.; Brewczyńska, A.; Zdanowski, R. Administration of Rhodiola kirilowii Extracts during Mouse Pregnancy and Lactation Stimulates Innate but Not Adaptive Immunity of the Offspring. *J. Immunol. Res.* **2017**, *2017*, 8081642. [CrossRef] [PubMed]

33. Lewicki, S.; Bałan, B.J.; Skopińska-Różewska, E.; Zdanowski, R.; Stelmasiak, M.; Szymański, Ł.; Stankiewicz, W. Modulatory effects of feeding pregnant and lactating mice Rhodiola kirilowii extracts on the immune system of offspring. *Exp. Ther. Med.* **2016**, *12*, 3450–3458. [CrossRef] [PubMed]

34. Lewicki, S.; Orłowski, P.; Krzyżowska, M.; Kiepura, A.; Skopińska-Różewska, E.; Zdanowski, R. The effect of feeding mice during gestation and nursing with Rhodiola kirilowii extracts or epigallocatechin on CD4 and CD8 cells number and distribution in the spleen of their progeny. *Cent. Eur. J. Immunol.* **2017**, *42*, 10–16. [CrossRef] [PubMed]

35. Bień, K.; Lewicki, S.; Zdanowski, R.; Skopińska-Różewska, E.; Krzyżowska, M. Feeding Pregnant and Lactating Mice Rhodiola kirilowii Extracts helps to Preserve Thymus Function of their Adult Progeny. *Pol. J. Vet. Sci.* **2016**, *19*, 581–587. [CrossRef] [PubMed]

36. Dabbou, S.; Rotolo, L.; Kovitvadhi, A.; Bergagna, S.; Dezzutto, D.; Barbero, R.; Rubiolo, P.; Schiavone, A.; De Marco, M.; Helal, A.N.; et al. Rabbit dietary supplementation with pale purple coneflower. 1. Effects on the reproductive performance and immune parameters of does. *Animal* **2016**, *10*, 1101–1109. [CrossRef] [PubMed]

37. Maass, N.; Bauer, J.; Paulicks, B.R.; Böhmer, B.M.; Roth-Maier, D.A. Efficiency of *Echinacea* purpurea on performance and immune status in pigs. *J. Anim. Physiol. Anim. Nutr.* **2005**, *89*, 244–252. [CrossRef] [PubMed]

38. Chow, G.; Johns, T.; Miller, S.C. Dietary *Echinacea* purpurea during murine pregnancy: Effect on maternal hemopoiesis and fetal growth. *Biol. Neonatol.* **2006**, *89*, 133–138. [CrossRef] [PubMed]

39. Barcz, E.; Sommer, E.; Nartowska, J.; Balan, B.; Chorostowska-Wynimko, J.; Skopińska-Rózewska, E. Influence of *Echinacea* purpurea intake during pregnancy on fetal growth and tissue angiogenic activity. *Folia Histochem. Cytobiol.* **2007**, *45* (Suppl. 1), S35–S39.

40. Kovitvadhi, A.; Gai, F.; Dabbou, S.; Ferrocino, I.; Rotolo, L.; Falzone, M.; Vignolini, C.; Gennero, M.S.; Bergagna, S.; Dezzutto, D.; et al. Rabbit dietary supplementation with pale purple coneflower. 2. Effects on the performances, bacterial community, blood parameters and immunity of growing rabbits. *Animal* **2016**, *10*, 1110–1117. [CrossRef] [PubMed]

41. Heitmann, K.; Havnen, G.C.; Holst, L.; Nordeng, H. Pregnancy outcomes after prenatal exposure to *Echinacea*: The Norwegian Mother and Child Cohort Study. *Eur. J. Clin. Pharmacol.* **2016**, *72*, 623–630. [CrossRef] [PubMed]

42. Gallo, M.; Sarkar, M.; Au, W.; Pietrzak, K.; Comas, B.; Smith, M.; Jaeger, T.V.; Einarson, A.; Koren, G. Pregnancy outcome following gestational exposure to *Echinacea*: A prospective controlled study. *Arch. Intern. Med.* **2000**, *160*, 3141–3143. [CrossRef]

43. Perri, D.; Dugoua, J.-J.; Mills, E.; Koren, G. Safety and efficacy of *Echinacea* (*Echinacea* angustafolia, e. purpurea and e. pallida) during pregnancy and lactation. *Can. J. Clin. Pharm.* **2006**, *13*, e262–e267.

44. Xi, Q.-Y.; Jiang, Y.; Zhao, S.; Zeng, B.; Wang, F.; Wang, L.-N.; Jiang, Q.-Y.; Zhang, Y.-L. Effect of ginseng polysaccharides on the immunity and growth of piglets by dietary supplementation during late pregnancy and lactating sows. *Anim. Sci. J.* **2017**, *88*, 863–872. [CrossRef] [PubMed]

45. Concha, C.; Hu, S.; Holmberg, O. The proliferative responses of cow stripping milk and blood lymphocytes to pokeweed mitogen and ginseng in vitro. *Vet. Res.* **1996**, *27*, 107–115. [PubMed]

46. Hu, S.; Concha, C.; Johannisson, A.; Meglia, G.; Waller, K.P. Effect of subcutaneous injection of ginseng on cows with subclinical Staphylococcus aureus mastitis. *J. Vet. Med. B Infect. Dis. Vet. Public Health* **2001**, *48*, 519–528. [CrossRef] [PubMed]

47. Kim, Y.O.; Lee, H.-Y.; Won, H.; Nah, S.-S.; Lee, H.-Y.; Kim, H.-K.; Kwon, J.-T.; Kim, H.-J. Influence of Panax ginseng on the offspring of adult rats exposed to prenatal stress. *Int. J. Mol. Med.* **2015**, *35*, 103–109. [CrossRef] [PubMed]

48. Saadeldin, I.M.; Hussein, M.A.; Suleiman, A.H.; Abohassan, M.G.; Ahmed, M.M.; Moustafa, A.A.; Moumen, A.F.; Abdel-Aziz Swelum, A. Ameliorative effect of ginseng extract on phthalate and bisphenol A reprotoxicity during pregnancy in rats. *Environ. Sci. Pollut. Res. Int.* **2018**, *25*, 21205–21215. [CrossRef] [PubMed]

49. Wanderley, M.I.; Saraiva, K.L.A.; César Vieira, J.S.B.; Peixoto, C.A.; Udrisar, D.P. Foetal exposure to Panax ginseng extract reverts the effects of prenatal dexamethasone in the synthesis of testosterone by Leydig cells of the adult rat. *Int. J. Exp. Pathol.* **2013**, *94*, 230–240. [CrossRef] [PubMed]

50. Belanger, D.; Calder, M.D.; Gianetto-Berruti, A.; Lui, E.M.; Watson, A.J.; Feyles, V. Effects of American Ginseng on Preimplantation Development and Pregnancy in Mice. *Am. J. Chin. Med.* **2016**, *44*, 981–995. [CrossRef]

51. Hachul, A.C.L.; Boldarine, V.T.; Neto, N.I.P.; Moreno, M.F.; Carvalho, P.O.; Sawaya, A.C.H.F.; Ribeiro, E.B.; do Nascimento, C.M.O.; Oyama, L.M. Effect of the consumption of green tea extract during pregnancy and lactation on metabolism of mothers and 28d-old offspring. *Sci. Rep.* **2018**, *8*, 1869. [CrossRef]

52. Matsumoto, E.; Kataoka, S.; Mukai, Y.; Sato, M.; Sato, S. Green tea extract intake during lactation modified cardiac macrophage infiltration and AMP-activated protein kinase phosphorylation in weanling rats from undernourished mother during gestation and lactation. *J. Dev. Orig. Health Dis.* **2017**, *8*, 178–187. [CrossRef]

53. Dey, A.; Gomes, A.; Dasgupta, S.C. Black Tea (Camellia sinensis) Extract Induced Prenatal and Postnatal Toxicity in Experimental Albino rats. *Pharm. Mag.* **2017**, *13*, S769–S774.

54. Dey, A.; Gomes, A.; Dasgupta, S.C. Black Tea (Camellia sinensis) Extract Induced Changes in Blood and Liver Parameters on Pregnant and Lactating Experimental Albino Rats. *Proc. Zool. Soc.* **2019**, *72*, 25–31. [CrossRef]

55. Otake, M.; Sakurai, K.; Watanabe, M.; Mori, C. Association Between Serum Folate Levels and Caffeinated Beverage Consumption in Pregnant Women in Chiba: The Japan Environment and Children's Study. *J. Epidemiol.* **2018**, *28*, 414–419. [CrossRef] [PubMed]

56. Shi, D.-D.; Guo, J.-J.; Zhou, L.; Wang, N. Epigallocatechin gallate enhances treatment efficacy of oral nifedipine against pregnancy-induced severe pre-eclampsia: A double-blind, randomized and placebo-controlled clinical study. *J. Clin. Pharm. Ther.* **2018**, *43*, 21–25. [CrossRef]

57. Wei, S.-Q.; Xu, H.; Xiong, X.; Luo, Z.-C.; Audibert, F.; Fraser, W.D. Tea consumption during pregnancy and the risk of pre-eclampsia. *Int. J. Gynaecol Obstet.* **2009**, *105*, 123–126. [CrossRef]

58. Okubo, H.; Miyake, Y.; Tanaka, K.; Sasaki, S.; Hirota, Y. Maternal total caffeine intake, mainly from Japanese and Chinese tea, during pregnancy was associated with risk of preterm birth: The Osaka Maternal and Child Health Study. *Nutr. Res.* **2015**, *35*, 309–316. [CrossRef]

59. Yang, J.; Chen, M.J.; Wang, X.X.; Sun, X.; Wang, X.; Wang, X.R.; Xia, Y.K. Association between maternal tea consumption in pregnancy and birth outcomes. *Chin. J. Prev. Med.* **2018**, *52*, 1013–1017.

60. Hachul, A.C.L.; Boldarine, V.T.; Neto, N.I.P.; Moreno, M.F.; Ribeiro, E.B.; do Nascimento, C.M.O.; Oyama, L.M. Maternal consumption of green tea extract during pregnancy and lactation alters offspring's metabolism in rats. *PLoS ONE* **2018**, *13*, e0199969. [CrossRef] [PubMed]

61. Zhang, H.; Su, S.; Yu, X.; Li, Y. Dietary epigallocatechin 3-gallate supplement improves maternal and neonatal treatment outcome of gestational diabetes mellitus: A double-blind randomised controlled trial. *J. Hum. Nutr. Diet.* **2017**, *30*, 753–758. [CrossRef] [PubMed]

62. Logsdon, A.L.; Herring, B.J.; Lockard, J.E.; Miller, B.M.; Kim, H.; Hood, R.D.; Bailey, M.M. Exposure to green tea extract alters the incidence of specific cyclophosphamide-induced malformations. *Birth Defects Res. B Dev. Reprod. Toxicol.* **2012**, *95*, 231–237. [CrossRef] [PubMed]

63. Zdanowski, R.; Skopińska-Różewska, E.; Wasiutyński, A.; Skopiński, P.; Siwicki, A.K.; Sobiczewska, E.; Lewicki, S.; Buchwald, W.; Kocik, J.; Stankiewicz, W. The effect of Rhodiola kirilowii extracts on tumor-induced angiogenesis in mice. *Cent. Eur. J. Immunol.* **2012**, *37*, 131–139.

64. Grace, M.H.; Yousef, G.G.; Kurmukov, A.G.; Raskin, I.; Lila, M.A. Phytochemical Characterization of an Adaptogenic Preparation from Rhodiola heterodonta. *Nat. Prod. Commun.* **2009**, *4*, 1053–1058. [CrossRef] [PubMed]

65. Zhou, J.-T.; Li, C.-Y.; Wang, C.-H.; Wang, Y.-F.; Wang, X.-D.; Wang, H.-T.; Zhu, Y.; Jiang, M.-M.; Gao, X.-M. Phenolic Compounds from the Roots of Rhodiola crenulata and Their Antioxidant and Inducing IFN-γ Production Activities. *Molecules* **2015**, *20*, 13725–13739. [CrossRef] [PubMed]

66. Grech-Baran, M.; Pietrosiuk, A.; Sykłowska-Baranek, K.; Giebułtowicz, J. Activity of tyrosol glucosyltransferase in Rhodiola kirilowii transgenic root cultures. *Planta Med.* **2012**, *78*, PI228. [CrossRef]

67. Mishra, K.P.; Ganju, L.; Singh, S.B. Anti-cellular and immunomodulatory potential of aqueous extract of Rhodiola imbricata rhizome. *Immunopharmacol. Immunotoxicol.* **2012**, *34*, 513–518. [CrossRef]

68. Cui, J.-L.; Guo, T.-T.; Ren, Z.-X.; Zhang, N.-S.; Wang, M.-L. Diversity and antioxidant activity of culturable endophytic fungi from alpine plants of Rhodiola crenulata, R. angusta, and R. sachalinensis. *PLoS ONE* **2015**, *10*, e0118204. [CrossRef]

69. Wójcik, R.; Siwicki, A.K.; Skopińska-Różewska, E.; Wasiutyński, A.; Sommer, E.; Furmanowa, M. The effect of Chinese medicinal herb Rhodiola kirilowii extracts on cellular immunity in mice and rats. *Pol. J. Vet. Sci.* **2009**, *12*, 399–405.

70. Zdanowski, R.; Lewicki, S.; Skopińska-Różewska, E.; Buchwald, W.; Mrozikiewicz, P.M.; Stankiewicz, W. Alcohol- and water-based extracts obtained from Rhodiola rosea affect differently the number and metabolic activity of circulating granulocytes in Balb/c mice. *Ann. Agric. Environ. Med.* **2014**, *21*, 120–123.

71. Bany, J.; Zdanowska, D.; Skopińska-Różewska, E.; Sommer, E.; Siwicki, A.K.; Wasiutyński, A. The effect of Rhodiola rosea extracts on the bacterial infection in mice. *Cent. Eur. J. Immunol.* **2009**, *34*, 35–37.

72. Zuo, G.; Li, Z.; Chen, L.; Xu, X. Activity of compounds from Chinese herbal medicine Rhodiola kirilowii (Regel) Maxim against HCV NS3 serine protease. *Antivir. Res.* **2007**, *76*, 86–92. [CrossRef] [PubMed]

73. Wong, Y.-C.; Zhao, M.; Zong, Y.-Y.; Chan, C.-Y.; Che, C.-T. Chemical constituents and anti-tuberculosis activity of root of Rhodiola kirilowii. *China J. Chin. Mater. Med.* **2008**, *33*, 1561–1565.

74. Khanna, K.; Mishra, K.P.; Ganju, L.; Singh, S.B. Golden root: A wholesome treat of immunity. *Biomed. Pharmacother.* **2017**, *87*, 496–502. [CrossRef] [PubMed]

75. Barman, D.; Nen, P.; Mandal, S.C.; Kumar, V. Immunostimulants for Aquaculture Health Management. *J. Mar. Sci. Res. Dev.* **2013**, *3*, 134. [CrossRef]

76. Lewicki, S.; Skopińska-Różewska, E.; Bałan, B.J.; Kalicki, B.; Patera, J.; Wilczak, J.; Wasiutyński, A.; Zdanowski, R. Morphofunctional Renal Alterations in Progeny of Mice Fed Rhodiola kirilowii Extracts or Epigallocatechin During Pregnancy and Lactation. *J. Med. Food* **2017**, *20*, 86–92. [CrossRef] [PubMed]

77. Blumenthal, M.; Farnsworth, N.R. Echinacea angustifolia in rhinovirus infections. *N. Engl. J. Med.* **2005**, *353*, 1971–1972. [PubMed]

78. Barnes, J.; Anderson, L.A.; Gibbons, S.; Phillipson, J.D. Echinacea species (*Echinacea* angustifolia (DC.) Hell., *Echinacea* pallida (Nutt.) Nutt., *Echinacea purpurea* (L.) Moench): A review of their chemistry, pharmacology and clinical properties. *J. Pharm. Pharmacol.* **2005**, *57*, 929–954. [CrossRef] [PubMed]

79. Schoop, R.; Klein, P.; Suter, A.; Johnston, S.L. Echinacea in the prevention of induced rhinovirus colds: A meta-analysis. *Clin. Ther.* **2006**, *28*, 174–183. [CrossRef]

80. Shah, S.A.; Sander, S.; White, C.M.; Rinaldi, M.; Coleman, C.I. Evaluation of Echinacea for the prevention and treatment of the common cold: A meta-analysis. *Lancet Infect. Dis.* **2007**, *7*, 473–480. [CrossRef]

81. Cheminat, A.; Zawatzky, R.; Becker, H.; Brouillard, R. Caffeoyl conjugates from *Echinacea* species: Structures and biological activity. *Phytochemistry* **1988**, *27*, 2787–2794. [CrossRef]

82. Melchart, D.; Clemm, C.; Weber, B.; Draczynski, T.; Worku, F.; Linde, K.; Weidenhammer, W.; Wagner, H.; Saller, R. Polysaccharides isolated from *Echinacea* purpurea herba cell cultures to counteract undesired effects of chemotherapy—A pilot study. *Phytother. Res.* **2002**, *16*, 138–142. [CrossRef] [PubMed]

83. Luettig, B.; Steinmüller, C.; Gifford, G.E.; Wagner, H.; Lohmann-Matthes, M.L. Macrophage activation by the polysaccharide arabinogalactan isolated from plant cell cultures of *Echinacea* purpurea. *J. Natl. Cancer Inst.* **1989**, *81*, 669–675. [CrossRef] [PubMed]

84. Forman, H.J.; Torres, M. Redox signaling in macrophages. *Mol. Asp. Med.* **2001**, *22*, 189–216. [CrossRef]

85. Hobbs, A.J.; Higgs, A.; Moncada, S. Inhibition of nitric oxide synthase as a potential therapeutic target. *Annu. Rev. Pharmacol. Toxicol.* **1999**, *39*, 191–220. [CrossRef] [PubMed]

86. Zhai, Z.; Haney, D.; Wu, L.; Solco, A.; Murphy, P.A.; Wurtele, E.S.; Kohut, M.L.; Cunnick, J.E. Alcohol extracts of *Echinacea* inhibit production of nitric oxide and tumor necrosis factor-alpha by macrophages in vitro. *Food Agric. Immunol.* **2007**, *18*, 221–236. [CrossRef] [PubMed]

87. Brüne, B.; Götz, C.; Meßmer, U.K.; Sandau, K.; Hirvonen, M.-R.; Lapetina, E.G. Superoxide Formation and Macrophage Resistance to Nitric Oxide-mediated Apoptosis. *J. Biol. Chem.* **1997**, *272*, 7253–7258. [CrossRef] [PubMed]

88. Chang, C.Y.; Tucci, M.; Baker, R.C. Lipopolysaccharide-stimulated nitric oxide production and inhibition of cell proliferation is antagonized by ethanol in a clonal macrophage cell line. *Alcohol* **2000**, *20*, 37–43. [CrossRef]

89. Facino, R.M.; Carini, M.; Aldini, G.; Saibene, L.; Pietta, P.; Mauri, P. Echinacoside and caffeoyl conjugates protect collagen from free radical-induced degradation: A potential use of *Echinacea* extracts in the prevention of skin photodamage. *Planta Med.* **1995**, *61*, 510–514. [CrossRef]

90. Hu, C.; Kitts, D.D. Studies on the antioxidant activity of *Echinacea* root extract. *J. Agric. Food Chem.* **2000**, *48*, 1466–1472. [CrossRef]

91. Pellati, F.; Benvenuti, S.; Magro, L.; Melegari, M.; Soragni, F. Analysis of phenolic compounds and radical scavenging activity of *Echinacea* spp. *J. Pharm. Biomed. Anal.* **2004**, *35*, 289–301. [CrossRef]

92. Dalby-Brown, L.; Barsett, H.; Landbo, A.-K.R.; Meyer, A.S.; Mølgaard, P. Synergistic antioxidative effects of alkamides, caffeic acid derivatives, and polysaccharide fractions from *Echinacea* purpurea on in vitro oxidation of human low-density lipoproteins. *J. Agric. Food Chem.* **2005**, *53*, 9413–9423. [CrossRef] [PubMed]

93. Choi, K. Botanical characteristics, pharmacological effects and medicinal components of Korean Panax ginseng C A Meyer. *Acta Pharmacol. Sin.* **2008**, *29*, 1109–1118. [CrossRef] [PubMed]

94. Baek, S.-H.; Bae, O.-N.; Park, J.H. Recent methodology in ginseng analysis. *J. Ginseng Res.* **2012**, *36*, 119–134. [CrossRef] [PubMed]

95. Rhule, A.; Navarro, S.; Smith, J.R.; Shepherd, D.M. Panax notoginseng attenuates LPS-induced pro-inflammatory mediators in RAW264.7 cells. *J. Ethnopharmacol.* **2006**, *106*, 121–128. [CrossRef] [PubMed]

96. Lee, J.-Y.; Shin, J.-W.; Chun, K.-S.; Park, K.-K.; Chung, W.-Y.; Bang, Y.-J.; Sung, J.-H.; Surh, Y.-J. Antitumor promotional effects of a novel intestinal bacterial metabolite (IH-901) derived from the protopanaxadiol-type ginsenosides in mouse skin. *Carcinogenesis* **2005**, *26*, 359–367. [CrossRef] [PubMed]

97. Lee, I.-A.; Hyam, S.R.; Jang, S.-E.; Han, M.J.; Kim, D.-H. Ginsenoside Re ameliorates inflammation by inhibiting the binding of lipopolysaccharide to TLR4 on macrophages. *J. Agric. Food Chem.* **2012**, *60*, 9595–9602. [CrossRef] [PubMed]

98. Kim, S.-J.; Murthy, H.N.; Hahn, E.-J.; Lee, H.L.; Paek, K.-Y. Parameters affecting the extraction of ginsenosides from the adventitious roots of ginseng (Panax ginseng C.A. Meyer). *Sep. Purif. Technol.* **2007**, *56*, 401–406. [CrossRef]

99. Byeon, S.E.; Lee, J.; Kim, J.H.; Yang, W.S.; Kwak, Y.-S.; Kim, S.Y.; Choung, E.S.; Rhee, M.H.; Cho, J.Y. Molecular mechanism of macrophage activation by red ginseng acidic polysaccharide from Korean red ginseng. *Mediat. Inflamm.* **2012**, *2012*, 732860. [CrossRef] [PubMed]

100. Baek, S.-H.; Lee, J.G.; Park, S.Y.; Bae, O.N.; Kim, D.-H.; Park, J.H. Pectic polysaccharides from Panax ginseng as the antirotavirus principals in ginseng. *Biomacromolecules* **2010**, *11*, 2044–2052. [CrossRef] [PubMed]

101. Kim, Y.O.; Kim, Y.; Lee, K.; Na, S.W.; Hong, S.P.; Valan Arasu, M.; Yoon, Y.W.; Kim, J. Panax ginseng Improves Functional Recovery after Contusive Spinal Cord Injury by Regulating the Inflammatory Response in Rats: An In Vivo Study. *Evid. Based Complement. Altern. Med.* **2015**, *2015*, 817096. [CrossRef] [PubMed]

102. Khalid, S.; Tahir, M.; Shoro, A.A. Ginseng Induced Fetal Skeletal Malformations. 2008. Available online: http://www.pjmhsonline.com/ginseng_induced_fetal_skeletal_m.htm (accessed on 29 June 2019).

103. Kim, M.-H.; Byon, Y.-Y.; Ko, E.-J.; Song, J.-Y.; Yun, Y.-S.; Shin, T.; Joo, H.-G. Immunomodulatory activity of ginsan, a polysaccharide of panax ginseng, on dendritic cells. *Korean J. Physiol. Pharmacol.* **2009**, *13*, 169–173. [CrossRef] [PubMed]

104. Shin, J.-Y.; Song, J.-Y.; Yun, Y.-S.; Yang, H.-O.; Rhee, D.-K.; Pyo, S. Immunostimulating effects of acidic polysaccharides extract of Panax ginseng on macrophage function. *Immunopharmacol. Immunotoxicol.* **2002**, *24*, 469–482. [CrossRef] [PubMed]

105. Jie, Y.H.; Cammisuli, S.; Baggiolini, M. Immunomodulatory effects of Panax Ginseng C.A. Meyer in the mouse. *Agents Actions* **1984**, *15*, 386–391. [CrossRef] [PubMed]

106. Ahn, J.-Y.; Song, J.-Y.; Yun, Y.-S.; Jeong, G.; Choi, I.-S. Protection of Staphylococcus aureus-infected septic mice by suppression of early acute inflammation and enhanced antimicrobial activity by ginsan. *FEMS Immunol. Med. Microbiol.* **2006**, *46*, 187–197. [CrossRef] [PubMed]

107. Chan, L.Y.; Kwok, H.H.; Chan, R.W.Y.; Peiris, M.J.S.; Mak, N.K.; Wong, R.N.S.; Chan, M.C.W.; Yue, P.Y.K. Dual functions of ginsenosides in protecting human endothelial cells against influenza H9N2-induced inflammation and apoptosis. *J. Ethnopharmacol.* **2011**, *137*, 1542–1546. [CrossRef] [PubMed]

108. Chattopadhyay, C.; Chakrabarti, N.; Chatterjee, M.; Mukherjee, S.; Sarkar, K.; Chaudhuri, A.R. Black tea (Camellia sinensis) decoction shows immunomodulatory properties on an experimental animal model and in human peripheral mononuclear cells. *Pharmacogn. Res.* **2012**, *4*, 15–21. [CrossRef] [PubMed]

109. Kuo, C.-L.; Chen, T.-S.; Liou, S.-Y.; Hsieh, C.-C. Immunomodulatory effects of EGCG fraction of green tea extract in innate and adaptive immunity via T regulatory cells in murine model. *Immunopharmacol. Immunotoxicol.* **2014**, *36*, 364–370. [CrossRef] [PubMed]

110. McKay, D.L.; Blumberg, J.B. The role of tea in human health: An update. *J. Am. Coll. Nutr.* **2002**, *21*, 1–13. [CrossRef] [PubMed]

111. Chen, Z.; Zhu, Q.Y.; Tsang, D.; Huang, Y. Degradation of green tea catechins in tea drinks. *J. Agric. Food Chem.* **2001**, *49*, 477–482. [CrossRef]

112. Chen, N.; Bezzina, R.; Hinch, E.; Lewandowski, P.A.; Cameron-Smith, D.; Mathai, M.L.; Jois, M.; Sinclair, A.J.; Begg, D.P.; Wark, J.D.; et al. Green tea, black tea, and epigallocatechin modify body composition, improve glucose tolerance, and differentially alter metabolic gene expression in rats fed a high-fat diet. *Nutr. Res.* **2009**, *29*, 784–793. [CrossRef] [PubMed]

113. Graham, H.N. Green tea composition, consumption, and polyphenol chemistry. *Prev. Med.* **1992**, *21*, 334–350. [CrossRef]

114. Anderson, R.A.; Polansky, M.M. Tea enhances insulin activity. *J. Agric. Food Chem.* **2002**, *50*, 7182–7186. [CrossRef] [PubMed]

115. Kawai, K.; Tsuno, N.H.; Kitayama, J.; Okaji, Y.; Yazawa, K.; Asakage, M.; Hori, N.; Watanabe, T.; Takahashi, K.; Nagawa, H. Epigallocatechin gallate attenuates adhesion and migration of CD8+ T cells by binding to CD11b. *J. Allergy Clin. Immunol.* **2004**, *113*, 1211–1217. [CrossRef] [PubMed]

116. Williamson, M.P.; McCormick, T.G.; Nance, C.L.; Shearer, W.T. Epigallocatechin gallate, the main polyphenol in green tea, binds to the T-cell receptor, CD4: Potential for HIV-1 therapy. *J. Allergy Clin. Immunol.* **2006**, *118*, 1369–1374. [CrossRef] [PubMed]

117. Tripathi, S.; Bruch, D.; Gatto, L.A.; Kittur, D.S. Green tea extract prolongs allograft survival as an adjunctive therapy along with low dose cyclosporine A. *J. Surg. Res.* **2009**, *154*, 85–90. [CrossRef] [PubMed]

118. Hamer, M. The beneficial effects of tea on immune function and inflammation: A review of evidence from in vitro, animal, and human research. *Nutr. Res.* **2007**, *27*, 373–379. [CrossRef]

119. Donà, M.; Dell'Aica, I.; Calabrese, F.; Benelli, R.; Morini, M.; Albini, A.; Garbisa, S. Neutrophil restraint by green tea: Inhibition of inflammation, associated angiogenesis, and pulmonary fibrosis. *J. Immunol.* **2003**, *170*, 4335–4341. [CrossRef] [PubMed]

120. Frei, B.; Higdon, J.V. Antioxidant activity of tea polyphenols in vivo: Evidence from animal studies. *J. Nutr.* **2003**, *133*, 3275S–3284S. [CrossRef] [PubMed]

121. Datta, P.; Sarkar, A.; Biswas, A.K.; Gomes, A. Anti arthritic activity of aqueous extract of Indian black tea in experimental and clinical study. *Orient. Pharm. Exp. Med.* **2012**, *12*, 265–271. [CrossRef]

122. Isbrucker, R.A.; Edwards, J.A.; Wolz, E.; Davidovich, A.; Bausch, J. Safety studies on epigallocatechin gallate (EGCG) preparations. Part 3: Teratogenicity and reproductive toxicity studies in rats. *Food Chem. Toxicol.* **2006**, *44*, 651–661. [CrossRef] [PubMed]

123. Wang, D.; Meng, J.; Xu, K.; Xiao, R.; Xu, M.; Liu, Y.; Zhao, Y.; Yao, P.; Yan, H.; Liu, L. Evaluation of oral subchronic toxicity of Pu-erh green tea (camellia sinensis var. assamica) extract in Sprague Dawley rats. *J. Ethnopharmacol.* **2012**, *142*, 836–844. [CrossRef] [PubMed]

124. Kayiran, S.M.; Ince, D.A.; Aldemir, D.; Gurakan, B. Investigating the effect of black tea consumption during pregnancy on the oxidant/antioxidant status of breastmilk. *Breastfeed. Med.* **2013**, *8*, 187–190. [CrossRef] [PubMed]

125. Jochum, F.; Alteheld, B.; Meinardus, P.; Dahlinger, N.; Nomayo, A.; Stehle, P. Mothers' Consumption of Soy Drink But Not Black Tea Increases the Flavonoid Content of Term Breast Milk: A Pilot Randomized, Controlled Intervention Study. *Ann. Nutr. Metab.* **2017**, *70*, 147–153. [CrossRef] [PubMed]

126. Chong, S.K.; Oberholzer, V.G. Ginseng–is there a use in clinical medicine? *Postgrad Med. J.* **1988**, *64*, 841–846. [CrossRef] [PubMed]

127. Takagi, K.; Saito, H.; Tsuchiya, M. Pharmacological studies of Panax Ginseng root: Pharmacological properties of a crude saponin fraction. *Jpn. J. Pharmacol.* **1972**, *22*, 339–346. [CrossRef] [PubMed]

128. Kim, H.J.; Kim, P.; Shin, C.Y. A comprehensive review of the therapeutic and pharmacological effects of ginseng and ginsenosides in central nervous system. *J. Ginseng Res.* **2013**, *37*, 8–29. [CrossRef] [PubMed]

129. Kacprzak, K.M. Chemistry and Biology of Cinchona Alkaloids. In *Natural Products*; Ramawat, K.G., Mérillon, J.-M., Eds.; Springer: Berlin/Heidelberg, Germany, 2013; pp. 605–641. ISBN 978-3-642-22143-9.

130. Karle, J.M.; Bhattacharjee, A.K. Stereoelectronic features of the cinchona alkaloids determine their differential antimalarial activity. *Bioorg. Med. Chem.* **1999**, *7*, 1769–1774. [CrossRef]

131. Druilhe, P.; Brandicourt, O.; Chongsuphajaisiddhi, T.; Berthe, J. Activity of a combination of three cinchona bark alkaloids against Plasmodium falciparum in vitro. *Antimicrob. Agents Chemother.* **1988**, *32*, 250–254. [CrossRef]

132. Bałan, B.J.; Skopińska-Różewska, E.; Skopiński, P.; Zdanowski, R.; Leśniak, M.; Kiepura, A.; Lewicki, S. Morphometric abnormalities in the spleen of the progeny of mice fed epigallocatechin during gestation and nursing. *Pol. J. Vet. Sci.* **2017**, *20*, 5–12. [CrossRef]

133. World Health Organization (Ed.) *National Policy on Traditional Medicine and Regulation of Herbal Medicines: Report of a WHO Global Survey*; World Health Organization: Geneva, Switzerland, 2005; ISBN 978-92-4-159323-6.

134. Chan, K. Some aspects of toxic contaminants in herbal medicines. *Chemosphere* **2003**, *52*, 1361–1371. [CrossRef]

135. Bouterfas, K.; Mehdadi, Z.; Elaoufi, M.M.; Latreche, A.; Benchiha, W. Antioxidant activity and total phenolic and flavonoids content variations of leaves extracts of white Horehound (Marrubium vulgare Linné) from three geographical origins. *Ann. Pharm. Fr.* **2016**, *74*, 453–462. [CrossRef] [PubMed]

136. Arnold, T.; Tanner, C.; Hatch, W. Phenotypic variation in polyphenolic content of the tropical brown alga Lobophora variegata as a function of nitrogen availability. *Mar. Ecol. Prog. Ser.* **1995**, *123*, 177–183. [CrossRef]

137. Marrassini, C.; Peralta, I.; Anesini, C. Comparative study of the polyphenol content-related anti-inflammatory and antioxidant activities of two Urera aurantiaca specimens from different geographical areas. *Chin. Med.* **2018**, *13*, 22. [CrossRef] [PubMed]

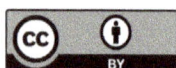

nutrients

MDPI

Review

The Impact of Mediterranean Dietary Patterns During Pregnancy on Maternal and Offspring Health

Federica Amati *, Sondus Hassounah and Alexandra Swaka

Department of Primary Care and Public Health, Imperial College London, London W6 8RP, UK;
s.hassounah@imperial.ac.uk (S.H.); a.swaka@imperial.ac.uk (A.S.)
* Correspondence: f.amati@imperial.ac.uk; Tel.: +44-207-594-2341

Received: 8 April 2019; Accepted: 13 May 2019; Published: 17 May 2019

Abstract: (1) Background: Pregnancy outcomes for both mother and child are affected by many environmental factors. The importance of pregnancy for 'early life programming' is well established and maternal nutrition is an important factor contributing to a favourable environment for developing offspring. We aim to assess whether following a Mediterranean Diet during pregnancy is beneficial for maternal and offspring outcomes; (2) Methods: a systematic review was performed using standardized reporting guidelines with the National Heart Lung and Blood Iinstitute quality assessment tool for selection and extraction; (3) Results: results show that being on a Mediterranean Diet during pregnancy is associated with favourable outcomes for both maternal and offspring health, particularly for gestational diabetes in mothers and congenital defects in offspring (4) Conclusions: Following a Mediterranean dietary pattern during gestation is beneficial for the health of both the mother and offspring. Pregnant women and those trying to conceive should be advised to follow a Mediterranean Diet to potentially decrease, for example, the likelihood of atopy (OR 0.55) in the offspring and Gestational Diabetes Mellitus in the mother (OR 0.73).

Keywords: maternal nutrition; Mediterranean diet; offspring health

---

1. Introduction

The maternal diet before conception and during pregnancy has long-term implications for maternal and offspring health, from placental development [1], risk of developing gestational diabetes [2], birth complications [3], birth weight [4] and risk of developing allergies in childhood [5–8]. Exposure to an unfavourable environment in early pregnancy is known to significantly increase the risk of diseases in adult life; this is known as 'early life programming' and one of the most important factors is the maternal diet [9]. Pregnancy presents an opportune time window for healthcare professionals' intervention to improve health for both the mother and child, making the evidence surrounding maternal diet an important tool for the healthcare practice.

Maternal diet is a blueprint for the diet which children are likely to follow into adolescence. This is due to the fact that, typically, mothers are responsible for feeding their children. Without intervention, pregnant women who do not follow a healthy diet or lifestyle choices are unlikely to change their patterns of behaviour. Sometimes obstacles to changes in behaviour can present themselves even for well-known harmful habits such as smoking during pregnancy, but as a unique window of opportunity, focusing health service efforts to impact the behaviour of pregnant women is crucial.

The Mediterranean Diet (MD) and Mediterranean Diet Adherence (MDA) is characterized by a high intake of fruits, vegetables, whole grain cereals, legumes, fish and nuts; low-to-moderate consumption of dairy products and limited amounts of red meat and red wine. It is low in saturated fats and high in antioxidants, fibre and mono and polyunsaturated fatty acids mainly derived from extra virgin olive oil (evoo) (MUFAs) and oily fish (n-3 PUFAs). The MD is known to have many beneficial effects for longevity and disease prevention, demonstrated in numerous high-quality studies, reviews and meta-analyses, making it the most widely studied and evidence-based dietary approach to healthy eating and disease prevention [10–13]. The unique synergy of various health benefitting nutrients makes MD an effective approach to improving health [11].

Recording dietary patterns through food diaries and food frequency questionnaires (FFQs) is a valuable tool to analyse eating behaviours and better understand which foods and food groups are consumed. Individual foods, such as extra virgin olive oil (evoo), as well as food groups, such as pulses, provide an insight to the nutrients consumed in the recorded foods, such as monounsaturated fatty acids (MUFAs) and fibre, respectively. Asking an individual to recount specific nutrient amounts is more complex than recounting what foods were consumed as part of the daily diet, making dietary pattern analysis more attainable for patients and crucial for research.

Evidence on the impact of diet during pregnancy on health outcomes focusses on either individual nutrients, such as folic acid, or the Mediterranean Diet for their impact on specific disease outcomes such as neural tube defects [14] or leukaemia [15]. The degree of evidence available for the impact of specific nutrients in pregnancy on outcomes for offspring health is more powerful than that for dietary patterns. For instance, the necessity for appropriate levels of folic acid during gestation is well-documented in the prevention of neural tube defects, and the mechanism by which folic acid prevents neural tube defects is well understood and documented. Whereas supplements are the quicker and easier way to address certain nutritional deficiencies of individual nutrients [11], dietary patterns are a useful way of studying the effects of dietary exposure, in turn, making recommended diets a potential health improvement intervention alongside appropriate and necessary supplementation in pregnancy.

The Mediterranean Diet is well established as beneficial in the literature [16]. Previous reviews of the evidence where several dietary patterns have been evaluated highlight that maternal dietary patterns are important factors in early life programming. Maternal dietary patterns which reflect the MD showed consistent associations with a lower risk for allergic disease in children [17], appropriate infant birthweight [18], and lower risk of pre-eclampsia and preterm birth [19]. This Review investigates and presents current evidence exclusively on the Mediterranean Diet's multifactorial impact on overall health outcomes for both the mother and offspring, as the sole dietary pattern of interest.

Our results indicate that the Mediterranean Diet has a significantly positive impact on maternal and offspring health, strengthening the evidence base to encourage its adoption as a preventive measure against diseases throughout the life course and especially in pregnancy when the outcome of two or more individuals can be positively impacted.

2. Materials and Methods

2.1. Data Sources and Search Strategy

This systematic review was performed using a predetermined, unpublished protocol and in accordance with standardized reporting guidelines [20]. Search terms identification and classification were guided by previous comprehensive relevant reviews [21]. One reviewer (FA) performed searches in the following online electronic databases (Medline, Embase, Web of Science, Scopus, Maternity & infant care and Cochrane). The search of online databases is up to date to February 2019. The search was not restricted by language or date.

The search was broken down into four main categories. To identify the relevant population, the first Boolean search was done using the term "OR" to explode (search by subject heading) and map (search by keyword) the following MeSH headings "child health" or "offspring" or "newborn" or "neonate" or "child" or "baby" or "gestation" or "pregnancy" or "pregnant woman" or "perinatal period" or "prenatal exposure" or "prenatal". To identify relevant interventions the second Boolean search used the term "OR" to explode and map "Mediterranean diet" or "fruit" or "vegetable" or "legume" or "nut" or "olive oil" or "evoo" or "oily fish" or "seafood" or "tomato". The third category of

MeSH headings was also related to the intervention and included ((low or little or medium or moderate or less or decrease or reduce or restrict) (intake or consumption or consume or eat or amount)) AND ("dairy product" or "red meat" or "processed meat" or "red wine"). Finally, the fourth group of key terms was used to identify the study design whereby a Boolean search using the term "OR" was used to explode and map the keywords "randomized controlled trial" or "controlled clinical trial" or "placebo" or "Retrospective Studies" or "Cohort Studies". The four search categories were then combined using the Boolean operator "AND". The hand searching of results in the Maternity & infant care database for a Mediterranean diet highlighted that using the terminology of 'child health' was not capturing some relevant papers, thus, the papers which were the result of searching for a Mediterranean diet in this database were hand-searched instead. For a full list of the search terms in each database please see Appendix A.

2.2. Study Selection

Three reviewers (FA, AS and SH) independently evaluated articles for eligibility in a three-stage procedure. In stage one, all identified titles and abstracts were reviewed. In stage two, a full-text review was performed on all the articles that met the predefined inclusion criteria as well as all articles for which there was uncertainty as to eligibility. In stage three, full texts were re-evaluated for data extraction.

2.3. Inclusion/Exclusion Criteria

Studies, publications or reports in the English-language describing an association between the Mediterranean diet during pregnancy and infant development were eligible for inclusion. Studies, publications or reports were included for analysis if they included the following:

1. Exposure: Comprehensive dietary assessment: Food frequency questionnaire (FFQ), 24 h diet recall, food record, diet history, Use of a priori dietary score or index;

2. Outcome: Clinical neonatal outcome, disorders assessed by study staff, medical records or clinician diagnosed (for example, Foetal growth restriction (FGR) and preterm delivery (PTD)), developmental issues assessed by validated scale/questionnaire;

3. Design: Observational studies (cross-sectional, cohort, case-control), Interventional studies (clinical trials);

4. Population: Pregnant women (at any gestational age).

Articles were excluded if they investigated pregnant women with other dietary complications (non-gestational diabetes, obesity, anorexia, malnourishment) and/or if they explored a specific nutrient impact as opposed to a dietary pattern (e.g., Omega-3 supplementation as a feature of the Med Diet.)

2.4. Data Extraction and Quality Assessment

Two reviewers (FA and AS) independently extracted data from all studies that satisfied the inclusion criteria. Any disagreement in data extraction and/or study inclusion was resolved through discussion between the two reviewers and, when necessary, a third reviewer (SH).

The primary outcome was the impact on maternal and offspring health. A number of other study characteristics were also extracted including geographic location, description of the study population, primary outcomes, description of intervention and control, and results. Furthermore, data pertaining to sample size, number, and features of the intervention were also extracted.

2.5. Quality Assessment

The methodological quality of studies was assessed and scored independently by two reviewers (FA and AS) using the validated National Heart, Lung, and Blood Institute (NHLBI) study Quality Assessment Tool [22] (see Appendix B Table A1). Disagreements were resolved through discussion. The summary score for each study was calculated (minimum: 1, maximum: 10) and categorised into three categories. Studies with a score of 8 or above were considered of high-quality, studies with a score of 5–7 were considered of fair quality and studies with a score of 4 or below were considered of poor quality. These categories were used to evaluate whether outcomes significantly varied according to study quality and to determine which weight studies should be given in the synthesis of the findings.

2.6. Data Synthesis and Presentation

Since exploring heterogeneity is one of the main aims of an SLR/MA, a descriptive synthesis approach was used instead of meta-analytic procedures. Our review includes studies with diverse designs and all shared comprehensive dietary assessment tools to measure MD adherence, with neonatal and maternal clinical markers as outcomes. The results of the quality assessment are presented in Table 1. As the narrative synthesis was used to analyse and present the findings, the results of data abstraction are summarized in Table 2, which outlines the type, objective and target of intervention, and measurement of effect for each intervention. Study results are summarized in Table 3 according to categories/themes and whether the MD was found to have a Protective, Null or Negative effect on outcomes.

3. Results

3.1. Literature Selection

Our initial database search is outlined in Figure 1, showing that a total of 125 articles were initially identified based on our search criteria, 14 duplicates were removed, leaving 111 articles for title and abstract screening, of which 67 were excluded for the title (25 were the wrong type of article for this review, 19 targetted the non-objective population, 8 were studies that included dietary complications or risk factors, and 15 focused on a specific nutrient impact); 16 at abstract following the inclusion/exclusion criteria (9 were the wrong type of article for this review, 3 targetted a non-objective population, 3 for studies that included dietary complications or risk factors, and 2 focused on specific nutrient impact); and 6 after full text screening, included in the Appendix C (2 were the wrong type of article for this review, 3 targetted a non-objective population, and 1 focused on specific nutrient impact), for a total of 22 articles reviewed and included in this paper.

The studies included all used a comprehensive dietary assessment tool to measure MD adherence, with neonatal and maternal clinical markers as outcomes. The selected studies included observational, interventional studies, randomized trials, and all studies included a population of pregnant women at any gestational age with neonatal or child follow-ups. Table 1 shows our quality assessment results and Appendix C Figure A1 shows papers excluded after full text review.

Table 1. The quality assessment score values: <4 = Low, 4–7 = Medium, 8–10 = High.

Author	Design	Score (1–10)	Quality Assessment
Assaf-Balut, C; Garcia de la Torre, N; A Duran et al. [23]	Prospective randomized interventional study	8	High
Assaf-Balut, Carla; Garcia de la Torre, et al. [24]	Prospective randomized controlled trial (The St Carlos GDM prevention study)	9	High
Botto, Lorenzo D.; Krikov, Sergey; et al. [25]	Multicentre population-based case-control study	9	High
Chatzi, L.; Rifas-Shiman, S.; [26]	Prospective Cohort study (Project Viva + Rhea Study)	9	High
Chatzi L.; Torrent, M.; et al. [27]	Prospective Cohort study	7	High
Chatzi, L.; Garcia, R.; et. al. [28]	Cohort study (INMA and Rhea Study)	9	High
E, Parlapani; et al. [29]	Cohort study	7	Medium
Fernandez-Barres, S.; et al. [30]	Birth Cohort study (INMA)	8	High
Gesteiro, E.; Rodriguez B., et al. [31]	Cohort study	7	Medium
Gesteiro, E.; Bastida S., et al. [32]	Cross-sectional study	7	Medium
Gonzalez-Nahm, S. et al. [33]	Cohort study	8	High
Haugen, M.; et al. [34]	Prospective Cohort study (MoBa)	8	High
House, J.; et al. [35]	Prospective Cohort study	9	High
Castro-Rodriguez, J.; et al. [36]	Cohort study	7	Medium

Table 1. *Cont.*

Author	Design	Score (1–10)	Quality Assessment
Lange, N. [37]	Longitudinal pre-birth cohort study	9	High
Mantzoros, C.; et al. [38]	Prospective cohort study (Project Viva)	8	High
Monteagudo, C.; et al. [39]	Cohort study	8	High
Peraita-Costa, I. et al. [40]	Retrospective cross-sectional population-based study	7	Medium
Saunders, L.; et al. [41]	Cohort study (TIMOUN)	8	High
Steenweg-de Graaff, J.; et al. [42]	Population-based cohort (The Generation R Study)	9	High
Vujkovic, M.; et al. [43]	Case-control study	7	Medium
Smith, L.; et al. [44]	Population-based cohort study	7	Medium

GDM = gestational diabetes mellitus, INMA = INfancia y Medio Ambiente study, TIMOUN= French Caribeean Mother Child cohort study.

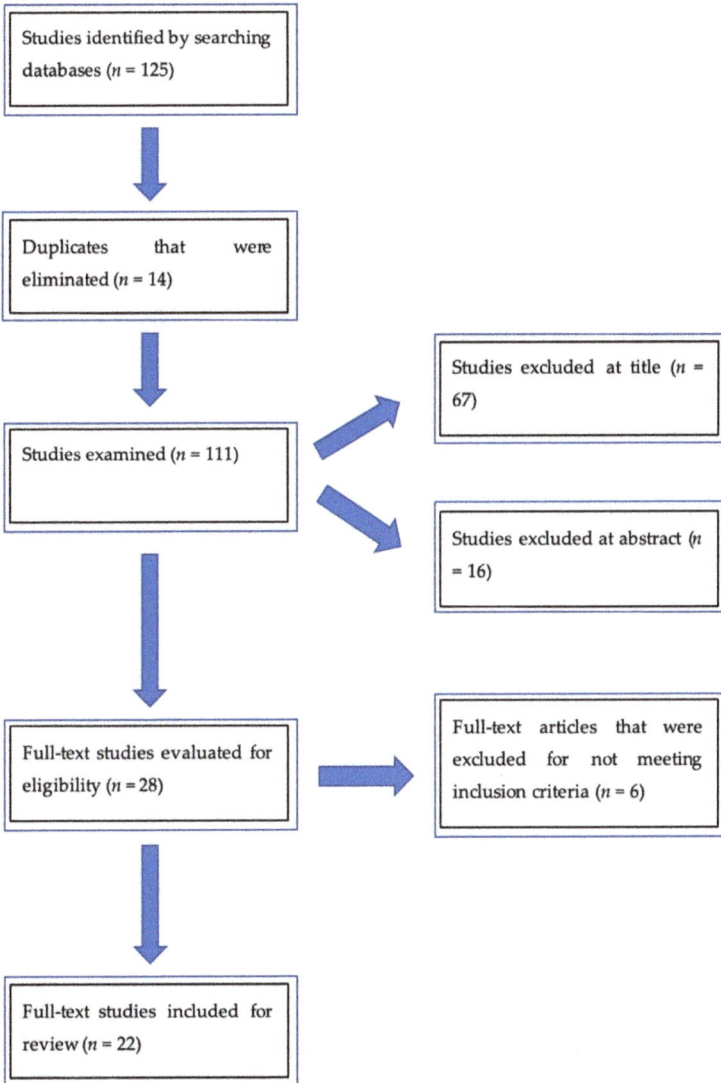

Studies identified by searching databases (*n* = 125)

Duplicates that were eliminated (*n* = 14)

Studies examined (*n* = 111)

Studies excluded at title (*n* = 67)

Studies excluded at abstract (*n* = 16)

Full-text studies evaluated for eligibility (*n* = 28)

Full-text articles that were excluded for not meeting inclusion criteria (*n* = 6)

Full-text studies included for review (*n* = 22)

Figure 1. The flow diagram of the process for study selection.

Table 2. The outcomes and effect estimates for the included studies.

Authors	Design and Cohort	Included Participants and Gestational Age	Intervention Type and Comparator	Results
Assaf-Balut, C; Garcia de la Torre, N; A Duran et al. [23] Spain	Prospective randomized interventional study	874; First Trimester	MD nutritional therapy	As an early nutritional intervention, MD reduces the incidence of GDM. Comparison of HbA$_{1c}$ levels at 24–28 weeks in women with GDM and normal glucose tolerance: $p = 0.001$. Values became similar at 36–38 gestational weeks with intervention.
Assaf-Balut, Carla; Garcia de la Torre, et al. [24] Spain	Prospective randomized controlled trial	874; intervention group (IG), $n = 434$ control group (CG), $n = 440$; 8–12 gestational weeks (First Trimester)	MD nutritional therapy with additional evoo and pistachios	Supplemented MD reduces the incidence of GDM as an early nutritional intervention. IG showed reduced rates of insulin-treated GDM: $p = < 0.05$
Botto, Lorenzo D.; Krikov, Sergey; et al. [25] USA	Multicentre population-based case-control study	Mothers of babies with major non-syndromic congenital heart defects ($n = 9885$); mothers with unaffected babies ($n = 9468$); maternal diet assessed in the year before pregnancy	A priori defined MDS with Quartiles 1–4 (worst to best)	Better diet quality is associated with a reduced occurrence of some conotruncal and septal heart defects. Overall conotruncal defects: OR 0.63, 95% CI 0.49 to 0.80 Overall tetralogy of Fallot: OR 0.76, 95% CI 0.64 to 0.91 Overall septal defects: OR 0.77, 95% CI 0.63 to 0.94 Overall atrial septal defects: OR 0.86, 95% CI 0.75 to 1.00
Chatzi, L.; Rifas-Shiman, S.; [26] USA, Greece	Cohort study; Project Viva	Mother–child pairs from USA: 997 Greece: 569 MDA measured during pregnancy with follow-up at median 4.2 and 7.7 years	MDA with a priori defined MDS through FFQ	Greater adherence to MD during pregnancy may protect against excess offspring cardiometabolic risk. For each 3-point increase in MDS, offspring BMI decreased by 0.14 units (95% confidence interval, −0.15 to −0.13)
Chatzi L.; Torrent, M.; et al. [27] Spain	Cohort study	507 mothers during the gestational period; 460 children at 6.5 years post-gestational follow-up	Impact of MDA during pregnancy on asthma and atopy in childhood using a priori defined MDS	Adherence to Med Diet during pregnancy support protective effect against asthma-like symptoms and atopy in childhood Persistent wheeze: OR 0.22; 95% CI 0.08 to 0.90 Atopic wheeze: OR 0.30; 95% CI 0.10 to 0.90 Atopy: (OR 0.55; 95% CI 0.31 to 0.97
Chatzi, L.; Garcia, R.; et al. [28] Spain, Greece	Cohort study; INMA (Spain) RHEA (Greece)	During pregnancy with follow-up within 1 year post-gestational; 1771 mother-newborn pairs (Spain); 745 pairs (Greece)	MDA calculated through completed FFQ	High meat intake during pregnancy may increase the risk of a wheeze in the first year of life; high dairy intake may decrease it RR 0.83, 95% CI 0.72, 0.96
E, Parlapani; et al. [29] Greece	Cohort study	82 women delivering preterm singletons ≤34 weeks	FFQ and MDA	High adherence to MD, may favourably affect intrauterine growth (IUGR), premature birth and maternal hypertension (HTN); Low-MDA neonates group had a higher rate of IUGR: OR 3.3 Low-MDA mothers had a higher rate of prematurity: OR 1.6 Low-MDA mothers had a higher gestational HTN: OR 3.8
Fernandez-Barres, S.; et al. [30] Spain	Cohort study; INMA	1827 mother-child pairs, assessed during pregnancy	FFQ and MDA	Adherence to MD during pregnancy not associated with a risk of childhood obesity, but is linked to a lower waist circumference; p-value for trend = 0.009

Table 2. *Cont.*

Authors	Design and Cohort	Included Participants and Gestational Age	Intervention Type and Comparator	Results
Gesteiro, E.; Rodriguez, B., et al. [31] Spain	Cohort study	35 women with 'adequate' or 'inadequate' diets according to HEI (healthy eating index) and MDA score; 1st trimester	13 point MDA score via FFQ	Maternal diets during the 1st trimester with low HEIs or adherence to MD have a negative effect on insulin markers at birth; Low MDA-score diets had low-fasting glycaemia: $p = 0.025$ and delivered infants with high insulinaemia: $p = 0.049$
Gesteiro, E.; Sanchez-Muiz FJ, et al. [32] Spain	Cross-sectional study	53 mother-neonate pairs; GDM screening at 24–28 gestational weeks	Maternal MDA and offspring lipoprotein profile	Neonates of mothers who consumed low adherence of MD during pregnancy presented impaired lipoprotein and higher homocysteine levels; Mothers' diet in the nAA + AT x mTT group (neonates carrying FTO rs9939609 T allele x Mothers homozygous for FTO rs9939609 T allele) had a significantly lower MDA score: $p = 0.05$
Gonzalez-Nahm, S. et al. [33] USA	Cohort study	390 women whose infants had DNA methylation cord blood data available; FFQ at preconception or 1st trimester	MDA via FFQ	Suggests that maternal diet can have a sex-specific impact on infant DNA methylation at specific imprinted DMRs; OR = 7.40, 95% CI 1.88–20.09
Haugen, M.; et al. [34] Norway	Cohort study; MoBa	MD criteria met: 569 women; 1–4 criteria met: 25,397 women; 0 MD criteria met: 159 women; 18–24 gestational weeks	MDA via FFQ	Women who adhered to the MD criteria did not have a reduced risk of preterm birth compared to women who met none of the criteria; OR: 0.73, 95% CI: 0.32, 1.68 Intake of fish twice a week or more associated with lower preterm birth; OR: 0.84; 95% CI: 0.74, 0.95
House, J.; et al. [35] USA	Cohort study; NEST	325 mother-infant pairs; 1st trimester; follow-up at 2 years post-gestation	MDA via FFQ	Offspring of women with high MDA less likely to exhibit neurobehavioural effects: Depression; OR = 0.28 Anxiety; OR = 0.42 Social relatedness; OR = 2.38
Castro-Rodriguez, J.; et al. [36] Spain, Chile	Cohort study	Gestational period; follow-up in 1000 preschoolers (at 1.5 yrs and 4 yrs)	MDA via FFQ	Low fruit and high meat consumption by the child had a negative effect on allergic responses (wheezing, rhinitis, or dermatitis); as did the high consumption of pasta and potatoes by the mother
Lange, N. [37] USA	Longitudinal prebirth cohort study; Project Viva	1376 mother-infant pairs; 1st and 2nd trimesters with follow-up at 3 years post-gestation	MDA via FFQ	Dietary pattern during pregnancy not associated with recurrent wheeze; OR per 1-point increase in MD: 0.98, 95% CI, 0.98–1.08
Mantzoros, C.; et al. [38] USA	Prospective cohort study; Project Viva	780 women; 1st and 2nd trimesters; post-gestational cord blood	MDA	Adherence to MD during pregnancy not associated with cord blood leptin or adiponectin; p-value = 0.38
Monteagudo, C.; et al. [39] Spain	Cohort study	320 umbilical cord serum samples	MDS-p (med diet score adapted to pregnancy)	Adherence to the MD and folic acid supplementation during pregnancy may indicate being overweight in newborns; OR = 3.33 (p = 0.019)

Table 2. *Cont.*

Authors	Design and Cohort	Included Participants and Gestational Age	Intervention Type and Comparator	Results
Peraita-Costa, I. et al. [40] Spain	Retrospective cross-sectional population-based study	492 mother-child pairs; immediately post-delivery and for 6 months thereafter	MDA with two groups identified: low and high adherence	Low adherence to an MD was not associated with a higher risk of a low birthweight newborn; aOR = 1.68; 95% CI 1.02–5.46
Saunders, L.; et al. [41] French West Indies	Cohort study; TIMOUN	728 pregnant women who delivered liveborn singletons with no malformations	Semi-quantitative FFQ analysed for MDA	Results suggest that adherence to a Caribbean diet may include benefits of MD, contributing to a reduction in preterm delivery in overweight women; A OR: 0.7, 95% CI 0.6, 0.9
Steenweg-de Graaff, J.; et al. [42] The Netherlands	Population-based cohort; Generation R Study	During pregnancy at median 13.5 weeks; Post-gestation in 3104 children at 1.5, 3, and 6 years of age	MDA via FFQ	High adherence to traditional Dutch diet and low adherence to MD are linked to an increased risk of child externalizing problems; OR per SD in MDS: 0.90, 95% CI: 0.83–0.97 OR per SD in Traditionally Dutch Score: 1.11, 95% CI: 1.03–1.21
Vujkovic, M.; et al. [43] The Netherlands	Case-control study	50 mothers of children with Spinal Bifida; 81 control mothers post-gestation	Dietary assessment via FFQ	MD seems to show an association with reducing the risk of offspring being affected by SB; Weak MDA; OR: 2.7 (95% CI 1.2–6.1) High MDA; OR: 3.5 (95% CI 1.5–7.9)
Smith, L.; et al. [44] United Kingdom	Population-based cohort study	922 LMPT; 965 term births; 32–36 weeks gestation (3rd Trimester)	Maternal interview for dietary factors: MDA, low fruit and vegetable intake, use of folic acid supplements	Women with 0 adherence to MD were nearly twice as likely to deliver LMPT; RR 1.81 (1.04 to 3.14) Smokers and low consumption of fruit and vegetables had a particularly high risk; RR 1.81 (1.29 to 2.53)

MD = Mediterranean Diet, MDS = Mediterranean Diet Score, MDA = Mediterranean Diet Adherence, FFQ = Food Frequency Questionnaire, HEI = Healthy Eating Index.

3.2. Study Characteristics

The studies included (*n* = 22) were published between 2008 and 2018 and were conducted in 8 countries, which included Spain, USA, Greece, Holland, Norway, Chile, French West Indies, and the United Kingdom. The common dietary measurements used were the adherence to the Mediterranean Diet Score (MDS) and an adapted MDS for pregnancy (MDS-p).

The MDS is an a priori defined score developed to measure compliance to a high intake of Mediterranean Diet foods with a score ranging from 0 to 9, where 9 indicates greater adherence to the diet [13]. The MDS-p is a scoring system that was designed by Montegaudo et al. [45] for pregnant women to better quantify the micronutrients in their diets such as calcium, folic acid, and iron, which are especially relevant in pregnancy [39].

Of the included studies, 16 were cohort studies, 1 was a randomized interventional study, 1 was a randomized controlled trial, 2 were case-control studies, and 2 were cross-sectional studies. All studies were conducted during the gestational period with follow-ups after birth. Table 2 shows the summarized characteristics of the studies including design, measures used, and results reported. The total number of participants for all of the studies is 63,336.

3.3. MAIN RESULTS

3.3.1. Allergic Disorders

Four studies focused on the relationship between maternal adherence to a Mediterranean Diet during pregnancy and neonatal or childhood outcomes of asthma and atopy. A cohort study by Chatzi, L; Torrent, M.; et al. [27] found that adherence to the MD during pregnancy supports a protective effect against asthma-like symptoms and atopy in childhood at 6.5 years old. Chatzi, L.; Garcia, R.; et al. [28] found that while adherence to the MD was not associated with the risk of wheeze and eczema in any cohort, high meat intake during pregnancy might increase the risk of wheeze during the first year of life. Through questionnaires of epidemiological factors, maternal diet during pregnancy, and childhood diet, Castro-Rodriguez, J.; M. Ramirez-Hernandez et al. [36], found that wheezing, rhinitis or dermatitis were negatively affected by high potato and pasta consumption by the mother and subsequent low fruit and high meat consumption by the child. Lange, N. et al. [37] however, examined 1376 mother-infant pairs and found that the dietary pattern is not associated with recurrent wheeze.

3.3.2. Premature Birth, Birth Weight, Childhood Obesity

Six studies examined the implications of the diet on premature birth, gestational diabetes (please see Table 3), birth weight, and/or childhood obesity. Parlapani, E. et al. [29] found that neonates of mothers with low adherence to the MD had significantly higher intrauterine growth restriction and lower birth weights. Haugen, M. et al. [34] investigated the association between women who met the MD adherence criteria and those who did not. The study showed that those who met the MD criteria of fish ≥2 times a week, fruit and vegetables ≥5 times a day, use of olive/canola oil, red meat intake ≤2 times a week, and ≤2 cups of coffee a day, did not have a lower risk of preterm birth compared to women who met none of the criteria. A population-based cohort study involving 922 late and moderate preterm births (LMPT) by Smith, L. et al. [44], identified that women who did not include any aspects of the MD during pregnancy were nearly twice as likely to have LMPT in comparison to higher adherence mothers. Fernandez-Barres, et al. [30] evaluated associates between adherence to the MD during pregnancy, but found no risk to childhood obesity, however, it was associated with a lower waist circumference, which is related to abdominal obesity and is an important health marker. Peraita-Costa et al. [40] administered the "Kidmed" questionnaire to collect dietary information from mothers on adherence to the MD. Of the 492 women, 40.2% showed low adherence to the MD, but this study did not directly correlate the results to low birth weight due to potentially confounding factors including smoking, low education levels, and low dairy intake. Saunders, L. et al. [41] found that low adherence to the MD could implicate a positive correlation between maternal diet and small birth weight.

Table 3. A summary of findings from our review of the evidence.

Health Outcomes	Impact of Maternal MD		
Outcome Variable	Protective	Negative	Inconclusive
Allergic Disorders	3 (27,28,36)		1 (37)
Premature birth, birth weight, childhood obesity	5 (29,30,39,41,44)		2 (30,36)
Cardiometabolic and congenital defects	3 (25,26,43)		
Gestational diabetes & pre-eclampsia	2 (23,24,29)		
DNA Methylation	2 (33,35)		
Biomarkers	2 (31,32)		1(38)
Behavioural development	1 (42)		

3.3.3. Cardiometabolic and Congenital Defects

Three studies examined the link between better maternal diet quality with congenital heart defects or metabolic factors. Chatzi, L.; Rifas-Shiman, S.; et al. [26] studied 997 mother-child pairs, finding that improved adherence to the MD during pregnancy showed lower systolic and diastolic blood pressures and may protect offspring against cardiometabolic risk. Botto, L. [25] et al. found, in a high-quality study, that diet quality was a factor of reduced conotruncal and atrial septal heart defects. Vujkovic, M. et al. [43] found that because of the higher levels of serum and RBC folate, Vitamin B12 and lower plasma homocysteine contained in the MD, offspring have a reduced risk of spina bifida.

3.3.4. Gestational Diabetes and Pre-Eclampsia

Two studies found that gestational nutrition based on the MD reduces the incidence of Gestational Diabetes (GDM). In a prospective randomized interventional study by A Duran, [24] 177 women out of 874 were diagnosed with GDM and found that with early intervention using the MD, gestational outcomes were improved. Likewise, the results of a randomized controlled trial conducted by Assaf-Balut, C. et al. [24] show that the incidence of GDM was reduced by early dietary intervention with a diet rich in EVOO and pistachios. Parlapani et al. [29] found that MDA was an independent predictor of gestational hypertension and pre-eclampsia.

3.3.5. DNA Methylation

Two studies examined the association between maternal adherence to the MD and DNA methylation in infants. One study conducted by Gonzalez-Nahm et al. [33] showed evidence that maternal diet of low MD adherence had an increased risk of female sex-linked hypo-methylation at the MEG3-IG differentially methylated region. House, J. et al. [35] also found an association between maternal adherence to the MD and female sex-linked methylation at MEG3, IGF2, and SGCE/PEG10 DMRs, and identified an association between MD and favourable neurobehavioral outcomes in early childhood.

3.3.6. Biomarkers

Four studies were associated with adherence to the MD and subsequent repercussions on biomarkers and implications of the pregnancy and on the newborn. Gesteiro, E. et al. [31] aimed to determine the relationship between diet within the first trimester and biomarkers of insulin resistance at birth. They found that women consuming low MD adherence diets had low-fasting glycaemia and delivered infants with high insulinaemia. A follow up cross-sectional study by Gasteiro, E., Bastida, S. et al. [32] aiming to identify the relationship between diet quality during pregnancy and serum lipid, arylesterase and homocysteine values at birth identified that neonates whose mothers had low adherence to the MD presented impaired levels of the referenced biomarkers. In a cohort study by Mantzoros et al. [38], multivariable linear regression was used to analyse the correlation between maternal diet during the 1st and 2nd trimesters and cord blood levels of leptin and adiponectin. High adherence to the MD was not found to be associated with these levels. Conversely, a study by Monteagudo et al. [39] on the exposure to organochlorine pesticides and maternal diet indicated that higher folic acid supplementation and greater exposure to the endocrine-disrupting residues were related to higher newborn weight.

3.3.7. Behavioural Development

One cohort study by Steenweg-de Graaff et al. [42], examining the pregnancies and follow-up of the 3104 children born, found that the MD was not associated with internalizing problems such as anxiety or depression, while low adherence to the MD was positively associated with increased child externalizing problems, such as aggression or inattention.

Of the 22 studies included, 18 found that adherence to the Mediterranean Diet during pregnancy had protective factors on the health of the newborn and 4 of the studies were inconclusive or showed no correlation. None of the studies showed a negative association between the MD and the outcomes.

4. Discussion

The mechanisms by which the MD exerts its effect on fetal development and maternal health are complex and need further research. By reviewing the available literature focusing specifically on MD interventions/exposure, as opposed to all dietary patterns as in previous reviews, we have a good overview of how the MD pattern effects mothers and their offspring on a variety of outcomes. Particularly interesting insights can be gleaned from the numerical values associated with some of the risk factors. The studies in this review are of good quality and represent a combined study population >63,000.

The observed heterogeneity of interventions, study populations and outcomes measured, allows for a big picture view of how the MD diet exerts its effects at all gestational ages and in the early years of life. For instance, when looking at behavioural outcomes, this review concluded that adherence to the MD in pregnancy has a statistically significant impact on decreasing the likelihood of offspring exhibiting depressive behaviours (OR 0.28) [35] in an ethnically diverse cohort, and another study added to this with a reduced OR of 0.90 [42] for developing externalising behaviours (such as aggression) for offspring of mothers with a high MDA.

Though some of the outcome categories we have identified only have 2 or 3 studies, they give a good starting point for future research to build on the current knowledge. Berti et al.'s comprehensive literature review of early life nutritional exposures on life-long health splits its findings into 'sections' [46] which, again, give a big picture overview on the vast impact that maternal, early life and even pre-conceptional nutrition can have. Unlike some more focused reviews, investigating the impact of maternal diet on allergic diseases [47], for instance, we hope that our review's heterogeneity contributes to a wider understanding of maternal dietary impact.

This review brings together some ideas of how the MD may be contributing to in-utero development through specific mechanistic pathways. The methylation of specific sites in two of the studies (see Table 3) present results on how the MD, as opposed to specific nutrients, contribute to this very time-sensitive window of change of DNA methylation during fetal development.

The results on atopy, asthma and eczema highlight that whilst the MD is not always protective, it is associated with a reduced likelihood of allergic disorders as a result of maternal MD diet adherence and compounded further by offspring MD adherence. This type of follow up warrants attention; further investigation into the impacts which MD adherence for offspring of mothers who had high adherence to the MD during pregnancy and lactation, compared to non-MD adherent mother-child pairs would allow for dietary recommendations to be evidence-based through the course of pregnancy and early life as a one-time course. Intuitively, this would be a good way to approach dietary recommendations for improving health, as most children adopt their mother's dietary choices as the main provider of food in early life.

With regards to premature birth, low birth weight and childhood obesity, the evidence is more mixed. The studies that found no association between the MD and decreased likelihood of premature birth were of high quality. Some of the uncertainty is due to the limitations of the studies, some not controlling for confounders of specific outcomes like intrauterine growth, such as smoking. Despite this, the studies that were inconclusive on the impact of the MD on their primary chosen outcome, for instance the INMA birth cohort study for childhood obesity [30] and Parlapani et al.'s work [29] on birth complications and prematurity, still found statistically significant positive associations between MD adherence and other health outcomes in their results, such as waist circumference and likelihood of pre-eclampsia and necrotizing enterocolitis for each study, respectively.

A strong case for the positive impact of the MD can be seen in the results of the studies focusing on cardiometabolic and congenital defects, GDM and DNA methylation. Though these studies investigated hugely different markers and outcomes, it is clear that the MD has a protective effect on them all. The evidence presented here regarding DNA methylation and biomarkers reflects a novel way to measure the impact of dietary changes and contributes to the understanding of the mechanisms behind the long-term impacts which 'early-life programming' has. The nature of DNA methylation in the fetal development time-course makes it possible to observe the impact which specific intra-uterine exposures have on offspring DNA methylations 20, 30 or 40 years later. For example, studies on the impact of intra-uterine exposure to famine showed that lower methylation of 5 CpG dinucleotides within the insulin-like growth factor-II differentially methylated region (DMR) [48] was detected in affected offspring decades later. Thus, the potential for future research on the impact of the MD on methylation sites of interest is vast, as dietary exposure has such a large impact.

The pattern of MD that may influence the reduction of adverse effects most appears to be one where there is purposefully added evoo and nuts. As seen in the present literature, increased vegetables and oily fish and decreased processed foods delivered positive results, and the effects are seen both in metabolically healthy and compromised gestation, indicating that the MD could be a diet with beneficial outcomes for GDM and metabolically healthy pregnancies.

The results of this review add to the growing body of evidence that the Mediterranean Diet is a beneficial dietary recommendation throughout the life course. By collating the evidence on outcomes of the MD for the mother and child, we highlight the broad range of effects this dietary intervention has. The limitations of this work are the small number of studies per outcome group, with the biggest group here being 'premature birth and birth weight' at only 7 studies total. Regular updates of this review are important as research around the topic is growing, and with an expanding evidence base, the possibility of meta-analysis for each category is likely. The biggest strength of this review is that, even with small numbers of studies, it highlights the impact which MDA in pregnancy and early childhood can have on several different health outcomes. The implications for clinical practice are great, as prescribing an MD pattern to women of reproductive age is a simple intervention, with important clinical potential for both the mother and offspring.

5. Conclusions

The Mediterranean Diet in pregnancy and early infancy is safe and beneficial for a wide range of maternal and offspring outcomes. Further research to ascertain the relationship and mechanisms maternal MD has with health outcomes of interest in different populations is needed to position it as a public health intervention for all populations.

Funding: This research received no external funding.

Acknowledgments: This article presents independent research commissioned by the National Institute for Health Research (NIHR) under the Collaborations for Leadership in Applied Health Research and Care (CLAHRC) programme for North West London. The views expressed in this publication are those of the authors and not necessarily those of the NHS, NIHR or the Department of Health.

Conflicts of Interest: The authors declare no conflict of interest.

Appendix A Search Strategy

Database: MEDLINE <1946 to February 04, 2019>:

1. exp Fruit/ or Fruit.mp. (131831)
2. edible grain/ or exp vegetables/ (42391)
3. Leguminosae.mp. or exp Fabaceae/ (69062)
4. nut.mp. or Nuts/ (6941)
5. exp Olive Oil/ or evoo.mp. (4609)
6. extra virgin olive oil.mp. (931)
7. monounsaturated fatty acids.mp. or exp Fatty Acids, Monounsaturated/ (45287)
8. Fishes/ or oily fish.mp. or Fatty Acids, Omega-3/ or Seafood/ (75289)
9. Lycopersicon esculentum/ or tomato*.mp. (23549)
10. ((high or more or increase* or elevat* or much or rais*) adj6 (intake or consumption or consume or eat* or amount*)).tw. (179734)
11. 1 or 2 or 3 or 4 or 5 or 6 or 7 or 8 or 9 (348823)
12. 10 and 11 (14459)
13. Milk/ or exp Dairy Products/ or dairy.mp. (120218)
14. red meat.mp. or exp Red Meat/ (4259)
15. Meat Products/ or processed meat.mp. (7285)
16. Wine/ or red wine.mp. (11501)
17. 13 or 14 or 15 or 16 (141175)
18. ((low or little or medium or moderate or less or decrease* or reduc* or restrict*) adj6 (intake or consumption or consume or eat* or amount*)).tw. (177151)
19. 17 and 18 (6736)
20. Mediterranean Diet.mp. or exp Diet, Mediterranean/ (4636)
21. exp Pregnancy/ or pregnan*.mp. (966432)
22. maternal diet.mp. (1885)
23. prenatal.mp. or Prenatal Nutritional Physiological Phenomena/ or Prenatal Exposure Delayed Effects/ (161569)
24. 21 or 22 or 23 (994947)
25. child health.mp. or Child/ or Child Health/ (1617258)
26. newborn.mp. or exp Infant, Newborn/ (717150)
27. 25 or 26 (2178391)
28. exp animals/ not humans.sh. (4543138)
29. randomized controlled trial.mp. or Randomized Controlled Trial/ (498499)
30. controlled clinical trial.mp. or Controlled Clinical Trial/ (105353)
31. placebo.de. (0)
32. trial.mp. (1103671)
33. Retrospective Studies/ or Cohort Studies/ or cohort stud*.mp. (994814)
34. 29 or 30 or 31 or 32 or 33 (2049754)
35. 34 not 28 (1998518)
36. ((12 and 19) or 20) and 24 and 27 and 35 (22)

Database: Embase Classic+Embase <1947 to 2019 February 04>:

1. exp Fruit/ (127584)
2. fruit.mp. (110586)

3. vegetable*.mp. or leafy vegetable/ or vegetable/ (128062)
4. exp legume/ or legume.mp. (79855)
5. exp nut/ or nut*.mp. (670576)
6. extra virgin olive oil/ or olive oil/ or evoo.mp. (12921)
7. monounsaturated fatty acids.mp. or exp monounsaturated fatty acid/ (8992)
8. exp fish/ or oily fish.mp. or omega 3 fatty acid/ (240566)
9. sea food/ (9239)
10. tomato*.mp. or tomato/ (24952)
11. ((high or more or increase* or elevat* or much or rais*) adj6 (intake or consumption or consume or eat* or amount*)).tw. (242744)
12. 1 or 2 or 3 or 4 or 5 or 6 or 7 or 8 or 9 or 10 (1171930)
13. 11 and 12 (49587)
14. exp dairy product/ (111325)
15. red meat/ or red meat.mp. (5486)
16. processed meat.mp. or exp processed meat/ (2238)
17. red wine.mp. or exp red wine/ (5583)
18. 14 or 15 or 16 or 17 (122438)
19. ((low or little or medium or moderate or less or decrease* or reduc* or restrict*) adj6 (intake or consumption or consume or eat* or amount*)).tw. (234104)
20. 18 and 19 (7553)
21. Mediterranean Diet.mp. or exp Mediterranean diet/ (7990)
22. gestation*.mp. (314747)
23. maternal diet.mp. or maternal nutrition/ (11842)
24. pregnancy/ or pregnant woman/ or pregnant.mp. or pregnancy.mp. (1002075)
25. perinatal.mp. or perinatal period/ (133359)
26. prenatal period/ or prenatal exposure/ or prenatal.mp. (242919)
27. 22 or 23 or 24 or 25 or 26 (1257012)
28. child health.mp. or child health/ (76176)
29. offspring.mp. or progeny/ (100561)
30. newborn.mp. or newborn/ (696375)
31. neonat*.mp. (351653)
32. child/ (1815590)
33. baby.mp. or exp baby/ (71511)
34. 28 or 29 or 30 or 31 or 32 or 33 (2643576)
35. (exp animal/ or nonhuman/) not exp human/ (6800562)
36. clinical trial.de. (974978)
37. randomized controlled trial.de. (537435)
38. randomization.de. (81390)
39. single blind procedure.de. (33905)
40. double blind procedure.de. (160469)
41. crossover procedure.de. (58496)
42. placebo.de. (340801)
43. prospective study.de. (502412)
44. (randomi?ed controlled adj1 trial*).mp. [mp=title, abstract, heading word, drug trade name, original title, device manufacturer, drug manufacturer, device trade name, keyword, floating subheading word, candidate term word] (744347)
45. rct.mp. (32969)

46. (random* adj1 allocat*).mp. [mp=title, abstract, heading word, drug trade name, original title, device manufacturer, drug manufacturer, device trade name, keyword, floating subheading word, candidate term word] (37316)
47. (single adj1 blind*).mp. [mp=title, abstract, heading word, drug trade name, original title, device manufacturer, drug manufacturer, device trade name, keyword, floating subheading word, candidate term word] (45468)
48. (double adj1 blind*).mp. [mp=title, abstract, heading word, drug trade name, original title, device manufacturer, drug manufacturer, device trade name, keyword, floating subheading word, candidate term word] (245874)
49. ((treble or triple) adj1 (blind* or placebo*)).mp. [mp=title, abstract, heading word, drug trade name, original title, device manufacturer, drug manufacturer, device trade name, keyword, floating subheading word, candidate term word] (1080)
50. 36 or 37 or 38 or 39 or 40 or 41 or 42 or 43 or 44 or 45 or 46 or 47 or 48 or 49 (2093989)
51. (exp animal/ or nonhuman/) not exp human/ (6800562)
52. ((13 and 20) or 21) and 27 and 34 and 50 (26)
53. 52 not 51 (26)

Database: Web of Science to February 04, 2019

1. (fruit*) (263,892)
2. (vegetable*) (112,459)
3. (legume*) (36,972)
4. (nut or nuts) (23,002)
5. ("olive oil*") (20,491)
6. (evoo) (626)
7. (oily fish) (417)
8. (seafood or "sea food") (11,311)
9. (tomato*) (71,792)
10. 9 or 8 or 7 or 6 or 5 or 4 or 3 or 2 or 1 (461,691)
11. ((high*or more or increase* or elevat* or raise*) Near/2 (intake* or consumption or cosume* or eat* or amount)) (263,946)
12. 11 and 10 (21,325)
13. (dairy) (120,668)
14. ("red meat*") (3894)
15. ("processed meat*") (2493)
16. ("red wine*") (12,350)
17. 16 or 15 or 14 or 13 (138,033)
18. ((low* or little or moderate or less or decrease* or reduc* or restric*) Near/2 (intake of consumption of consume or eat* or amount*)) (278,089)
19. 18 and 17
20. 19 and 12 (960)
21. (Mediterranean Near/2 diet*) (7.892)
22. 21 or 20 (8715)
23. (pregnancy or pregnant) (448,186)
24. (gestation) (97,107)
25. (maternal near/2 nutrition*) (3839)
26. (maternal near/2 diet*) (4936)
27. (perinatal) (65,900)
28. 27 or 26 or 25 or 24 or 23 (529,985)

29. (child* near/2 health*) (73,055)
30. (offspring) (84,383)
31. (baby or babies) (62,022)
32. (newborn*) (139,175)
33. (f?ctus*) (6686)
34. 33 or 32 or 31 or 30 or 29 (347,022)
35. 34 and 28 (76,415)
36. 35 and 22 (76)

Cochrane: <xx to February 04, 2019>:
TITLE-ABS-KEY ("Mediterranean Diet" AND (pregnan* OR prenatal OR perinatal OR pregnan* OR maternal) AND (offspring OR baby OR child AND health OR newborn))

Appendix B

Table A1. The based on National Institutes of Health (NIH) study quality assessment tools for controlled trials [1].

Criteria	Yes	No	Other
Cohort/cross-sectional studies			(CD, NR, NA) *
1. Was the research question or objective in this paper clearly stated?			
2. Was the study population clearly specified and defined?			
3. Was the participation rate of eligible persons at least 50%?			
4. Were all the subjects selected or recruited from the same or similar populations (including the same time period)? Were inclusion and exclusion criteria for being in the study prespecified and applied uniformly to all participants?			
5. Was a sample size justification, power description, or variance and effect estimates provided?			
6. For the analyses in this paper, were the exposure(s) of interest measured prior to the outcome(s) being measured?			
7. Was the timeframe sufficient so that one could reasonably expect to see an association between exposure and outcome if it existed?			
8. For exposures that can vary in amount or level, did the study examine different levels of the exposure as related to the outcome (e.g., categories of exposure, or exposure measured as continuous variable)?			
9. Were the exposure measures (independent variables) clearly defined, valid, reliable, and implemented consistently across all study participants?			
10. Was the exposure(s) assessed more than once over time?			
11. Were the outcome measures (dependent variables) clearly defined, valid, reliable, and implemented consistently across all study participants?			
12. Were the outcome assessors blinded to the exposure status of participants?			
13. Was loss to follow-up after baseline 20% or less?			
14. Were key potential confounding variables measured and adjusted statistically for their impact on the relationship between exposure(s) and outcome(s)?			
Quality Rating (Good, Fair, or Poor)			
Rater #1 FA:			
Rater #2 AS:			
Additional Comments (If POOR, please state why):			
Randomized Control Trials			
1. Was the study described as randomized, a randomized trial, a randomized clinical trial, or an RCT?			
2. Was the method of randomization adequate (i.e., use of randomly generated assignment)?			
3. Was the treatment allocation concealed (so that assignments could not be predicted)?			
4. Were study participants and providers blinded to the treatment group assignment?			
5. Were the people assessing the outcomes blinded to the participants' group assignments?			
6. Were the groups similar at baseline on important characteristics that could affect outcomes (e.g., demographics, risk factors, co-morbid conditions)?			
7. Was the overall drop-out rate from the study at endpoint 20% or lower of the number allocated to treatment?			
8. Was the differential drop-out rate (between treatment groups) at the endpoint 15 percentage points or lower?			
9. Was there high adherence to the intervention protocols for each treatment group?			
10. Were other interventions avoided or similar in the groups (e.g., similar background treatments)?			
11. Were outcomes assessed using valid and reliable measures, implemented consistently across all study participants?			
12. Did the authors report that the sample size was sufficiently large to be able to detect a difference in the main outcome between groups with at least 80% power?			
13. Were outcomes reported or subgroups analyzed prespecified (i.e., identified before analyses were conducted)?			

Table A1. *Cont.*

Criteria	Yes	No	Other
14. Were all randomized participants analyzed in the group to which they were originally assigned, i.e., did they use an intention-to-treat analysis?			
Quality Rating (Good, Fair, or Poor)			
Rater #1 initials:			
Rater #2 initials:			
Additional Comments (If POOR, please state why):			

* CD, cannot determine; NA, not applicable; NR, not reported; [1] National Heart, Lung, and Blood Institute (NHLBI). Study Quality Assessment Tools. NHLBI. Available at: https://www.nhlbi.nih.gov/health-topics/study-quality-assessment-tools.

Appendix C

The studies excluded after full text screening:

Schulpis, Kleopatra H.; Gavrili, Stavroula; Vlachos, George; Karikas, George A.; Michalakakou, Kelly; Demetriou, Elisabeth; Papassotiriou, Ioannis	2006	The effect of nutritional habits on maternal-neonatal lipid and lipoprotein serum levels in three different ethnic groups	Annals of Nutrition and Metabolism
Rasmussen, Morten Arendt; Maslova, Ekaterina; Halldorsson, Thorhallur Ingi; Olsen, Sjurdur Frodi	2014	Characterization of Dietary Patterns in the Danish National Birth Cohort in Relation to Preterm Birth	Plos One
Cuervo, Marta; Sayon-Orea, Carmen; Santiago, Susana; Alfredo Martinez, Jose	2014	Dietary and Health Profiles of Spanish Women in Preconception, Pregnancy and Lactation	Nutrients
Balci, Yasemin Isik; Ergin, Ahmet; Karabulut, Aysun; Polat, Aziz; Dogan, Mustafa; Kucuktasci, Kazim	2014	Serum Vitamin B12 and Folate Concentrations and the Effect of the Mediterranean Diet on Vulnerable Populations	Pediatric Hematology and Oncology
Andrusaityte, Sandra; Grazuleviciene, Regina; Petraviciene, Inga	2017	Effect of diet and maternal education on allergies among preschool children: A case-control study	Environmental Research
Haggarty, Paul; Campbell, Doris M.; Duthie, Susan; Andrews, Katherine; Hoad, Gwen; Piyathilake, Chandrika; McNeill, Geraldine	2009	Diet and deprivation in pregnancy	British Journal of Nutrition

Figure A1. The papers excluded after full-text screening.

References

1. Reijnders, I.F.; Mulders, A.G.M.G.J.; van der Windt, M.; Steegers, E.A.P.; Steegers-Theunissen, R.P.M. The impact of periconceptional maternal lifestyle on clinical features and biomarkers of placental development and function: A systematic review. *Hum. Reprod. Update* **2019**, *25*, 72–94. [CrossRef] [PubMed]
2. Kampmann, U.; Madsen, L.R.; Skajaa, G.O.; Iversen, D.S.; Moeller, N.; Ovesen, P. Gestational diabetes: A clinical update. *World J. Diabetes* **2015**, *6*, 1065–1072. [CrossRef] [PubMed]
3. Kind, K.L.; Moore, V.M.; Davies, M.J. Diet around conception and during pregnancy – effects on fetal and neonatal outcomes. *Reprod. Biomed. Online* **2006**, *12*, 532–541. [CrossRef]

4. Zerfu, T.A.; Pinto, E.; Baye, K. Consumption of dairy, fruits and dark green leafy vegetables is associated with lower risk of adverse pregnancy outcomes (APO): A prospective cohort study in rural Ethiopia. *Nutr. Diabetes* **2018**, *8*, 52. [CrossRef] [PubMed]
5. Sewell, D.A.; Hammersley, V.S.; Devereux, G.; Robertson, A.; Stoddart, A.; Weir, C.; Worth, A.; Sheikh, A. Investigating the effectiveness of the Mediterranean diet in pregnant women for the primary prevention of asthma and allergy in high-risk infants: Protocol for a pilot randomised controlled trial. *Trials Electron. Resour.* **2013**, *14*, 173. [CrossRef] [PubMed]
6. Seyedrezazadeh, E.; Moghaddam, M.P.; Ansarin, K.; Vafa, M.R.; Sharma, S.; Kolahdooz, F. Fruit and vegetable intake and risk of wheezing and asthma: A systematic review and meta-analysis. *Nutr. Rev.* **2014**, *72*, 411–428. [CrossRef]
7. Nurmatov, U.; Devereux, G.; Sheikh, A. Nutrients and foods for the primary prevention of asthma and allergy: Systematic review and meta-analysis. *J. Allergy Clin. Immunol.* **2011**, *127*, 724–733. [CrossRef]
8. Venter, C.; Brown, K.R.; Maslin, K.; Palmer, D.J. Maternal dietary intake in pregnancy and lactation and allergic disease outcomes in offspring. *Pediatr. Allergy Immunol.* **2017**, *28*, 135–143. [CrossRef] [PubMed]
9. Moody, L.; Chen, H.; Pan, Y.-X. Early-Life Nutritional Programming of Cognition—The Fundamental Role of Epigenetic Mechanisms in Mediating the Relation between Early-Life Environment and Learning and Memory Process12. *Adv. Nutr.* **2017**, *8*, 337–350. [CrossRef] [PubMed]
10. Estruch, R.; Martínez-González, M.A.; Corella, D.; Salas-Salvadó, J.; Ruiz-Gutiérrez, V.; Covas, M.I.; Fiol, M.; Gómez-Gracia, E.; López-Sabater, M.C.; Vinyoles, E.; et al. Effects of a Mediterranean-style diet on cardiovascular risk factors: A randomized trial. *Ann. Int. Med.* **2006**, *145*, 1–11. [CrossRef]
11. Jacobs, D.R.; Gross, M.D.; Tapsell, L.C. Food synergy: An operational concept for understanding nutrition. *Am. J. Clin. Nutr.* **2009**, *89*, 1543S–1548S. [CrossRef] [PubMed]
12. Reduction in the Incidence of Type 2 Diabetes with the Mediterranean Diet | Diabetes Care. Available online: http://care.diabetesjournals.org/content/34/1/14.short (accessed on 6 March 2019).
13. Widmer, R.J.; Flammer, A.J.; Lerman, L.O.; Lerman, A. The Mediterranean Diet, its Components, and Cardiovascular Disease. *Am. J. Med.* **2015**, *128*, 229–238. [CrossRef]
14. Fischer, M.; Stronati, M.; Lanari, M. Mediterranean diet, folic acid, and neural tube defects. *J. Pediatr.* **2017**, *43*, 74. [CrossRef] [PubMed]
15. Dessypris, N.; Karalexi, M.A.; Ntouvelis, E.; Diamantaras, A.-A.; Papadakis, V.; Baka, M.; Polychronopoulou, S.; Sidi, V.; Stiakaki, E.; Petridou, E.T. Association of maternal and index child's diet with subsequent leukemia risk: A systematic review and meta analysis. *Cancer Epidemiol.* **2017**, *47*, 64–75. [CrossRef]
16. Sofi, F.; Abbate, R.; Gensini, G.F.; Casini, A. Accruing evidence on benefits of adherence to the Mediterranean diet on health: An updated systematic review and meta-analysis. *Am. J. Clin. Nutr.* **2010**, *92*, 1189–1196. [CrossRef] [PubMed]
17. Netting, M.J.; Middleton, P.F.; Makrides, M. Does maternal diet during pregnancy and lactation affect outcomes in offspring? A systematic review of food-based approaches. *Nutrition* **2014**, *30*, 1225–1241. [CrossRef]
18. Grieger, J.A.; Clifton, V.L. A Review of the Impact of Dietary Intakes in Human Pregnancy on Infant Birthweight. *Nutrients* **2014**, *7*, 153–178. [CrossRef] [PubMed]
19. Chen, X.; Zhao, D.; Mao, X.; Xia, Y.; Baker, P.N.; Zhang, H. Maternal Dietary Patterns and Pregnancy Outcome. *Nutrients* **2016**, *8*, 351. [CrossRef]
20. Liberati, A.; Altman, D.G.; Tetzlaff, J.; Mulrow, C.; Gøtzsche, P.C.; Ioannidis, J.P.A.; Clarke, M.; Devereaux, P.J.; Kleijnen, J.; Moher, D. The PRISMA Statement for Reporting Systematic Reviews and Meta-Analyses of Studies That Evaluate Health Care Interventions: Explanation and Elaboration. *PLoS Med.* **2009**, *6*, e1000100. [CrossRef] [PubMed]
21. Rees, K.; Hartley, L.; Flowers, N.; Clarke, A.; Hooper, L.; Thorogood, M.; Stranges, S. "Mediterranean" dietary pattern for the primary prevention of cardiovascular disease. *Cochrane Database Syst. Rev.* **2013**, *12*, CD009825. [CrossRef]
22. National Heart, Lung, and Blood Institute (NHLBI). Study Quality Assessment Tools. Available online: https://www.nhlbi.nih.gov/health-topics/study-quality-assessment-tools (accessed on 23 March 2019).

23. Assaf-Balut, C.; Garcia de la Torre, N.; Durán, A.; Fuentes, M.; Bordiú, E.; del Valle, L.; Valerio, J.; Familiar, C.; Jiménez, I.; Herraiz, M.A.; et al. Medical nutrition therapy for gestational diabetes mellitus based on Mediterranean Diet principles: A subanalysis of the St Carlos GDM Prevention Study. *BMJ Open Diabetes Res. Care* **2018**, *6*, e000550. [CrossRef] [PubMed]

24. Assaf-Balut, C.; Garcia de la Torre, N.; Duran, A.; Fuentes, M.; Bordiu, E.; Del Valle, L.; Familiar, C.; Ortolá, A.; Jiménez, I.; Herraiz, M.A.; et al. A Mediterranean diet with additional extra virgin olive oil and pistachios reduces the incidence of gestational diabetes mellitus (GDM): A randomized controlled trial: The St. Carlos GDM prevention study. *PLoS ONE* **2017**, *12*, e0185873. [CrossRef] [PubMed]

25. Botto, L.D.; Krikov, S.; Carmichael, S.L.; Munger, R.G.; Shaw, G.M.; Feldkamp, M.L. Lower rate of selected congenital heart defects with better maternal diet quality: A population-based study. *Arch. Dis. Child. Fetal Neonatal Ed.* **2016**, *101*, 43–49. [CrossRef] [PubMed]

26. Chatzi, L.; Rifas-Shiman, S.L.; Georgiou, V.; Joung, K.E.; Koinaki, S.; Chalkiadaki, G.; Margioris, A.; Sarri, K.; Vassilaki, M.; Vafeiadi, M.; et al. Adherence to the Mediterranean diet during pregnancy and offspring adiposity and cardiometabolic traits in childhood. *Pediatr. Obes.* **2017**, *12*, 47–56. [CrossRef] [PubMed]

27. Chatzi, L.; Torrent, M.; Romieu, I.; Garcia-Esteban, R.; Ferrer, C.; Vioque, J.; Kogevinas, M.; Sunyer, J. Mediterranean diet in pregnancy is protective for wheeze and atopy in childhood. *Thorax* **2008**, *63*, 507–513. [CrossRef] [PubMed]

28. Chatzi, L.; Kogevinas, M. Prenatal and childhood Mediterranean diet and the development of asthma and allergies in children. *Public Health Nutr.* **2009**, *12*, 1629–1634. [CrossRef] [PubMed]

29. Parlapani, E.; Agakidis, C.; Karagiozoglou-Lampoudi, T.; Sarafidis, K.; Agakidou, E.; Athanasiadis, A.; Diamanti, E. The Mediterranean diet adherence by pregnant women delivering prematurely: Association with size at birth and complications of prematurity. *J. Mater. Fetal Neonatal Med.* **2017**, *13*, 1–8. [CrossRef]

30. Fernandez-Barres, S.; Romaguera, D.; Valvi, D.; Martinez, D.; Vioque, J.; Navarrete-Munoz, E.M.; Amiano, P.; Gonzalez-Palacios, S.; Guxens, M.; Pereda, E.; et al. Mediterranean dietary pattern in pregnant women and offspring risk of overweight and abdominal obesity in early childhood: The INMA birth cohort study. *Pediatr. Obes.* **2016**, *11*, 491–499. [CrossRef] [PubMed]

31. Gesteiro, E.; Rodriguez Bernal, B.; Bastida, S.; Sanchez-Muniz, F.J. Maternal diets with low healthy eating index or Mediterranean diet adherence scores are associated with high cord-blood insulin levels and insulin resistance markers at birth. *J. Clin. Nutr.* **2012**, *66*, 1008–1015. [CrossRef]

32. Gesteiro, E.; Sanchez-Muniz, F.J.; Ortega-Azorin, C.; Guillen, M.; Corella, D.; Bastida, S. Maternal and neonatal FTO rs9939609 polymorphism affect insulin sensitivity markers and lipoprotein profile at birth in appropriate-for-gestational-age term neonates. *J. Physiol.* **2016**, *72*, 169–181. [CrossRef]

33. Gonzalez-Nahm, S.; Mendez, M.; Robinson, W.; Murphy, S.K.; Hoyo, C.; Hogan, V.; Diane, R. Low maternal adherence to a Mediterranean diet is associated with increase in methylation at the MEG3-IG differentially methylated region in female infants. *Environ. Epigenetics* **2017**, *3*. [CrossRef]

34. Haugen, M.; Meltzer, H.M.; Brantsaeter, A.L.; Mikkelsen, T.; Osterdal, M.L.; Alexander, J.; Olsen, S.F.; Bakketeig, L. Mediterranean-type diet and risk of preterm birth among women in the Norwegian Mother and Child Cohort Study (MoBa): A prospective cohort study. *Acta Obstet. Gynecol. Scand.* **2008**, *87*, 319–324. [CrossRef]

35. House, J.S.; Mendez, M.; Maguire, R.L.; Gonzalez-Nahm, S.; Huang, Z.; Daniels, J.; Susan KMurphy, B.; Fuemmeler, F.A.; Wright, C.H. Periconceptional Maternal Mediterranean Diet Is Associated with Favorable Offspring Behaviors and Altered CpG Methylation of Imprinted Genes. *Front. Cell Dev. Biol.* **2018**, *6*. [CrossRef]

36. Castro-Rodriguez, J.A.; Ramirez-Hernandez, M.; Padilla, O.; Pacheco-Gonzalez, R.M.; Pérez-Fernández, V.; Garcia-Marcos, L. Effect of foods and Mediterranean diet during pregnancy and first years of life on wheezing, rhinitis and dermatitis in preschoolers. *Allergol. Immunopathol. (Madr)* **2016**, *44*, 400–409. [CrossRef]

37. Lange, N.E.; Rifas-Shiman, S.L.; Camargo, C.A.; Gold, D.R.; Gillman, M.W.; Litonjua, A.A. Maternal dietary pattern during pregnancy is not associated with recurrent wheeze in children. *J. Allergy Clin. Immunol.* **2010**, *126*, 250–255. [CrossRef]

38. Mantzoros, C.S.; Sweeney, L.; Williams, C.J.; Oken, E.; Kelesidis, T.; Rifas-Shiman, S.L.; Gillman, M.W. Maternal diet and cord blood leptin and adiponectin concentrations at birth. *Clin. Nutr.* **2010**, *29*, 622–626. [CrossRef]

39. Monteagudo, C.; Mariscal-Arcas, M.; Heras-Gonzalez, L.; Ibanez-Peinado, D.; Rivas, A.; Olea-Serrano, F. Effects of maternal diet and environmental exposure to organochlorine pesticides on newborn weight in Southern Spain. *Chemosphere* **2016**, *1*, 135–142. [CrossRef]

40. Peraita-Costa, I.; Llopis-Gonzalez, A.; Perales-Marin, A.; Sanz, F.; Llopis-Morales, A.; Morales-Suarez-Varela, M. A Retrospective Cross-Sectional Population-Based Study on Prenatal Levels of Adherence to the Mediterranean Diet: Maternal Profile and Effects on the Newborn. *J. Environ. Res.* **2018**, *15*, 1530. [CrossRef]

41. Saunders, L.; Guldner, L.; Costet, N.; Kadhel, P.; Rouget, F.; Monfort, C.; Thomé, J.P.; Multigner, L. Cordier S.Effect of a Mediterranean diet during pregnancy on fetal growth and preterm delivery: Results from a French Caribbean Mother-Child Cohort Study (TIMOUN). *Paediatr. Perinat. Epidemiol.* **2014**, *28*, 235–244. [CrossRef]

42. Steenweg-de Graaff, J.; Tiemeier, H.; Steegers-Theunissen, R.P.M.; Hofman, A.; Jaddoe, V.W.V.; Verhulst, F.C.; Roza, S.J. Maternal dietary patterns during pregnancy and child internalising and externalising problems. The Generation R Study. *Clin. Nutr.* **2014**, *33*, 115–121. [CrossRef]

43. Vujkovic, M.; Steegers, E.A.; Looman, C.W.; Ocké, M.C.; Spek, P.; van der Steegers-Theunissen, R.P. The maternal Mediterranean dietary pattern is associated with a reduced risk of spina bifida in the offspring. *BJOG Int. J. Obstet. Gynaecol.* **2009**, *116*, 408–415. [CrossRef]

44. Smith, L.K.; Draper, E.S.; Evans, T.A.; Field, D.J.; Johnson, S.J.; Manktelow, B.N.; Seaton, S.E.; Marlow, N.; Petrou, S.; Boyle, E.M. Associations between late and moderately preterm birth and smoking, alcohol, drug use and diet: A population-based case-cohort study. *Arch. Dis. Child. Fetal Neonatal Ed.* **2015**, *100*, F486–F491. [CrossRef]

45. Mariscal-Arcas, M.; Rivas, A.; Monteagudo, C.; Granada, A.; Cerrillo, I.; Olea-Serrano, F. Proposal of a Mediterranean diet index for pregnant women. *J. Nutr.* **2009**, *102*, 744–749. [CrossRef]

46. Berti, C.; Agostoni, C.; Davanzo, R.; Hyppönen, E.; Isolauri, E.; Meltzer, H.M.; Steegers-Theunissen, R.P.; Cetin, I. Early-life nutritional exposures and lifelong health: Immediate and long-lasting impacts of probiotics, vitamin D, and breastfeeding. *Nutr. Rev.* **2017**, *75*, 83–97. [CrossRef]

47. Beckhaus, A.A.; Garcia-Marcos, L.; Forno, E.; Pacheco-Gonzalez, R.M.; Celedón, J.C.; Castro-Rodriguez, J.A. Maternal nutrition during pregnancy and risk of asthma, wheeze, and atopic diseases during childhood: A systematic review and meta-analysis. *Allergy* **2015**, *70*, 1588–1604. [CrossRef]

48. Heijmans, B.T.; Tobi, E.W.; Stein, A.D.; Putter, H.; Blauw, G.J.; Susser, E.S.; Slagboom, P.E.; Lumey, L.H. Persistent epigenetic differences associated with prenatal exposure to famine in humans. *Proc. Natl. Acad. Sci. USA* **2008**, *105*, 17046–17049. [CrossRef]

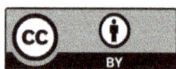

Review

The Impact of Maternal Eating Disorders on Dietary Intake and Eating Patterns during Pregnancy: A Systematic Review

Annica F. Dörsam [1,*], Hubert Preißl [2], Nadia Micali [3], Sophia B. Lörcher [1], Stephan Zipfel [1] and Katrin E. Giel [1]

[1] Department of Psychosomatic Medicine and Psychotherapy, Medical University Hospital Tübingen, 72076 Tübingen, Germany; Sophia.Loercher@med.uni-tuebingen.de (S.B.L.); Stephan.Zipfel@med.uni-tuebingen.de (S.Z.); Katrin.Giel@med.uni-tuebingen.de (K.E.G.)
[2] Institute for Diabetes Research and Metabolic Diseases of the Helmholtz Center Munich at the University of Tübingen; fMEG Center; German Center for Diabetes Research (DZD), 72076 Tübingen, Germany; Hubert.Preissl@uni-tuebingen.de
[3] Department of Psychiatry, Faculty of Medicine, University of Geneva, 1205 Geneva, Switzerland; nadia.micali@hcuge.ch
* Correspondence: Annica.Doersam@med.uni-tuebingen.de; Tel.: +49-7071-29-85467

Received: 19 March 2019; Accepted: 10 April 2019; Published: 13 April 2019

Abstract: Maternal nutrition in pregnancy has a key influence on optimum fetal health. Eating disorders (EDs) during pregnancy may have detrimental effects on fetal growth and the child's early development. There is limited knowledge concerning the eating behavior, dietary intake and derived nutritional biomarkers as well as the nutrient supplementation in women with EDs during pregnancy. We performed a systematic review according to the PRISMA statement to synthesize current evidence in this field. Of $N = 1203$ hits, 13 full-texts were included in the qualitative synthesis. While women with current Binge Eating Disorder (BED) showed higher energy and fat intakes during pregnancy, women with a lifetime Anorexia Nervosa (AN), Bulimia Nervosa (BN) or both (AN + BN) had similar patterns of nutrient intake and dietary supplement use as healthy women. There is evidence, that women with a history of EDs have a sufficient diet quality and are more likely to be vegetarian. Dieting and bingeing improved substantially with pregnancy. The highlighted differences in the consumption of coffee/caffeine and artificially sweetened beverages as well as the elevated prevalence of iron deficiency anemia in women with a past or active ED during pregnancy might have an important impact on fetal development.

Keywords: anorexia nervosa; bulimia nervosa; binge eating disorder; diet; eating behavior; eating disorders; nutrition; pregnancy; purging

1. Introduction

In pregnancy, a lifestyle characterized by regular exercise and a balanced and diverse diet is a significant determinant of the course of pregnancy, the child's development, and the short- and long-term health of the mother and child [1]. In relation to the slight increase in energy intake in the last months of pregnancy, the demand for some vitamins and minerals (including trace elements) increases significantly more [1], usually from the 4th month of pregnancy on [2]. For the nutrients folate and iodine, a markedly increased intake is recommended from the beginning of pregnancy or, ideally, before conception [2]. There is substantial interest in nutrition during pregnancy, due to the extensive research in the area of early nutrition programming [3], arisen from the initial work by Barker ('Fetal Origins of Adult Disease'; FOAD) [4]. Barker's initial concept was later modified to the 'Developmental Origins of Health and Disease' (DOHaD) [5], which postulates that exposure to certain environmental influences during critical periods of development (e.g., intrauterine deficiency or oversupply of nutrients) and growth may have a significant impact on the development of non-communicable diseases (NCDs), such as obesity, diabetes mellitus, cardiovascular and mental disorders, as well as cancer in later life [5–7].

Given that eating disorders (EDs) are characterized by dysfunctional eating behaviors (e.g., caloric restriction, purging behavior), which may result in specific maternal macro- and micronutrient deficiencies, one would predict negative consequences of maternal EDs on the health, growth, and development of the fetus and the newborn infant. Research suggests that up to 7.5% of pregnant women are affected by an ED [8]. EDs include Anorexia Nervosa (AN), Bulimia Nervosa (BN), Binge Eating Disorder (BED) and 'Other Specified Feeding or Eating Disorders' (OSFED) [9]. AN is characterized by an excessive restriction of energy intake, which leads to severe weight loss with a pathological fear of weight gain and a distorted body image [9]. BN is defined by regular episodes of binge eating followed by inappropriate compensatory behaviors such as self-induced vomiting, abuse of laxatives, fasting or excessive exercise to avoid weight gain [9]. BED is associated with recurring episodes of eating significantly more food in a short period of time than most people would eat under comparable conditions, accompanied by feelings of lack of control, guilt, embarrassment or disgust [9].

There is increasing evidence from large cohort studies and register data showing that maternal disordered eating behavior and dysregulated body weight have detrimental effects on the course of pregnancy and birth outcomes. Pregnant women with an active ED are at increased risk of experiencing antepartum hemorrhage [10], hyperemesis gravidarum [11], higher rates of miscarriage [12], caesarean sections, and postpartum depression [13]. The literature on fetal outcomes of women with EDs displays lower [14] and higher birth weights [15,16], intrauterine growth restriction [10], small head circumferences [17], neurobehavioral dysregulations early after birth [18] as well as premature deliveries and perinatal mortality [15]. Disturbances and dysfunctions related to nutrition and eating behaviors which are core symptoms of EDs might contribute to these adverse pregnancy outcomes seen in women with EDs. On the other hand, given that affected women are often unduly preoccupied by eating and weight-control practices, they might have a higher nutritional knowledge, especially in terms of nutrient sources [19]. Therefore, one could also assume that at least subgroups of women with EDs might have a higher diet quality during pregnancy. Although most studies report an improvement in the ED symptomatology during pregnancy [20–23], there is limited knowledge about the actual food intake and overall dietary behavior of pregnant women with EDs.

The present systematic review aims to provide a synthesis of evidence regarding overall nutrition and related issues of pregnant women with a history of EDs. The main research questions are:

1. Do pregnant women with a history of EDs show different dietary intakes and patterns as compared to healthy pregnant women?
2. Do pregnant women with a history of EDs deviate from international dietary recommendations guidelines for pregnancy?
3. Do pregnant women with a history of EDs differ from healthy pregnant women with regard to nutritional biomarkers and dietary supplement intake?
4. Do pregnant women with a history of EDs show dysfunctional eating behaviors, i.e., restrictive eating, dieting, binge eating? Here, we will focus exclusively on behavioral *eating* aspects (which also represent ED symptoms), but not solely on ED symptoms with no direct connection to food intake (e.g., self-induced vomiting).

2. Methods

The review process was conducted according to the 'Preferred Reporting Items for Systematic Reviews and Meta-Analyses' (PRISMA) [24]. Papers were searched on PubMed and PsycInfo and covered a period ranging from 1987 to November 2018. The approach of this systematic review was specified in advance and documented in a protocol.

2.1. Search Strategy

Studies were identified by searching electronic databases and scanning reference lists of articles for relevant studies. The search was applied using the scientific databases PubMed and PsycInfo. In addition, we handsearched contents pages of 'The International Journal of Eating Disorders', the 'Journal of Eating Disorders', the 'European Eating Disorders Review', 'Eating Disorders: The Journal of Treatment and Prevention' and 'Nutrients'.

Until November 2018, a search of two databases was performed using the terms 'nutrition', 'food intake', 'eating behavior', 'pregnancy', and 'eating disorders'. As an example, for the PubMed search, the search term was defined as follows:

'(((("nutritional status"[MeSH Terms] OR ("nutritional"[All Fields] AND "status"[All Fields]) OR "nutritional status"[All Fields] OR "nutrition"[All Fields] OR "nutritional sciences"[MeSH Terms] OR ("nutritional"[All Fields] AND "sciences"[All Fields]) OR "nutritional sciences"[All Fields]) OR ("eating"[MeSH Terms] OR "eating"[All Fields] OR ("food"[All Fields] AND "intake"[All Fields]) OR "food intake"[All Fields])) OR ("eating behaviour"[All Fields] OR "feeding behavior"[MeSH Terms] OR ("feeding"[All Fields] AND "behavior"[All Fields]) OR "feeding behavior"[All Fields] OR ("eating"[All Fields] AND "behavior"[All Fields]) OR "eating behavior"[All Fields])) AND ("pregnancy"[MeSH Terms] OR "pregnancy"[All Fields])) AND ("feeding and eating disorders"[MeSH Terms] OR ("feeding"[All Fields] AND "eating"[All Fields] AND "disorders"[All Fields]) OR "feeding and eating disorders"[All Fields] OR ("eating"[All Fields] AND "disorders"[All Fields]) OR "eating disorders"[All Fields]) AND "humans"[MeSH Terms]'.

The first stage of study selection included the removal of duplicate studies, conducted by the paper's first author (A.F.D.). The first and the fourth author (S.B.L.) roughly screened the remaining studies by scanning article titles and abstracts. In the next step, the same two authors performed full text examinations of potentially relevant studies according to the defined eligibility criteria. Disagreements were resolved by discussion between the two investigators; if no agreement could be reached, the last review author (K.E.G.) was consulted.

The first author then extracted information from each included study using a specifically designed data collection sheet. The data collection sheet sought the following variables: (i) study characteristics (including study design, follow-up period, study size, country, funding sources), and the trial's inclusion and exclusion criteria; (ii) characteristics of trial participants (including method of ED diagnosis, gestational week); (iii) type of outcome measures (including dietary quantity and quality, eating patterns, dietary supplement use, nutritional biomarkers, and eating behavior in general), and results (including limitations, strengths, clinical implications and conclusions).

2.2. Eligibility Criteria

Eligibility criteria were based on the five PICOS dimensions, i.e., participants (P), interventions (I), comparators (C), outcome (O) and study design (S) [25].

2.2.1. Participants

Participants included pregnant women of any age with a past or current ED. Eating disorders were defined as AN, BN, BED and OSFED, previously known as 'Eating Disorder Not Otherwise Specified' (EDNOS), according to DSM criteria. Pica, an eating disorder that involves the persistent eating of substances that are not food and do not provide nutritional value, was defined as exclusion criterion for this review, as Pica is often described inaccurately as a part of culturally supported or socially normative practices [26]. Pregnant women with additional severe mental disorders (e.g., dementia, schizophrenia) as well as somatic syndromes influencing weight or eating behavior (e.g., diabetes mellitus, epilepsy, Prader-Willi syndrome), or virus infections (e.g., malaria) were excluded from this review.

2.2.2. Interventions

Trials assessing the dietary intake and eating patterns of pregnant women with a history of EDs in comparison to pregnant women without EDs. Dietary intake includes dietary quality, dietary supplement use, and eating behavior in general. Additionally, this review includes studies reporting on nutritional biomarkers of under- or malnutrition.

2.2.3. Comparators

Studies were eligible if a control group was included that consisted of pregnant women without any EDs. If there was no control group assessed, international dietary recommendation guidelines for pregnancy were used as a comparator [1,27,28].

2.2.4. Outcome

Primary outcome measures: Dietary intake in terms of food quantity and food quality, eating patterns regarding different forms of nutrition (e.g., vegetarianism, veganism), dietary supplement use (e.g., vitamin supplements), and nutritional biomarkers (e.g., ferritin). *Secondary outcome measures:* eating behavior in general (e.g., dieting or binge eating).

2.2.5. Study design

Cross-sectional and longitudinal observational studies assessing the dietary intake and eating patterns of pregnant women with a history of EDs. No publication date restrictions were imposed. Unpublished material and abstracts were included; publications in form of book chapters, reviews, case reports/series or dissertations were excluded. This review was limited to studies in English, French or German language.

3. Results

A total of 13 studies were identified for inclusion in this review. Interrater reliability was good, with κ = 0.71. See the flow diagram for an overview of the study selection process (Figure 1).

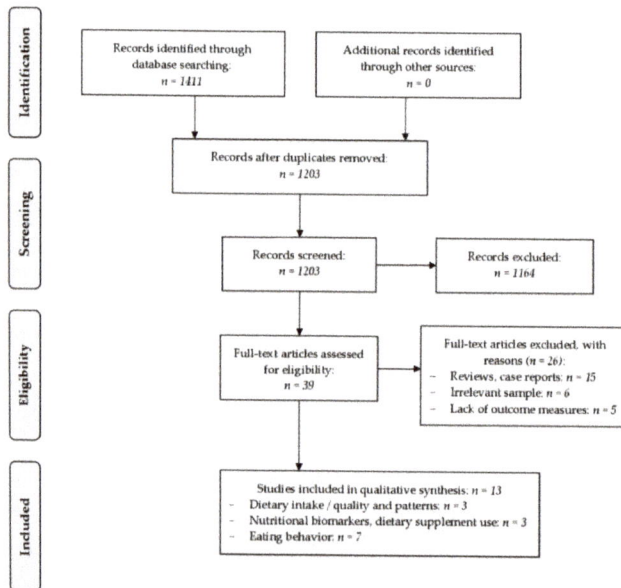

Figure 1. PRISMA flow chart for study inclusion.

We clustered the 13 studies according to the following topics concerning pregnant women with EDs:

1. Dietary intake/quality and patterns (*n* = 3)
2. Nutritional biomarkers and dietary supplement use (*n* = 3)
3. Eating behavior (*n* = 7)

3.1. Studies Investigating Dietary Intake and Patterns in Pregnant Women with Eating Disorders

We identified three studies which investigated dietary intakes in pregnancy in women with lifetime EDs [29–31]. All three studies were cross-sectional analyses, using data from large population-based cohort studies (see Table 1). Women with lifetime EDs were compared with control women free of any EDs before or during pregnancy. Maternal history of lifetime EDs was assessed during pregnancy [31] with self-reported questionnaires, either at gestational week (GW) 12 [29], or at six months prior to pregnancy and at GW 18.1 [30]. Dietary information was collected via food frequency questionnaires (FFQs) in the first half of the pregnancy [30,31] and in the third trimester [29]. The FFQ determines the frequency of consumption and the portion size of a wide variety of foods and drinks. Additionally, Micali et al. [29] and Siega-Riz et al. [30] combined related foods into different food groups (e.g., red meat, poultry, sausages/burgers, pies/pasties = 'meat'). Two of the three studies [29,30] examined the exact dietary intake of pregnant women across the ED spectrum in comparison to pregnant women without EDs. Siega-Riz et al. [30] focused on nutrient and food group intakes of pregnant women with BED and BN in the second trimester. Micali et al. [29] examined the dietary intake as well as dietary patterns of pregnant women with AN, BN or both (AN + BN) in the third trimester.

In terms of macronutrient intake, there were no differences to healthy pregnant women in energy, carbohydrate, fat and protein consumption of pregnant women with AN, BN or both in the third trimester [29]. In contrast, women with BED before and during pregnancy showed a higher consumption of total energy and total fat (monounsaturated fatty acids, MUFA; saturated fatty acids, SFA) in the second trimester [30]. Women who developed BED during pregnancy also had a higher total energy and SFA intake [30].

With regard to micronutrient intake through diet, there was very little difference in pregnancy in women with EDs compared with control women [29,30]. In particular, women in the second trimester with BED before and during pregnancy had lower intakes of folate, potassium and vitamin C [30]. This is reflected in the food group consumption, showing lower intakes of fruit and juices in those women [30]. In the third trimester, women with AN and AN + BN had higher folate and potassium intakes; women with AN + BN showed higher intakes of calcium, phosphorus, zinc, and vitamin C and women with BN had a slightly higher vitamin E intake compared to control women [29]. In general, the average mineral and vitamin intakes were satisfying in women with EDs throughout pregnancy [27,28].

In relation to food group consumption, women with BED before and during pregnancy had higher intakes of overall fat (butter, margarines, and oils) and milk desserts in the second trimester [30]. Pregnant women with AN, BN or both in the third trimester were less likely to use butter and drink full-fat milk in favor of skimmed and soya milk [29]. Those women also consumed less meat and fewer potatoes; however, they had a higher intake of soya products and pulses compared to the referent group [29]. Similarly, women with BN before and during pregnancy had a lower intake of high-fat meats in the second trimester [30]. Moreover, a higher consumption of artificially sweetened beverages among women with active and past BN and BED was observed [30]. Women with an active BED showed a slight increase in mean coffee consumption and women with lifetime AN and AN + BN reported a significantly higher coffee consumption (>355 mg caffeine/week) during pregnancy [29,30].

Regarding dietary patterns, women with lifetime EDs scored higher on the vegetarian dietary pattern (high intakes of meat substitutes, pulses, nuts and herbal teas, and high negative intakes of red meat and poultry), which corresponds to their self-report as being vegetarian [29]. Women with a lifetime AN scored higher on the 'traditional' dietary pattern (high loadings for all types of vegetables and red meat and poultry); women with a lifetime AN + BN scored higher on the 'health conscious' (high intake of salad, fruit, rice, pasta, oat and bran-based breakfast cereals, fish, pulses, fruit juices and non-white bread) and the 'traditional' dietary pattern [29].

Nguyen et al. [31] calculated a diet quality score with the data of the FFQs on the basis of the Dutch national dietary guidelines, including 15 components and cut-offs (e.g., vegetables (≥200 g/day), dairy (≥300 g/day), and red meat (≤375 g/week)). After adjustment for socioeconomic and lifestyle factors (maternal age, ethnicity, educational level, BMI, household income, psychiatric symptoms), women with a history of EDs had a significantly higher diet quality score than women unexposed [31].

3.2. Studies Investigating Maternal Biomarkers of Nutrition and Dietary Supplement Use in Pregnant Women with Eating Disorders

We identified two studies which assessed maternal biomarkers of nutrition in pregnant women with a history of EDs [15,32], and one study which focused on the dietary supplement use in those women [33] (see Table 2).

Koubaa et al. [32] examined biomarkers of nutrition and stress during early pregnancy in a cohort of women with a previous history of AN or BN in comparison to healthy women. Women with a history of AN showed a significantly higher frequency of anemia (hemoglobin, Hb < 110 g/L), which was related to low levels of maternal serum ferritin in early pregnancy compared to controls ($p < 0.01$). In their large register search study ($n = 4299$), Linna et al. [15] also found an increased occurrence of anemia in women with AN compared to healthy controls.

Regarding dietary supplement use, Dellava et al. [33] performed a cross-sectional analysis of the Norwegian Mother and Child Cohort Study (MoBa). Over 90% of women with an ED diagnosis as well as women without EDs used dietary supplements during pregnancy. Folic acid supplementation was the most common dietary supplement. After adjusting for covariates (maternal age, parity, smoking, household income, and educational level), no significant differences existed across groups for the use of any dietary supplement during pregnancy. However, women with EDNOS-P (purging subtype) were significantly more likely to take iron supplements during pregnancy ($p < 0.04$) [33].

3.3. Studies Investigating Eating Behavior in Pregnant Women with EDs

Concerning dysfunctional eating behaviors in pregnant women with a history of EDs, we identified seven relevant studies [20,23,34–38]. These studies provide evidence for a general improvement in dysfunctional eating behaviors during pregnancy in women with a recent or past ED (see Table 3). Women who actively suffered from BN during pregnancy reported an improvement of objective binge episodes with each passing trimester [36,37]. In particular, the frequency of objective binge eating in pregnant women with full or partial AN, BN or BED decreased to 2.9 episodes per 28 days intrapartum compared to 8.7 episodes prepartum [23]. 65% of pregnant women with an active BN, AN or mixed symptoms (AN + BN) who restricted their intake reported that they improved nutritionally or stopped restricting entirely; 56% of those who binged improved during pregnancy [38]. Blais et al. [20] also found a decrease in binge frequency in women with an active BN intrapartum, but no significant differences for binge frequencies and restrictive eating were seen in women with an active AN. For pregnant women with an active AN, BN or both, there was also evidence that bingeing became worse in pregnancy (18%) and that increased impulsivity within food intake resulted in overeating in 12% of those women [38]. Cross-sectional analyses of the Avon Longitudinal Study of Parents and Children (ALSPAC) revealed that 11.3% of women with a recent ED and 4.4% of women with a past ED dieted in late pregnancy, compared to 8% of obese and 2.5% of nonobese control women [34]. Regarding the question of whether they felt a loss of control over eating (LOC) during pregnancy, 72.5% of women with a recent ED and 42.8% of women with a past ED as well as 33.8% of healthy obese women and 36.1% of healthy nonobese women confirmed this question. Especially women with a recent BN were more likely to report LOC in pregnancy compared to all other groups [34].

Table 1. Studies investigating dietary intake/quality/patterns in pregnant women with eating disorders.

Source	Study Design	Country	Sample	ED Diagnosis	n	Prevalence of EDs	Outcome	Dietary Information
Nguyen et al., 2017 [31]	Cross-sectional analysis of the Generation R study	Netherlands	Pregnant women with and without a history of any ED	Self-reported questionnaire and clinical diagnoses (subsample; n = 928) during pregnancy	6196	9.5% (n = 591)	Diet quality score, including 15 components and cut-offs (e.g., vegetables (≥200 g/day), dairy (≥300 g/day), red meat (≤375 g/week))	Semi-quantitative modified 293-item FFQ at 13.6 weeks of gestation (12.4–16.2)
Main findings	Women with a history of EDs had a higher diet quality score than women without EDs							
Micali et al., 2012 [29]	Cross-sectional analysis of the ALSPAC study	United Kingdom	Pregnant women with and without a lifetime AN, BN, and AN + BN (exclusion: non-singleton pregnancies, miscarriage)	Self-reported questionnaire at 12 weeks of gestation	10,137	4.1% (n = 414); AN (n = 151); BN (n = 186); AN + BN (n = 77)	Frequency of consumption of various food groups, daily nutrient intakes (macronutrients), and dietary patterns	FFQ at 32 weeks of gestation; 14 food groups, 5 dietary patterns
Main findings (compared to control women)	1. Women with lifetime ED: - 2.8 times more likely to describe themselves as vegetarian - ↑ scoring on 'vegetarian' dietary pattern - ↓ meat, potatoes, SFA (AN, AN + BN) - ↑ soya products, pulses, skimmed and soya milk, fiber - ↓ butter, full-fat milk - ↑ caffeine (>355 mg/day) (esp. AN, AN + BN)					2. Women with a lifetime AN: - ↑ scoring on 'traditional' dietary pattern 3. Women with a lifetime BN: - ↑ bread (1.1 slices/d more), PUFA - ↓ sugar, non-milk extrinsic sugar 4. Women with a lifetime AN + BN: - ↑ scoring on 'health conscious' and 'traditional' dietary pattern		
Siega-Riz et al., 2008 [30]	Cross-sectional analysis of the MoBa study	Norway	Pregnant women with and without lifetime BN and BED	Self-reported questionnaire 6 month before and during pregnancy (18.1 week of gestation)	30,040	6.1% lifetime ED (n = 1840); 4.6% active ED (n = 1393); BN/BN (n = 99); BN/BED (n = 60); BED/BED (n = 650); none/BED (n = 624)	Nutrient and food group intakes	Semi-quantitative FFQ at gestational weeks 15–22; 255 questions, 20 food groups
Main findings (compared to control women)	1. Women with BED before + during pregnancy: - ↑ total energy (2459.0 ± 30.2 kcal vs. 2348.3 ± 4.6 kcal) - ↑ total fat (87.5 ± 1.2 g vs. 80.8 ± 0.2 g) - ↑ MUFA (27.8 ± 0.4 g vs. 26.6 ± 0.1 g) - ↑ SFA (34.2 ± 0.5 g vs. 31.3 ± 0.1 g) - ↑ folate (268.9 ± 3.8 µg vs. 273.4 ± 0.7 µg) - ↑ potassium (4008.1 ± 49 mg vs. 4018.6 ± 7.6 mg) - ↓ vitamin C (155.5 ± 3.7 mg vs. 167.5 ± 0.6 mg) - ↑ butter, margarines, oils, milk desserts, candy, coffee - ↓ fruit, juices, chicken					2. Women with incident BED during pregnancy: - ↑ total energy (2544.1 ± 41.2 kcal vs. 2348.3 ± 4.6 kcal) - ↑ SFA (34.9 ± 0.6 g vs. 31.3 ± 0.1 g) - ↑ cakes, candy, milk desserts, coffee; ↓ juices 3. Women with BN before and during pregnancy: - ↑ yogurt, cheeses - ↓ sweetened beverages, high-fat meats		

Abbreviations: ED: eating disorder; AN: Anorexia Nervosa; BN: Bulimia Nervosa; BED: Binge Eating Disorder; ALSPAC: Avon Longitudinal Study of Parents and Children: MoBa: Norwegian Mother and Child Cohort Study; FFQ: Food Frequency Questionnaire; ↑: higher (consumption); ↓: lower (consumption); SFA: saturated fatty acids; MUFA: monounsaturated fatty acids; PUFA: polyunsaturated fatty acids; BN/BN = BN before and during pregnancy; BN/BED = BN before, BED during pregnancy; BED/BED = BED before and during pregnancy; none/BED = no ED before, BED during pregnancy.

Table 2. Studies investigating nutritional biomarkers and dietary supplement use in pregnant women with eating disorders.

Source	Study Design	Country	Sample	ED Diagnosis	n	Prevalence of EDs	Outcome	Main Findings
Koubaa et al., 2015 [32]	Longitudinal cohort study (follow-up period: 1 year)	Sweden	Pregnant, nulliparous non-smoking women with and without a history of AN and BN	Interview according to DSM-IV diagnostic criteria; medical records	96	38.5% (n = 37); AN (active AN: n = 8; past AN: n = 12); BN (active BN: n = 1; past BN: n = 16)	Maternal serum biomarkers of nutrition and stress at 10 weeks of gestation within a routine blood sample (ferritin, cortisol, TSH, T4, insulin, IGF-I and IGFBP1)	Women with previous AN: - ↑ frequency (70%) of anemia (Hb < 110 g/L) compared to controls (12%) 1. ↓ serum ferritin levels compared to controls
Linna et al., 2014 [15]	Register search study	Finland	Female ED patients and unexposed controls	Attending physicians at the clinic with ICD-10 (AN, BN, atypical AN/BN) and DSM-IV (BED) criteria	4299	15.3% (n = 657); AN (n = 182); BN (n = 436); BED (n = 39)	Pregnancy complications (obtained from Medical Birth Register): gestational diabetes mellitus, initiation of insulin treatment, anemia, antenatal corticosteroid treatment, pregnancy-related ICD-10 diagnoses	Anemia was more frequent among women with AN (3.97%) compared with unexposed women (1.54%)
Dellava et al., 2013 [33]	Cross-sectional analysis of the MoBA study	Norway	Pregnant women across eating disorder subtypes compared with a referent group	Self-reported questionnaire at GW 19	37,307	6.3% (n = 2348); AN (n = 34); BN (n = 326); BED (n = 1944); EDNOS-P (n = 44)	Use of dietary supplements (checklist including 22 specific nutrients, at three time points prior to pregnancy (≥9 weeks), 8–5 weeks and 4–1 week before conception) and eight time periods during pregnancy (GW 1–4, 5–8, 9–12 13–16, 17–20, 21–24, 25–28, and 29+)	Dietary supplement use during pregnancy was as follows (between group differences were not statistically significant): - 91.2% of women with AN - 92.2% of women with BN - 93.2% of women with EDNOS-P (↑ intake of Fe-containing supplements) - 90.6% of women with BED - 93.5% of the women without EDs

Abbreviations: ED: eating disorder; AN: Anorexia Nervosa; BN: Bulimia Nervosa; BED: Binge Eating Disorder; EDNOS-P: Eating Disorder Not Otherwise Specified – Purging subtype; MoBa: Norwegian Mother and Child Cohort Study; TSH: Thyroid-Stimulating Hormone; T4: Free Thyroxine (T4); IGF-I: Insulin-Like Growth Factor I; IGFBP1: IGF Binding Protein 1; Hb: Hemoglobin; Fe: Iron; DSM: Diagnostic and Statistical Manual of Mental Disorders; ICD-10: International Statistical Classification of Diseases and Related Health Problems; GW: gestational week; ↑: higher; ↓: lower.

Table 3. Studies investigating eating behavior in pregnant women with eating disorders.

Source	Study Design	Country	Sample	ED Diagnosis	n	Prevalence of EDs	Outcome	Main Findings
Crow et al., 2008 [23]	Cross-sectional analysis of the McKnight Longitudinal Study of Eating Disorders	United States of America	Pregnant women with full/subthreshold AN, BN or BED	EDE	42	AN (n = 5; 11.9%); BN (n = 15; 35.7%); BED (n = 4; 9.5%); partial AN (n = 5; 11.9%); partial BN (n = 10; 23.8%); partial BED (n = 3; 7.1%)	Eating behaviors and disordered eating cognitions over the course of pregnancy	Frequency of objective binge eating episodes per 28 days intrapartum: 2.9 (vs. 8.7 prepartum)
Micali et al., 2007 [34]	Cross-sectional analysis of the ALSPAC study	United Kingdom	Pregnant women with and without recent/past AN, BN, AN + BN	Self-reported questionnaire at 12 weeks of gestation	12,252	0.5% recent ED (n = 57; 6 AN, 51 BN); 3.2% past ED (n = 395; 167 AN, 158 BN, 70 AN + BN)	18 GW: Self-induced vomiting, laxative use, exercise behavior, shape and weight concern; 32 GW: appraisals about weight gain during pregnancy, dieting, LOC	Dieting in pregnancy: - recent ED: 11.3% - past ED: 4.4% - nonobese controls: 2.5% LOC: - recent ED: 72.5% - past ED: 42.8% - nonobese controls: 36.1% Women with recent BN were more likely to report LOC in pregnancy compared to all other groups
Crow et al., 2004 [35]	Cross-sectional analysis of a longitudinal study (follow-up period: 10 – 15 years)	United States of America	Pregnant women with BN	EDI; SCID; Eating Disorders Questionnaire; self-report of BN symptoms	129	all BN	Bulimic symptoms, alcohol, drug, and tobacco use during pregnancy	Frequency of binge eating during pregnancy was rated as: - decreased by 59.6% - increased by 7.4% - unchanged by 33.0% The prevalence of alcohol use decreased after pregnancy was recognized (35% vs. 14%)
Blais et al., 2000 [20]	Longitudinal Study	United States of America	Pregnant women with AN and BN	LIFE-EAT II every 6 month	82	31.7% AN (AN-R: n = 7; AN-BP: n = 19); 68.3% BN (n = 56)	Pregnancy outcome (live birth, therapeutic/spontaneous abortion), ED symptomatology (restrictive eating, binging, etc.)	BN subjects: ↓ frequency of binging from prepregnancy to post-pregnancy AN subjects: No significant differences were seen for binging frequency and restrictive eating

Table 3. *Cont.*

Source	Study Design	Country	Sample	ED Diagnosis	n	Prevalence of EDs	Outcome	Main Findings
Morgan et al., 1999 [37]	Retrospective analysis	United Kingdom	Pregnant women actively suffering from BN	EDE, SCID	94	all BN	Symptoms of bulimia nervosa and associated psychopathology at conception, each trimester and postnatally	Objective binge episodes improved with each passing trimester of pregnancy
Lemberg, et al., 1989 [38]	Longitudinal study	United States of America	Pregnant women with an active AN, BN or mixed symptoms	Retrospective, 55-item questionnaire on ED symptoms and course of pregnancy	43	57% AN-R; 77% BN; 16% combination of both	Eating behaviors both antenatal and postnatal	Women who restricted their intake (*n* = 36): - 65% reported improved nutrition or stopping restricting // complete cessation: 7% Women who binged (*n* = 41): - improvement: 56% // worsening: 18.6% // complete cessation: 14% All women: 12% ↑ impulsivity with food by overeating
Lacey et al., 1987 [36]	Longitudinal study	United Kingdom	Pregnant untreated BN women	St George's Hospital eating disorder unit; DSM-III	20	all BN	Impact of pregnancy on dietary difficulties of the bulimic woman	19 of the 20 subjects reduced frequency of binge eating over the course of pregnancy; only 5 patients were binge eating during the 3rd trimester; 75% having a complete cessation of bingeing by the 3rd trimester

Abbreviations: ED: eating disorder; AN: Anorexia Nervosa; AN-R: Anorexia Nervosa Restrictive subtype; AN-BP: Anorexia Nervosa Binge-Purge subtype; BN: Bulimia Nervosa; BED: Binge Eating Disorder; LOC: Loss of control over eating; ALSPAC: Avon Longitudinal Study of Parents and Children; EDE: Eating Disorder Examination; EDI: Eating Disorder Inventory; Structured Clinical Interview for DSM Axis I Disorders (SCID); LIFE-EAT II: Eating Disorders Longitudinal Interval Follow-up Evaluation; DSM: Diagnostic and Statistical Manual of Mental Disorders; GW: gestational week; ↑: higher; ↓: lower.

4. Discussion

This systematic review analyzed diet quality, nutritional biomarkers and dietary supplement use as well as dysfunctional eating behaviors in women with a current or past ED during pregnancy. Given the fact that, up to now, only three studies have investigated dietary intake and diet quality in women with EDs during pregnancy [29–31], and only one study has investigated nutritional biomarkers [32] and dietary supplement use [33] in pregnant women with EDs, a clear finding of our review is that more research in this area is urgently needed.

4.1. Dietary Intake and Patterns in Pregnant Women with Eating Disorders

Summarizing the current findings of the three relevant studies, there is congruent evidence for an adequate diet in pregnant women with EDs, although there are specific subgroup differences [29–31].

The strengths of these studies are their population-based, longitudinal design, and therefore very large sample sizes. However, all cited studies have a general limitation regarding the examination of food intake with the use of food frequency questionnaires, as they rely on memory and reported intakes, which are subject to measurement errors [39]. Moreover, the items of the FFQ are adapted on the specific diet of a country; thus, carefulness is required regarding participants with different ethnic backgrounds [31]. Another weakness is the use of standard portion sizes to assess nutrient intakes from the FFQs, resulting in imprecise estimates of the actual food quantity [29,30]. It remains unclear whether the FFQ is a valid tool for the dietary assessment in pregnant women with EDs who experience worries and feelings of guilt or embarrassment for not caring for their unborn children, as they may under- or over-report specific food items (e.g., energy-dense foods) [31]. However, several studies conclude that the FFQ is a valid tool for ranking women in accordance with their nutrient intakes during pregnancy [40–42].

Nguyen et al. calculated a higher diet quality score for women with a history of EDs, not differentiating the disorder into active, past or type of ED [31]. Furthermore, the exact dietary data was not presented in the article. Micali et al. examined nutrient and food group intakes of pregnant women with lifetime AN, BN and both [29]; Siega-Riz et al. investigated those of women with active BN and active BED [30]. Consequently, except for the BN group, the other subgroups cannot be compared on the basis of uniform diagnoses between those studies. Nevertheless, the data on dietary intake in pregnant women with a history of AN, BN and AN + BN suggests a relatively good diet quality, supported by a vegetarian dietary pattern with lower intakes of meat and similar protein, fat and carbohydrate intakes compared to controls. However, these results can also be the result of persistent ED symptoms during pregnancy [31]. More precisely, women whose ED cognitions are present in pregnancy might have made more informed choices about a 'healthy' diet that included low caloric foods (e.g., vegetables, skimmed milk) to prevent further weight gain [31] or to avoid 'fattening' foods during an interval when purging episodes may be reduced [30]. If so, those women would have scored higher on the diet quality. An alternative explanation for better nutrition in women with a history of AN, BN or both is an improvement in the ED symptoms during pregnancy, which is suggested by the majority of previous studies in this field [20–23]. This is supported by the notion that, especially during pregnancy, expectant mothers are often highly motivated to optimize their lifestyle [1]. However, women with BED before and during pregnancy showed higher energy and overall fat intakes and lower intakes of some nutrients compared to controls. For women with BED, pregnancy could be a trigger for the continuation or even deterioration of symptoms [22].

The higher consumption of artificially sweetened beverages among women with active and past BN and BED [24] might be a reflection of their ED pattern in reducing added sugars. Summarized data from three very large prospective cohort studies showed several risks which were associated with the consumption of artificially sweetened beverages by pregnant women, including prematurity and the diagnosis of asthma in their children up to the age of seven years [43].

Similarly, the high consumption of caffeine (>355 mg/day), especially in women with AN and AN + BN, is of high concern, since caffeine and coffee consumption during pregnancy might be associated with spontaneous abortion at daily levels of 300 mg caffeine and above in a dose-dependent way (7–19% for every increase in caffeine intake of 100–150 mg/day) [44,45]. Based on limited data, a Cochrane meta-analysis was unable to conclude on the effectiveness of the abstention from caffeine on birth weight or other relevant endpoints [46]. In a clinical sample of ED patients, the main reasons for consuming caffeinated beverages were appetite suppression, feeling of fullness, facilitation with purging, and increasing the metabolic rate to enhance energy expenditure [47]. There is evidence that habitual coffee consumption plays a possible role in weight loss (increased metabolic rate, energy expenditure, lipid oxidation, and lipolytic and thermogenic activities) [48]. However, the American College of Obstetricians (ACOG) and the European Food Safety Authority (EFSA) recommend that pregnant women should drink no more than 200 mg of caffeine per day [49,50].

Lastly, the average intake of all nutrients was sufficient for women with active and past EDs, except for potassium and phosphorus being very high and iron and folate being much lower than recommended in the analyses by Siega-Riz et al. [30]. However, nutrient intakes from supplement use were not included in the analyses.

4.2. Maternal Biomarkers of Nutrition and Dietary Supplement Use in Pregnant Women with Eating Disorders

Both studies that identified nutritional biomarkers during pregnancy showed an increased risk of maternal iron deficiency anemia (IDA) for women with AN during early pregnancy [15,32]. However, data of the nutritional biomarkers throughout pregnancy was not available, since the determination was performed only in one blood sample in early pregnancy [32]. The etiology of anemia is multifactorial and includes insufficient dietary intake of folate, vitamin B_{12} and A, along with iron, which is the most common nutritional cause [51]. According to previous World Health Organization (WHO) reports, on average, about 50% of all cases of anemia in pregnancy were due to iron deficiency [52]. During pregnancy, there is an increased need for iron, because more iron is required for the fetus, placenta and 20% increased erythrocytes in the expectant mother [1]. Iron deficiency in pregnancy increases the risk of premature birth, low birth weight and irreversible or partially reversible neurobehavioral and cognitive impairments [32,51,53–55]. For instance, Koubaa et al. found that maternal serum levels of ferritin in women with a history of AN correlated strongly with impaired memory function in their children at five years of age [32]. Linna et al. did not relate maternal iron status with newborn outcomes, but they reported that maternal AN was associated with several adverse perinatal outcomes (e.g., slow fetal growth, very premature birth, small for gestational age, low birth weight), which could be mediated by low folate or iron intakes during pregnancy [15]. If an IDA is medically diagnosed, iron supplementation in addition to sufficient intake of iron-rich foods is recommended [1]. Therefore, pregnant women with a history of EDs, and particularly of AN, should be closely monitored in terms of nutrient deficiencies.

To our knowledge, the study by Dellava et al. is the only study to date that examined the dietary supplement intake in pregnant women with EDs compared to control women [26]. Unfortunately, it was not possible to determine if women with EDs consumed more or less micronutrients from dietary supplements than women without EDs, since information of the amount of each item contained in the dietary supplements was not collected [26]. It would also be important to know whether women with EDs were instructed by their gynecologist to take dietary supplements [26]. Over 90% of women with EDs used dietary supplements during pregnancy, with folic acid being the most commonly used supplement. Folic acid supplement use was higher during pregnancy than periconceptional for all women [26]. Numerous epidemiological studies and subsequent meta-analyses have shown that a periconceptional folic acid supplementation of 400 µg (alone or in combination with other micronutrients) can reduce the risk of childhood malformations of the nervous system (neural tube defects) [56,57]. However, in the study by Dellava et al., the increase in folic acid supplementation prior to pregnancy in women with and without EDs was likely too late to prevent birth defects associated with folate deficiency according to the Norwegian recommendations [26]. Therefore, involved specialists should motivate women with EDs to supplement critical nutrients (e.g., folate, iron, iodine). Supplements could easily be accepted by these women, as they are not associated with caloric intake [26]. However, in women with purging behavior, it is questionable as to how many supplemented nutrients might be absorbed at the intestinal absorption site.

4.3. Dysfunctional Eating Behavior in Pregnant Women with EDs

In terms of behavioral aspects of eating, pregnancy is associated with an overall improvement in the severity of dysfunctional eating behavior for most women [20,23,34–38]. Reasons for the improvement in eating behavior may include the relief of a sense of responsibility for body weight and shape and the woman's worries about its harming effects on her unborn child [37]. However, pregnancy might also be a trigger for the deterioration of bingeing and overeating [22,38]. After all, every tenth pregnant woman with a recent ED reports restrictive intake, which is worrisome [34]. Reasons for the intensification of dysfunctional eating behaviors may include increased anxiety over weight gain [38]. Furthermore, physiological changes in the course of pregnancy, such as changes in satiety associated with an altered leptin level, may have important influences on eating behavior [58]. The increased rates of LOC, both in women with and without EDs, might be correlated with general ravenous appetite experienced in pregnancy. Interestingly, in the study by Blais et al., pregnancy outcomes (lower live birth rates, higher therapeutic abortion rates) of women with AN and BN were not associated with the maternal age, or the presence of ED symptoms at conception [20].

Additionally, in the postpartum phase, the improvement seems to decline, and dysfunctional eating behaviors tend to return toward prepregnancy levels [29]. Therefore, pregnant women with eating disorders need enhanced intrapartum *and* postnatal support. From a nutritional point of view, the latter is of great importance regarding (breast)feeding practices in women with EDs. For example, in a study with 20 bulimic women, three mothers reported that they restricted the dietary intake of their children within the first year of life [36].

4.4. Strengths and Limitations

This is the first systematic review that has examined pregnancy nutrition and related issues in women with a history of EDs. The strengths of this review are its methodical procedure according to the PRISMA statement and the focus on nutritional aspects of eating disorders during pregnancy. Thus, this review draws attention to important gaps in the eating disorder research.

Given the fact that the studies eligible for this review were very heterogeneous, a quality rating and meta-analysis could not be performed. The articles were ranging over a time span of 30 years; consequently, consistent diagnostic criteria for EDs were not applied. Another major issue is the inadequate diagnostic identification of EDs through self-report in some of the reviewed studies. Therefore, a reporter bias and misclassification of EDs cannot be ruled out. Furthermore, women who reported an ED might have a milder form of ED, since women who suffer from a severe ED might not participate in research studies or might not report their ED accordingly due to potential feelings of sorrow and guilt. Consequently, the prevalence of women with ED and differences in dietary intake might be underestimated. Moreover, it was not possible to ascertain between active and lifetime ED during pregnancy in some studies, resulting in mixed study samples of reduced comparability. There is a limited generalizability in studies that extracted data from the MoBa study, since differences exist between the study sample and the general population in terms of educational level and multivitamin consumption. From the seven studies investigating dysfunctional eating behavior of pregnant women with EDs, three studies had small sample sizes [23,36,38], two studies relied on retrospective recall [35,37] and, unfortunately, only one study included a control group of women without EDs [34].

5. Conclusions and Future Directions

Based on our four research questions investigated in the present systematic review, our main findings are as follows: (1) considering the drawback that dietary intakes were assessed by self-report, pregnant women with a history of EDs show a similar dietary intake to healthy pregnant women; there is evidence that women with EDs have a sufficient diet quality and are more likely to follow a vegetarian dietary pattern. Women with BED seem to be an exception as they show inadequate energy and fat intakes; (2) the startling caffeine and coffee consumption, especially in pregnant women with AN and AN + BN, and the use of artificially sweetened beverages in pregnant women with active and past BN and BED is of high concern and needs further investigation in relation to fetal outcomes; (3) women with AN were at increased risk of experiencing iron deficiency anemia in pregnancy; anyhow, women with EDs did not differ in overall dietary supplement use compared to healthy women; (4) dysfunctional eating behaviors (bingeing, dieting) improved substantially with pregnancy.

We feel that the issue of EDs in pregnancy is still an understudied field. There is still no consistent answer to the underlying biological mechanisms that might explain the increased risk for adverse perinatal outcomes in women with EDs. As outlined above, most of the current evidence in the field is derived from self-report data, which is prone to biases, e.g., due to influences of social desirability or memory gaps. This highlights the need for method combinations, integrating data from self-report, observational data, and in order to elucidate consequences of nutrition practices for fetal development, ideally also from neuropsychological and neurobiological methods [32,59]. For example, fetal magnetoencephalography (fMEG) is a non-invasive method to study fetal brain activity, which has previously revealed evidence that the maternal metabolism might program the fetal brain [60,61]. However, the first step is the adequate assessment and identification of EDs through medical professionals (general practitioner, gynecologist, or fertility specialist), ideally before pregnancy [62]. Paslakis and de Zwaan [62] recently provided clinical recommendations and specific algorithms for the management of pregnant females with EDs and for females with EDs seeking fertility treatment, underlining the importance of an interdisciplinary approach.

Regarding the research gaps concerning pregnant women with EDs, nutrition quality/food intake (including the adherence to a vegan diet), gestational weight gain, gestational diabetes, and dysfunctional behaviors (including substance misuse) are just a few topics which urgently require further investigation. Especially during pregnancy, women with EDs might be highly motivated to change their behavior in favor of their developing child. Therefore, studies on the treatment of EDs during pregnancy are urgently needed to ensure an optimal development of the fetus and to contribute to the prevention of intergenerational transmission of EDs.

Based on the evidence available, the assessment of maternal nutritional status is complex, but especially needed for vulnerable groups like women with EDs during pregnancy. With the exception of women with BED, food intake seems sufficient during pregnancy and dysfunctional eating habits are improved, which is an encouraging finding. Particularly women with active EDs might need nutritional counselling and close monitoring of nutrient deficits. More research is needed to confirm previous studies and to identify treatment interventions that support lasting improvements in eating behaviors and dietary intake in the postpartum phase.

Author Contributions: K.E.G., N.M. and A.F.D. conceived the review topic and research questions. K.E.G. and A.F.D. developed search terms and eligibility criteria. A.F.D. and S.B.L. screened, reviewed and selected the search results, K.E.G. served as a third reviewer for study inclusion. A.F.D. analyzed the included studies and drafted the manuscript. K.E.G., N.M., H.P. and S.Z. critically revised the manuscript.

Acknowledgments: This work was supported by a grant within the fortüne program from the Medical Faculty Tübingen (Project no. F1292064). We acknowledge support by Deutsche Forschungsgemeinschaft and Open Access Publishing Fund of University of Tübingen.

Conflicts of Interest: The authors declare no conflict of interest.

References

1. Koletzko, B.; Cremer, M.; Flothkötter, M.; Graf, C.; Hauner, H.; Hellmers, C.; Kersting, M.; Krawinkel, M.; Przyrembel, H.; Röbl-Mathieu, M.; et al. Diet and lifestyle before and during pregnancy—Practical recommendations of the germany-wide healthy start—Young family network. *Geburtshilfe Frauenheilkd.* **2018**, *78*, 1262–1282. [CrossRef]

2. Berti, C.; Biesalski, H.K.; Gärtner, R.; Lapillonne, A.; Pietrzik, K.; Poston, L.; Redman, C.; Koletzko, B.; Cetin, I. Micronutrients in pregnancy: Current knowledge and unresolved questions. *Clin. Nutr.* **2011**, *30*, 689–701. [CrossRef]

3. Lucas, A. Long-term programming effects of early nutrition—Implications for the preterm infant. *J. Perinatol.* **2005**, *25*, S2. [CrossRef]

4. Barker, D.J. The fetal and infant origins of adult disease. *BMJ (Clin. Res. Ed.)* **1990**, *301*, 1111. [CrossRef]

5. Hoffman, D.J.; Reynolds, R.M.; Hardy, D.B. Developmental origins of health and disease: Current knowledge and potential mechanisms. *Nutr. Rev.* **2017**, *75*, 951–970. [CrossRef]

6. Barker, D.J.P. The origins of the developmental origins theory. *J. Intern. Med.* **2007**, *261*, 412–417. [CrossRef] [PubMed]

7. Gluckman, P.D.; Hanson, M.A.; Cooper, C.; Thornburg, K.L. Effect of in utero and early-life conditions on adult health and disease. *New Engl. J. Med.* **2008**, *359*, 61–73. [CrossRef]

8. Easter, A.; Bye, A.; Taborelli, E.; Corfield, F.; Schmidt, U.; Treasure, J.; Micali, N. Recognising the symptoms: How common are eating disorders in pregnancy? *Eur. Eat. Disord. Rev.* **2013**, *21*, 340–344. [CrossRef] [PubMed]

9. APA. *Diagnostic and Statistical Manual of Mental Disorders*, 5th ed.; APA: Washington, DC, USA, 2013.

10. Eagles, J.M.; Lee, A.J.; Raja, E.A.; Millar, H.R.; Bhattacharya, S. Pregnancy outcomes of women with and without a history of anorexia nervosa. *Psychol. Med.* **2012**, *42*, 2651–2660. [CrossRef]

11. Koubaa, S.; Hallstrom, T.; Lindholm, C.; Hirschberg, A.L. Pregnancy and neonatal outcomes in women with eating disorders. *Obstet. Gynecol.* **2005**, *105*, 255–260. [CrossRef] [PubMed]

12. Micali, N.; Simonoff, E.; Treasure, J. Risk of major adverse perinatal outcomes in women with eating disorders. *Br. J. Psychiatry* **2007**, *190*, 255–259. [CrossRef]

13. Franko, D.L.; Blais, M.A.; Becker, A.E.; Delinsky, S.S.; Greenwood, D.N.; Flores, A.T.; Ekeblad, E.R.; Eddy, K.T.; Herzog, D.B. Pregnancy complications and neonatal outcomes in women with eating disorders. *Am. J. Psychiatry* **2001**, *158*, 1461–1466. [CrossRef]

14. Solmi, F.; Sallis, H.; Stahl, D.; Treasure, J.; Micali, N. Low birth weight in the offspring of women with anorexia nervosa. *Epidemiol. Rev.* **2014**, *36*, 49–56. [CrossRef]

15. Linna, M.S.; Raevuori, A.; Haukka, J.; Suvisaari, J.M.; Suokas, J.T.; Gissler, M. Pregnancy, obstetric, and perinatal health outcomes in eating disorders. *Am. J. Obstet. Gynecol.* **2014**, *211*, e391–e398. [CrossRef]

16. Bulik, C.M.; Von Holle, A.; Siega-Riz, A.M.; Torgersen, L.; Lie, K.K.; Hamer, R.M.; Berg, C.K.; Sullivan, P.; Reichborn-Kjennerud, T. Birth outcomes in women with eating disorders in the norwegian mother and child cohort study (moba). *Int. J. Eat. Disord.* **2009**, *42*, 9–18. [CrossRef]

17. Koubaa, S.; Hallstrom, T.; Hagenas, L.; Hirschberg, A.L. Retarded head growth and neurocognitive development in infants of mothers with a history of eating disorders: Longitudinal cohort study. *BJOG Int. J. Obstet. Gynaecol.* **2013**, *120*, 1413–1422. [CrossRef]

18. Barona, M.; Taborelli, E.; Corfield, F.; Pawlby, S.; Easter, A.; Schmidt, U.; Treasure, J.; Micali, N. Neurobehavioural and cognitive development in infants born to mothers with eating disorders. *J. Child Psychol. Psychiatry* **2017**, *58*, 931–938. [CrossRef]

19. HO, A.S.L.; SOH, N.L.; WALTER, G.; TOUYZ, S. Comparison of nutrition knowledge among health professionals, patients with eating disorders and the general population. *Nutr. Diet.* **2011**, *68*, 267–272. [CrossRef]

20. Blais, M.A.; Becker, A.E.; Burwell, R.A.; Flores, A.T.; Nussbaum, K.M.; Greenwood, D.N.; Ekeblad, E.R.; Herzog, D.B. Pregnancy: Outcome and impact on symptomatology in a cohort of eating-disordered women. *Int. J. Eat. Disord.* **2000**, *27*, 140–149. [CrossRef]

21. Micali, N.; Treasure, J. Biological effects of a maternal ed on pregnancy and foetal development: A review. *Eur. Eat. Disord. Rev.* **2009**, *17*, 448–454. [CrossRef]

22. Bulik, C.M.; Von Holle, A.; Hamer, R.; Knoph Berg, C.; Torgersen, L.; Magnus, P.; Stoltenberg, C.; Siega-Riz, A.M.; Sullivan, P.; Reichborn-Kjennerud, T. Patterns of remission, continuation and incidence of broadly defined eating disorders during early pregnancy in the norwegian mother and child cohort study (moba). *Psychol. Med.* **2007**, *37*, 1109–1118. [CrossRef]

23. Crow, S.J.; Agras, W.S.; Crosby, R.; Halmi, K.; Mitchell, J.E. Eating disorder symptoms in pregnancy: A prospective study. *Int. J. Eat. Disord.* **2008**, *41*, 277–279. [CrossRef]

24. Moher, D.; Liberati, A.; Tetzlaff, J.; Altman, D.G.; The, P.G. Preferred reporting items for systematic reviews and meta-analyses: The prisma statement. *PLoS Med.* **2009**, *6*, e1000097. [CrossRef]

25. Liberati, A.; Altman, D.G.; Tetzlaff, J.; et al. The prisma statement for reporting systematic reviews and meta-analyses of studies that evaluate health care interventions: Explanation and elaboration. *Ann. Intern. Med.* **2009**, *151*, W-65–W-94. [CrossRef]

26. NEDA. PICA. Available online: https://www.nationaleatingdisorders.org/learn/by-eating-disorder/other/pica (accessed on 8 January 2019).

27. Procter, S.B.; Campbell, C.G. Position of the academy of nutrition and dietetics: Nutrition and lifestyle for a healthy pregnancy outcome. *J. Acad. Nutr. Diet.* **2014**, *114*, 1099–1103. [CrossRef]

28. Maternal and Child Nutrition. Public Health Guideline [ph11]. Available online: https://www.nice.org.uk/guidance/qs98/resources/maternal-and-child-nutrition-pdf-2098975759045 (accessed on 8 January 2019).

29. Micali, N.; Northstone, K.; Emmett, P.; Naumann, U.; Treasure, J.L. Nutritional intake and dietary patterns in pregnancy: A longitudinal study of women with lifetime eating disorders. *Br. J. Nutr.* **2012**, *108*, 2093–2099. [CrossRef]

30. Siega-Riz, A.M.; Haugen, M.; Meltzer, H.M.; Von Holle, A.; Hamer, R.; Torgersen, L.; Knopf-Berg, C.; Reichborn-Kjennerud, T.; Bulik, C.M. Nutrient and food group intakes of women with and without bulimia nervosa and binge eating disorder during pregnancy. *Am. J. Clin. Nutr.* **2008**, *87*, 1346–1355. [CrossRef]

31. Nguyen, A.N.; de Barse, L.M.; Tiemeier, H.; Jaddoe, V.W.V.; Franco, O.H.; Jansen, P.W.; Voortman, T. Maternal history of eating disorders: Diet quality during pregnancy and infant feeding. *Appetite* **2017**, *109*, 108–114. [CrossRef]

32. Koubaa, S.; Hallstrom, T.; Brismar, K.; Hellstrom, P.M.; Hirschberg, A.L. Biomarkers of nutrition and stress in pregnant women with a history of eating disorders in relation to head circumference and neurocognitive function of the offspring. *BMC Pregnancy Childbirth* **2015**, *15*, 318. [CrossRef]

33. Dellava, J.E.; Von Holle, A.; Torgersen, L.; Reichborn-Kjennerud, T.; Haugen, M.; Meltzer, H.M.; Bulik, C.M. Dietary supplement use immediately before and during pregnancy in norwegian women with eating disorders. *Int. J. Eat. Disord.* **2011**, *44*, 325–332. [CrossRef]

34. Micali, N.; Treasure, J.; Simonoff, E. Eating disorders symptoms in pregnancy: A longitudinal study of women with recent and past eating disorders and obesity. *J. Psychosom. Res.* **2007**, *63*, 297–303. [CrossRef]

35. Crow, S.J.; Keel, P.K.; Thuras, P.; Mitchell, J.E. Bulimia symptoms and other risk behaviors during pregnancy in women with bulimia nervosa. *Int. J. Eat. Disord.* **2004**, *36*, 220–223. [CrossRef]

36. Lacey, J.H.; Smith, G. Bulimia nervosa: The impact of pregnancy on mother and baby. *Br. J. Psychiatry* **1987**, *150*, 777–781. [CrossRef]

37. Morgan, J.F.; Lacey, J.H.; Sedgwick, P.M. Impact of pregnancy on bulimia nervosa. *Br. J. Psychiatry* **1999**, *174*, 135–140. [CrossRef]

38. Lemberg, R.; Phillips, J. The impact of pregnancy on anorexia nervosa and bulimia. *Int. J. Eat. Disord.* **1989**, *8*, 285–295. [CrossRef]

39. Rodrigo, C.P.; Aranceta, J.; Salvador, G.; Varela-Moreiras, G. Food frequency questionnaires. *Nutr. Hosp.* **2015**, *31*, 49–56.

40. Pinto, E.; Severo, M.; Correia, S.; Dos Santos Silva, I.; Lopes, C.; Barros, H. Validity and reproducibility of a semi-quantitative food frequency questionnaire for use among portuguese pregnant women. *Matern. Child Nutr.* **2010**, *6*, 105–119. [CrossRef]

41. Brantsæter, A.L.; Haugen, M.; Alexander, J.; Meltzer, H.M. Validity of a new food frequency questionnaire for pregnant women in the norwegian mother and child cohort study (moba). *Matern. Child Nutr.* **2008**, *4*, 28–43. [CrossRef]

42. McGowan, C.A.; Curran, S.; McAuliffe, F.M. Relative validity of a food frequency questionnaire to assess nutrient intake in pregnant women. *J. Hum. Nutr. Diet.* **2014**, *27*, 167–174. [CrossRef]

43. Bernardo, W.; Simões, R.; Buzzini, R.; Nunes, V.; Glina, F. Adverse effects of the consumption of artificial sweeteners—Systematic review. *Rev. Da Assoc. Médica Bras.* **2016**, *62*, 120–122. [CrossRef]

44. Li, J.; Zhao, H.; Song, J.-M.; Zhang, J.; Tang, Y.-L.; Xin, C.-M. A meta-analysis of risk of pregnancy loss and caffeine and coffee consumption during pregnancy. *Int. J. Gynecol. Obstet.* **2015**, *130*, 116–122. [CrossRef] [PubMed]

45. Chen, L.-W.; Wu, Y.; Neelakantan, N.; Chong, M.F.-F.; Pan, A.; van Dam, R.M. Maternal caffeine intake during pregnancy and risk of pregnancy loss: A categorical and dose–response meta-analysis of prospective studies. *Public Health Nutr.* **2016**, *19*, 1233–1244. [CrossRef]

46. Jahanfar, S.; Jaafar, S.H. Effects of restricted caffeine intake by mother on fetal, neonatal and pregnancy outcomes. *Cochrane Database Syst. Rev.* **2015**. [CrossRef]

47. Hart, S.; Abraham, S.; Franklin, R.C.; Russell, J. The reasons why eating disorder patients drink. *Eur. Eat. Disord. Rev.* **2011**, *19*, 121–128. [CrossRef]

48. Cano-Marquina, A.; Tarín, J.J.; Cano, A. The impact of coffee on health. *Maturitas* **2013**, *75*, 7–21. [CrossRef] [PubMed]

49. EFSA NDA Panel (EFSA Panel on Dietetic Products, Nutrition and Allergies). Scientific opinion on the safety of caffeine. *EFSA J.* **2015**, *13*, 4102.

50. ACOG. Committee opinion no. 462: Moderate caffeine consumption during pregnancy. *Obstet. Gynecol.* **2010**, *116*, 467–468. [CrossRef] [PubMed]

51. Scholl, T.O. Maternal iron status: Relation to fetal growth, length of gestation, and iron endowment of the neonate. *Nutr. Rev.* **2011**, *69*, S23–S29. [CrossRef]

52. McLean, E.; Cogswell, M.; Egli, I.; Wojdyla, D.; de Benoist, B. Worldwide prevalence of anaemia, who vitamin and mineral nutrition information system, 1993–2005. *Public Health Nutr.* **2009**, *12*, 444–454. [CrossRef]

53. Milman, N. Oral iron prophylaxis in pregnancy: Not too little and not too much! *J. Pregnancy* **2012**, *2012*, 8. [CrossRef]

54. Menon, K.C.; Ferguson, E.L.; Thomson, C.D.; Gray, A.R.; Zodpey, S.; Saraf, A.; Das, P.K.; Skeaff, S.A. Effects of anemia at different stages of gestation on infant outcomes. *Nutrition* **2016**, *32*, 61–65. [CrossRef]

55. Scholl, T.O.; Hediger, M.L.; Fischer, R.L.; Shearer, J.W. Anemia vs iron deficiency: Increased risk of preterm delivery in a prospective study. *Am. J. Clin. Nutr.* **1992**, *55*, 985–988. [CrossRef]

56. De-Regil, L.M.; Peña-Rosas, J.P.; Fernández-Gaxiola, A.C.; Rayco-Solon, P. Effects and safety of periconceptional oral folate supplementation for preventing birth defects. *Cochrane Database Syst. Rev.* **2015**, *12*, 1–254. [CrossRef] [PubMed]

57. U.S. Preventive Services Task Force. Folic acid supplementation for the prevention of neural tube defects: Us preventive services task force recommendation statement. *JAMA* **2017**, *317*, 183–189. [CrossRef] [PubMed]

58. Henson, M.C.; Castracane, V.D. Leptin in pregnancy: An update1. *Biol. Reprod.* **2006**, *74*, 218–229. [CrossRef]

59. Easter, A.; Taborelli, E.; Bye, A.; Zunszain, P.A.; Pariante, C.M.; Treasure, J.; Schmidt, U.; Micali, N. Perinatal hypothalamic-pituitary-adrenal axis regulation among women with eating disorders and their infants. *Psychoneuroendocrinology* **2017**, *76*, 127–134. [CrossRef] [PubMed]

60. Schleger, F.; Linder, K.; Walter, L.; Heni, M.; Brändle, J.; Brucker, S.; Pauluschke-Fröhlich, J.; Weiss, M.; Häring, H.-U.; Preissl, H.; et al. Family history of diabetes is associated with delayed fetal postprandial brain activity. *Front. Endocrinol.* **2018**, *9*, 673. [CrossRef]

61. Fehlert, E.; Willmann, K.; Fritsche, L.; Linder, K.; Mat-Husin, H.; Schleger, F.; Weiss, M.; Kiefer-Schmidt, I.; Brucker, S.; Häring, H.-U.; et al. Gestational diabetes alters the fetal heart rate variability during an oral glucose tolerance test: A fetal magnetocardiography study. *BJOG Int. J. Obstet. Gynaecol.* **2017**, *124*, 1891–1898. [CrossRef]

62. Paslakis, G.; de Zwaan, M. Clinical management of females seeking fertility treatment and of pregnant females with eating disorders. *Eur. Eat. Disord. Rev.* **2019**, 1–9. [CrossRef]

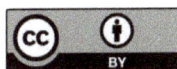

![nutrients logo] *nutrients*

MDPI

Article

Can a Simple Dietary Screening in Early Pregnancy Identify Dietary Habits Associated with Gestational Diabetes?

Laufey Hrolfsdottir [1,2,*], Ingibjorg Gunnarsdottir [1], Bryndis Eva Birgisdottir [1], Ingibjorg Th Hreidarsdottir [3], Alexander Kr. Smarason [2], Hildur Hardardottir [3,4] and Thorhallur I. Halldorsson [1,5]

[1] Unit for Nutrition Research, Landspitali University Hospital and Faculty of Food Science and Nutrition, University of Iceland, Eiríksgata 29 101 Reykjavik, Iceland
[2] Institution of Health Science Research, University of Akureyri and Akureyri Hospital, Eyrarlandsvegi, 600 Akureyri, Iceland
[3] Department of Obstetrics and Gynecology, Landspitali University Hospital, Hringbraut, 101 Reykjavík, Iceland
[4] Faculty of Medicine, University of Iceland, Vatnsmýrarvegi 16, 101 Reykjavík, Iceland
[5] Centre for Fetal Programming, Department of Epidemiology Research, Statens Serum Institut, Artillerivej 5, 2300 Copenhagen, Denmark
* Correspondence: laufeyh@sak.is; Tel.: +354-69599898

Received: 11 July 2019; Accepted: 9 August 2019; Published: 11 August 2019

Abstract: Gestational diabetes mellitus (GDM) is predominantly a lifestyle disease, with diet being an important modifiable risk factor. A major obstacle for the prevention in clinical practice is the complexity of assessing diet. In a cohort of 1651 Icelandic women, this study examined whether a short 40-item dietary screening questionnaire administered in the 1st trimester could identify dietary habits associated with GDM. The dietary variables were aggregated into predefined binary factors reflecting inadequate or optimal intake and stepwise backward elimination was used to identify a reduced set of factors that best predicted GDM. Those binary factors were then aggregated into a risk score (range: 0–7), that was mostly characterised by frequent consumption of soft drinks, sweets, cookies, ice creams and processed meat. The women with poor dietary habits (score ≥ 5, n = 302), had a higher risk of GDM (RR = 1.38; 95%CI = 3, 85) compared with women with a more optimal diet (score ≤ 2, n = 407). In parallel, a pilot (n = 100) intervention was conducted among overweight and obese women examining the effect of internet-based personalized feedback on diet quality. Simple feedback was given in accordance with the answers provided in the screening questionnaire in 1st trimester. At the endpoint, the improvements in diet quality were observed by, as an example, soft drink consumption being reduced by ~1 L/week on average in the intervention group compared to the controls. Our results suggest that a simple dietary screening tool administered in the 1st trimester could identify dietary habits associated with GMD. This tool should be easy to use in a clinical setting, and with simple individualized feedback, improvements in diet may be achieved.

Keywords: dietary habits; maternal nutrition; gestational diabetes; food frequency questionnaire; dietary screening

---

1. Introduction

Gestational diabetes mellitus (GDM) is a major pregnancy complication, defined as glucose intolerance with onset during pregnancy. The prevalence of GDM in European countries ranges from 2 to 22% with a median of 6% [1]. GDM has been associated with several adverse outcomes [2], including offspring macrosomia [3] and the mothers' increased risk of the development of type 2 diabetes postpartum [4]. Longitudinal studies also suggest that offspring of mothers diagnosed with GDM are more prone to metabolic abnormalities later in life [5].

High pre-pregnancy BMI is one of the strongest risk factors for GDM and it is commonly used to identify pregnant women at risk for further monitoring [6]. The use of BMI to identify women at GDM risk does, however, have its limitations as high BMI alone is by no means an indicator for unhealthy dietary habits or a lifestyle that may influence GDM risk. Improvements in weight are also difficult to achieve in the short term and during pregnancy, other modifiable risk factors, such as diet, must be prioritised.

Recent observational studies indicate that unhealthy dietary habits before [7,8] and during pregnancy [9–12] are associated with a higher risk of GDM. Despite the observational nature, the link between poor carbohydrate and fat quality observed in these studies is both biologically plausible and in line with the established risk factors for type 2 diabetes [13]. However, an important limitation for targeting dietary habits of pregnant women is that the dietary assessment methods, developed for research purposes, are time-consuming and difficult to use in maternal care [14]. The complexity of diet is also challenging in terms of focusing efforts. To bypass this challenge, previous intervention studies have often focused on adherence to relatively strict dietary regimes aimed at achieving major changes [15–17]. These strategies have generally resulted in limited compliance and unclear benefits, highlighting the need to explore more targeted and flexible approaches.

The aim of this study was to examine if a short dietary screening questionnaire administered in weeks 11–14 of gestation could be used to identify unhealthy dietary habits associated with GMD and, in parallel, to investigate if a simple personalized web-based feedback tool could result in improvement in dietary habits in pregnancy.

2. Materials and Methods

This study was based on two studies of different designs that recruited pregnant women in Iceland from 2015 to 2017. In a cohort setting, this study examined, in a set of 1651 women, the association between dietary habits recorded in early pregnancy and the risk of GDM. In parallel, a pilot ($n = 100$) intervention study was conducted to test to what extent dietary changes could be achieved in the study population. In terms of the prevention and use in a clinical setting, an association between dietary habits and pregnancy complications such as GDM is limited on its own, unless there are indications that changes in those dietary factors can be modified using low intensity and cost-effective measures. This is the logic behind conducting these studies and to combine them in one paper.

2.1. The Cohort Study

The PREWICE cohort (PREgnant Women of ICEland) has been described elsewhere [18]. All women ($n = 2734$) with singleton pregnancies who attended a routine early ultrasound (11–14 week of gestation) at the prenatal diagnostic unit at Landspitali University Hospital in Reykjavik, South Iceland between 1 October, 2015 to 31 September, 2016, were invited to take part in the study. In total, 2113 women, (~50% of all births in Iceland during the study period) agreed to participate, whereof 417 (~20%) had missing hospital records, most likely as they gave birth outside Landspitali University Hospital. The additional 26 women who had multiple births and another 19 who had missing dietary data were excluded, resulting in 1651 women being eligible for analyses. No major differences were found in the baseline characteristics or dietary measures among those who were included in the full analysis and those who were excluded because of missing data [18].

2.1.1. The Outcome Variable

The information regarding GDM cases was retrieved from maternal hospital records (ICD-10 codes O24.4 and O24.9, but O24.9 is used at Landspitali GDM treated with medications). The criteria for GDM diagnoses was according to the 2010 International Association of Diabetes and Pregnancy Study Groups (IADPSG) Consensus Panel [6].

2.1.2. The Dietary Assessment and the Dietary Risk Score

The details about the dietary assessment and construction of the dietary risk score have been described in detail elsewhere [18]. In short, the dietary screening questionnaire consisted of a 40-item list of common foods and food groups for which the frequency of consumption was recorded (see Supplemental File S1). The list was designed to give a rough overview of the participant's general diet in comparison to current food-based dietary guidelines. The dietary data collected was converted to frequency per week for all food groups, which was then transformed into 13 predefined dietary risk factors for inadequate diet (Figure 1). The 13 factors used to construct the risk score are based on the Nordic [19] and Icelandic dietary recommendations [20] and supported by evidence from studies conducted in pregnant women [21–25].

Risk factors for inadequate diet	
1. Not eating a varied diet	8. Sugar and artificially sweetened beverages ≥5 times/week
2. Vegetables and fruits<5 times/day	9. Sweets, ice cream, cakes, cookies ≥2.5 times/week
3. Fish intake <2 times/week	10. French fries and fried potatoes ≥1 time/week
4. Dairy intake <2 times/day	11. High dairy intake ≥5 times/day
5. Wholegrain products <2 times/day	12. Processed meat products ≥1 time/week
6. Beans, nuts, seeds <3.5 times/week	13. Quality of fat - using butter (or other unsaturated fat sources) rather than oil (≥50%)
7. Vitamin-D <5 times/week	

Figure 1. The predefined dietary risk factors for inadequate diet. The risk factors were mainly based on the Nordic Nutrition Recommendations [19] and the Icelandic Food-Based Dietary Recommendations [20]. If the women excluded/avoided any of the main food groups (cereal, vegetables/fruits, fish, meat, eggs, high-fat foods or dairy), they were categorized to the group of not eating a varied diet.

Using these 13 predefined dietary risk factors as inputs, a stepwise backward elimination was used to identify a reduced set of variables with the highest maximum likelihood that best predicted GDM. The model performance was assessed by Nagelkerke's R^2. The following set of seven dietary risk factors (predictors) were included in the final model: Non-varied diet; sugar/artificially sweetened beverages ≥5 times/week; sweets, ice cream, cakes, cookies ≥2.5 times/week; processed meat products ≥1 time/week; whole grain products <2 times/day; dairy <2 times/day and vitamin D intake <5 times/week. The set of seven variables was then used to calculate a combined dietary risk score. Each participant got 1 score for fulfilling the risk criteria, and 0 for not fulfilling the risk criteria. The scores of the dietary risk factors were then summed up, ranging from 0 to 7.

To verify the the stability of our findings in terms of variable selection, comparable risk scores were created based on either a fewer or a larger number of dietary factors being retained in the model. The associations between these different scores in relation to GDM risk are shown in Table A1 (Appendix A).

2.2. The Pilot Intervention Study

For the pilot intervention study, 100 women with pre-pregnancy body mass ≥25 kg/m^2, attending prenatal care at the Health Care Institution of North Iceland were recruited. At recruitment, i.e., at the first antenatal care visit, the women answered the same dietary questionnaire as described above for the cohort study. The participants were then randomized into a control group receiving the habitual care of brochures on the recommended diet during pregnancy according to clinical guidelines (n = 50; 9 dropouts), and an intervention group (n = 50; 3 dropouts), receiving personalized feedback on their diet quality through an interactive website [26]. This website was designed to give each woman simple personalized feedback, aimed at improving diet quality, in accordance with the answers provided by the dietary questionnaire. At baseline, a nutritionist showed the participants in the intervention group the website and went through the personalized feedback with them. Dietary intake in gestation weeks 24–26 and 35–38 was assessed by two 24-h recalls. These recalls were performed by another nutritionist who was blinded to the intervention assignment.

2.3. Statistical Analyses

The students t-tests were used to compare the normally distributed continuous variables, whereas, for skewed and categorical variables, the Mann-Whitney U test and Chi-square tests were used, respectively.

For the cohort study, the associations between the diet reported at baseline and GDM was assessed using multivariable Poisson log-linear regression. The covariates included in the adjusted models were selected, a priori, based on their potential influence on dietary habits and GDM [27–31]. The covariates included in the regression analyses were: Maternal pre-pregnancy BMI (<25, 25–29.99, ≥30 kg/m^2); maternal age (quartiles); parity (nulliparous versus primi/multiparous); education (elementary schooling, high school and/or technical school, university education, and higher academic education); maternal smoking during pregnancy (yes/no) and family history of type 2 diabetes. The information on these covariates was recorded at recruitment with the exception of maternal age and family history of type 2 diabetes, which was retrieved from hospital records. The missing values for covariates (maternal pre-pregnancy BMI (0.7%), parity (1.2%), educational level (0.9%), and maternal smoking during pregnancy (1.5%) were assumed to be missing at random and were imputed using multiple imputations as implemented in *proc MI* in SAS v9.2 8. Statistical significance was accepted at $p < 0.05$.

2.4. Ethics

The ethics committee of Landspitali University Hospital approved the study protocol (21/2015) for the cohort study. For the intervention study, ethical approval was received from The National Bioethics committee (VSN-15-111-S1). Written consent was obtained from all participants in both studies.

3. Results

The characteristics of the PREWICE cohort are presented in Table 1. The mean age was 30 years, and most (94%) participants were non-smokers, 39% were nulliparous and 58% of the women had a university education or higher academic degree. In total, 16% (n = 265) were diagnosed with GDM during pregnancy. Stratified by pre-pregnancy weight, the prevalence of GDM among women of normal weight (BMI < 25 kg/m^2), overweight (BMI 25–29.99 kg/m^2) or obesity (BMI ≥ 30 kg/m^2) was 5%, 15% and 49%, respectively. The mothers who developed GDM were also more likely to be older, Primi/multiparous and have a lower educational level (Table 1).

Table 1. Birth outcomes and characteristics of mothers at baseline in relation to gestational diabetes mellitus diagnoses.

	All [a] (n = 1651)	GDM [a,b] (16%)	No GDM [a] (84%)	p Value [c]
Maternal age (year)	30.3 ± 5.2	31.8 ± 5.4	30.0 ± 5.1	<0.01 [d]
Height (cm)	167.5 ± 6.1	166.5 ± 6.3	167.7 ± 6.1	<0.01 [d]
Birth weight (g)	3670 ± 552	3686 ± 587	3667± 545	0.64 [d]
Gestational age (weeks)	40.0 (1.0)	39.0 ± 2.0	40.0 ± 2.0	<0.01 [e]
Pre-pregnancy weight (kg)	68.0 (20.0)	85.0 (19.5)	66.0 (16.0)	<0.01 [e]
Pre-pregnancy BMI (kg/m^2)	24.2 (6.7)	30.5 (7.6)	23.5 (5.3)	<0.01 [e]
Pre-pregnancy BMI (groups)				<0.01 [f]
<18.5 kg/m^2 (%)	3	1	4	
18.5–24.99 kg/m^2 (%)	54	17	61	
25–29.99 kg/m^2 (%)	24	24	23	
≥30 kg/m^2 (%)	19	59	11	
Exc. GWG (%)	36	33	36	0.38 [f]
Parity (%)				<0.01 [f]
Nulliparous	39	31	41	
Primi/multiparous	61	69	59	
Single (%)	6	7	5	0.34 [f]
Smoking during pregnancy (%)	6	7	6	0.74 [f]
Family history of type 2 diabetes (%)	18	15	39	<0.01 [f]
Education (%)				<0.01 [f]
Elementary schooling	13	18	12	
High sch. and technical sch.	30	32	29	
University education	34	37	34	
Higher academic	24	14	26	

Abbreviations: BMI, body mass index; GDM, gestational diabetes mellitus; GWG, gestational weight gain. [a] Values are mean ± standard deviation or median (IQR) for continuous variables and percentages for categorical variables; [b] The criteria that was used [6] [c] Differences between GDM and no GDM. [d] F-test (Type III) of differences among groups. [e] Mann-Whitney U test of differences among groups. [f] Chi-square test of differences among groups.

The number of women who fulfilled the risk criteria for each of the identified dietary risk factors is shown in Table 2. In total, 21% reported that they had a nonvaried diet, i.e., that they avoided or excluded some food groups. In total, 28% frequently consumed sugar and artificially sweetened beverages (≥5 times/week), 59% had a frequent intake of sweets, ice creams, cakes and cookies (≥2.5 times/week), and 31% ate processed meat products weekly (≥1 time/week). Most women did neither meet the public recommendations for whole grain intake of at least two portions per day (91%) nor the two recommended dairy portions per day (78%), and 30% of the women reported intake of vitamin D supplements less than <5 times per week. A higher proportion of women with GDM fulfilled the risk criteria for the consumption of sugar and artificially sweetened beverages ($p \leq 0.01$) and processed meat products ($p = 0.04$) compared with women with no GDM. The other dietary risk factors did not differ significantly (Table 2).

Table 2. Percent of women fulfilling the predefined risk criteria.

Risk factors	All (n = 1651)	GDM [a] (16%)	No GDM (84%)	p [b]
Not eating a varied diet	21%	23%	21%	0.43
Sugar and artificially sweetened beverages ≥5 times/week	28%	37%	27%	<0.01
Sweet, ice cream, cakes, cookies ≥2.5 times/week	59%	63%	58%	0.14
Processed meat products ≥1 time/week	31%	37%	30%	0.04
Whole grain products <2 times/day	91%	93%	91%	0.26
Dairy <2 times/day	78%	81%	77%	0.18
Vitamin D intake <5 times/week	30%	34%	29%	0.12

[a] The criteria that was used [6]. [b] Chi-square test of differences among groups (GDM vs. no GDM).

In Table 3, the results for the multivariable association between the dietary risk score and GDM are presented. When dichotomizing the exposure, women with a high (≥5, $n = 302$) versus low (≤2, $n = 407$) dietary risk scores had 38% higher relative risk (RR) (95%CI: 3, 85%) of being diagnosed with GDM. The effect modification by pre-pregnancy BMI was formally tested. This was done by including the dietary risk score (continuous variable), BMI (continuous variable) and an interaction term between the two in the logistic regression model, along with the remaining covariates. An interaction was not observed ($p = 0.81$). In accordance to these results, similar results were found when comparing those with a high versus low dietary risk score among women with BMI < 25 (RR = 1.11 95%CI: 0.90, 1.36) vs. BMI ≥ 25 (RR = 1.09 95%CI: 1.002, 1.19).

Table 3. The association between the dietary risk score and gestational diabetes [a].

	Cases (%)/n	RR (95% CI) [b]	
		Crude	Adjusted [c]
Dichotomized score			
≤2 scores	49 (12%)/407	ref	ref
3 scores	76 (15%)/503	1.26 (0.90, 1.75)	0.96 (0.72, 1.30)
4 scores	69 (16%)/439	1.31 (0.93, 1.83)	1.00 (0.74, 1.37)
≥5 scores	71 (24%)/302	1.95 (1.40, 2.72)	1.38 (1.03, 1.85)
p for trend		<0.01	0.02
Stratified analyses, continuous score			
All women	265 (16%)/1651	1.20 (1.10, 1.32)	1.10 (1.02, 1.20)
BMI < 25 kg/m² [d]	51 (5%)/947	1.20 (0.96, 1.52)	1.11 (0.90, 1.36)
BMI ≥ 25 kg/m² [d]	214 (30%)/704	1.12 (1.02, 1.23)	1.09 (1.002, 1.19)

Abbreviations: BMI, body mass index; [a] The criteria that was used [6]. [b] Logistic regression model reflecting the odds of GDM. [c] Adjusted for maternal pre-pregnancy BMI, age, parity, smoking during pregnancy, educational level and family history of type 2 diabetes. [d] Pre-pregnancy BMI not included as a covariate.

Table 4. Baseline characteristics and dietary habits at the endpoint among pregnant women participating in the pilot intervention.

	Control ($n = 41$) [a]	Intervention ($n = 47$) [a]	p-Value [b]
Baseline Characteristics			
Pre-pregnancy BMI (kg/m²)	28.7 (27.1–31.5)	29.4 (27.5–35.2)	0.40
Gestational length at baseline (weeks)	15.0 ± 2.5	14.8 ± 2.7	0.83
Age			0.27
18–24, n (%)	10 (24)	10 (21)	
25–34, n (%)	28 (68)	28 (60)	
≥35, n (%)	3 (7)	9 (19)	
Parity			0.27
Nulliparous, n (%)	13 (32)	10 (21)	
Primi/multiparous, n (%)	28 (68)	37 (79)	
Smoking during pregnancy, n (%)	5 (12)	5 (11)	0.82
Dietary habits at endpoint [c]			
Milk and cultured milk products (g/d)	217 (138–396)	247 (102–376)	0.91
Vegetables (g/d)	91 (23–148)	101 (57–135)	0.18
Fruits and berries (g/d)	105 (73–220)	150 (70–215)	0.67
Fish ≥300g/week (%)	22%	32%	0.30
Processed meat (g/d)	14 (0–42)	10 (0–25)	0.69
Soft drinks (g/d)	125 (25–365)	75 (0–200)	0.03
French fries or chips ≥100g/week (%)	27%	19%	0.38
Cakes, biscuits, and/or sweets (g/d)	62 (19–114)	37 (18–88)	0.25

[a] Values are mean ± standard deviation or median (25th–75th centiles) for continuous variables and percentages for categorical variables. [b] F test (Type III) or Mann-Whitney U test was used to assess differences among groups for continuous variables and Chi-square test for categorical variables. [c] Mean of two 24 h recalls in gestational weeks 24–26. and 35–38.

In the pilot study, neither differences in the background variables (Table 4) nor dietary intake at baseline (Table A2) were observed. In total, 88 women completed both 24 h recalls (47 in the intervention group and 41 in the control group). Table 4 shows the median intake of selected food groups based on the two 24 h recalls. At the endpoint, soft drink consumption was significantly lower in the intervention group compared with the control group, corresponding to approximately one liter less consumption per week. Other differences in dietary intake between the groups were not statistically significant.

4. Discussion

This study found that a dietary risk score, partly characterized by frequent consumption of sugar/artificially sweetened beverages, sweets, cookies, ice creams and processed meat products, was associated with GDM diagnoses. The most pronounced differences in dietary habits of GDM versus non-GDM cases, as recorded at baseline, was excessive (≥5 times/week) consumption of soft drinks. The pilot intervention study, conducted in parallel, showed that internet-based personalized feedback on diet, reported early in pregnancy, could substantially reduce soft drink consumption. Whether such reduction can reduce GDM risks needs to be explored further in an intervention setting.

The results of this study are in line with previous studies using more detailed dietary assessment methods. For example, a recent Icelandic study showed that women who were overweight or obese but had a healthy diet were not at higher risk of gestational diabetes in comparison to women with normal weight [9]. Moreover, unhealthy dietary patterns, soft drinks and the intake of foods high in added sugar have previously been linked to a higher risk of GDM [10–12,32,33]. The regular intake of processed meat products has also commonly been associated with a higher risk of Type 2 diabetes [34,35] and GDM [8,12] and there are some indications that poor vitamin D status, commonly observed at Northern latitudes, may also be important for glucose homeostasis [36].

The Finnish Gestational Diabetes Prevention Study (RADIEL) [37] succeeded in reducing the overall incidence of GDM. However, here the focus was on obese women (and women with previous history of gestational diabetes) without taking into account the baseline dietary habits. Although high pre-pregnancy BMI status is a strong risk factor for GDM, not all overweight or obese women develop GDM [28] and as a substantial proportion of the general population is overweight and obese [38] more precise cost-effective risk assessment is needed.

Apart from GDM, a healthy diet in pregnancy has also been associated with a decreased risk for several other pregnancy and birth outcomes [23,24,39–45]. However, the translation and implementation of these results into clinical practice is still a challenge. One reason for this is that dietary assessment tools used in research settings are very time-consuming and not suitable for use in maternal care. The motivation for the studies reported here was to develop and test a diet screening questionnaire to be used in combination with a web-based platform that automatically gives users feedback on their diet during pregnancy [26]. This application is currently being tested for integration into the National Citizen Health Portal in Iceland. The portal is a centralized web-application where all citizens have secure, digital access to their own health information (e.g., maternal records) and official eHealth services currently available in the country. The inclusion of dietary screening into the portal may increase the feasibility of implementing dietary screening in early pregnancy on a national level and for use in clinical practice. To the authors' best knowledge, information on dietary intake (other than supplement use) is not recorded anywhere in national prenatal health registries, but valid information about diet quality in early pregnancy might change the way women in need for dietary support during pregnancy are defined.

The main strengths of our cohort study include prospective data collection, high participation rates (77%), and information on GDM retrieved from medical records. However, as with all observational studies, the role of confounding cannot be excluded. It is important to note that the methodology used in our cohort study is based on both predefined and data-driven methods, tested in Iceland. The observed association with GDM might therefore not apply directly to other populations. However, this approach, i.e., to use a short FFQ (that takes into consideration population's dietary habits) and to identify the potential risk factors based on existing recommendations, can be used in other settings to generate comparable (but perhaps not identical) results valuable for use in clinical practice. Using the same methodology as used in the present study, the authors have previously identified a dietary risk score that predicts the risk of excessive gestational weight gain and giving birth to a child weighing >4500 g (defined as macrosomia) independent of other known risk factors [18]. These findings need to be tested further in well-powered intervention settings. The short dietary screening questionnaire has been validated against 4-day weighed food records in a pilot study among 25 pregnant women (Spearman's correlation >+0.3). The validation against biochemical analysis is part of an ongoing project (PREWICE II). Its ability to rank subjects according to consumption will be assessed, as well as its ability to detect the risk of predefined nutrient deficiency.

The pilot study had several limitations including a few participants. Moreover, the intervention consisted only of one contact with the participants at baseline. More frequent conversations about the results of the diet screening might have resulted in a greater difference between the groups [43,44]. However, the strength of this approach was its simplicity. This study showed that a simple intervention can result in dietary changes, i.e., lower soft drink consumption, in a population where excessive soft drink intake (≥5 times/week) was relatively common (~28%). While there was a trend towards improvement for other factors, no significant differences were observed. However, in the context of the result from the cohort study, these results are important as the most pronounced difference in the diet between GDM and non GDM cases was excessive consumption of soft drink (see Table 2). Previous intervention studies aimed at encouraging lifestyle changes to reduce the risk of GDM have often selected participants and tested interventions [46] regardless of the participants baseline diet and other lifestyle habits. The results from our studies here and recent work [47] suggest that a sensible way forward would be to select participants based on their baseline diet or other lifestyle factors that can be improved. Prioritizing and identifying a few factors to focus on might also be more attainable for women and more practicable in the clinical setting.

In summary, our results showed that a simple dietary screening tool administered in the 1st trimester could be used to identify dietary habits associated with GMD. This approach could be used to identify women in more need of support and diet counselling. Moreover, the results from the pilot intervention indicate that improvements in dietary quality can be achieved using low intensity and cost-effective measures. This procedure might strengthen preventative measures and enable targeted intervention among individuals most likely to benefit.

Supplementary Materials: The following are available online at http://www.mdpi.com/2072-6643/11/8/1868/s1, File S1: The dietary screening questionnaire (English translation).

Author Contributions: Conceptualization, I.G., L.H. and T.I.H.; data curation, L.H., I.G. and T.I.H. formal analysis, L.H. and T.I.H.; funding acquisition, I.G., T.I.H. and L.H.; investigation, L.H., I.G., B.E.B., I.T.H., A.K.S., H.H. and T.I.H.; methodology, I.G., L.H. and T.I.H.; project administration, I.G.; resources, I.G., H.H., I.T.H. and T.I.H.; supervision, I.G. and L.H.; visualization, I.G., L.H. and T.I.H.; writing—original draft, L.H. and T.I.H.; writing—review and editing, L.H., I.G., B.E.B., I.T.H., A.K.S., H.H. and T.I.H.

Funding: This research was funded by the Doctoral Grants of the University of Iceland Research Fund, The Technology Development Fund, The Icelandic Centre for Research (RANNIS) and the University of Iceland Research Fund.

Acknowledgments: We are particularly grateful to the women who participated in the studies. We would also like to acknowledge the work of the PREWICE staff and the great staff at the Ultrasound Department at Landspitali National University Hospital and the Health Care Institution of North Iceland who made the study possible.

Conflicts of Interest: IG is the owner of a nonprofit company behind the website www.nmb.is that includes the questionnaire used in the present study. The website is run as a non for profit NGO. LH, BEB, ITH, AS, HH and TIH have no conflicts of interest to declare. The funders had no role in the design of the study; in the collection, analyses, or interpretation of data; in the writing of the manuscript, or in the decision to publish the results.

Appendix A

As the use of backward elimination for selecting factors that predict gestational diabetes involves some arbitrary decisions in terms of where to stop the elimination process, we examined the stability of our findings by creating standardized risk scores based on fewer and more dietary factors being retained in the model (Table A1).

SCORE-1 included two dietary risk factors, i.e., the factors most strongly associated with GDM in the multivariable model: sugar and artificially sweetened beverages ≥5 times/week and processed meat products ≥1 time/week.

SCORE-2 included seven dietary risk factors, i.e., a non-varied diet, sugar and artificially sweetened beverages ≥5 times/week, sweet, ice cream, cakes, cookies ≥2.5 times/week, processed meat products ≥1 time/week, whole grain products <2 times/day, dairy <2 times/day and vitamin D intake <5 times/week.

SCORE-3 included all 13 dietary risk factors, i.e., not eating a varied diet, vegetables and fruits <5 times/day, fish intake <2 times/day, dairy intake <2 times/day, whole grain products <2 times /day, beans, nuts, seeds <3.5 times/week, vitamin D <5 times/week, quality of fat—using butter rather than oil (≥50%), french fries and fried potatoes ≥1 time/week, sweets, ice cream, cakes, cookies ≥2.5 times/week, sugar and artificially sweetened beverages ≥5 times/week, dairy intake ≥5 times/day, processed meat products ≥1 time/week.

As can be seen in Table A1, The combination of the seven dietary risk factors resulted in the most significant association.

Table A1. Different combinations of the dietary risk score and the risk of gestational diabetes mellitus (GDM) [a].

	Crude [b] RR (95%CI)	Adjusted [b,c] RR (95%CI)
SCORE-1	1.23 (1.10, 1.36)	1.11 (1.00, 1.22)
SCORE-2	1.26 (1.13, 1.40)	1.13 (1.02, 1.25)
SCORE-3	1.22 (1.09, 1.36)	1.10 (0.99, 1.22)

[a] The criteria that was used [6]. [b] Standardized coefficient reflecting the risk of GDM per standard deviation increase in the dietary risk score. [c] Adjusted for maternal pre-pregnancy BMI, age, parity, smoking during pregnancy, educational level and family history of type 2 diabetes.

Table A2. Baseline dietary intake (frequency per week) of subjects in the pilot study.

5	Control (*n* = 41) [a]	Intervention (*n* = 47) [a]	*p* Value [b]
Milk	5.3 (2.2–7.6)	5.4 (2.1–14.4)	0.289
Cultured milk	5.0 (1.0–5.0)	2.5 (1.0–5.0)	0.876
Beans, nuts and/or seeds	0.5 (0.1–1.0)	0.5 (0.1–2.5)	0.244
Vegetables	7.0 (3.8–7.0)	7.0 (2.5–14)	0.202
Fruits and berries	14.0 (7.0–14)	7.0 (5.0–14)	0.655
Fish	1.1 (1.0–2.8)	1.5 (0.8–2.8)	0.803
Processed meat	0.5 (0.3–0.8)	0.5 (0.3–1.0)	0.158
Soft drinks	2.0 (0.6–5.0)	2.0 (0.6–3.5)	0.556
French fries or chips	0.5 (0.5–1.0)	0.5 (0.5–1.0)	0.554
Cakes, biscuits, ice and sweets	3.5 (1.5–6.0)	2.7 (1.5–5.0)	0.058

[a] Values are median (25th–75th centiles). [b] Mann-Whitney U test was used to assess differences among groups.

References

1. Zhu, Y.; Zhang, C. Prevalence of Gestational Diabetes and Risk of Progression to Type 2 Diabetes: A Global Perspective. *Curr. Diabetes Rep.* **2016**, *16*, 7. [CrossRef] [PubMed]
2. Wendland, E.M.; Torloni, M.R.; Falavigna, M.; Trujillo, J.; Dode, M.A.; Campos, M.A.; Duncan, B.B.; Schmidt, M.I. Gestational diabetes and pregnancy outcomes—A systematic review of the World Health Organization (WHO) and the International Association of Diabetes in Pregnancy Study Groups (IADPSG) diagnostic criteria. *BMC Pregnancy Childbirth* **2012**, *12*, 23. [CrossRef] [PubMed]
3. Alberico, S.; Montico, M.; Barresi, V.; Monasta, L.; Businelli, C.; Soini, V.; Erenbourg, A.; Ronfani, L.; Maso, G. The role of gestational diabetes, pre-pregnancy body mass index and gestational weight gain on the risk of newborn macrosomia: Results from a prospective multicentre study. *BMC Pregnancy Childbirth* **2014**, *14*, 23. [CrossRef] [PubMed]

4. Bellamy, L.; Casas, J.P.; Hingorani, A.D.; Williams, D. Type 2 diabetes mellitus after gestational diabetes: A systematic review and meta-analysis. *Lancet* **2009**, *373*, 1773–1779. [CrossRef]
5. Vohr, B.R.; Boney, C.M. Gestational diabetes: The forerunner for the development of maternal and childhood obesity and metabolic syndrome? *J. Matern. Fetal Neonatal Med.* **2008**, *21*, 149–157. [CrossRef] [PubMed]
6. Metzger, B.E.; Gabbe, S.G.; Persson, B.; Buchanan, T.A.; Catalano, P.A.; Damm, P.; Dyer, A.R.; Leiva, A.; Hod, M.; Kitzmiler, J.L.; et al. International association of diabetes and pregnancy study groups recommendations on the diagnosis and classification of hyperglycemia in pregnancy. *Diabetes Care* **2010**, *33*, 676–682. [CrossRef] [PubMed]
7. Donazar-Ezcurra, M.; Lopez-Del Burgo, C.; Martinez-Gonzalez, M.A.; Basterra-Gortari, F.J.; de Irala, J.; Bes-Rastrollo, M. Pre-pregnancy adherences to empirically derived dietary patterns and gestational diabetes risk in a Mediterranean cohort: The Seguimiento Universidad de Navarra (SUN) project. *Br. J. Nutr.* **2017**, *118*, 715–721. [CrossRef] [PubMed]
8. Zhang, C.; Schulze, M.B.; Solomon, C.G.; Hu, F.B. A prospective study of dietary patterns, meat intake and the risk of gestational diabetes mellitus. *Diabetologia* **2006**, *49*, 2604–2613. [CrossRef] [PubMed]
9. Tryggvadottir, E.A.; Medek, H.; Birgisdottir, B.E.; Geirsson, R.T.; Gunnarsdottir, I. Association between healthy maternal dietary pattern and risk for gestational diabetes mellitus. *Eur. J. Clin. Nutr.* **2016**, *70*, 237–242. [CrossRef] [PubMed]
10. He, J.R.; Yuan, M.Y.; Chen, N.N.; Lu, J.H.; Hu, C.Y.; Mai, W.B.; Zhang, R.F.; Pan, Y.H.; Qiu, L.; Wu, Y.F.; et al. Maternal dietary patterns and gestational diabetes mellitus: A large prospective cohort study in China. *Br. J. Nutr.* **2015**, *113*, 1292–1300. [CrossRef] [PubMed]
11. Shin, D.; Lee, K.W.; Song, W.O. Dietary Patterns during Pregnancy Are Associated with Risk of Gestational Diabetes Mellitus. *Nutrients* **2015**, *7*, 9369–9382. [CrossRef] [PubMed]
12. Schoenaker, D.A.; Mishra, G.D.; Callaway, L.K.; Soedamah-Muthu, S.S. The Role of Energy, Nutrients, Foods, and Dietary Patterns in the Development of Gestational Diabetes Mellitus: A Systematic Review of Observational Studies. *Diabetes Care* **2016**, *39*, 16–23. [CrossRef] [PubMed]
13. Hu, F.B.; Manson, J.E.; Stampfer, M.J.; Colditz, G.; Liu, S.; Solomon, C.G.; Willett, W.C. Diet, lifestyle, and the risk of type 2 diabetes mellitus in women. *N. Engl. J. Med.* **2001**, *345*, 790–797. [CrossRef] [PubMed]
14. Shim, J.S.; Oh, K.; Kim, H.C. Dietary assessment methods in epidemiologic studies. *Epidemiol. Health* **2014**, *36*, e2014009. [CrossRef] [PubMed]
15. Walsh, J.M.; McGowan, C.A.; Mahony, R.; Foley, M.E.; McAuliffe, F.M. Low glycaemic index diet in pregnancy to prevent macrosomia (ROLO study): Randomised control trial. *BMJ* **2012**, *345*, e5605. [CrossRef]
16. Khoury, J.; Henriksen, T.; Christophersen, B.; Tonstad, S. Effect of a cholesterol-lowering diet on maternal, cord, and neonatal lipids, and pregnancy outcome: A randomized clinical trial. *Am. J. Obstet. Gynecol.* **2005**, *193*, 1292–1301. [CrossRef] [PubMed]
17. Briley, A.L.; Barr, S.; Badger, S.; Bell, R.; Croker, H.; Godfrey, K.M.; Holmes, B.; Kinnunen, T.I.; Nelson, S.M.; Oteng-Ntim, E.; et al. A complex intervention to improve pregnancy outcome in obese women; the UPBEAT randomised controlled trial. *BMC Pregnancy Childbirth* **2014**, *14*, 74. [CrossRef]
18. Hrolfsdottir, L.; Halldorsson, T.I.; Birgisdottir, B.E.; Hreidarsdottir, I.T.; Hardardottir, H.; Gunnarsdottir, I. Development of a dietary screening questionnaire to predict excessive weight gain in pregnancy. *Matern. Child Nutr.* **2018**, e12639. [CrossRef]
19. Nordic Nutrition Recommendations. *Integrating Nutrition and Physical Activity*; Nordic Council of Ministers: Copenhagen, Denmark, 2014.
20. Embætti Landlæknis. *Grundvöllur Ráðlegginga um Mataræði og Ráðlagðir Dagskammtar Næringarefna*; Embætti Landlæknis: Reykjavík, Iceland, 2016.
21. Gunnarsdottir, I.; Tryggvadottir, E.A.; Birgisdottir, B.E.; Halldorsson, T.I.; Medek, H.; Geirsson, R.T. Diet and nutrient intake of pregnant women in the capital area in Iceland. *Laeknabladid* **2016**, *102*, 378–384.
22. Olsen, S.F.; Halldorsson, T.I.; Willett, W.C.; Knudsen, V.K.; Gillman, M.W.; Mikkelsen, T.B.; Olsen, J. Milk consumption during pregnancy is associated with increased infant size at birth: Prospective cohort study. *Am. J. Clin. Nutr.* **2007**, *86*, 1104–1110. [CrossRef]
23. Renault, K.M.; Carlsen, E.M.; Norgaard, K.; Nilas, L.; Pryds, O.; Secher, N.J.; Olsen, S.F.; Halldorsson, T.I. Intake of Sweets, Snacks and Soft Drinks Predicts Weight Gain in Obese Pregnant Women: Detailed Analysis of the Results of a Randomised Controlled Trial. *PLoS ONE* **2015**, *10*, e0133041. [CrossRef]

24. Englund-Ogge, L.; Brantsaeter, A.L.; Haugen, M.; Sengpiel, V.; Khatibi, A.; Myhre, R.; Myking, S.; Meltzer, H.M.; Kacerovsky, M.; Nilsen, R.M.; et al. Association between intake of artificially sweetened and sugar-sweetened beverages and preterm delivery: A large prospective cohort study. *Am. J. Clin. Nutr.* **2012**, *96*, 552–559. [CrossRef]

25. Zhu, Y.; Olsen, S.F.; Mendola, P.; Halldorsson, T.I.; Rawal, S.; Hinkle, S.N.; Yeung, E.H.; Chavarro, J.E.; Grunnet, L.G.; Granstrom, C.; et al. Maternal consumption of artificially sweetened beverages during pregnancy, and offspring growth through 7 years of age: A prospective cohort study. *Int. J. Epidemiol.* **2017**, *46*, 1499–1508. [CrossRef]

26. Nutrition Mother and Baby; In Icelandic Næring Móðir og Barn. Available online: https://nmb.is/ (accessed on 1 April 2019).

27. White, S.L.; Lawlor, D.A.; Briley, A.L.; Godfrey, K.M.; Nelson, S.M.; Oteng-Ntim, E.; Robson, S.C.; Sattar, N.; Seed, P.T.; Vieira, M.C.; et al. Early Antenatal Prediction of Gestational Diabetes in Obese Women: Development of Prediction Tools for Targeted Intervention. *PLoS ONE* **2016**, *11*, e0167846. [CrossRef]

28. Torloni, M.R.; Betran, A.P.; Horta, B.L.; Nakamura, M.U.; Atallah, A.N.; Moron, A.F.; Valente, O. Prepregnancy BMI and the risk of gestational diabetes: A systematic review of the literature with meta-analysis. *Obes. Rev.* **2009**, *10*, 194–203. [CrossRef]

29. Bouthoorn, S.H.; Silva, L.M.; Murray, S.E.; Steegers, E.A.; Jaddoe, V.W.; Moll, H.; Hofman, A.; Mackenbach, J.P.; Raat, H. Low-educated women have an increased risk of gestational diabetes mellitus: The Generation R Study. *Acta Diabetol.* **2015**, *52*, 445–452. [CrossRef]

30. England, L.J.; Levine, R.J.; Qian, C.; Soule, L.M.; Schisterman, E.F.; Yu, K.F.; Catalano, P.M. Glucose tolerance and risk of gestational diabetes mellitus in nulliparous women who smoke during pregnancy. *Am. J. Epidemiol.* **2004**, *160*, 1205–1213. [CrossRef]

31. Lawlor, D.A.; Emberson, J.R.; Ebrahim, S.; Whincup, P.H.; Wannamethee, S.G.; Walker, M.; Smith, G.D. Is the association between parity and coronary heart disease due to biological effects of pregnancy or adverse lifestyle risk factors associated with child-rearing? Findings from the British Women's Heart and Health Study and the British Regional Heart Study. *Circulation* **2003**, *107*, 1260–1264.

32. Donazar-Ezcurra, M.; Lopez-Del Burgo, C.; Martinez-Gonzalez, M.A.; Basterra-Gortari, F.J.; de Irala, J.; Bes-Rastrollo, M. Soft drink consumption and gestational diabetes risk in the SUN project. *Clin. Nutr.* **2018**, *37*, 638–645. [CrossRef]

33. Ruiz-Gracia, T.; Duran, A.; Fuentes, M.; Rubio, M.A.; Runkle, I.; Carrera, E.F.; Torrejon, M.J.; Bordiu, E.; Valle, L.D.; Garcia de la Torre, N.; et al. Lifestyle patterns in early pregnancy linked to gestational diabetes mellitus diagnoses when using IADPSG criteria. The St Carlos gestational study. *Clin. Nutr.* **2016**, *35*, 699–705. [CrossRef]

34. Battaglia Richi, E.; Baumer, B.; Conrad, B.; Darioli, R.; Schmid, A.; Keller, U. Health Risks Associated with Meat Consumption: A Review of Epidemiological Studies. *Int. J. Vitam. Nutr. Res.* **2015**, *85*, 70–78. [CrossRef]

35. Boada, L.D.; Henriquez-Hernandez, L.A.; Luzardo, O.P. The impact of red and processed meat consumption on cancer and other health outcomes: Epidemiological evidences. *Food Chem. Toxicol.* **2016**, *92*, 236–244. [CrossRef]

36. Zhang, Y.; Gong, Y.; Xue, H.; Xiong, J.; Cheng, G. Vitamin D and gestational diabetes mellitus: A systematic review based on data free of Hawthorne effect. *BJOG* **2018**, *125*, 784–793. [CrossRef]

37. Koivusalo, S.B.; Rono, K.; Klemetti, M.M.; Roine, R.P.; Lindstrom, J.; Erkkola, M.; Kaaja, R.J.; Poyhonen Alho, M.; Tiitinen, A.; Huvinen, E.; et al. Gestational Diabetes Mellitus Can Be Prevented by Lifestyle Intervention: The Finnish Gestational Diabetes Prevention Study (RADIEL): A Randomized Controlled Trial. *Diabetes Care* **2016**, *39*, 24–30. [CrossRef]

38. NCD Risk Factor Collaboration (NCD-RisC). Trends in adult body-mass index in 200 countries from 1975 to 2014: A pooled analysis of 1698 population-based measurement studies with 19.2 million participants. *Lancet* **2016**, *387*, 1377–1396.

39. Assaf-Balut, C.; Garcia de la Torre, N.; Duran, A.; Fuentes, M.; Bordiu, E.; Del Valle, L.; Familiar, C.; Valerio, J.; Jimenez, I.; Herraiz, M.A.; et al. A Mediterranean Diet with an Enhanced Consumption of Extra Virgin Olive Oil and Pistachios Improves Pregnancy Outcomes in Women Without Gestational Diabetes Mellitus: A Sub-Analysis of the St. Carlos Gestational Diabetes Mellitus Prevention Study. *Ann. Nutr. Metab.* **2019**, *74*, 69–79. [CrossRef]

40. Chen, L.W.; Aris, I.M.; Bernard, J.Y.; Tint, M.T.; Chia, A.; Colega, M.; Gluckman, P.D.; Shek, L.P.; Saw, S.M.; Chong, Y.S.; et al. Associations of Maternal Dietary Patterns during Pregnancy with Offspring Adiposity from Birth Until 54 Months of Age. *Nutrients* **2016**, *9*, 2. [CrossRef]

41. Brantsaeter, A.L.; Haugen, M.; Samuelsen, S.O.; Torjusen, H.; Trogstad, L.; Alexander, J.; Magnus, P.; Meltzer, H.M. A dietary pattern characterized by high intake of vegetables, fruits, and vegetable oils is associated with reduced risk of preeclampsia in nulliparous pregnant Norwegian women. *J. Nutr.* **2009**, *139*, 1162–1168. [CrossRef]

42. Hillesund, E.R.; Bere, E.; Haugen, M.; Overby, N.C. Development of a New Nordic Diet score and its association with gestational weight gain and fetal growth—A study performed in the Norwegian Mother and Child Cohort Study (MoBa). *Public Health Nutr.* **2014**, *17*, 1909–1918. [CrossRef]

43. Martin, C.L.; Sotres-Alvarez, D.; Siega-Riz, A.M. Maternal Dietary Patterns during the Second Trimester Are Associated with Preterm Birth. *J. Nutr.* **2015**, *145*, 1857–1864. [CrossRef]

44. Wolff, S.; Legarth, J.; Vangsgaard, K.; Toubro, S.; Astrup, A. A randomized trial of the effects of dietary counseling on gestational weight gain and glucose metabolism in obese pregnant women. *Int. J. Obes. (Lond.)* **2008**, *32*, 495–501. [CrossRef]

45. Haby, K.; Glantz, A.; Hanas, R.; Premberg, A. Mighty Mums—An antenatal health care intervention can reduce gestational weight gain in women with obesity. *Midwifery* **2015**, *31*, 685–692. [CrossRef]

46. Rogozinska, E.; Marlin, N.; Jackson, L.; Rayanagoudar, G.; Ruifrok, A.E.; Dodds, J.; Molyneaux, E.; van Poppel, M.N.; Poston, L.; Vinter, C.A.; et al. Effects of antenatal diet and physical activity on maternal and fetal outcomes: Individual patient data meta-analysis and health economic evaluation. *Health Technol. Assess. (Winch. Engl.)* **2017**, *21*, 1–158. [CrossRef]

47. Guo, X.Y.; Shu, J.; Fu, X.H.; Chen, X.P.; Zhang, L.; Ji, M.X.; Liu, X.M.; Yu, T.T.; Sheng, J.Z.; Huang, H.F. Improving the effectiveness of lifestyle interventions for gestational diabetes prevention: A meta-analysis and meta-regression. *BJOG* **2019**, *126*, 311–320. [CrossRef]

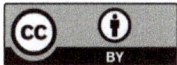

![nutrients logo]

MDPI

Communication

Maternal Omega-3 Nutrition, Placental Transfer and Fetal Brain Development in Gestational Diabetes and Preeclampsia

Prasad P. Devarshi *, Ryan W. Grant, Chioma J. Ikonte and Susan Hazels Mitmesser

Science and Technology, Pharmavite, LLC, West Hills, CA 91304, USA; rgrant@pharmavite.net (R.W.G.); cikonte@pharmavite.net (C.J.I.); smitmesser@pharmavite.net (S.H.M.)
* Correspondence: pdevarshi@pharmavite.net; Tel.: +1-818-221-6420

Received: 1 April 2019; Accepted: 14 May 2019; Published: 18 May 2019

Abstract: Omega-3 fatty acids, particularly docosahexaenoic fatty acid (DHA), are widely recognized to impact fetal and infant neurodevelopment. The impact of DHA on brain development, and its inefficient synthesis from the essential alpha-linolenic acid (ALA), has led to recommended DHA intakes of 250–375 mg eicosapentaenoic acid + DHA/day for pregnant and lactating women by the Dietary Guidelines for Americans. Despite these recommendations, the intake of omega-3s in women of child-bearing age in the US remains very low. The low maternal status of DHA prior to pregnancy could impair fetal neurodevelopment. This review focuses on maternal omega-3 status in conditions of gestational diabetes mellitus (GDM) and preeclampsia, and the subsequent impact on placental transfer and cord blood concentration of omega-3s. Both GDM and preeclampsia are associated with altered maternal omega-3 status, altered placental omega-3 metabolism, reduced cord blood omega-3 levels and have an impact on neurodevelopment in the infant and on brain health later in life. These findings indicate lower DHA exposure of the developing baby may be driven by lower placental transfer in both conditions. Thus, determining approaches which facilitate increased delivery of DHA during pregnancy and early development might positively impact brain development in infants born to mothers with these diseases.

Keywords: DHA; gestational diabetes; preeclampsia; placental transport

1. Introduction

Eicosapentaenoic acid (EPA, C20:5) and docosahexaenoic acid (DHA, C22:6) are omega-3 polyunsaturated fatty acids that are well-studied in humans [1–3]. Because they can be synthesized in the body from their precursor, alpha-linolenic acid (ALA, C18:3), EPA and DHA are not considered essential fatty acids. However, inefficient conversion of ALA to EPA and DHA [4,5] has led to recommendations to include food and dietary supplements as sources of EPA and DHA.

Wide recognition of the importance of EPA and DHA in infant development has led to recommendations for pregnant and lactating women from many regulatory bodies [6–10] and medical/scientific societies [11–17]. In the US, the American Academy of Pediatrics, American College of Obstetricians and Gynecologists, and March of Dimes recommend an intake of fish or omega-3 fatty acids resulting in ~200 mg DHA/day, and the Dietary Guidelines for Americans (DGA) recommends ~250–375 mg EPA + DHA/day. Despite these recommendations to promote the intake of omega-3 fatty acids, consumption of omega-3 fatty acids remains low across the US population [18], specifically in child-bearing-age, pregnant and lactating women [19]. Up to 95% of child-bearing-age and pregnant women do not meet the DGA recommendations for EPA + DHA intake [19]. Because of the impact DHA has on fetal development, the gap between the recommended and the actual DHA intake is concerning.

It is well established that DHA is an important structural component of the human brain and retina [20]. In the retina, DHA represents ~80% of all polyunsaturated fatty acids, while 60% of the dry weight of the brain is fatty acids, of which DHA is the major omega-3 fatty acid [21,22]. Omega-3 fatty acid deficiency leads to low levels of DHA in the cerebral cortex of the offspring and affects learning ability in animal models [23,24]. During fetal and infant development, membranes of the retina and brain grey matter become enriched with DHA [20]. During the third trimester, DHA selectively accumulates in the brain at a higher rate than other fatty acids [25]. This incorporation of DHA continues at these high rates until age 2 [26]. The first two years of life are an essential period of neurodevelopment for infants [27]. In the brain, DHA plays many important roles, including cell signaling, regulation of gene expression and neurotransmission [28–30]. In 60-day old rats, a diet deficient in omega-3 fatty acids led to altered physiology of neurotransmitters such as serotonin and dopamine, which are important for brain function [31]. Additionally, DHA deficiency led to decreased neuron size in various areas of the brain such as the hypothalamus and the hippocampus in animal models [32]. Normal neuron size is essential for their function in the brain [32]. Moreover, it was shown that maternal omega-3 deficiency not only affects neuronal size, but also neurogenesis in animals [33]. A lower rate of neurogenesis may affect cognitive function later in life [33]. Human studies have demonstrated that maternal omega-3 fatty acid supplementation increases maternal as well as fetal levels of DHA. DHA supplementation (200 mg/day) starting at the 21st week of gestation through lactation showed an increase in maternal red blood cells (RBCs) DHA at 37 weeks gestation and 3 months post birth. Additionally, this led to increased DHA in human milk and RBC DHA in the infant [34]. The benefits of omega-3 fatty acid supplementation during pregnancy have been well documented in the infant. After 1500 mg/week supplementation of DHA (as a functional food) during pregnancy, 9-month-old infants had improved performance on problem-solving tasks compared to the non-supplemented group [35]. Fish oil supplementation (2200 mg DHA and 1100 mg EPA per day) starting at 20 weeks gestation until birth showed an improvement in hand and eye coordination in the children at two and half years of age [36]. Additionally, hand and eye coordination scores positively correlated with omega-3 fatty acid levels in cord blood RBCs [36]. Supplementation of 600 mg/day of DHA from 14.5 weeks of gestation until birth, led to high levels of sustained attention in infants at 4, 6 and 9 month of age, while sustained attention declined in the control group during this period [37], suggesting the importance of omega-3 fatty acids in fetal brain development and function.

Despite the importance of omega-3 fatty acid intake on fetal brain development [38], most pregnant and child-bearing age women in the US are consuming less than the recommended amount [19]. While it is known that socioeconomic status influences infant cognitive development and nutrition [39,40], this review focuses on the effect of low placental omega-3 transfer in gestational diabetes mellitus (GDM) and preeclampsia on neurodevelopment. In addition to the low omega-3 fatty acid intake among pregnant women, in women with GDM and preeclampsia the transfer of DHA through the placenta to the fetus is compromised [41,42]. GDM is defined as impaired glucose tolerance first detected during pregnancy and is associated with various implications for fetal growth [43,44]. Preeclampsia is defined as systolic blood pressure of ≥140 mm Hg or diastolic blood pressure ≥90 mm Hg on two occasions at least 4 h apart, along with proteinuria, thrombocytopenia, renal insufficiency, impaired liver function, pulmonary edema, or cerebral or visual symptoms after 20 weeks of gestation [45]. Both GDM and preeclampsia are pregnancy disorders that have effects on fetal growth and development [43,44,46]. Due to the importance of omega-3 fatty acids in fetal brain development, it is important to understand the underlying mechanisms likely responsible for the reduced transfer of DHA to the fetus in GDM and preeclampsia. Here, we review the association of GDM and preeclampsia with maternal omega-3 fatty acid status, the impact of these disorders on the transfer of omega-3 fatty acids to the fetus, and subsequent effects on fetal brain development.

2. Gestational Diabetes

2.1. Maternal and Fetal Effects

In the course of gestation in all pregnancies, including normal pregnancies, insulin resistance increases progressively and is highest in the third trimester [47]. In normal pregnancies, the pancreatic beta cells produce higher levels of insulin which prevents hyperglycemia, whereas, in GDM, the response of these beta cells is inadequate, leading to hyperglycemia [47]. GDM is defined as impaired glucose tolerance first detected during pregnancy and is associated with various implications for fetal growth [43,44]. According to the 2014 analysis by the Centers for Disease Control and Prevention, GDM affects 9.2% of all pregnancies in the US [48]. Mechanisms involving progesterone and glucocorticoids and their effect on insulin sensitivity have been suggested to be responsible for the increase of insulin resistance during gestation [49,50]. Progesterone secretion increases during pregnancy and it has been shown to decrease the ability of insulin to suppress synthesis of glucose in the liver [49]. Cortisol is a glucocorticoid that increases during pregnancy and has have been shown to affect skeletal muscle insulin signaling [50,51]. Glucocorticoids reduce phosphorylation of the insulin receptor and reduce the content of insulin receptor substrate-1, which is involved in insulin signaling, in the skeletal muscle [50]. Women with GDM have higher levels of insulin resistance compared to normal pregnancy controls [52]. The combination of elevated insulin resistance and inadequate beta cells response both likely contribute to hyperglycemia in GDM [47,52,53]. GDM has a complicated etiology involving numerous metabolic and genetic factors with many underlying mechanisms [54]. A large prospective cohort study found that aging, obesity, non-white ethnicity, family history of diabetes and smoking increases the risk for developing GDM [55]. In addition, the development of GDM during pregnancy increases the risk of GDM in future pregnancies [56].The etiology of GDM is complex and comprises lifestyle and genetic risk factors, with many potential mechanisms.

GDM leads to adverse long-term effects including a higher risk of developing metabolic diseases in the mother and the child [57,58]. In addition to these adverse effects, the presence of diabetes during pregnancy is associated with impaired neurodevelopment [59–64]. Infants of mothers with GDM showed lower mental and psychomotor development indexes compared to infants of non-GDM mothers at 6 months of age [59]. Similarly, children below 9 years of age, of mothers with GDM, had lower verbal IQ scores than children of non-GDM mothers [60]. These children also scored low compared to children of non-GDM mothers in the Pollack tapper test, which is used to detect learning disabilities [60]. GDM also affects language development during childhood [61]. Children (18 and 30 months) of GDM mothers had lower expressive vocabulary and grammar scores compared to children of non-GDM mothers [61]. These children were at a 2.2-fold higher risk of having impaired language development [61]. In children of GDM mothers at 8 years of age, a trend towards lower IQ scores compared to children of non-GDM mothers was seen [64]. As DHA is an important nutrient for fetal brain development [38], it has been suggested that the effects on neurodevelopment may be as a result of low cord blood levels of DHA seen in GDM [59]. Additionally, in animal models, it has been suggested that inflammation due to GDM can lead to adverse effects on neurodevelopment in the offspring [65]. In totality, these studies demonstrate the influence of GDM on neurodevelopment.

2.2. Placental Transfer of Omega-3 Fatty Acids in GDM

The negative neurodevelopment effects observed in children of mothers with GDM could be a result of lower omega-3 fatty acid transfer from the mother to the fetus [66]. Maternal DHA is the primary source of DHA for the fetus as it cannot be synthesized in the fetus or the placenta [41]. The placenta preferentially absorbs DHA for transfer to the fetus during pregnancy and this is demonstrated by higher cord vein DHA levels compared to maternal blood DHA levels [67]. In GDM pregnancies, cord vein blood levels of DHA are lower than the levels in normal pregnancies [59,66,68]. Specifically, maternal DHA levels have been shown to be 11–44% higher in GDM, while cord blood levels were lower compared to normal pregnancies, indicating a possibility of reduced placental transfer of DHA to the fetus in GDM [69]. Thomas et al. similarly found that cord vein DHA was lower in GDM versus normal pregnancy [68]. Wijendran et al. observed that GDM mothers had a higher intake of omega-3 fatty acids during the third trimester of pregnancy compared to normal pregnancy controls [66]. Due to higher dietary intake, GDM mothers also had significantly higher maternal DHA erythrocyte content [66]. However, in spite of higher DHA intake and maternal DHA erythrocyte levels, DHA in cord vein erythrocytes was significantly lower (37% lower) than in normal pregnancy controls [66]. In this study, maternal plasma DHA positively correlated with DHA in fetal erythrocytes in the normal pregnancy control group, however this correlation was not present in GDM mothers [66]. Moreover, maternal hemoglobin A1c (HbA1C) levels were inversely related to fetal erythrocyte DHA content in GDM mothers, which suggests a relation between GDM and transfer of DHA to the fetus [66].

Several mechanisms have been proposed for the reduction in placental transfer of DHA in GDM. Peroxisome proliferator-activated receptor (PPAR)-alpha and PPAR-gamma belong to the family of nuclear receptors that control various fatty acid metabolism related genes, including genes related to fatty acid transport [70]. PPAR-alpha mainly controls fatty acid oxidation related genes and PPAR-gamma controls adipogenesis related genes [70]. PPAR-alpha was downregulated in GDM placentae compared to uncomplicated term placentae [71]. Also, PPAR-gamma had lower gene and protein expression in GDM placenta [71]. Lipoprotein lipase (LPL), which is expressed in the microvillous plasma membrane of the placenta, is needed to release free fatty acids from triglycerides in circulating lipoproteins, leading to uptake by the placenta [72]. In pregnancies complicated by type-1 diabetes, LPL activity in the microvillous plasma membrane of the placenta was increased by 39% compared to the normal pregnancy control, but no difference was seen in GDM pregnancies indicating that LPL is not involved in mechanisms related to reduced placental transfer of DHA in GDM [72,73]. The transport of fatty acid through the placenta is orchestrated by a number of proteins, including: Fatty acid transfer proteins such as fatty acid transport protein (FATP)-1-6, cluster of differentiation 36 (CD-36), fatty-acid-binding protein (FABP)-pm, placental-FABP-pm in the plasma membrane and FABP-1, 3, 4, 5, 7 [74]. In GDM placenta, it was seen that expression of FATP-1 and FATP-4 were decreased, while expression of CD-36 and FATP-6 were increased compared to normal pregnancy controls [75]. The major facilitator superfamily domain-containing protein 2A (MFSD2A) was identified as a brain choline and DHA transporter [76]. It was seen that MFSD2A was significantly reduced in GDM placentae [77]. DHA percentage in the cord vein blood correlated with levels of MFSD2A, suggesting a possible role in placental transfer of DHA to the fetus [77]. These alterations could be possibly responsible for reduced DHA transfer across the placenta.

Some studies have investigated the effect of omega-3 fatty acid supplementation during pregnancy on GDM [78–80]. Zhou et al. investigated the effect of DHA supplementation on the incidence of GDM [81]. DHA intake of 800 mg/day did not affect risk of developing GDM [81]. In GDM women, 800 mg/day of DHA supplementation starting at 17–33 weeks of gestation, increased DHA in maternal plasma and RBCs, but failed to increase DHA in cord vein plasma and RBCs. More studies investigating the effects of early DHA supplementation on placental expression of fatty acid metabolism-related genes and fetal outcomes are needed.

3. Preeclampsia

3.1. Maternal and Fetal Effects

Preeclampsia occurs in ~3% of pregnancies and negatively impacts both maternal and fetal health outcomes [45]. The American College of Obstetricians and Gynecologists defines preeclampsia as a systolic blood pressure of ≥140 mm Hg or diastolic blood pressure ≥90 mm Hg on two occasions at least 4 h apart, which co-occurs with proteinuria, thrombocytopenia, renal insufficiency, impaired liver function, pulmonary edema, or cerebral or visual symptoms after 20 weeks of gestation [45]. Although preeclampsia typically develops during the second trimester of pregnancy, its disease pathogenesis likely begins in the first trimester during implantation. Delivery of nutrients from the mother to the fetus depends on placental vasculature. Placental vascular development requires remodeling of the uterine spiral arteries from narrow vessels to wider, low resistance vessels [82]. Impairment of vascular remodeling during early gestation is thought to result in the later development of preeclampsia. Proposed mechanisms leading to preeclampsia include impairment of endothelial function and a maternal immune response to the invading trophoblast cells that remodel the spiral arteries [82]. During pregnancy, the maternal immune system develops tolerance to cells of the fetus [83]. Defects in the development of tolerance and activation of a pro-inflammatory response may be contributing factors to the development of preeclampsia [83].

Impairment of placental vascularization during preeclampsia limits efficient delivery of nutrients and oxygen to the fetus. Low oxygen levels lead to increased rates of neuronal apoptosis in experimental models of preeclampsia and perinatal asphyxia [84]. In addition to the sensitivity of neurons to low oxygen levels, hypoxia can drive tissue inflammatory responses. Preeclampsia upregulates placental expression of proinflammatory cytokines (tumor necrosis factor-α, Interleukin-1 (IL-1), and IL-18) and downregulates the anti-inflammatory cytokine IL-10 [85]. Indeed, human term placental explants exposed to low oxygen levels had increased production of tumor necrosis factor-α, IL-1α and β [86]. In ischemic brain injury, there is upregulation of both IL-1β and IL-18. Mice that lack production of IL-18 or were treated with an intracerebroventricular injection of an IL-1 receptor antagonist have reduced ischemic brain injury [87,88]. Hypoxia additionally promotes the production of reactive oxygen species and the development of oxidative stress, which can also contribute to neuronal apoptosis [89]. The impact of hypoxia on neuronal apoptosis, inflammation and oxidative stress likely function together to negatively impact brain development. In children, prenatal hypoxia is a known contributor to impaired cognitive development [90]. Specifically, preeclampsia negatively impacts several aspects of cognitive function including verbal reasoning and executive function during early childhood [91]. Preeclampsia may also impact brain health later in life. Children from mothers with preeclampsia had higher depression symptoms during adulthood [91]. These findings suggest that preeclampsia may impact the brain across the lifespan. To establish a link between preeclampsia and brain function, some studies have analyzed brain structure. Initial studies have demonstrated that children from preeclamptic pregnancies exhibit differences in the structure and connectivity of limbic system components, an area of the brain linked with mood, behavior and cognition [91]. Although the underlying factors that drive preeclampsia are not completely understood, evidence indicates that preeclampsia impacts maternal and fetal health, as well as long-term development.

3.2. Placental Transfer of Omega-3 Fatty Acids in Preeclampsia

Omega-3 fatty acids, and particularly DHA, are critical to the structure and function of developing nervous system cells. Several factors influence the availability of DHA and EPA to fetal tissues, including: Dietary intake, endogenous synthesis from alpha-linolenic acid, transport within the blood for delivery to placental tissues, placental tissue uptake and transfer to cord blood. Several case-controlled studies have demonstrated that during the third trimester or postpartum, blood levels of omega-3 fatty acids are reduced in mothers with preeclampsia compared to normal pregnancy. An initial study of postpartum mothers indicated that women in the lowest tertile of erythrocyte omega-3 fatty acid content were 7.6 times more likely to have preeclampsia compared with those in the highest tertile [92]. Kulkarni et al. found that at delivery, plasma DHA levels were reduced in preeclamptic vs. normotensive pregnancy, and this difference was also reflected in infant cord blood samples [93]. An additional study found that third trimester levels of omega-3 fatty acids were reduced in mothers with preeclampsia or intrauterine growth restriction (IUGR) compared to normal pregnancy [94]. Cord blood taken from these subjects also indicates a reduction in total omega-3 fatty acids and DHA compared to normal pregnancy [94]. Although differences in maternal omega-3 fatty acids during the third trimester are apparent, they don't account for exposure across the duration of pregnancy. A more recent study examined longitudinal changes of serum fatty acid proportions in normotensive and preeclamptic pregnant women. This study demonstrated reduced circulation of total omega-3 fatty acids, DHA and arachidonic acid at 16–20 weeks but not at 26–30 weeks or at delivery in preeclamptic pregnant women [95]. This study did confirm lower cord blood levels of both DHA and total omega-3 fatty acids at delivery with preeclampsia, which were similar to the differences found by Kulkarni et al. [95]. This study also revealed significant correlation of maternal plasma DHA with cord plasma DHA across all three time points [95], highlighting reduced maternal omega-3 fatty acids during preeclampsia.

Given that maternal blood levels of omega-3 fatty acids are low during preeclampsia, a key question is whether the placenta can compensate by upregulating the trafficking, synthesis and/or transfer of omega-3 fatty acids. The fatty acid composition of placentas from mothers with preeclampsia is different from those with normal pregnancies. Wang et al. demonstrated that placentas from preeclamptic women have reduced total non-esterified polyunsaturated fatty acids, including lower total omega-3 fatty acids and DHA compared to placenta from normal pregnant women [96]. The observation of reduced placental DHA has been confirmed by other studies [95,97,98]. An initial study comparing omega-3 fatty acid composition in different areas of the placenta indicates regional differences between normotensive controls, term pregnancy with preeclampsia and preterm pregnancy with preeclampsia. DHA and total omega-3 fatty acid concentrations were consistently lower in the central fetal and maternal areas of the placenta in mothers with preeclampsia and preterm delivery [97]. Additionally, in the central fetal area there were higher concentrations of ALA with preterm delivery and preeclampsia, indicating a possibility of inefficient conversion of ALA to DHA [97]. Because there were no matched normotensive preterm controls, it is unclear whether these changes are driven by gestational time or the severity of disease.

The placenta transports omega-3 fatty acids and expresses enzymes which contribute to the metabolism of ALA into EPA and DHA. Thus far, studies do not indicate increased capability for EPA + DHA synthesis or transport in preeclampsia. The expression of genes responsible for placental lipid transport (FATP 1 and 4) and fatty acid elongation (fatty acid desaturase 1) were reduced with preeclampsia, while others (fatty acid desaturase 2 and FABP-3) were not altered [95]. This indicates that during preeclampsia there may be a down regulation of the capacity to transport lipid in the placenta, and potentially a reduced capacity to synthesize DHA from ALA in placental tissue. Placental mRNA expression of MFSD2A, a DHA transporter in the brain, is reduced during severe preeclampsia compared to normotensive pregnancy [99]. However, it is unknown what the impact of this reduction is on fetal development. Collectively, these observations indicated altered transport and metabolism of omega-3 fatty acids during preeclampsia. These results are supported by reduced omega-3 fatty acids in placental tissue and cord blood from mothers with preeclampsia versus normal pregnancy. It is currently unknown whether cord blood DHA levels are responsive to increased dietary intake during preeclampsia.

A number of intervention trials were conducted to understand if supplemental omega-3 fatty acids from fish oil could impact maternal outcomes associated with preeclampsia. These studies have been largely ineffective [100] and vary widely in dose and composition of omega-3 fatty acids, as well as gestational age at the onset of the intervention [101]. Although studies have focused on the mother, this does not preclude impact on the baby. It was noted by Kulkarni et al. that cord blood DHA levels were correlated with serum DHA levels in mothers with preeclampsia. This raises the possibility that increasing maternal omega-3 fatty acid status may increase omega-3 fatty acid exposure of the developing baby. Future studies are needed to determine whether increased maternal prenatal omega-3 fatty acid intake can improve cord blood DHA and developmental outcomes in babies born to mothers with preeclampsia.

4. Conclusions

Despite the recommendations from various authorities, 95% of pregnant and child-bearing-age women do not consume enough omega-3 fatty acids [19,38]. Transfer of omega-3 fatty acids through the placenta to the cord blood and fetus is impaired in GDM and preeclampsia [41,42,75,77,95]. This is reflected in both conditions by lower cord vein DHA levels compared to normal pregnancies [66,93]. Given the role DHA plays in fetal neurodevelopment, lower DHA transfer to the fetus may contribute to impaired neurodevelopment.

Although it is apparent that GDM and preeclampsia are associated with lower cord blood levels of DHA, the impact of DHA and omega-3 fatty acid supplementation on fetal neurodevelopment in this population remains unclear. In GDM, increasing DHA intake later in pregnancy did not increase cord blood levels, possibly due to impaired DHA placental transfer [102]. Future studies in both GDM and preeclampsia need to focus on very early interventions. Such studies could elucidate the time course of serum fatty acids during pregnancy and the impact of DHA supplementation on maternal blood, placental and cord vein DHA levels. Additionally, there is a need to further link infant neurodevelopmental outcomes to omega-3 fatty acid intake. One factor that may influence the effects of omega-3 fatty acids on neurodevelopment may be socioeconomic status. Most of the studies discussed did not evaluate the impact of socioeconomic status on offspring neurodevelopment. This is a limitation, as socioeconomic status has been suggested to affect neurodevelopment and omega-3 nutrition [39,40]. Future studies are needed to determine the effect of socioeconomic status on maternal nutritional interventions and offspring neurodevelopment. While DHA intake prior to and during pregnancy is important, postnatal DHA intake could be an impactful opportunity to increase delivery of DHA to the breast-fed new born baby. Interventions supporting increased DHA consumption might positively impact neurodevelopmental outcomes associated with GDM and preeclampsia.

Author Contributions: Conceptualization, P.P.D. and R.W.G.; writing—original draft preparation, P.P.D. and R.W.G.; and writing—review and editing, C.J.I. and S.H.M.

Funding: This research received no external funding.

Conflicts of Interest: P.P.D., R.W.G., C.J.I. and S.H.M. are employed at Pharmavite LLC.

References

1. Mozaffarian, D.; Wu, J.H.Y. Omega-3 Fatty Acids and Cardiovascular Disease. *J. Am. Coll. Cardiol.* **2011,** *58,* 2047. [CrossRef] [PubMed]
2. Lorente-Cebrián, S.; Costa, A.G.V.; Navas-Carretero, S.; Zabala, M.; Martínez, J.A.; Moreno-Aliaga, M.J. Role of omega-3 fatty acids in obesity, metabolic syndrome, and cardiovascular diseases: A review of the evidence. *J. Physiol. Biochem.* **2013,** *69,* 633–651. [CrossRef]
3. Ruxton, C.H.S.; Reed, S.C.; Simpson, M.J.A.; Millington, K.J. The health benefits of omega-3 polyunsaturated fatty acids: A review of the evidence. *J. Hum. Nutr. Diet.* **2004,** *17,* 449–459. [CrossRef] [PubMed]
4. Goyens, P.L.; Spilker, M.E.; Zock, P.L.; Katan, M.B.; Mensink, R.P. Compartmental modeling to quantify alpha-linolenic acid conversion after longer term intake of multiple tracer boluses. *J. Lipid Res.* **2005,** *46,* 1474–1483. [CrossRef] [PubMed]
5. Hussein, N.; Ah-Sing, E.; Wilkinson, P.; Leach, C.; Griffin, B.A.; Millward, D.J. Long-chain conversion of [13C]linoleic acid and alpha-linolenic acid in response to marked changes in their dietary intake in men. *J. Lipid Res.* **2005,** *46,* 269–280. [CrossRef] [PubMed]
6. Fats and fatty acids in human nutrition. Report of an expert consultation. *FAO Food Nutr. Pap.* **2010,** *91,* 1–166.
7. Koletzko, B.; Lien, E.; Agostoni, C.; Bohles, H.; Campoy, C.; Cetin, I.; Decsi, T.; Dudenhausen, J.W.; Dupont, C.; Forsyth, S.; et al. The roles of long-chain polyunsaturated fatty acids in pregnancy, lactation and infancy: Review of current knowledge and consensus recommendations. *J. Perinat. Med.* **2008,** *36,* 5–14. [CrossRef]
8. Koletzko, B.; Cetin, I.; Brenna, J.T.; Perinatal Lipid Intake Working Group; Child Health Foundation; Diabetic Pregnancy Study Group; European Association of Perinatal Medicine; European Society for Clinical Nutrition and Metabolism; European Society for Paediatric Gastroenterology, Hepatology and Nutrition; Committee on Nutrition; et al. Dietary fat intakes for pregnant and lactating women. *Br. J. Nutr.* **2007,** *98,* 873–877. [CrossRef]

9. Scientific Opinion on Dietary Reference Values for fats, including saturated fatty acids, polyunsaturated fatty acids, monounsaturated fatty acids, trans fatty acids, and cholesterol. *EFSA J.* **2010**, *8*, 1461. [CrossRef]

10. Simopoulos, A.P.; Leaf, A.; Salem, N., Jr. Workshop on the Essentiality of and Recommended Dietary Intakes for Omega-6 and Omega-3 Fatty Acids. *J. Am. Coll. Nutr.* **1999**, *18*, 487–489. [CrossRef]

11. Nesheim, M.; Yaktine, A. (Eds.) Analysis of the balancing of benefits and risks of seafood consumption. In *Seafood Choices: Balancing Benefits and Risks*; National Academies Press: Washington, DC, USA, 2007; pp. 195–216.

12. Carlson, S.E. Docosahexaenoic acid supplementation in pregnancy and lactation. *Am. J. Clin. Nutr.* **2009**, *89*, 678S–684S. [CrossRef] [PubMed]

13. Coletta, J.M.; Bell, S.J.; Roman, A.S. Omega-3 Fatty acids and pregnancy. *Rev. Obstet. Gynecol.* **2010**, *3*, 163–171. [CrossRef] [PubMed]

14. Dimes, M.O. Vitamins and Other Nutrients During Pregnancy. Available online: https://www.marchofdimes. org/pregnancy/vitamins-and-other-nutrients-during-pregnancy.aspx (accessed on 1 March 2019).

15. Pediatrics, A.A.O. Breastfeeding and the use of human milk. *Pediatrics* **2012**, *129*, e827–e841. [CrossRef]

16. US Department of Health and Human Services. 2015–2020 Dietary Guidelines for Americans. Available online: https://health.gov/dietaryguidelines/2015/resources/2015-2020_Dietary_Guidelines.pdf (accessed on 4 March 2019).

17. 2017 EPA-FDA Advice about Eating Fish and Shellfish. Available online: https://www.epa.gov/fish-tech/2017-epa-fda-advice-about-eating-fish-and-shellfish (accessed on 1 March 2019).

18. Papanikolaou, Y.; Brooks, J.; Reider, C.; Fulgoni, V.L. US adults are not meeting recommended levels for fish and omega-3 fatty acid intake: Results of an analysis using observational data from NHANES 2003–2008. *Nutr. J.* **2014**, *13*, 31. [CrossRef] [PubMed]

19. Zhang, Z.; Fulgoni, V.L.; Kris-Etherton, P.M.; Mitmesser, S.H. Dietary Intakes of EPA and DHA Omega-3 Fatty Acids among US Childbearing-Age and Pregnant Women: An Analysis of NHANES 2001-2014. *Nutrients* **2018**, *10*, 416. [CrossRef] [PubMed]

20. Innis, S.M. Perinatal biochemistry and physiology of long-chain polyunsaturated fatty acids. *J. Pediatrics* **2003**, *143*, S1–S8. [CrossRef]

21. Giusto, N.M.; Pasquare, S.J.; Salvador, G.A.; Castagnet, P.I.; Roque, M.E.; Ilincheta de Boschero, M.G. Lipid metabolism in vertebrate retinal rod outer segments. *Prog. Lipid Res.* **2000**, *39*, 315–391. [CrossRef]

22. Bradbury, J. Docosahexaenoic acid (DHA): An ancient nutrient for the modern human brain. *Nutrients* **2011**, *3*, 529–554. [CrossRef]

23. Neuringer, M.; Connor, W.E.; Lin, D.S.; Barstad, L.; Luck, S. Biochemical and functional effects of prenatal and postnatal omega 3 fatty acid deficiency on retina and brain in rhesus monkeys. *Proc. Natl. Acad. Sci. USA* **1986**, *83*, 4021–4025. [CrossRef]

24. Yamamoto, N.; Hashimoto, A.; Takemoto, Y.; Okuyama, H.; Nomura, M.; Kitajima, R.; Togashi, T.; Tamai, Y. Effect of the dietary alpha-linolenate/linoleate balance on lipid compositions and learning ability of rats. II. Discrimination process, extinction process, and glycolipid compositions. *J. Lipid Res.* **1988**, *29*, 1013–1021.

25. Cetin, I.; Alvino, G.; Cardellicchio, M. Long chain fatty acids and dietary fats in fetal nutrition. *J. Physiol.* **2009**, *587*, 3441–3451. [CrossRef]

26. Lauritzen, L.; Brambilla, P.; Mazzocchi, A.; Harsløf, L.B.S.; Ciappolino, V.; Agostoni, C. DHA Effects in Brain Development and Function. *Nutrients* **2016**, *8*, 6. [CrossRef]

27. Schwarzenberg, S.J.; Georgieff, M.K. Advocacy for Improving Nutrition in the First 1000 Days to Support Childhood Development and Adult Health. *Pediatrics* **2018**, *141*, e20173716. [CrossRef]

28. Kitajka, K.; Puskas, L.G.; Zvara, A.; Hackler, L., Jr.; Barcelo-Coblijn, G.; Yeo, Y.K.; Farkas, T. The role of n-3 polyunsaturated fatty acids in brain: Modulation of rat brain gene expression by dietary n-3 fatty acids. *Proc. Natl. Acad. Sci. USA* **2002**, *99*, 2619–2624. [CrossRef] [PubMed]

29. Stillwell, W.; Shaikh, S.R.; Zerouga, M.; Siddiqui, R.; Wassall, S.R. Docosahexaenoic acid affects cell signaling by altering lipid rafts. *Reprod. Nutr. Dev.* **2005**, *45*, 559–579. [CrossRef]

30. Chalon, S. Omega-3 fatty acids and monoamine neurotransmission. *Prostaglandins Leukot. Essent. Fat. Acids* **2006**, *75*, 259–269. [CrossRef]

31. Delion, S.; Chalon, S.; Herault, J.; Guilloteau, D.; Besnard, J.C.; Durand, G. Chronic dietary alpha-linolenic acid deficiency alters dopaminergic and serotoninergic neurotransmission in rats. *J. Nutr.* **1994**, *124*, 2466–2476. [CrossRef]

32. Ahmad, A.; Moriguchi, T.; Salem, N. Decrease in neuron size in docosahexaenoic acid-deficient brain. *Pediatric Neurol.* **2002**, *26*, 210–218. [CrossRef]

33. Coti Bertrand, P.; O'Kusky, J.R.; Innis, S.M. Maternal dietary (n-3) fatty acid deficiency alters neurogenesis in the embryonic rat brain. *J. Nutr.* **2006**, *136*, 1570–1575. [CrossRef]

34. Bergmann, R.L.; Haschke-Becher, E.; Klassen-Wigger, P.; Bergmann, K.E.; Richter, R.; Dudenhausen, J.W.; Grathwohl, D.; Haschke, F. Supplementation with 200 mg/day docosahexaenoic acid from mid-pregnancy through lactation improves the docosahexaenoic acid status of mothers with a habitually low fish intake and of their infants. *Ann. Nutr. Metab.* **2008**, *52*, 157–166. [CrossRef]

35. Judge, M.P.; Harel, O.; Lammi-Keefe, C.J. Maternal consumption of a docosahexaenoic acid-containing functional food during pregnancy: Benefit for infant performance on problem-solving but not on recognition memory tasks at age 9 mo. *Am. J. Clin. Nutr.* **2007**, *85*, 1572–1577. [CrossRef] [PubMed]

36. Dunstan, J.A.; Simmer, K.; Dixon, G.; Prescott, S.L. Cognitive assessment of children at age 2(1/2) years after maternal fish oil supplementation in pregnancy: A randomised controlled trial. *Arch. Dis. Child. Fetal Neonatal Ed.* **2008**, *93*, F45–F50. [CrossRef]

37. Colombo, J.; Gustafson, K.M.; Gajewski, B.J.; Shaddy, D.J.; Kerling, E.H.; Thodosoff, J.M.; Doty, T.; Brez, C.C.; Carlson, S.E. Prenatal DHA supplementation and infant attention. *Pediatric Res.* **2016**, *80*, 656–662. [CrossRef]

38. Innis, S.M. Dietary omega 3 fatty acids and the developing brain. *Brain Res.* **2008**, *1237*, 35–43. [CrossRef]

39. Nordgren, T.M.; Lyden, E.; Anderson-Berry, A.; Hanson, C. Omega-3 Fatty Acid Intake of Pregnant Women and Women of Childbearing Age in the United States: Potential for Deficiency? *Nutrients* **2017**, *9*, 197. [CrossRef]

40. Chin-Lun Hung, G.; Hahn, J.; Alamiri, B.; Buka, S.L.; Goldstein, J.M.; Laird, N.; Nelson, C.A.; Smoller, J.W.; Gilman, S.E. Socioeconomic disadvantage and neural development from infancy through early childhood. *Int. J. Epidemiol.* **2015**, *44*, 1889–1899. [CrossRef]

41. Gil-Sánchez, A.; Demmelmair, H.; Parrilla, J.; Koletzko, B.; Larqué, E. Mechanisms Involved in the Selective Transfer of Long Chain Polyunsaturated Fatty Acids to the Fetus. *Front. Genet.* **2011**, *2*, 57. [CrossRef]

42. Wadhwani, N.; Patil, V.; Joshi, S. Maternal long chain polyunsaturated fatty acid status and pregnancy complications. *Prostaglandins Leukot. Essent. Fat. Acids* **2018**, *136*, 143–152. [CrossRef] [PubMed]

43. Ornoy, A. Prenatal origin of obesity and their complications: Gestational diabetes, maternal overweight and the paradoxical effects of fetal growth restriction and macrosomia. *Reprod. Toxicol.* **2011**, *32*, 205–212. [CrossRef] [PubMed]

44. Gestational Diabetes Mellitus. *Diabetes Care* **2004**, *27*, s88. [CrossRef] [PubMed]

45. American College of Obstetricians and Gynecologists. Hypertension in pregnancy. Report of the American College of Obstetricians and Gynecologists' task force on hypertension in pregnancy. *Obstet. Gynecol.* **2013**, *122*, 1122.

46. Backes, C.H.; Markham, K.; Moorehead, P.; Cordero, L.; Nankervis, C.A.; Giannone, P.J. Maternal preeclampsia and neonatal outcomes. *J. Pregnancy* **2011**, *2011*, 214365. [CrossRef] [PubMed]

47. Di Cianni, G.; Miccoli, R.; Volpe, L.; Lencioni, C.; Del Prato, S. Intermediate metabolism in normal pregnancy and in gestational diabetes. *Diabetes/Metab. Res. Rev.* **2003**, *19*, 259–270. [CrossRef] [PubMed]

48. DeSisto, C.L.; Kim, S.Y.; Sharma, A.J. Prevalence estimates of gestational diabetes mellitus in the United States, Pregnancy Risk Assessment Monitoring System (PRAMS), 2007–2010. *Prev. Chronic Dis.* **2014**, *11*, E104. [CrossRef] [PubMed]

49. Nelson, T.; Shulman, G.; Grainger, D.; Diamond, M.P. Progesterone administration induced impairment of insulin suppression of hepatic glucose production. *Fertil. Steril.* **1994**, *62*, 491–496. [CrossRef]

50. Giorgino, F.; Almahfouz, A.; Goodyear, L.J.; Smith, R.J. Glucocorticoid regulation of insulin receptor and substrate IRS-1 tyrosine phosphorylation in rat skeletal muscle in vivo. *J. Clin. Investig.* **1993**, *91*, 2020–2030. [CrossRef]

51. Buss, C.; Davis, E.P.; Shahbaba, B.; Pruessner, J.C.; Head, K.; Sandman, C.A. Maternal cortisol over the course of pregnancy and subsequent child amygdala and hippocampus volumes and affective problems. *Proc. Natl. Acad. Sci. USA* **2012**, *109*, E1312–E1319. [CrossRef]

52. Xiang, A.H.; Peters, R.K.; Trigo, E.; Kjos, S.L.; Lee, W.P.; Buchanan, T.A. Multiple metabolic defects during late pregnancy in women at high risk for type 2 diabetes. *Diabetes* **1999**, *48*, 848–854. [CrossRef]

53. Kautzky-Willer, A.; Prager, R.; Waldhausl, W.; Pacini, G.; Thomaseth, K.; Wagner, O.F.; Ulm, M.; Streli, C.; Ludvik, B. Pronounced insulin resistance and inadequate beta-cell secretion characterize lean gestational diabetes during and after pregnancy. *Diabetes Care* **1997**, *20*, 1717–1723. [CrossRef]

54. Johns, E.C.; Denison, F.C.; Norman, J.E.; Reynolds, R.M. Gestational Diabetes Mellitus: Mechanisms, Treatment, and Complications. *Trends Endocrinol. Metab. TEM* **2018**, *29*, 743–754. [CrossRef] [PubMed]

55. Solomon, C.G.; Willett, W.C.; Carey, V.J.; Rich-Edwards, J.; Hunter, D.J.; Colditz, G.A.; Stampfer, M.J.; Speizer, F.E.; Spiegelman, D.; Manson, J.E. A prospective study of pregravid determinants of gestational diabetes mellitus. *Jama* **1997**, *278*, 1078–1083. [CrossRef]

56. Kim, C.; Berger, D.K.; Chamany, S. Recurrence of gestational diabetes mellitus: A systematic review. *Diabetes Care* **2007**, *30*, 1314–1319. [CrossRef]

57. Metzger, B.E. Long-term outcomes in mothers diagnosed with gestational diabetes mellitus and their offspring. *Clin. Obstet. Gynecol.* **2007**, *50*, 972–979. [CrossRef]

58. West, N.A.; Crume, T.L.; Maligie, M.A.; Dabelea, D. Cardiovascular risk factors in children exposed to maternal diabetes in utero. *Diabetologia* **2011**, *54*, 504–507. [CrossRef]

59. Zornoza-Moreno, M.; Fuentes-Hernandez, S.; Carrion, V.; Alcantara-Lopez, M.V.; Madrid, J.A.; Lopez-Soler, C.; Sanchez-Solis, M.; Larque, E. Is low docosahexaenoic acid associated with disturbed rhythms and neurodevelopment in offsprings of diabetic mothers? *Eur. J. Clin. Nutr.* **2014**, *68*, 931–937. [CrossRef]

60. Ornoy, A.; Wolf, A.; Ratzon, N.; Greenbaum, C.; Dulitzky, M. Neurodevelopmental outcome at early school age of children born to mothers with gestational diabetes. *Arch. Disease Child. Fetal Neonatal Ed.* **1999**, *81*, F10–F14. [CrossRef]

61. Dionne, G.; Boivin, M.; Seguin, J.R.; Perusse, D.; Tremblay, R.E. Gestational diabetes hinders language development in offspring. *Pediatrics* **2008**, *122*, e1073–e1079. [CrossRef]

62. Dahlquist, G.; Kallen, B. School marks for Swedish children whose mothers had diabetes during pregnancy: A population-based study. *Diabetologia* **2007**, *50*, 1826–1831. [CrossRef]

63. DeBoer, T.; Wewerka, S.; Bauer, P.J.; Georgieff, M.K.; Nelson, C.A. Explicit memory performance in infants of diabetic mothers at 1 year of age. *Dev. Med. Child Neurol.* **2005**, *47*, 525–531. [CrossRef]

64. Fraser, A.; Nelson, S.M.; Macdonald-Wallis, C.; Lawlor, D.A. Associations of existing diabetes, gestational diabetes, and glycosuria with offspring IQ and educational attainment: The Avon Longitudinal Study of Parents and Children. *Exp. Diabetes Res.* **2012**, *2012*, 963735. [CrossRef]

65. Vuong, B.; Odero, G.; Rozbacher, S.; Stevenson, M.; Kereliuk, S.M.; Pereira, T.J.; Dolinsky, V.W.; Kauppinen, T.M. Exposure to gestational diabetes mellitus induces neuroinflammation, derangement of hippocampal neurons, and cognitive changes in rat offspring. *J. Neuroinflamm.* **2017**, *14*, 80. [CrossRef]

66. Wijendran, V.; Bendel, R.B.; Couch, S.C.; Philipson, E.H.; Cheruku, S.; Lammi-Keefe, C.J. Fetal erythrocyte phospholipid polyunsaturated fatty acids are altered in pregnancy complicated with gestational diabetes mellitus. *Lipids* **2000**, *35*, 927–931. [CrossRef]

67. Berghaus, T.M.; Demmelmair, H.; Koletzko, B. Essential fatty acids and their long-chain polyunsaturated metabolites in maternal and cord plasma triglycerides during late gestation. *Biol. Neonate* **2000**, *77*, 96–100. [CrossRef]

68. Thomas, B.A.; Ghebremeskel, K.; Lowy, C.; Offley-Shore, B.; Crawford, M.A. Plasma fatty acids of neonates born to mothers with and without gestational diabetes. *Prostaglandins Leukot. Essent. Fat. Acids* **2005**, *72*, 335–341. [CrossRef]

69. Leveille, P.; Rouxel, C.; Plourde, M. Diabetic pregnancy, maternal and fetal docosahexaenoic acid: A review of existing evidence. *J. Matern. Fetal Neonatal Med.* **2018**, *31*, 1358–1363. [CrossRef]

70. Grygiel-Górniak, B. Peroxisome proliferator-activated receptors and their ligands: Nutritional and clinical implications-a review. *Nutr. J.* **2014**, *13*, 17. [CrossRef]

71. Holdsworth-Carson, S.J.; Lim, R.; Mitton, A.; Whitehead, C.; Rice, G.E.; Permezel, M.; Lappas, M. Peroxisome proliferator-activated receptors are altered in pathologies of the human placenta: Gestational diabetes mellitus, intrauterine growth restriction and preeclampsia. *Placenta* **2010**, *31*, 222–229. [CrossRef] [PubMed]

72. Magnusson, A.L.; Waterman, I.J.; Wennergren, M.; Jansson, T.; Powell, T.L. Triglyceride hydrolase activities and expression of fatty acid binding proteins in the human placenta in pregnancies complicated by intrauterine growth restriction and diabetes. *J. Clin. Endocrinol. Metab.* **2004**, *89*, 4607–4614. [CrossRef]

73. Barrett, H.L.; Kubala, M.H.; Scholz Romero, K.; Denny, K.J.; Woodruff, T.M.; McIntyre, H.D.; Callaway, L.K.; Nitert, M.D. Placental Lipases in Pregnancies Complicated by Gestational Diabetes Mellitus (GDM). *PLoS ONE* **2014**, *9*, e104826. [CrossRef]

74. Gil-Sanchez, A.; Koletzko, B.; Larque, E. Current understanding of placental fatty acid transport. *Curr. Opin. Clin. Nutr. Metab. Care* **2012**, *15*, 265–272. [CrossRef]

75. Segura, M.T.; Demmelmair, H.; Krauss-Etschmann, S.; Nathan, P.; Dehmel, S.; Padilla, M.C.; Rueda, R.; Koletzko, B.; Campoy, C. Maternal BMI and gestational diabetes alter placental lipid transporters and fatty acid composition. *Placenta* **2017**, *57*, 144–151. [CrossRef] [PubMed]

76. Nguyen, L.N.; Ma, D.; Shui, G.; Wong, P.; Cazenave-Gassiot, A.; Zhang, X.; Wenk, M.R.; Goh, E.L.; Silver, D.L. Mfsd2a is a transporter for the essential omega-3 fatty acid docosahexaenoic acid. *Nature* **2014**, *509*, 503–506. [CrossRef] [PubMed]

77. Prieto-Sanchez, M.T.; Ruiz-Palacios, M.; Blanco-Carnero, J.E.; Pagan, A.; Hellmuth, C.; Uhl, O.; Peissner, W.; Ruiz-Alcaraz, A.J.; Parrilla, J.J.; Koletzko, B.; et al. Placental MFSD2a transporter is related to decreased DHA in cord blood of women with treated gestational diabetes. *Clin. Nutr.* **2017**, *36*, 513–521. [CrossRef]

78. Samimi, M.; Jamilian, M.; Asemi, Z.; Esmaillzadeh, A. Effects of omega-3 fatty acid supplementation on insulin metabolism and lipid profiles in gestational diabetes: Randomized, double-blind, placebo-controlled trial. *Clin. Nutr.* **2015**, *34*, 388–393. [CrossRef]

79. Jamilian, M.; Samimi, M.; Kolahdooz, F.; Khalaji, F.; Razavi, M.; Asemi, Z. Omega-3 fatty acid supplementation affects pregnancy outcomes in gestational diabetes: A randomized, double-blind, placebo-controlled trial. *J. Matern. -Fetal Neonatal Med.* **2016**, *29*, 669–675. [CrossRef]

80. Jamilian, M.; Samimi, M.; Mirhosseini, N.; Afshar Ebrahimi, F.; Aghadavod, E.; Taghizadeh, M.; Asemi, Z. A Randomized Double-Blinded, Placebo-Controlled Trial Investigating the Effect of Fish Oil Supplementation on Gene Expression Related to Insulin Action, Blood Lipids, and Inflammation in Gestational Diabetes Mellitus-Fish Oil Supplementation and Gestational Diabetes. *Nutrients* **2018**, *10*, 163. [CrossRef]

81. Zhou, S.J.; Yelland, L.; McPhee, A.J.; Quinlivan, J.; Gibson, R.A.; Makrides, M. Fish-oil supplementation in pregnancy does not reduce the risk of gestational diabetes or preeclampsia. *Am. J. Clin. Nutr.* **2012**, *95*, 1378–1384. [CrossRef] [PubMed]

82. Armaly, Z.; Jadaon, J.E.; Jabbour, A.; Abassi, Z.A. Preeclampsia: Novel Mechanisms and Potential Therapeutic Approaches. *Front. Physiol.* **2018**, *9*, 973. [CrossRef]

83. Jafri, S.; Ormiston, M.L. Immune regulation of systemic hypertension, pulmonary arterial hypertension, and preeclampsia: Shared disease mechanisms and translational opportunities. *Am. J. Physiol. Regul. Integr. Comp. Physiol.* **2017**, *313*, R693–R705. [CrossRef]

84. Cosar, H.; Ozer, E.; Topel, H.; Kahramaner, Z.; Turkoglu, E.; Erdemir, A.; Sutcuoglu, S.; Bagriyanik, A.; Ozer, E.A. Neuronal apoptosis in the neonates born to preeclamptic mothers. *J. Matern. Fetal Neonatal Med.* **2013**, *26*, 1143–1146. [CrossRef]

85. Raghupathy, R. Cytokines as key players in the pathophysiology of preeclampsia. *Med. Princ. Pract.* **2013**, *22* (Suppl. 1), 8–19. [CrossRef]

86. Benyo, D.F.; Miles, T.M.; Conrad, K.P. Hypoxia stimulates cytokine production by villous explants from the human placenta. *J. Clin. Endocrinol. Metab.* **1997**, *82*, 1582–1588. [CrossRef] [PubMed]

87. Loddick, S.A.; Rothwell, N.J. Neuroprotective effects of human recombinant interleukin-1 receptor antagonist in focal cerebral ischaemia in the rat. *J. Cereb. Blood Flow Metab.* **1996**, *16*, 932–940. [CrossRef]

88. Hedtjarn, M.; Leverin, A.L.; Eriksson, K.; Blomgren, K.; Mallard, C.; Hagberg, H. Interleukin-18 involvement in hypoxic-ischemic brain injury. *J. Neurosci.* **2002**, *22*, 5910–5919. [CrossRef]

89. Blomgren, K.; Leist, M.; Groc, L. Pathological apoptosis in the developing brain. *Apoptosis* **2007**, *12*, 993–1010. [CrossRef]

90. Nalivaeva, N.N.; Turner, A.J.; Zhuravin, I.A. Role of Prenatal Hypoxia in Brain Development, Cognitive Functions, and Neurodegeneration. *Front. Neurosci.* **2018**, *12*, 825. [CrossRef]

91. Figueiro-Filho, E.A.; Mak, L.E.; Reynolds, J.N.; Stroman, P.W.; Smith, G.N.; Forkert, N.D.; Paolozza, A.; Ratsep, M.T.; Croy, B.A. Neurological function in children born to preeclamptic and hypertensive mothers—A systematic review. *Pregnancy Hypertens.* **2017**, *10*, 1–6. [CrossRef]

92. Williams, M.; Zingheim, R.W.; King, I.B.; Zebelman, A.M. Omega-3 fatty acids in maternal erythrocytes and risk of preeclampsia. *Epidemilogy* **1995**, *6*, 232–237. [CrossRef]

93. Kulkarni, A.V.; Mehendale, S.S.; Yadav, H.R.; Kilari, A.S.; Taralekar, V.S.; Joshi, S.R. Circulating angiogenic factors and their association with birth outcomes in preeclampsia. *Hypertens. Res. Off. J. Jpn. Soc. Hypertens.* **2010**, *33*, 561–567. [CrossRef] [PubMed]

94. Mackay, V.A.; Huda, S.S.; Stewart, F.M.; Tham, K.; McKenna, L.A.; Martin, I.; Jordan, F.; Brown, E.A.; Hodson, L.; Greer, I.A.; et al. Preeclampsia is associated with compromised maternal synthesis of long-chain polyunsaturated fatty acids, leading to offspring deficiency. *Hypertension* **2012**, *60*, 1078–1085. [CrossRef] [PubMed]

95. Wadhwani, N.; Patil, V.; Pisal, H.; Joshi, A.; Mehendale, S.; Gupte, S.; Wagh, G.; Joshi, S. Altered maternal proportions of long chain polyunsaturated fatty acids and their transport leads to disturbed fetal stores in preeclampsia. *Prostaglandins Leukot. Essent. Fat. Acids (PLEFA)* **2014**, *91*, 21–30. [CrossRef]

96. Wang, Y.; Walsh, S.W.; Kay, H.H. Placental tissue levels of nonesterified polyunsaturated fatty acids in normal and preeclamptic pregnancies. *Hypertens. Pregnancy* **2005**, *24*, 235–245. [CrossRef]

97. Rani, A.; Chavan-Gautam, P.; Mehendale, S.; Wagh, G.; Joshi, S. Differential regional fatty acid distribution in normotensive and preeclampsia placenta. *BBA Clin.* **2015**, *4*, 21–26. [CrossRef] [PubMed]

98. Kulkarni, A.V.; Mehendale, S.S.; Yadav, H.R.; Joshi, S.R. Reduced placental docosahexaenoic acid levels associated with increased levels of sFlt-1 in preeclampsia. *Prostaglandins Leukot. Essent. Fat. Acids* **2011**, *84*, 51–55. [CrossRef]

99. Toufaily, C.; Vargas, A.; Lemire, M.; Lafond, J.; Rassart, E.; Barbeau, B. MFSD2a, the Syncytin-2 receptor, is important for trophoblast fusion. *Placenta* **2013**, *34*, 85–88. [CrossRef] [PubMed]

100. Makrides, M.; Duley, L.; Olsen, S.F. Marine oil, and other prostaglandin precursor, supplementation for pregnancy uncomplicated by pre-eclampsia or intrauterine growth restriction. *Cochrane Database Syst. Rev.* **2006**, *3*, CD003402. [CrossRef] [PubMed]

101. Burchakov, D.I.; Kuznetsova, I.V.; Uspenskaya, Y.B. Omega-3 Long-Chain Polyunsaturated Fatty Acids and Preeclampsia: Trials Say "No," but Is It the Final Word? *Nutrients* **2017**, *9*, 1364. [CrossRef] [PubMed]

102. Min, Y.; Djahanbakhch, O.; Hutchinson, J.; Eram, S.; Bhullar, A.S.; Namugere, I.; Ghebremeskel, K. Efficacy of docosahexaenoic acid-enriched formula to enhance maternal and fetal blood docosahexaenoic acid levels: Randomized double-blinded placebo-controlled trial of pregnant women with gestational diabetes mellitus. *Clin. Nutr.* **2016**, *35*, 608–614. [CrossRef]

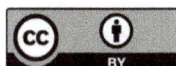

nutrients

MDPI

Review

Preterm Birth: A Narrative Review of the Current Evidence on Nutritional and Bioactive Solutions for Risk Reduction

Tinu M. Samuel [1], Olga Sakwinska [1], Kimmo Makinen [1], Graham C. Burdge [2], Keith M. Godfrey [3] and Irma Silva-Zolezzi [4,*]

[1] Nestlé Research, 1000 Lausanne, Switzerland
[2] School of Human Development and Health, Faculty of Medicine, University of Southampton, Southampton SO16 6YD, UK
[3] MRC Lifecourse Epidemiology Unit and NIHR Southampton Biomedical Research Centre, University of Southampton & University Hospital Southampton NHS Foundation Trust, Southampton SO16 6YD, UK
[4] Nestlé Research, Singapore 618802, Singapore
* Correspondence: irma.silvazolezzi@rdsg.nestle.com; Tel.: +65-8833-33714

Received: 12 July 2019; Accepted: 2 August 2019; Published: 6 August 2019

Abstract: Preterm birth (PTB) (<37 weeks of gestation) is the leading cause of newborn death and a risk factor for short and long-term adverse health outcomes. Most cases are of unknown cause. Although the mechanisms triggering PTB remain unclear, an inappropriate increase in net inflammatory load seems to be key. To date, interventions that reduce the risk of PTB are effective only in specific groups of women, probably due to the heterogeneity of its etiopathogenesis. Use of progesterone is the most effective, but only in singleton pregnancies with history of PTB. Thus, primary prevention is greatly needed and nutritional and bioactive solutions are a promising alternative. Among these, docosahexaenoic acid (DHA) is the most promising to reduce the risk for early PTB. Other potential nutrient interventions include the administration of zinc (possibly limited to populations with low nutritional status or poor zinc status) and vitamin D; additional preliminary evidence exists for vitamin A, calcium, iron, folic acid, combined iron-folate, magnesium, multiple micronutrients, and probiotics. Considering the public health relevance of PTB, promising interventions should be studied in large and well-designed clinical trials. The objective of this review is to describe, summarize, and discuss the existing evidence on nutritional and bioactive solutions for reducing the risk of PTB.

Keywords: preterm birth; preterm labor; etiology; nutrition; DHA; probiotics

1. Introduction

Preterm birth (PTB) is defined as birth at <37 weeks of gestation or at <259 days since the first day of a woman's last menstruation, and it is broadly classified into extremely preterm (PT) (<28 weeks), very PT (28 to <32 weeks), and moderate PT (32 to <37 completed weeks of gestation). Moderate PTB is further categorized as early PTB (EPTB) and late PTB (LPTB) depending on whether the infant was born <34 weeks or between 34 and <37 weeks of gestation, respectively [1]. PTB is a risk factor for adverse short and long-term health outcomes. Short term, it is the leading cause of neonatal death and the second cause of all under-5 mortality [2]. Long term, it is associated with increased risks of hypertension, cardiovascular and cerebrovascular diseases, type 2 diabetes, chronic kidney disease, asthma and abnormalities in pulmonary function, and neurocognitive disorders [3,4]. In addition, PTB is associated with increased health care costs [5] and socioeconomic disadvantages in adulthood [6].

Estimates based on most recent data from 107 countries suggest that in 2014 an estimated 10.6% of livebirths worldwide (14.84 million) were preterm, with 81.1% occurring in Asia and sub-Saharan

Africa. There are also significant disparities in PTB rates between countries (8.7% in Europe vs. 13.55% in North Africa) [7]. PTB rates have been increasing in most countries with reliable data, attributed to factors including but not limited to, better detection, older maternal age, multiple pregnancies from assisted reproductive technologies, and higher rates of underlying conditions such as diabetes and hypertensive disorders [8]. The reported prevalence may be an underestimate due to lack of routine collection, and within and between country comparisons are challenging due to inconsistencies in reporting pregnancy outcomes and utilizing standard definitions of PTB.

A series of maternal factors have been identified that impact the risk of PTB. Of these, some are non-modifiable, such as history of PTB, extremes in maternal age (<19 and >35 years) [9–11], multiple pregnancies [12], short cervical length (CL) [13], uterine abnormalities, prior cervical excision [14], dilation/curettage [15], ethnicity and family history [16], and genetic factors [17–20]. In addition, some are modifiable, such as nutrition, low socioeconomic status, low body mass index (BMI), obesity, poor pregnancy weight gain, smoking, substance abuse, short inter-pregnancy interval, periodontal disease, bacterial vaginosis, late or no prenatal care, untreated antenatal depression, and the use of assisted reproductive technologies [21].

The clinical presentation of PTB is either "spontaneous" (70%) or "indicated". Spontaneous PTB is characterized by preterm labor (PTL) with cervical dilation or preterm premature rupture of membranes (PPROM), while indicated PTB is initiated by obstetricians due to complications in absence of labor or PPROM [22,23]. Recent evidence indicates that etiologist of spontaneous and indicated LPTB overlap and are often characterized by placental vascular mal-perfusion lesions. However, the etiologies of EPTB differ, with indicated PTB typically characterized by placental vascular mal-perfusion lesions and spontaneous PTB by placental infectious inflammatory lesions [24]. This suggests that the underlying molecular mechanisms associated with EPTB differ to those of LPTB and thus potentially efficacy of preventive interventions may differ between EPTB and LPTB.

Differential mechanisms underlying PTB are also inherent to a series of clinical conditions that trigger labor and have been associated with PTB (see Figure 1): (1) decidual hemorrhage caused by placental abruption [25], possibly triggered by infection, inflammation, hypoxia, or oxidative stress [26]; (2) uterine factors such as cervical insufficiency [27] and uterine distension or stretch [21]; (3) maternal mood and distress involving activation of the hypothalamic–pituitary–adrenal axis [28–30] and increased production of prostaglandins (e.g., prostaglandin E2) [31,32]; (4) extra and intra-uterine infections [33], as well as intra-amniotic infection (IAI) [34,35], including intrauterine and systemic viral infections [36]; (5) inflammation in the absence of infection (e.g., via production of parturition-triggering cytokines) [37]; and (6) PPROM [38] representing a common final pathway to PTB associated with other of these clinical conditions [39].

Although the molecular mechanisms underlying labor onset remain puzzling, it is generally accepted that a "parturition cascade" triggers spontaneous PTL by premature stimulation of pro-inflammatory pathways within the uterus triggered by different clinical conditions (see Figure 1) [33,40,41]. At a molecular level, this cascade is mediated by progesterone and involves the coordinated activation of progesterone receptor-B (PR-B) and its truncated and much less active nuclear PR isoform progesterone receptor-A (PR-A) (see Figure 1) [41]. The balance between inflammation and progesterone activity seems key for timing of delivery.

Novel approaches to reduce the risk of PTB are needed due to the very limited success of different medical strategies to achieve this goal. For example, for women experiencing PTL, tocolytics (cyclooxygenase inhibitors, calcium channel blockers, or betamimetics) are used to stop contractions and delay delivery; unfortunately, these do not remove the underlying stimulus that initiated parturition or reverse parturition [42]. Thus, early identification of risk factors, as well as effective preventive interventions, are needed. Currently, screening, while imperfect, is done based on measuring CL (the strongest clinical predictor of PTB in asymptomatic women), as well as fetal fibronectin levels and CL assessment, the latter in singleton pregnancies with acute PTL symptoms. These approaches remain to be proven in multiple pregnancies [43]. Stopping smoking early in pregnancy has also been shown to reduce the risk of PTB, and other more specific strategies exist for scenarios of low- and high-risk pregnancies [9,44].

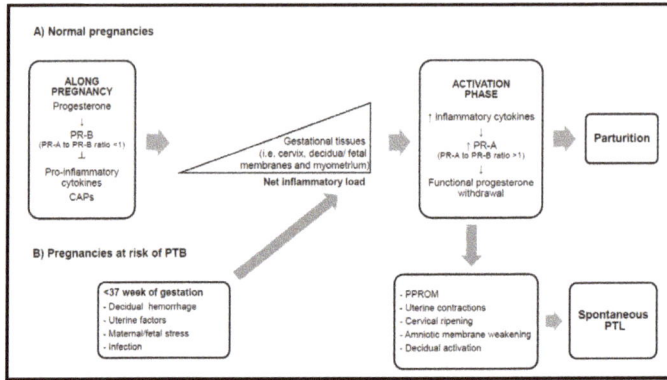

Figure 1. Parturition cascade in normal term and preterm pregnancies. PR-A and PR-B: progesterone receptors A and B, respectively; CAPs: contraction-associated proteins, PTL: preterm labor; PTB: preterm birth; PPROM: preterm premature rupture of membranes.

In asymptomatic pregnancies with a shortened cervix (CL ≤25 mm) identified at mid-trimester, vaginal progesterone is efficacious for preventing PTB, particularly in multiple pregnancies [45,46]. In singleton at-risk pregnancies and those with history of PTB, vaginal progesterone administered from 16 to 36 weeks of gestation is efficacious [47]. Also, serial CL screening is indicated between 16 and 24 weeks of gestation. In pregnancies with a shortened cervix (CL ≤25 mm) or with history of PTB, vaginal progesterone is the preferred option, with tightening the cervix with a stitch (cerclage) and closing the cervix with a silicone ring (cervical pessary) being alternatives [47,48].

Although promising, no approach is uniformly effective as primary-prevention to lower PTB rates because most cases are of unknown cause [49]. Inadequate nutrition preconception and during pregnancy has been associated with the risk of PTB and intervention studies suggest roles for specific nutrients in reducing PTB risk and/or increasing the duration of gestation [50]. The aim of this review is to summarize the evidence on nutritional and bioactive solutions for reducing the risk of PTB.

2. Materials and Methods

Literature search and selection criteria: We conducted a narrative literature review and search using SCOPUS and PubMed databases limited to English language original research, literature reviews and conference abstracts/papers/presentations published before May 2019. For omega-3 fatty acids (with the largest body of evidence today), we reviewed intervention studies of either docosahexaenoic acid (DHA) or eicosapentaenoic acid (EPA) alone or using varying combinations of both, food-based intervention studies, and systematic reviews/meta-analyses. We only reviewed those studies in which long-chain polyunsaturated fatty acid (LC-PUFA) administration was started no later than 12–32 weeks of gestation. The key words used were LC-PUFA, omega 3, eicosapentaenoic acid (EPA) and docosahexaenoic acid (DHA), intervention studies, clinical trials, pregnancy, gestational age at birth, preterm birth, and early preterm birth. For all other macro and micronutrients, we summarized the evidence based on the latest systematic reviews and meta-analyses. The key words used were nutrients, systematic review, meta-analyses, pregnancy, gestational age at birth, preterm birth, and early preterm birth. For probiotics, we included studies that reported PTB as either the primary or secondary outcome, and those that reported outcomes relevant to PTB such as the gestational age at birth or vaginal health during pregnancy; we only included studies where probiotic administration was started no later than 12–32 weeks gestation.

3. Results

3.1. The Role of Nutrition in Reducing the Risk of PTB

In the preceding sections, while a broad overview of the pathophysiology of PTB has been presented, there is increasing evidence that infection and/or inflammation are the pathological process for which the molecular pathophysiology has been best defined and a causal link with PTB has been fairly well established [51]. It is therefore of significant relevance to evaluate whether specific diet patterns and nutritional/bioactive interventions targeted to modulate inflammation/infection can be efficacious in reducing the risk of PTB. In the following sections of this review we document the evidence of maternal diet patterns, nutrients, and bioactives on PTB risk reduction and/or increasing gestational age at birth, probably via an anti-inflammatory and/or an immunomodulatory effect.

3.1.1. Evidence from Dietary Pattern Analyses

Observational studies indicate that poor maternal nutrition preconception and during early pregnancy may influence PTB risk [12]. In observational studies, consumption of specific foods such as >1 serving/day of artificially sweetened and sugar-sweetened beverages have been associated with increased PTB risk (adjusted odds ratios: 1.11 and 1.24, respectively), [52], but other studies have found no association [53]. Assessment of dietary patterns found that high scores on a "prudent" dietary pattern (higher intakes of vegetables, salad, onion/leek/garlic, fruit and berries, nuts, vegetable oils, water as beverage, whole grain cereals, poultry, and fiber rich bread, as well as low intake of processed meat products, white bread, and pizza/tacos) was associated with significant reductions in the risk of PTB (by 12%) and spontaneous PTB (by 15%), comparing the highest and lowest thirds of the population. Several mechanisms are postulated through which a prudent diet may reduce PTB risk, including an anti-stressor effect of a low fat diet on the hypothalamic–pituitary–adrenal axis or an anti-inflammatory effect due to an increased antioxidant intake or attributable to a diet low in saturated fat [54]. Adherence to a Mediterranean diet has been linked with a reduced PTB risk. Among Danish women, intake of a Mediterranean diet (fish bi-weekly or more, using olive or rape seed oil, >5 portions of fruit and vegetables/day, meat other than poultry and fish at most twice a week, and at most 2 cups of coffee/day) lowered the risk of EPTB by 72%, although PTB risk was not significantly reduced [55]. Adherence to a dietary pattern similar to Mediterranean diet was associated with a 30% decreased risk of PTD specifically in overweight and obese pregnant women in a French Caribbean island where the population is largely of African descent [56]. Similarly, in a randomized controlled trial (RCT) in healthy Norwegian pregnant women, those adhering to a dietary pattern resembling the Mediterranean diet had a 90% reduction in PTB risk [57]. However, Norwegian women who met the Mediterranean Diet criteria (fish ≥2 times a week, fruit and vegetables ≥5 times/day, use of olive/canola oil, red meat intake ≤2 times/week, and ≤2 cups of coffee/day) did not have reduced risk of PTB [58]. In addition, a vegetarian diet or pre-dominantly plant-based diet, both low in vitamin B12, vitamin D, zinc [59], EPA and DHA [60], as well as marginal intakes or low status of these nutrients have been associated with increased PTB risk [61]. These observational studies are reinforced by three recent systematic reviews showing that a "healthy" dietary pattern during pregnancy higher in fruits, vegetables, legumes and whole grains is associated with a lower risk of PTB (21% to 25% reduced risk) [62–64].

3.1.2. Nutrient-Based Interventions

Omega 3 Fatty Acids

Omega-3 fatty acids are long-chain, polyunsaturated fatty acids (PUFAs) of plant and marine origin. Alpha linolenic acid (ALA) and linoleic acid (LA) cannot be synthesized by the human body and must be derived from dietary sources. ALA is the parent omega-3 fatty acid that can be converted into longer chain n-3 PUFA including EPA and DHA [65]. The conversion of ALA to EPA and DHA is inefficient in humans and varies markedly between individuals; only 8–12% ALA is converted to EPA and less than 0.05% to DHA [66]. The efficiency of the conversion is dependent on epigenetic and genetic processes influencing the transcription of the fatty acid desaturase (*FADS*) genes [67]. Dietary factors can reduce conversion efficiency. In particular, greater conversion is observed among women compared to men, probably due to the influence of estrogen or other hormones [65,66]. It is recommended to obtain EPA and DHA preformed from additional dietary sources including fish/seafood and oils from marine animals, such as fish oil and cod liver oil. DHA intake across the world is variable [68,69].

The following sections briefly describe the evidence relating to EPA and DHA and PTB risk reduction. The first evidence that omega 3 fatty acids may play a role in reducing the risk of PTB was observed in women from Faeroe Islands who consumed a diet high in fish and showed an increased duration of gestation (4 days) and birth weight (194 g) compared to Danish women [70]. Additional supportive observational evidence included a prospective study in pregnant women reporting that non-consumers of fish had a shorter gestational length and higher odds of PTB, compared to fish eaters [71], another showing that any intake of seafood was associated with a lower prevalence of PTB [72], and a dose–response relationship observed for the association between seafood intake and risk of PTB [73]. However, other large cohort studies in the United States [74] and the United Kingdom [75] did not support the association of n-3 PUFA intake and/or seafood intake with length of gestation or PTB risk.

Ten clinical trials have investigated the role of omega 3 fatty acids on the duration of gestation and/or the incidence of PTB and/or EPTB [76–85] (Table 1). Eight of these 10 trials were interventions constituting of either DHA or EPA alone or used varying combinations of both, and two were predominantly food based [84,85]. Only two trials were carried out among pregnant women from low or middle-income countries (Mexico and Chile) [78,84]. Three trials were conducted in women with high-risk pregnancies (history of PTB, history or high risk of developing intra-uterine growth restriction (IUGR), or pregnancy-induced hypertension (PIH), women diagnosed with pre-eclampsia in current pregnancy or twin pregnancies) [80–82]. While most of the trials started the intervention around mid-pregnancy and followed through to delivery, one trial recruited women as early as 12–14 weeks gestation [82], and another at approximately 30 weeks of gestation [83].

The Kansas DHA Outcome Study (KUDOS trial), demonstrated that a daily administration of 600 mg DHA/day in pregnant women improved gestation duration (2.9 days) [76], and while an overall reduction in PTB was not observed, there was a reduction in EPTB (<34 weeks gestation). The results of this study are in accordance with those of another very large Australian trial (DHA to Optimize Mother Infant Outcome, DOMInO) in which positive findings in secondary outcomes such as an increase in the duration of gestation (1 day) and a 51% reduced risk of EPTB were also observed [77]. A trial among Danish pregnant women also demonstrated an improvement in the duration of gestation (4 days) with fish oil supplementation (2.7 g n-3 fatty acids) compared to olive oil. In this study, the effect of supplementation on the length of gestation seemed to depend on the habitual intake of fish. Among women who had the highest intake of fish at randomization, no difference could be detected between the groups, while in the women with the lowest intake for fish; a significant difference of 7.4 day was observed [83]. In contrast, a large trial among predominantly middle-class Mexican women from urban areas with access to health care indicated no benefit of supplementation of 400 mg DHA/day on gestational age, incidence of PTB, birth weight, length, or head circumference [78]. The results from the Norway [79], United Kingdom [81] and the Netherlands [82] trials concurred with the Mexican trial and did not find that omega 3 fatty acids lengthened the duration of gestation or reduced the incidence of PTB or early PTB. Two food-based interventions have assessed the effect of a dairy product fortified with multiple micronutrients, ALA and LA [84] or DHA-enriched eggs [85], on the length of gestation and birth weight. Both these trials reported a lower incidence of EPTB and an increase in the length of gestation. The latter trial [85] demonstrated an increase of 6 days of gestation with as little as 133 mg DHA/day.

Table 1. Characteristics and efficacy of clinical trials investigating the role of omega-3 fatty acids in reducing risk of early and any PTB.

Ref.	Study				Main Results	Comments
	Objective	Design	Population/Sample Size	Duration	Ingredient, Daily Dosage	
Carlson et al. 2013 [76]	To assess if DHA supplementation can increase maternal and newborn DHA status, gestation duration, birth weight, and length	RCT, DB, PC.	Healthy pregnant women between 8 and 20 weeks of gestation from the USA, n = 350	<20 weeks of gestation until delivery	Intervention: 3 capsules/day of a marine algae-oil source of DHA (600 mg DHA/day) Placebo: 3 capsules containing half soybean and half corn oil	Compared to placebo, DHA supplementation resulted in: (1) Longer gestation duration (2.9 day; $p = 0.041$). (2) Fewer infants born <34 weeks of gestation ($p = 0.025$). EPTB reduced by 87.5%. (3) Shorter hospital stays for PT infants (40.8 compared with 8.9 day; $p = 0.026$). (4) Similar PTB incidence between groups, with more EPTB in the placebo group (4.8% vs. 0.6%; $p = 0.025$). (5) Greater birth weight (172 g; $p = 0.004$), length (0.7 cm; $p = 0.022$), and head circumference (0.5 cm; $p = 0.012$). (6) Higher maternal and cord Red Blood Cell-phospholipid-DHA (2.6%; $p < 0.001$).	Women taking supplements <300 mg DHA/day were not excluded. Dietary n–3 LC-PUFA intakes were not assessed. Many secondary variables were studied but without adjustment for multiple comparisons. Incidence of PTB and EPTB were secondary outcomes.
Makrides et al. 2010 [77]	To assess if DHA supplementation during the last half of pregnancy has a beneficial effect on maternal depressive symptoms and child neurodevelopment	RCT, DB, PC.	Healthy pregnant women <21 weeks gestation from Australia n = 2399	<21 weeks of gestation until delivery	Intervention: 3 capsules/day of DHA-rich fish oil concentrate (800 mg DHA/day A + 100 mg EPA/day) Placebo: 3 capsules/day of vegetable oil containing a blend of rapeseed, Sunflower, and palm oil	Compared to placebo, DHA+EPA supplementation resulted in (1) No differences in the rate of women with depressive symptoms, as well as the cognitive and language composite scores of their children. (2) A small to modest increase in the duration of gestation (precise estimate of effect size could not be determined due to obstetric interventions). (3) Fewer infants born <34 weeks gestation (1.09 % vs. 2.25% adjusted Relative Risk (RR), 0.49; $p = 0.03$), and association with fewer low birth weight infants and fewer admissions to neonatal intensive care. EPTB was reduced by 51.6%.	Dietary intake of n-3 LC-PUFAs was not assessed. The study failed to demonstrate an improvement in primary outcomes such as reduction in depressive symptoms among women and improvement in cognitive and language scores of their children.
Ramakrishnan et al. 2010 [78]	To assess if prenatal DHA supplementation increases gestational age and birth size	RCT, DB, PC.	Healthy pregnant women from 18 to 22 weeks of gestation from Mexico n = 1094	From 18 to 22 weeks of gestation until delivery	Intervention: 2 capsules/day of 200 mg of DHA derived from an algal source (400 mg DHA/day) Placebo: 2 capsules/day containing olive oil	Compared to placebo, DHA supplementation resulted in (1) No differences in mean gestational age, PTB, weight, length and head circumference at birth.	

Table 1. *Cont.*

Ref.	Study				Ingredient, Daily Dosage	Main Results	Comments
	Objective	Design	Population/Sample Size	Duration			
Helland et al. 2001 [79]	To evaluate the effect of n-3 or n-6 long-chain PUFAs on birth weight, gestational length, and infant development	RCT, DB, PC.	Healthy, nulli- or primiparous women in weeks 17 to 19 of pregnancy from Norway *n* = 590	17 to 19 weeks of gestation until 3 months after delivery	Intervention: 10 mL/day of cod liver oil, providing around 2 g daily of the long chain omega-3 fatty acids. Placebo: 10 mL/day of corn oil, providing around 5 g daily of omega-6 fatty acid linoleic acid.	In comparison with placebo, cod liver oil supplementation resulted in (1) No differences in gestational length or birth weight, length or head circumference. (2) Higher concentrations of n-3 fatty acids EPA, DHA, and DHA in umbilical plasma phospholipids. (3) Neonates with high concentration of DHA in umbilical plasma phospholipids (upper quartile) had longer gestational length than those with low concentration (lower quartile; 282.5 (8.5) vs. 275.4 (9.3) days).	Substantial numbers of women excluded from the two groups post randomization due to withdrawals. It does not mention gestational lengths to facilitate undertaking of an ITT analyses. In this population, baseline intake of long-chain n-3 fatty acids was estimated to be relatively high (0.5 g/day) and less than one 1% had a PTB.
Olsen et al. 2000 [80]	To test the preventive effects of dietary n-3 fatty acids on Pre-term delivery, Intrauterine growth retardation, and pregnancy-induced hypertension	Multicenter RCT, PC (4 prophylactic + 2 therapeutic trials)	High risk pregnancies from 19 hospitals in 7 different countries in Europe. Four prophylactic trials: previous pre-term (*n* = 232), IUGR (*n* = 280), PIH (*n* = 386) and twin pregnancies (*n* = 579) Two therapeutic trials: threatening pre-eclampsia (*n* = 79) and suspected IUGR (*n* = 63)	From ~20 weeks (prophylactic trials) or 33 weeks (therapeutic trials) until delivery.	Intervention: prophylactic trials (4 capsules/day of fish oil, 1.3 g EPA and 0.9 g DHA) and therapeutic trials (9 capsules/day of fish oil, 2.9 g EPA and 2.1g DHA) (32% EPA, 23% DHA, 2 mg tocopherol/mL) Placebo: identical looking capsules of olive oil (72% oleic acid, 12% linoleic acid)	Compared to placebo, fish oil supplementation resulted in the following among women with a previous Pre-term delivery in the prophylactic trial: (1) Reduced recurrence risk of PTB from 33% to 21% (Odds Ratio (OR) 0.54 (95% Confidence Interval (CI) 0.30–0.98) (2) Reduced recurrence risk of EPTB from 13.3% to 4.6% (OR 0.32 (95% CI 0.11–0.89)). (3) Longer mean gestational length by 8.5 day (95% CI 1.9–15.2. (4) No effect on PTB in twin pregnancies.	
Onwude et al. 1995 [81]	To determine whether n-3 fatty acid (EPA/DHA) prophylaxis is beneficial in high-risk pregnancies	RCT, DB, PC.	Pregnant women at high risk of developing PIH and asymmetrical IUGR from an antenatal clinic from UK *n* = 233	From around 25 weeks of gestation until 38 weeks of gestation	Intervention: 9 capsules/day of fish oil providing 2.7 g omega-3 fatty acids/day (1.62 g of EPA and 1.08 g of DHA) Placebo: matching air-filled capsules	Compared to placebo, fish oil supplementation resulted in (1) No difference in the duration of gestation or other outcomes such as proteinuric PIH, non-proteinuric PIH, or birth weight within the lowest 3% on the growth charts.	This study failed to support the hypothesis that fish oil supplementation improved pregnancy outcome in an at risk population for impaired fetal growth or PIH.
Bulstra Ramakers et al. 1995 [82]	To study the effects of adding 3 g/day of EPA to the diet, on recurrence rate of IUGR and PIH in a high-risk population	RCT, DB, PC.	Pregnant women with a history of IUGR with or without PIH in the previous pregnancy from the Netherlands *n* = 63	From 12 to 14 weeks of gestation until delivery	Intervention: 4 capsules 3 times daily, which corresponded to a daily dose of 3 g of EPA Placebo: Identical capsules with coconut oil	Compared to placebo, EPA supplementation resulted in (1) No difference in the rates of PTB	No information was provided about content of DHA No estimate of mean gestational length was provided

Table 1. *Cont.*

Ref.	Study Objective	Study Design	Study Population/Sample Size	Duration	Ingredient, Daily Dosage	Main Results	Comments
Olsen et al. 1992 [83]	To study the effect of a fish-oil supplement, a control olive-oil supplement, and no supplementation on pregnancy duration, birthweight, and birth length	RCT	Healthy pregnant women from Denmark n = 533	From gestation week 30 until delivery	Intervention: Four 1 g fish oil capsules/day containing 2.7 g n-3 fatty acids- 32% EPA, 23% DHA, 2 mg tocopherol Placebo: Four 1 g olive oil capsules/day No supplement group	Compared to placebo fish oil supplementation when all 3 groups were compared in a single analysis (fish oil, olive oil and no supplement: 283, 279.4 and 281.7 days respectively, $p = 0.006$). (2) On an average 4 days longer pregnancies in the fish-oil group compared to the olive oil group (95% CI: 1.5–6.4, $p = 0.005$). (3) The effect seemed to depend on the baseline intake of fish. -Among those 20% of the women who had the highest intake of fish at randomization, no difference could be detected between the oil groups. -In those 20% who had the lowest intake for fish, a difference of 7.4 days was observed (95% CI 2.2–12.6 days, $p = 0.01$). -In the middle 60%, the groups differed by 4.8 days (95 CI 1.8–7.8, $p = 0.005$).	Maternal baseline dietary intake could explain differences in the duration of gestation and higher intakes may have a saturating effect
Mardones et al. 2008 [84]	To study the effect of maternal food fortification with omega-3 fatty acids and multiple micronutrients on birth weight and gestation duration	Non-blinded, RCT, PC.	Healthy pregnant women up to 20 weeks Gestation from Chile n = 972	From up to 20 weeks of gestation until delivery	Intervention: 2 kg/month of powdered milk fortified with multiple micronutrients and both α-linolenic acid and linolenic acid; iron was supplied in an amino-chelated form Placebo: 2 kg/month powdered milk fortified with small amounts of iron sulphate, copper, zinc, and vitamin C.	Based on ITT analyses and in comparison with placebo, the intervention resulted in (1) Lower incidence of EPTB (0.4% vs. 2.1%; crude OR (95% CI): 5.26 (1.08–34.90), $p = 0.02$). (2) Increase in gestation duration (1.40 days difference, 95% CI: -0.02–2.82 d, $p = 0.05$). (3) Higher mean birth weight (65.4 g difference, 95% CI: 5–126 g; $p = 0.03$). (4) Higher infant length (0.37 cm difference, 95% CI: 0.06–0.68 cm, $p = 0.019$).	Impossibility to perform a blinded design and have strict control of compliance with the prescribed amounts of the products taken to the homes of the study subjects Slight difference in gestational age at recruitment Associations with gestation duration would need a larger sample size for confirmation (the statistical power reached only 0.61 in ITT analyses)
Smuts et al. 2003 [85]	To assess whether higher intake of DHA would increase duration of gestation and birth weight in US women	RCT, DB, PC.	Healthy pregnant women between the 24th and 28th week of pregnancy from the US (predominant black population) n = 291	From 24–28 weeks of gestation until delivery	Intervention: 1 DHA enriched egg/day (133 mg DHA) Placebo: 1 ordinary egg/day (33 mg DHA)	Compared to the placebo group, the supplementation with DHA-enriched egg resulted in (1) Increased duration of gestation (6.0 ± 2.3 days, $p = 0.009$) (based on analyses adjusted for maternal BMI at enrollment and number of prior pregnancies).	The unadjusted analysis showed a difference of 2.6 days (not statistically significant), while adjustment for maternal BMI at enrollment and number of prior pregnancies resulted in an increased duration of gestation by 6 days. The adjustments may have introduced a post hoc element into the interpretation of the result.

BMI: body mass index, DHA: docosahexaenoic acid, EPA: eicosapentanoic acid, EPTB: early PTB, PTB: preterm birth, IUGR: intrauterine growth retardation, LC-PUFA: long-chain polyunsaturated fatty acids, PIH: pregnancy-induced hypertension, RCT: randomized controlled trial, DB: double blind, PC: placebo controlled.

Many factors may influence the response to supplementation and variability in outcomes observed in these trials, including variability in the dose of n−3 LC-PUFA, differences in the source of DHA, population differences in gestation duration, PTB rates and birth weight within the control arm, differences in habitual intakes of DHA from food, differences in baseline n-3 fatty acid status, and high-risk pregnancies with a history of PTB. The role of *FADS* gene variants as determinants of PUFA levels should also be considered as depending on genetic variants, requirements of dietary PUFA or LC-PUFA intakes to achieve comparable biological effects may differ [86] In the Child, parent and health: lifestyle and genetic constitution (KOALA—acronym of the Dutch title) birth cohort, both maternal DHA intake and the maternal FADS rs174556 Single Nucleotide Polymorphism (SNP) genotype were associated with pregnancy duration, and women who were homozygous for the minor allele (indicating their lower n−3 LC-PUFA interconversion and hence higher dependence on dietary supply) had significantly shorter pregnancies (2 days) [87]. In all of the trials with DHA supplementation, PTB or EPTB was never a primary outcome, but rather a secondary or safety-related outcome. Two ongoing RCTs (Assessment of DHA On Reducing Early preterm birth, ADORE and Omega-3 fats to Reduce the Incidence of Prematurity, ORIP) will examine the efficacy and safety of high dose DHA supplementation to reduce early PTB as a primary outcome (1000 mg/day and 800 mg/day DHA, respectively) [88,89].

Six meta-analyses/systematic reviews/Cochrane reviews have evaluated the effect of EPA + DHA (n-3 LC-PUFA) supplementation during pregnancy on gestation duration and risk of PTB and found that supplementing pregnant women with n−3 LC-PUFA appears to be beneficial in reducing the risk of EPTB (magnitude of the effect ranging from 26% to 61%) [90–94]. However, the clinical relevance of a minor increment in gestation duration is questionable. The most recent Cochrane systematic review of RCTs comparing omega-3 fatty acids during pregnancy with placebo or no omega-3 showed a risk reduction of 42% for EPTB (nine RCTs, 5204 participants; high-quality evidence) and 11% for PTB (26 RCTs, 10,304 participants; high-quality evidence). The mean gestational length was also greater in women who received omega-3 LC-PUFA (mean difference (MD) 1.67 days, 41 trials, 12,517 participants; moderate-quality evidence) [95]. Another recent meta-analysis (nine RCTs) demonstrated that n-3 LC-PUFA are effective at reducing the risk of EPTB by 58%, any PTB by 17%, increasing the length of gestation by 1.95 weeks and increasing birth weight by 122.1 g, and that these effects did not differ according to the risk status of women or dose or timing of the intervention [93]. Evidence from recent trials that have used DHA alone (600 mg DHA/day) [76] or DHA as the main n-3 fatty acid in terms of dose (800 mg DHA/day + 100 mg EPA/day) [77] also showed reduction of the risk of EPTB (magnitude of the effect from 51.6% to 87.5%). It also appears that higher doses of DHA (≥600 mg DHA/day) may be needed to have a protective effect, as trials providing <600 mg DHA/day have not found a reduction in EPTB, and ongoing studies will test the efficacy of doses up to 1000 mg DHA/day.

It could be hypothesized that DHA supplementation reduces the inflammation responsible for both cervical ripening and spontaneous EPTB [87] or that it increases circulating EPA through enhanced biosynthesis via retro conversion from supplemented DHA [96]. Other mechanisms may explain a lengthened duration of gestation. EPA competes with arachidonic acid (ARA), which is the source of pro-constriction mediators such as the 2-series prostaglandins E2 and F2α that can cause contraction of myometrium and cervical ripening and result in an increase the production of prostacyclins (PGI2 and PGI3), with a relaxant effect on the myometrium [70]. Omega 3 fatty acids are also thought to have an "antiarrhythmic" effect on the myometrium that may delay the initiation of labor [97]. Increased intake of marine PUFA is hypothesized to attenuate inflammation by modifying the membrane phospholipid fatty acid composition, altering the physical properties of the cell membrane such as membrane fluidity, through its effects on cell signaling pathways or by altering the pattern of the lipid mediators produced [98].

Other Macro and Micronutrients

Zinc is key for protein synthesis, cellular division, and nucleic acid metabolism [99]. Inadequate intakes (diets lacking in animal food sources rich in zinc) coupled with the limited zinc absorption (high consumption of phytate from cereals) and chronic infections result in reduced maternal plasma concentrations, resulting in reduced supply of zinc to the fetus [100,101]. Zinc deficiency alters the circulating levels of a number of hormones associated with the onset of labor such as progesterone and prolactin [100]. Zinc supplementation has been proposed to reduce the incidence or the severity of maternal infections, and thereby lower the risk of PTB [102]. A Cochrane review (16 RCTs, 7637 women) demonstrated moderate quality evidence of a small but significant 14% reduction in PTB with antenatal supplementation of zinc alone or in combination with other micronutrients compared to placebo. However, this was not accompanied by a similar reduction in the proportion of low birth weight infants or a difference in the gestational age at birth. Most of the studies included women from low- and middle-income settings who had, or were likely to have, low zinc concentrations and overall low nutritional status, making these findings particularly relevant in low-income countries with high perinatal mortality [103]. To the contrary, a more recent systematic review found no association between maternal zinc status and spontaneous PTB, however the authors expressed uncertainty on the evidence due to the heterogeneity in the studies included and the need for further studies populations at increased risk of zinc deficiency [104].

The hormonal form of vitamin D3 (1α,25-dihydroxyvitamin D3) plays a role in the mineralization of the skeleton and regulation of parathyroid hormone, and affects physiological pathways involved in PTB, including inflammation, immunomodulation, and transcription of genes involved in placental function [105]. Vitamin D deficiency in reproductive-age women is widespread and low maternal vitamin D status during pregnancy is a risk factor for various adverse birth outcomes including PTB [106]. Vitamin D is suggested to have an effect on PTB due to its immunomodulatory role and anti-inflammatory effects [107,108]. Two recent meta-analyses of observational studies have shown that vitamin D deficiency as indicated by serum 25 hydroxyvitamin D (25-OHD) levels <50 nmol/L is associated with an increased risk of PTB (by an odds of 1.25 to 1.29 times) [109,110]. Another meta-analysis of observational studies found that 25(OH) D levels >50 nmol/L was associated with longer gestation duration (difference of 0.2 week) [111]. A Cochrane review showed that supplementation with vitamin D alone versus no intervention/placebo reduced the risk of PTB by 64% (three trials and 477 women, moderate quality evidence), while supplementation with vitamin D and calcium versus no treatment/placebo significantly increased the risk of PTB (3 trials and 798 women); however, most trials included were of low methodological quality [112] Recent high quality trials such as The Maternal Vitamin D Osteoporosis Study (MAVIDOS) [113] were not included in the review; in the MAVIDOS trial PTB was reported only as a safety-related outcome but there was no effect of vitamin D supplementation on PTB.

Magnesium is key in the regulation of body temperature, synthesis of nucleic acids and proteins, and maintenance of electrical potentials in nerves and muscle membranes. Ionized and total magnesium levels are shown to decrease with increasing gestational age [114]. Insufficient magnesium intake is common in women [115] and magnesium deficiency during pregnancy is associated with a higher risk of chronic hypertension, preeclampsia, placental dysfunction and premature labor [116]. Reduced placental vascular flow is considered responsible for placental insufficiency and fetal intra-uterus growth restriction and magnesium is believed to have an immediate effect on placental vascular flow [117]. A 2001 Cochrane review (seven trials, 2689 women) reported that oral magnesium supplementation starting before 25 weeks of gestation compared to placebo was associated with a 27% reduction in risk of PTB, without any effect on gestational age at birth. However, when one of the studies that had a cluster design was excluded, there was no effect of magnesium supplementation on any of the outcomes [118]. A recent update of this review reported no significant differences in outcomes such as gestational age at birth (five trials, 5564 women) and PTB (seven trials, 5981 women) between the magnesium supplemented group and the control group [119]. Overall, both reviews reported a lack of high quality evidence. Magnesium sulphate has been used as a tocolytic agent to inhibit uterine activity in women in the setting of preterm labor with the aim of preventing PTB. However, a Cochrane review (37 trials, 3571 women), concluded that magnesium sulphate is ineffective at delaying birth or preventing PTB, has no clear benefits on neonatal and maternal outcomes and may be associated with an increased risk of fetal, neonatal, or infant mortality [120]. A multicenter double-blind, placebo-controlled randomized clinical trial of oral magnesium citrate supplementation (the BRAzil MAGnesium (BRAMAG) trial) among high-risk pregnant women starting at 12 to 20 weeks of gestation through to delivery is currently ongoing [121], with the primary perinatal outcome being a composite of PTB < 37 weeks gestation, stillbirth >20 weeks gestation, neonatal death < 28 days, or Small for Gestational Age (SGA) birthweight <3rd percentile.

Calcium plays a role in nerve cell function, muscle contraction, enzyme and hormone actions, and bone mineralization. A recent Cochrane review suggested that there are no benefits of calcium supplementation during pregnancy in reducing the risk for either PTB or EPTB. The significant heterogeneity among studies (13 trials), led the investigators to perform sub-group analyses stratified by the total dose of calcium per day (<1000 mg/day or ≥1000 mg/day), starting time of calcium supplementation (before or after 20 weeks), and type of calcium (calcium carbonate, lactate and gluconate). There were no statistically significant differences between sub-groups for either the starting time of supplementation or the type of calcium [122]. The effects of baseline calcium intake ($n = 5$ trials) and risk for hypertensive disorders of pregnancy ($n = 4$ trials) have also been studied, however, no protective effect of calcium supplementation on PTB risk reduction was observed [123]. Iron is key for oxygen transport from lungs to tissues, in energy transfer and facilitating oxygen use and storage in muscles. Iron deficiency is the most common nutrient deficiency among pregnant women and results from an increased requirement for iron during pregnancy, a diet poor in absorbable iron, and parasitic infections [124]. Folate is essential for the synthesis of nucleic acid, amino acids, phospholipids and, consequently, lipoproteins, cell division, tissue growth, and DNA methylation. Supplementation with folic acid in the immediate period before and early in pregnancy reduces the risk of neural tube defects [125]. Observational studies show that both anemia [126] and iron deficiency [127] are associated with increased risk of PTB. Recent Cochrane reviews have analyzed the efficacy of a range of interventions containing iron alone, folic acid alone or iron and folic acid together on reduction of PTB. There were no reported differences in the number of women experiencing PTB receiving supplements with iron alone versus no treatment/placebo (six trials, 1713 women) [124], folic acid alone (three trials, 2959 women) [128], daily iron and folic acid supplements versus no treatment or placebo (three trials, 1497 women), or any supplements containing iron and folic acid versus same supplements without iron nor folic acid or placebo (three trials, 1497 women) [124,128]. The studies were of low quality and used a heterogeneous definition of PTB ranging from anywhere between 36 to 38 weeks.

Vitamin A plays a role in visual function and modulation of the expression of genes involved in immune function, reproduction, tissue growth and embryonic development. Vitamin A deficiency (low serum and breast milk vitamin A concentrations) is highly prevalent among pregnant women from Asia, South Asia, and Africa [129]. Vitamin A or beta carotene supplementation during pregnancy has been shown to improve hematologic status of women by improving hemoglobin levels and reducing the risk of anemia [130]. A large trial in Nepal demonstrated that vitamin A supplementation during pregnancy was associated with a 40% reduced risk for pregnancy-related maternal mortality [131]. However, a meta-analysis reported no significant effect of vitamin A supplementation either on PTB (five studies) or EPTB (two studies) risk reduction, and only one trial among South African women reported a significant 33% reduction in the prevalence of PTB and a 66% reduction in EPTB, but this effect disappeared after excluding multiple pregnancies [130].

Sub-optimal micronutrient intakes and micronutrient deficiencies during pregnancy are a global problem and have been associated with placental oxidative stress and complications of pregnancy such as PTB and preeclampsia [100,132]. Although mechanisms linking the use of multivitamins with PTB are not fully understood, they are thought to be involved in the process of normal placentation, and deficiencies in vitamin B12 and folate have been implicated in the development of defects within the placental vascular bed [133]. Impaired placentation has been associated with recurrent PTB [134]. Results from the Danish National Birth Cohort show that peri-conceptional multivitamin use was associated with a 16% reduced risk of PTBs, with a 20% risk reduction of preterm labor in non-overweight women [135]. However, a recent Cochrane review showed no significant differences in PTB between women who were supplemented with Multiple Micronutrient (MMN) containing iron and folic acid versus those receiving iron, with or without folic acid (15 trials, 90892 women, high quality evidence). A sub-group analysis, however, showed that MMN supplementation led to significantly fewer PTB in women with a BMI <20 kg/m^2 (RR 0.85, 95% CI 0.80–0.90, $n = 4$) [136].

Balanced protein-energy supplementation (protein <25% of the total energy content) was found to reduce the risk of intrauterine growth retardation (IUGR) (23% risk reduction) [137] and was associated with modest increases in maternal weight gain (on average 21 g/week), birth weight (on average 38 g) and a substantial 32% reduction in risk of small-for-gestational-age (SGA) [137]. However, evidence from five trials with 2436 pregnant women reported a non-significant reduction in PTB with balanced protein energy supplementation (without any effect on mean gestational age), possibly related to lack of data on gestational age or problems in gestational age measurement, highlighting the need for confirmatory trials in this area [138].

3.2. Role of Probiotics in Reducing the Risk for PTB

The main rationale for intervention with probiotics stems from observational data suggesting a link between vaginal infections, dysbiosis, and PTB [139]. It is universally accepted that a certain proportion of PTB is caused by ascending infections from vagina underlying the importance of vaginal health. Moreover, it has been suggested that vaginal dysbiosis (bacterial vaginosis, BV) could trigger an inflammatory cascade leading to PTB even in the absence of ascending infection. Antibiotics such as metronidazole are the standard of care treatment for BV, but there is conflicting evidence whether such treatment results in the risk reduction of PTB [140]. The modest, at best, efficacy of antibiotics is not be surprising, because bacterial vaginosis is characterized by the absence of lactobacilli in addition to the presence of specific pathogenic organisms, and antibiotics cannot restore the depleted lactobacilli. *Lactobacillus* probiotics could fulfill this role through the production of lactic acid, lowering vaginal pH and helping to prevent the growth of potentially pathogenic microorganisms through production of hydrogen peroxide, bacteriocins, and surface-binding proteins that inhibit adhesion of pathogens. Indeed, oral or vaginal administration of probiotics have improved vaginal microbiota composition or alleviated BV in several studies [141]. In addition, and independently of maintenance of vaginal health, oral probiotics may act directly in the gut, down-modulating local and systemic inflammation [142].

3.2.1. Probiotic Intervention studies

We identified 71 publications derived from 21 individual clinical studies that described health outcomes following the administration of probiotics during pregnancy. One reported PTB as the primary outcome and four as a secondary outcome. The rest reported other outcomes informative of PTB such as the gestational age at birth or vaginal health during pregnancy. Of the 21 studies, only eight, where probiotic administration was started no later than at 12–32 weeks of gestation, were considered here (Table 2).

3.2.2. The effect of Oral Probiotics on PTB Rates

Two studies (NCT00217308 and NCT00303082), were designed to test the effect of oral administration of *Lactobacillus rhamnosus* GR-1 and *Lactobacillus reuteri* RC-14 or placebo on the incidence of BV and PTB (co-primary outcomes [143]). Both were discontinued due to difficulties with recruitment, but the partial results were published [144]. The PTB rate was 1.6% in the treatment and 3.3% in the placebo group (RR:0.495; 95% CI: 0.17,1.43; $p = 0.14$). The overall PTB rate (2.5%) was lower than the national average for Brazil (9%) [8].

The same combination of probiotics was tested in a German study [145] with BV as the primary outcome, and PTB rate reported as a secondary outcome. The investigators expected BV rates of 28–42%, but only 6% at baseline was observed, decreasing to 2.5% by the end of the study. There were no differences in BV incidence between the probiotic and placebo groups. PTB rate (4%) was lower than the national average of 9.2% [8].

PTB rates were reported as a secondary outcome in two studies testing different combinations of probiotics. *Lactobacillus rhamnosus* GG and *Bifidobacterium lactis* Bb12 were tested in Finland [146], and *Lactobacillus rhamnosus* LPR and *Bifidobacterium lactis* NCC 2818 in the Philippines [147]. Both studies found PTB rates much lower than national averages reported by WHO, 1.7% vs. 5.5% in Finland and 2.4% vs. 15% in the Philippines [8].

In all the above studies, no firm conclusions could be drawn regarding the effect of probiotics on PTB due to its lower than expected rates, but also raised questions about causes of the observed low PTB rates. The enrollment biases resulting in inadvertent exclusion of women at highest risk is the likely explanation.

Four studies in which probiotic administration was started at 24–32 weeks of pregnancy reported that the gestational age and its range did not differ between the probiotic and the placebo groups [148]. However, because direct data on PTB rates were not reported and the statistical power of the studies with regards to PTB is unknown, no conclusions on the potential effect of probiotics on PTB can be drawn from them.

A prospective cohort study conducted based on Norwegian Mother and Child Cohort Study (MoBa) examined the consumption of probiotic milk during pregnancy and concluded that the intake in early pregnancy (around 17 weeks of gestation) was associated with reduced risk of preterm birth, while late intake (around 30 weeks of gestation) was not [149,150]. The main probiotic milks available in Norway at that time contained *Lactobacillus acidophilus* LA-5, *B. lactis* Bb12, and *L. rhamnosus* GG. Regarding systematic reviews and meta-analyses, a 2007 Cochrane review on the efficacy of probiotics for preventing preterm labor [151] concluded that there were insufficient data as only one study with PTB as an outcome (not primary) was found [146]. The review was updated in 2010 with unchanged conclusions. A recent systematic review and meta-analysis which included unpublished data from previous studies concluded that there was no evidence that taking probiotics or prebiotics in pregnancy decreases the risk of preterm birth [152]. However, even though thirteen studies with 2484 participants were included, the overall PTB rate was only 3.6%. Moreover, the probiotic administration was started in early pregnancy (before 18 weeks of gestation) in only two studies. A recent Cochrane review examined the impact of probiotics on prevention of morbidity and mortality in preterm infants, and the rate of PTB [153]. The overall conclusion was that there is insufficient evidence and more research is needed. Therefore, it appears that the question about potential benefits of probiotic administration in early pregnancy remains open.

3.2.3. The Effect of Vaginal Probiotics on Outcomes Related to PTB

Stojanovic et al. 2012 [154] reported a study testing the effect of a vaginal tablet containing *Lactobacillus rhamnosus* BMX 54 on vaginal health. However, the probiotic had a favorable impact on parameters considered indicative of increased risk of PTB or miscarriage, such as the length, consistency and dilatation of the cervix, the level of the presenting part of the fetus as well as the prevalence of pathogenic microorganisms in vaginal and/or cervical swabs, lower vaginal pH, and lower vaginal discharge "whiff test" positivity. Since the study did not follow the women until delivery, and no data on PTB or other birth outcomes are available but the improvement in parameters associated with PTB was observed. Two ongoing studies in US (NCT00635622, NCT02766023), conducted in non-pregnant women, are testing the benefits of vaginal application of *Lactobacillus crispatus* CTV-05 on BV, as recent data indicate that absence of *L. crispatus*, as opposed to any lactobacilli, is most strongly correlated with adverse vaginal health outcomes [155,156].

Table 2. Characteristics, efficacy and safety of clinical trials investigating the role of probiotics in reducing risk of any preterm delivery.

Ref.	Study Objective	Design	Population/ Sample Size	Duration	Ingredient, Daily Dose	Main Results	Comments
Gille et al. 2016 [145]	To assess whether probiotic supplementation with *Lactobacillus rhamnosus* GR-1 and *Lactobacillus reuteri* RC-14 can improve maternal vaginal microbiota	RCT, DB, PC	Healthy pregnant women (first trimester) from Germany, $n = 320$, 2010–2012	8 weeks to assess Nugent scores; entire pregnancy for PTB (secondary outcome)	Capsules with 10^9 CFU, once daily	Compared to placebo, DHA supplementation resulted in No effect on vaginal microbiota (improvement in Nugent scores). No effect on PTB rates.	Low rate of preterm of 4% Very low rate of bacterial vaginosis 3%. Trend increase on miscarriages in treated (7.7% vs. 3.1%, $p = 0.08$).
Luoto et al. 2010 [146]	To assess whether dietary counselling and probiotic supplementation with (*Lactobacillus rhamnosus* GG and *Bifidobacterium lactis* Bb12) can improve pregnancy outcomes	RCT, PC 3 groups: (1) Probiotics and dietary counselling vs. (2) Placebo and dietary counselling (DB); (3) Placebo without dietary counselling (SB)	Healthy pregnant women in the first trimester from Finland, $n = 256$, late 1990s	From the first antenatal visit to the end of pregnancy	Capsules with 10^{10} CFU, once daily	Compared to placebo, probiotic supplementation resulted in 1. No effect on PTB rate 2. No effect on duration of gestation.	Very low rate of PTB: 1.7%.
Kraus Silva 2011 [143]	To assess whether probiotic supplementation with (*L. rhamnosus* GR-1 and *L. reuteri* RC-14) can reduce BV and PTB	RCT, DB, PC	Pregnant women (8 to 20 weeks gestation). With asymptomatic BV: Vaginal pH >4.5, Nugent >4 from Brazil $n = 644$ randomized, late 1990s	<20 weeks gestation to 24 or 26 weeks	Capsules with 10^9 colony-forming units each, twice daily	Compared to placebo, probiotics supplementation resulted in no effect on PTB rate. However, the PTB rates were lower with treatment (ITT: 1.6%, 5 in 304; vs. 3.3% 10 in 301).	Low rate of PTB 2.5% Low probiotics dose Exclusion criteria were very broad: previous history of PTB, hypertension, diabetes, asthma, cervical incompetence, atypical vaginal bleeding, atypical vaginal secretion, HPV, gonorrhea, syphilis, dysuria, pruritus, burning, corticotherapy, recent antibiotic therapy (within 8 weeks prior to screening)
Rautava et al. 2012 [148]	The effect of maternal administration of probiotics on atopic disease in infants.	RCT, DB, PC.	Pregnant women with atopic sensitization and either a history of or active allergic disease from Finland $n = 241$	Probiotics given to the mother 8 weeks before and 8 weeks after delivery.	(1) Dietary food supplement with *Lactobacillus rhamnosus* LPR + *Bifidobacterium longum* NCC 3001 (10^9 CFU/day) (2) Dietary food supplement with *Lactobacillus paracasei* ST11 + NCC 3001 (10^9 CFU/day) (3) Placebo	No information on preterm birth rates. Gestational age in all groups was 39 weeks with a similar range (34–41 weeks).	Not possible to draw firm conclusions about effects on preterm delivery. However, papers seems to suggest lack of effect because gestational ages were similar between groups.
Kim et al. 2010 [157]	The effect of maternal and infant administration of probiotics on atopic disease in infants	RCT, DB, PC.	Pregnant women with a family history of allergic diseases day $n = 112$, and their infants. from Korea	Probiotic was given to mothers from 8 weeks before delivery until 3 months post-delivery, then to infants from 4 months until 6 months	(1) Bifido Inc mix (*Bifidobacterium bifidum* BGN4, *Bifidobacterium lactis* AD011, *Lactobacillus acidophilus* AD030), 1.6×10^9 CFU/day each, in powder (2) Placebo powder (maltodextrin and alpha-corn)	Infants delivered before 36 weeks were excluded. No difference observed in the number of infants removed between the two groups, suggesting no difference in PTB rates. In both groups the gestational ages were around 40 weeks, and birth weights were similar.	Not possible to draw conclusions about effects on PTB. However, papers seems to suggest lack of effect.

Table 2. Cont.

Ref.	Study			Duration	Ingredient, Daily Dose	Main Results	Comments
	Objective	Design	Population/ Sample Size				
Ou et al. 2012 [158]	The effect of maternal administration of probiotics on atopic disease in infants	RCT, DB, PC	Pregnant women with atopic diseases history and Total IgE >100 kU/L from Taiwan $n = 191$	From 24 weeks gestation until delivery. After delivery, administration was exclusively to breastfeeding mothers	(1) L. *rhamnosus* GG (Valio, ATCC 53103) 10^{10} CFU/day (2) Placebo (microcrystalline cellulose)	PTB rates were not reported. However, gestational age was 39 weeks in both groups (range 31–41 weeks in the L. *rhamnosus* GG group and 35–41 weeks in placebo group), which suggests lack of efficacy on PTB rates.	The study suggests that L. *rhamnosus* GG probably has no impact on PTB rates.
Vitali et al. 2012 [159]	The effect of probiotic supplementation during late pregnancy on vaginal microbiota and cytokine secretion	Non-randomized, controlled, pilot	Healthy pregnant women with no symptoms of vaginal or urinary tract infection from Italy $n = 27$	Probiotic was given during weeks 32–37 of gestation.	(1) Probiotic group: one sachet of VSL #3 (*Lactobacillus acidophilus, Lactobacillus plantarum, Lactobacillus casei, Lactobacillus delbrueckii ssp. bulgaricus, Bifidobacterium breve, Bifidobacterium longum, Bifidobacterium infantis, S. salivaris ssp. thermophilus*) ($n = 12$) 9×10^{11} total CFU/day (2) Control group: no supplementation ($n = 12$)	PTB rates were not reported, but the gestational ages were not different between the two groups. This suggests that the probiotic did had no effect on PTB rates. No significant changes were found in the amounts of the principal vaginal bacterial populations in women administered with VSL#3, but qPCR results suggested a potential role of the probiotic product in counteracting the decrease of *Bifidobacterium* and the increase of *Atopobium*, that occurred in control women during late pregnancy. Incidence of vaginal infections was not reported.	The study is too small to draw conclusions, but it did not show any effect of VSL3 on gestational age.
Stojanovic et al. 2012 [154]	The effect of probiotics on vaginal microflora, cervical length, cervical consistency, and fetal positioning.	Observational, randomized, prospective	Pregnant women	Probiotic was administered for 12 weeks during pregnancy	(1) untreated arm of the study ($n = 30$) (2) vaginal application of one tablet containing L. *rhamnosus* BMX 54 (Normogin™ ($n = 30$) once a week	No data on PTB rates as women were not followed until delivery. Increase in pathogenic microorganisms in the vaginal and/or cervical swabs of untreated women ($p < 0.05$), also in average pH values ($p < 0.05$), amount ($p < 0.05$) and "whiff test" positivity ($p < 0.05$) of vaginal discharge. Significant trend was also found for decrease in length ($p < 0.0001$) and increase in dilatation ($p < 0.05$) of cervix, as well as for lower position of the fetus ($p < 0.0001$). In the group treated with L. *rhamnosus* BMX 54, none of these values significantly changed throughout the observation period, with the exception of cervical length that was significantly decreased at T3 ($p < 0.01$).	Cannot conclude on PTB rates. However, it suggests that vaginally administered probiotic had a positive impact on parameters associated with PTB.

CFU: colony forming unit, RCT: randomized controlled trial, DB: double blind, PC: placebo controlled.

3.2.4. Ongoing Probiotic Studies

In an ongoing study (NCT02693041), *L. rhamnosus* GG or placebo is administered orally in pregnancy starting at 17 weeks gestation, to test the hypothesis that the probiotic decreases the rate of PTB and the incidence of pre-eclampsia (PE) by affecting the inflammatory state. In addition, several registered trials (NCT02430246, NCT02692820, NCT02150655) target the treatment of bacterial vaginosis in pregnancy, all with the combination of *L rhamnosus* GR-1 and *L. reuteri* RC-14. Even though PTB prevention is not a primary outcome in these trials, one of them will report it as a secondary outcome. All trials also refer, in their scientific rationale, to PTB prevention, which could be targeted in subsequent trials once the efficacy of probiotics to decrease BV during pregnancy is proven.

4. Conclusions

Worldwide about 15 million preterm babies are born annually, and despite intensive research the specific mechanisms triggering the PTB remain unclear. An increase in the net pro-inflammatory load has been proposed as main driver of progesterone withdrawal, leading to the onset of parturition. Progesterone has been shown to be the most effective pharmacological intervention to reduce the risk of PTB in singleton pregnancies among at-risk women with a previous PTB, but most approaches tested, mainly directed at at-risk pregnancies, have not proven effective at lowering the rate of PTB, probably because the majority of cases are of unknown cause. Though great effort has been placed on early diagnosis, only a small proportion of PTB are successfully predicted using CL measurements, alone and in combination with fetal fibronectin quantification. In the absence of predictive tests that are sensitive, specific, and feasible to implement, more general approaches for primary prevention are needed. In this respect, nutritional and bioactive interventions seem a promising alternative. This review provides a comprehensive overview of the existing literature on the role of nutritional approaches to reducing the risk of PTB. The beneficial effect of n−3 LC-PUFAs (combinations of EPA and DHA) in reducing the risk of EPTB has been demonstrated in large intervention studies and several meta-analyses. Also, the role of only DHA is supported by two large RCTs. Higher doses of DHA (doses ≥600 mg DHA/day) may be needed to have a protective effect, although the optimal dosage is yet to be determined. The evidence of n−3 LC PUFA and in particular DHA appears to be quite substantial, and the two large ongoing studies should provide further clarity and confirmation as to whether DHA could be brought into clinical practice and recommended for all pregnant women or specific populations at risk. Other nutrients that may help reduce the risk of PTB include zinc (effects might be limited to populations with low overall nutritional status or poor zinc status) and vitamin D (Table 3). The emerging evidence is promising; however, larger and well-designed studies with EPTB and/or PTB as primary outcome are needed before conclusions can be drawn or recommendations made. Current data do not permit any conclusions to be drawn for the efficacy of vitamin A, calcium, iron, folic acid, iron folate, MMN, and probiotics in reducing the risk of PTB. Ongoing studies will elucidate the role of magnesium supplementation and probiotics on reducing risk for PTB. Large-scale clinical trials of promising interventions are needed to provide sound evidence-based recommendations for clinical practice. Due to the heterogeneity in the etiology of PTB, we hypothesize that differential responses to treatment will be identified. Thus, it will be important to include a sufficiently wide and deep selection of high-throughput and comprehensive analyses of the host (e.g., genomics, metabolomics) as well as gut and vaginal microbiome (metagenomics, metabolomics) to allow for the identification of subpopulations and individual responses. If successful, it will be of utmost importance to develop implementation of targeted strategies that enable both practical and affordable scaling-up to cover gaps as well as evidence-based precision nutrition in antenatal care. This is central considering that PTB is a public health problem in both high- and low-income countries.

Table 3. Nutrients with known efficacy to reduce the risk of PTB.

Nutrient	Evidence for Efficacy	Dose	Duration	Comments
n–3 LC-PUFA (combinations of EPA and DHA)	26–61% reduction in the risk of early PTB	DHA: 133 to 2100 mg DHA/day EPA: 100 to 3000 mg EPA/day	Supplementation started between 12 to 30 weeks of gestation	Eight trials supplementing either DHA or EPA alone or using varying combinations of both (five trials in healthy pregnancies and three in at-risk pregnancies), two food-based interventions and 6 meta-analyses
DHA (predominantly DHA)	51.6% to 87.5% reduction in the risk of early PTB (<34 weeks)	600 to 800 mg DHA/day	Supplementation started <20 to 21 weeks of gestation	Two large RCTs available where PTB and EPTB were secondary outcomes and not the primary outcome.
Zinc	14% reduction in PTB	5 mg/day to 44 mg/day	Supplementations started from as early as before conception (one study) to at least starting before 26 weeks	Most studies were conducted in low income countries among women with poor nutritional status and likely to have low zinc concentrations. The reduction in PTB was not accompanied by reduction in LBW or a difference in the gestational age at birth.
Vitamin D	64% reduction in PTB	400 to 1000 IU/day (two trials), 60000–12000 IU (depending on baseline serum 25 (OH)D (one trial) cholecalciferol D3	Supplementation started between 20–30 weeks of gestation	The trials available were all of low quality.

DHA: docosahexaenoic acid, EPA: eicosapentanoic acid, EPTB: early PTB, PTB: preterm Birth, LBW: low birth weight.

Author Contributions: Conceptualization, T.M.S., O.S., I.S.-Z.; Investigation, T.M.S., O.S., K.M., I.S.-Z.; Original draft preparation, T.M.S., O.S., K.M., I.S.-Z.; Methodology, T.M.S., O.S.; Supervision, G.C.B., K.M.G., I.S.-Z.; critical appraisal, G.C.B. and K.M.G.; writing—review and editing, all authors.

Funding: This research received no specific funding either public or commercial.

Conflicts of Interest: T.M.S., O.S., K.M., I.S.Z. are employees of Société des Produits Nestlé SA (SPN). K.M.G. has received reimbursement for speaking at conferences sponsored by companies selling nutritional products, and is part of an academic consortium that has received research funding from Abbott Nutrition, Nestec and Danone. K.M.G. is supported by the UK Medical Research Council (MC_UU_12011/4), the National Institute for Health Research (NIHR Senior Investigator (NF-SI-0515-10042), NIHR Southampton 1000Days Plus Global Nutrition Research Group) and NIHR Southampton Biomedical Research Centre), the European Union (Erasmus+ Programme Early Nutrition eAcademy Southeast Asia-573651-EPP-1-2016-1-DE-EPPKA2-CBHE-JP), the US National Institute On Aging of the National Institutes of Health (Award No. U24AG047867), and the UK ESRC and BBSRC (Award No. ES/M00919X/1). GCB declares that there is no conflict of interest with this article.

References

1. Blencowe, H.; Cousens, S.; Chou, D.; Oestergaard, M.; Say, L.; Moller, A.B.; Kinney, M.; Lawn, J. Born Too Soon: The global epidemiology of 15 million preterm births. *Reprod. Health* **2013**, *10*, S2. [CrossRef] [PubMed]
2. Liu, L.; Johnson, H.L.; Cousens, S.; Perin, J.; Scott, S.; Lawn, J.E.; Rudan, I.; Campbell, H.; Cibulskis, R.; Li, M.; et al. Global, regional, and national causes of child mortality: An updated systematic analysis for 2010 with time trends since 2000. *Lancet* **2012**, *379*, 2151–2161. [CrossRef]
3. Raju, T.N.K.; Pemberton, V.L.; Saigal, S.; Blaisdell, C.J.; Moxey-Mims, M.; Buist, S. Long-Term Healthcare Outcomes of Preterm Birth: An Executive Summary of a Conference Sponsored by the National Institutes of Health. *J. Pediatr.* **2017**, *181*, 309–318. [CrossRef] [PubMed]
4. Luu, T.M.; Rehman Mian, M.O.; Nuyt, A.M. Long-Term Impact of Preterm Birth: Neurodevelopmental and Physical Health Outcomes. *Clin. Perinatol.* **2017**, *44*, 305–314. [CrossRef] [PubMed]
5. Jacob, J.; Lehne, M.; Mischker, A.; Klinger, N.; Zickermann, C.; Walker, J. Cost effects of preterm birth: A comparison of health care costs associated with early preterm, late preterm, and full-term birth in the first 3 years after birth. *Eur. J. Health* **2016**, *18*, 1041–1046. [CrossRef]
6. Heinonen, K.; Eriksson, J.G.; Kajantie, E.; Pesonen, A.K.; Barker, D.J.; Osmond, C.; Räikkönen, K. Late-Preterm Birth and Lifetime Socioeconomic Attainments: The Helsinki Birth Cohort Study. *Pediatrics* **2013**, *132*, 647–655. [CrossRef] [PubMed]

7. Chawanpaiboon, S.; Vogel, J.P.; Moller, A.-B.; Lumbiganon, P.; Petzold, M.; Hogan, D.; Landoulsi, S.; Jampathong, N.; Kongwattanakul, K.; Laopaiboon, M.; et al. Global, regional, and national estimates of levels of preterm birth in 2014, a systematic review and modelling analysis. *Lancet Glob. Health* **2018**, *7*, e37–e46. [CrossRef]

8. Blencowe, H.; Cousens, S.; Oestergaard, M.Z.; Chou, D.; Moller, A.B.; Narwal, R.; Adler, A.; Garcia, C.V.; Rohde, S.; Say, L.; et al. National, regional, and worldwide estimates of preterm birth rates in the year 2010 with time trends since 1990 for selected countries: A systematic analysis and implications. *Lancet* **2012**, *379*, 2162–2172. [CrossRef]

9. Van Zijl, M.D.; Koullali, B.; Mol, B.W.; Pajkrt, E.; Oudijk, M.A. Prevention of preterm delivery: Current challenges and future prospects. *Int. J. Womens Health* **2016**, *8*, 633–645. [CrossRef]

10. Leader, J.; Bajwa, A.; Lanes, A.; Hua, X.; White, R.R.; Rybak, N.; Walker, M. The Effect of Very Advanced Maternal Age on Maternal and Neonatal Outcomes: A Systematic Review. *J. Obstet. Gynaecol. Can.* **2018**, *40*, 1208–1218. [CrossRef]

11. Mayo, J.A.; Shachar, B.Z.; Stevenson, D.K.; Shaw, G.M. Nulliparous teenagers and preterm birth in California. *J. Périnat. Med.* **2017**, *45*, 959–967. [CrossRef] [PubMed]

12. Fuchs, F.; Senat, M.V. Multiple gestations and preterm birth. *Semin. Fetal Neonatal Med.* **2016**, *21*, 113–120. [CrossRef] [PubMed]

13. Berghella, V. Universal Cervical Length Screening for Prediction and Prevention of Preterm Birth. *Obstet. Gynecol. Surv.* **2012**, *67*, 653–657. [CrossRef] [PubMed]

14. Kyrgiou, M.; Koliopoulos, G.; Martin-Hirsch, P.; Arbyn, M.; Prendiville, W.; Paraskevaidis, E. Obstetric outcomes after conservative treatment for intraepithelial or early invasive cervical lesions: Systematic review and meta-analysis. *Lancet* **2006**, *367*, 489–498. [CrossRef]

15. Lemmers, M.; Verschoor, M.A.; Hooker, A.B.; Opmeer, B.C.; Limpens, J.; Huirne, J.A.; Ankum, W.M.; Mol, B.W. Dilatation and curettage increases the risk of subsequent preterm birth: A systematic review and meta-analysis. *Hum. Reprod. (Oxf. Engl.)* **2016**, *31*, 34–45. [CrossRef] [PubMed]

16. Smid, M.C.; Lee, J.H.; Grant, J.H.; Miles, G.; Stoddard, G.J.; Chapman, D.A.; Manuck, T.A. Maternal race and intergenerational preterm birth recurrence. *Am. J. Obstet. Gynecol.* **2017**, *217*, 480.e1–480.e9. [CrossRef] [PubMed]

17. Manuck, T.A. The genomics of prematurity in an era of more precise clinical phenotyping: A review. *Semin. Fetal Neonatal Med.* **2016**, *21*, 89–93. [CrossRef] [PubMed]

18. Strauss, J.F., 3rd; Romero, R.; Gomez-Lopez, N.; Haymond-Thornburg, H.; Modi, B.P.; Teves, M.E.; Pearson, L.N.; York, T.P.; Schenkein, H.A. Spontaneous Preterm Birth: Advances Toward the Discovery of Genetic Predisposition. *Am. J. Obstet. Gynecol.* **2017**, *218*, 294–314. [CrossRef] [PubMed]

19. Manuck, T.A. Racial and ethnic differences in preterm birth: A complex, multifactorial problem. *Semin. Perinatol.* **2017**, *41*, 511–518. [CrossRef]

20. Zhang, G.; Feenstra, B.; Bacelis, J.; Liu, X.; Muglia, L.M.; Juodakis, J.; Miller, D.E.; Litterman, N.; Jiang, P.P.; Russell, L.; et al. Genetic Associations with Gestational Duration and Spontaneous Preterm Birth. *N. Engl. J. Med.* **2017**, *377*, 1156–1167. [CrossRef]

21. Jarde, A.; Morais, M.; Kingston, D.; Giallo, R.; MacQueen, G.M.; Giglia, L.; Beyene, J.; Wang, Y.; McDonald, S.D. Neonatal Outcomes in Women With Untreated Antenatal Depression Compared With Women Without Depression. *JAMA Psychiatry* **2016**, *73*, 826–837. [CrossRef] [PubMed]

22. Rubens, C.E.; Sadovsky, Y.; Muglia, L.; Gravett, M.G.; Lackritz, E.; Gravett, C. Prevention of preterm birth: Harnessing science to address the global epidemic. *Sci. Transl. Med.* **2014**, *6*, 262sr5. [CrossRef] [PubMed]

23. Frey, H.A.; Klebanoff, M.A. The epidemiology, etiology, and costs of preterm birth. *Semin. Fetal Neonatal Med.* **2016**, *21*, 68–73. [CrossRef] [PubMed]

24. Nijman, T.A.; van Vliet, E.O.; Benders, M.J.; Mol, B.W.; Franx, A.; Nikkels, P.G.; Oudijk, M.A. Placental histology in spontaneous and indicated preterm birth: A case control study. *Placenta* **2016**, *48*, 56–62. [CrossRef] [PubMed]

25. Norman, S.M.; Odibo, A.O.; Macones, G.A.; Dicke, J.M.; Crane, J.P.; Cahill, A.G. Ultrasound-detected subchorionic hemorrhage and the obstetric implications. *Obstet. Gynecol.* **2010**, *116*, 311–315. [CrossRef] [PubMed]

26. Nagy, S.; Bush, M.; Stone, J.; Lapinski, R.H.; Gardo, S. Clinical significance of subchorionic and retroplacental hematomas detected in the first trimester of pregnancy. *Obstet. Gynecol.* **2003**, *102*, 94–100. [PubMed]

27. Vink, J.; Feltovich, H. Cervical etiology of spontaneous preterm birth. *Semin. Fetal Neonatal Med.* **2016**, *21*, 106–112. [CrossRef] [PubMed]

28. Staneva, A.; Bogossian, F.; Pritchard, M.; Wittkowski, A. The effects of maternal depression, anxiety, and perceived stress during pregnancy on preterm birth: A systematic review. *Women Birth* **2015**, *28*, 179–193. [CrossRef]

29. Robinson, B.G.; Emanuel, R.L.; Frim, D.M.; Majzoub, J.A. Glucocorticoid stimulates expression of corticotropin-releasing hormone gene in human placenta. *Proc. Natl. Acad. Sci. USA* **1988**, *85*, 5244–5248. [CrossRef]

30. Howland, M.A.; Sandman, C.A.; Glynn, L.M.; Crippen, C.; Davis, E.P. Fetal exposure to placental corticotropin-releasing hormone is associated with child self-reported internalizing symptoms. *Psychoneuroendocrinology* **2016**, *67*, 10–17. [CrossRef]

31. Sun, K.; Ma, R.; Cui, X.; Campos, B.; Webster, R.; Brockman, D.; Myatt, L. Glucocorticoids Induce Cytosolic Phospholipase A2 and Prostaglandin H Synthase Type 2 But Not Microsomal Prostaglandin E Synthase (PGES) and Cytosolic PGES Expression in Cultured Primary Human Amnion Cells. *J. Clin. Endocrinol. Metab.* **2003**, *88*, 5564–5571. [CrossRef] [PubMed]

32. Zhu, X.O.; Yang, Z.; Guo, C.M.; Ni, X.T.; Li, J.N.; Ge, Y.C.; Myatt, L.; Sun, K. Paradoxical stimulation of cyclooxygenase-2 expression by glucocorticoids via a cyclic AMP response element in human amnion fibroblasts. *Mol. Endocrinol.* **2009**, *23*, 1839–1849. [CrossRef] [PubMed]

33. Dunn, A.B.; Dunlop, A.L.; Hogue, C.J.; Miller, A.; Corwin, E.J. The Microbiome and Complement Activation: A Mechanistic Model for Preterm Birth. *Boil. Res. Nurs.* **2017**, *19*, 295–307. [CrossRef] [PubMed]

34. Romero, R.; Dey, S.K.; Fisher, S.J. Preterm Labor: One Syndrome, Many Causes. *Science* **2014**, *345*, 760–765. [CrossRef] [PubMed]

35. Kim, C.J.; Romero, R.; Chaemsaithong, P.; Chaiyasit, N.; Yoon, B.H.; Kim, Y.M. Acute chorioamnionitis and funisitis: Definition, pathologic features, and clinical significance. *Am. J. Obstet. Gynecol.* **2015**, *213*, S29–S52. [CrossRef] [PubMed]

36. Cappelletti, M.; Della Bella, S.; Ferrazzi, E.; Mavilio, D.; Divanovic, S. Inflammation and preterm birth. *J. Leukoc. Biol.* **2016**, *99*, 67–78. [CrossRef] [PubMed]

37. Romero, R.; Chaiworapongsa, T.; Alpay Savasan, Z.; Xu, Y.; Hussein, Y.; Dong, Z.; Kusanovic, J.P.; Kim, C.J.; Hassan, S.S. Damage-associated molecular patterns (DAMPs) in preterm labor with intact membranes and preterm PROM: A study of the alarmin HMGB1. *J. Matern. Fetal Neonatal Med.* **2011**, *24*, 1444–1455. [CrossRef] [PubMed]

38. Goldenberg, R.L.; Culhane, J.F.; Iams, J.D.; Romero, R. Epidemiology and causes of preterm birth. *Lancet* **2008**, *371*, 75–84. [CrossRef]

39. Lannon, S.M.R.; Vanderhoeven, J.P.; Eschenbach, D.A.; Gravett, M.G.; Waldorf, K.M.A. Synergy and Interactions Among Biological Pathways Leading to Preterm Premature Rupture of Membranes. *Reprod. Sci.* **2014**, *21*, 1215–1227. [CrossRef]

40. Norwitz, E.R.; Bonney, E.A.; Snegovskikh, V.V.; Williams, M.A.; Phillippe, M.; Park, J.S.; Abrahams, V.M. Molecular Regulation of Parturition: The Role of the Decidual Clock. *Cold Spring Harb. Perspect. Med.* **2015**, *5*, a023143. [CrossRef]

41. Menon, R.; Bonney, E.A.; Condon, J.; Mesiano, S.; Taylor, R.N. Novel concepts on pregnancy clocks and alarms: Redundancy and synergy in human parturition. *Hum. Reprod. Updat.* **2016**, *22*, 535–560. [CrossRef] [PubMed]

42. Navathe, R.; Berghella, V. Tocolysis for Acute Preterm Labor: Where Have We Been, Where Are We Now, and Where are We Going? *Am. J. Perinatol.* **2016**, *33*, 229–235. [PubMed]

43. Son, M.; Miller, E.S. Predicting preterm birth: Cervical length and fetal fibronectin. *Semin. Perinatol.* **2017**, *41*, 445–451. [CrossRef] [PubMed]

44. Koullali, B.; Oudijk, M.A.; Nijman, T.A.; Mol, B.W.; Pajkrt, E. Risk assessment and management to prevent preterm birth. *Semin. Fetal Neonatal Med.* **2016**, *21*, 80–88. [CrossRef] [PubMed]

45. Romero, R.; Conde-Agudelo, A.; El-Refaie, W.; Rode, L.; Brizot, M.L.; Cetingoz, E.; Serra, V.; Da Fonseca, E.; Abdelhafez, M.S.; Tabor, A.; et al. Vaginal progesterone decreases preterm birth and neonatal morbidity and mortality in women with a twin gestation and a short cervix: An updated meta-analysis of individual patient data. *Ultrasound Obstet. Gynecol.* **2017**, *49*, 303–314. [CrossRef]

46.   Romero, R.; Nicolaides, K.H.; Conde-Agudelo, A.; O'Brien, J.M.; Cetingoz, E.; Da Fonseca, E.; Creasy, G.W.; Hassan, S.S. Vaginal progesterone decreases preterm birth birth </=34 weeks of gestation in women with a singleton pregnancy and a short cervix: an updated meta-analysis including data from the OPPTIMUM study. *Ultrasound Obstet. Gynecol.* **2016**, *48*, 308–317. [CrossRef] [PubMed]

47.   Jarde, A.; Lutsiv, O.; Beyene, J.; McDonald, S.D. Vaginal progesterone, oral progesterone, 17-OHPC, cerclage and pessary for preventing preterm birth in singleton pregnancies: An updated systematic review and network meta-analysis. *BJOG Int. J. Obstet. Gynaecol.* **2019**, *126*, 556–567. [CrossRef]

48.   Jarde, A.; Lutsiv, O.; Park, C.K.; Beyene, J.; Dodd, J.M.; Barrett, J.; Shah, P.S.; Cook, J.L.; Saito, S.; Biringer, A.B.; et al.   Effectiveness of progesterone, cerclage and pessary for preventing preterm birth in singleton pregnancies: A systematic review and network meta-analysis. *BJOG Int. J. Obstet. Gynaecol.* **2017**, *124*, 1176–1189. [CrossRef]

49.   Newnham, J.P.; Kemp, M.W.; White, S.W.; Arrese, C.A.; Hart, R.J.; Keelan, J.A. Applying Precision Public Health to Prevent Preterm Birth. *Front. Public Health* **2017**, *5*, 66. [CrossRef]

50.   Bloomfield, F.H. How is maternal nutrition related to preterm birth? *Annu. Rev. Nutr.* **2011**, *31*, 235–261. [CrossRef]

51.   Romero, R.; Espinoza, J.; Goncalves, L.F.; Kusanovic, J.P.; Friel, L.; Hassan, S. The role of inflammation and infection in preterm birth. *Semin. Reprod. Med.* **2007**, *25*, 21–39. [CrossRef] [PubMed]

52.   Englund-Ögge, L.; Brantsæter, A.L.; Haugen, M.; Sengpiel, V.; Khatibi, A.; Myhre, R.; Myking, S.; Meltzer, H.M.; Kacerovsky, M.; Nilsen, R.M.; et al. Association between intake of artificially sweetened and sugar-sweetened beverages and preterm delivery: A large prospective cohort study123. *Am. J. Clin. Nutr.* **2012**, *96*, 552–559. [CrossRef] [PubMed]

53.   Englund-Ögge, L.; Birgisdóttir, B.E.; Sengpiel, V.; Brantsæter, A.L.; Haugen, M.; Myhre, R.; Meltzer, H.M.; Jacobsson, B. Meal frequency patterns and glycemic properties of maternal diet in relation to preterm delivery: Results from a large prospective cohort study. *PLoS ONE* **2017**, *12*, e0172896. [CrossRef] [PubMed]

54.   Englund-Ögge, L.; Brantsæter, A.L.; Sengpiel, V.; Haugen, M.; Birgisdottir, B.E.; Myhre, R.; Meltzer, H.M.; Jacobsson, B. Maternal dietary patterns and preterm delivery: Results from large prospective cohort study. *BMJ* **2014**, *348*, g1446. [CrossRef] [PubMed]

55.   Mikkelsen, T.B.; Osterdal, M.L.; Knudsen, V.K.; Haugen, M.; Meltzer, H.M.; Bakketeig, L.; Olsen, S.F. Association between a Mediterranean-type diet and risk of preterm birth among Danish women: A prospective cohort study. *Acta Obstet. Gynecol. Scand.* **2008**, *87*, 325–330. [CrossRef] [PubMed]

56.   Saunders, L.; Guldner, L.; Costet, N.; Kadhel, P.; Rouget, F.; Monfort, C.; Thomé, J.-P.; Multigner, L.; Cordier, S. Effect of a Mediterranean Diet during Pregnancy on Fetal Growth and Preterm Delivery: Results From a French Caribbean Mother-Child Cohort Study (TIMOUN). *Paediatr. Périnat. Epidemiol.* **2014**, *28*, 235–244. [CrossRef] [PubMed]

57.   Khoury, J.; Henriksen, T.; Christophersen, B.; Tonstad, S. Effect of a cholesterol-lowering diet on maternal, cord, and neonatal lipids, and pregnancy outcome: A randomized clinical trial. *Am. J. Obstet. Gynecol.* **2005**, *193*, 1292–1301. [CrossRef] [PubMed]

58.   Haugen, M.; Meltzer, H.M.; Brantsaeter, A.L.; Mikkelsen, T.; Osterdal, M.L.; Alexander, J.; Olsen, S.F.; Bakketeig, L. Mediterranean-type diet and risk of preterm birth among women in the Norwegian Mother and Child Cohort Study (MoBa): A prospective cohort study. *Acta Obstet. Gynecol. Scand.* **2008**, *87*, 319–324. [CrossRef]

59.   Position of the American Dietetic Association and Dietitians of Canada: Vegetarian diets. *J. Am. Diet. Assoc.* **2003**, *103*, 748–765. [CrossRef]

60.   Burdge, G.C.; Tan, S.Y.; Henry, C.J. Long-chain n-3 PUFA in vegetarian women: A metabolic perspective. *J. Nutr. Sci.* **2017**, *6*, e58. [CrossRef]

61.   Rogne, T.; Tielemans, M.J.; Chong, M.F.; Yajnik, C.S.; Krishnaveni, G.V.; Poston, L.; Jaddoe, V.W.; Steegers, E.A.; Joshi, S.; Chong, Y.S.; et al. Associations of Maternal Vitamin B12 Concentration in Pregnancy With the Risks of Preterm Birth and Low Birth Weight: A Systematic Review and Meta-Analysis of Individual Participant Data. *Am. J. Epidemiol.* **2017**, *185*, 212–223. [CrossRef] [PubMed]

62.   Raghavan, R.; Dreibelbis, C.; Kingshipp, B.L.; Wong, Y.P.; Abrams, B.; Gernand, A.D.; Rasmussen, K.M.; Siega-Riz, A.M.; Stang, J.O.; Casavale, K.; et al. Dietary patterns before and during pregnancy and birth outcomes: A systematic review. *Am. J. Clin. Nutr.* **2019**, *109*, 729S–756S. [CrossRef] [PubMed]

63. Chia, A.R.; Chen, L.W.; Lai, J.S.; Wong, C.H.; Neelakantan, N.; Van Dam, R.M.; Chong, M.F.F. Maternal Dietary Patterns and Birth Outcomes: A Systematic Review and Meta-Analysis. *Adv. Nutr.* **2019**, *10*, 685–695. [CrossRef] [PubMed]

64. Kibret, K.T.; Chojenta, C.; Gresham, E.; Tegegne, T.K.; Loxton, D. Maternal dietary patterns and risk of adverse pregnancy (hypertensive disorders of pregnancy and gestational diabetes mellitus) and birth (preterm birth and low birth weight) outcomes: A systematic review and meta-analysis. *Public Health Nutr.* **2018**, *22*, 506–520. [CrossRef] [PubMed]

65. Burdge, G.C.; Calder, P.C. Conversion of alpha-linolenic acid to longer-chain polyunsaturated fatty acids in human adults. *Reprod. Nutr. Dev.* **2005**, *45*, 581–597. [CrossRef] [PubMed]

66. Burdge, G.C.; Jones, A.E.; Wootton, S.A. Eicosapentaenoic and docosapentaenoic acids are the principal products of α-linolenic acid metabolism in young men. *Br. J. Nutr.* **2002**, *88*, 355–363. [CrossRef] [PubMed]

67. Baker, E.J.; Miles, E.A.; Burdge, G.C.; Yaqoob, P.; Calder, P.C. Metabolism and functional effects of plant-derived omega-3 fatty acids in humans. *Prog. Lipid Res.* **2016**, *64*, 30–56. [CrossRef] [PubMed]

68. Papanikolaou, Y.; Brooks, J.; Reider, C.; Fulgoni, V.L., 3rd. U.S. adults are not meeting recommended levels for fish and omega-3 fatty acid intake: Results of an analysis using observational data from NHANES 2003–2008. *Nutr. J.* **2014**, *13*, 31. [CrossRef]

69. Kuriki, K.; Nagaya, T.; Imaeda, N.; Tokudome, Y.; Fujiwara, N.; Sato, J.; Ikeda, M.; Maki, S.; Tokudome, S. Discrepancies in dietary intakes and plasma concentrations of fatty acids according to age among Japanese female dietitians. *Eur. J. Clin. Nutr.* **2002**, *56*, 524–531. [CrossRef]

70. Olsen, S.F.; Hansen, H.S.; Sorensen, T.I.; Jensen, B.; Secher, N.J.; Sommer, S.; Knudsen, L.B. Intake of marine fat, rich in (n-3)-polyunsaturated fatty acids, may increase birthweight by prolonging gestation. *Lancet (Lond. Engl.)* **1986**, *2*, 367–369. [CrossRef]

71. Olsen, S.F.; Østerdal, M.L.; Salvig, J.D.; Kesmodel, U.; Henriksen, T.B.; Hedegaard, M.; Secher, N.J. Duration of pregnancy in relation to seafood intake during early and mid pregnancy: Prospective cohort. *Eur. J. Epidemiol.* **2006**, *21*, 749–758. [CrossRef] [PubMed]

72. Brantsæter, A.L.; Englund-Ögge, L.; Haugen, M.; Birgisdottir, B.E.; Knutsen, H.K.; Sengpiel, V.; Myhre, R.; Alexander, J.; Nilsen, R.M.; Jacobsson, B.; et al. Maternal intake of seafood and supplementary long chain n-3 poly-unsaturated fatty acids and preterm delivery. *BMC Pregnancy Childbirth* **2017**, *17*, 61.

73. Olsen, S.F.; Secher, N.J. Low Consumption of Seafood in Early Pregnancy as a Risk Factor for Preterm Delivery: Prospective Cohort Study. *Obstet. Gynecol. Surv.* **2002**, *57*, 651–652. [CrossRef]

74. Oken, E.; Kleinman, K.P.; Olsen, S.F.; Rich-Edwards, J.W.; Gillman, M.W. Associations of Seafood and Elongated n-3 Fatty Acid Intake with Fetal Growth and Length of Gestation: Results from a US Pregnancy Cohort. *Am. J. Epidemiol.* **2004**, *160*, 774–783. [CrossRef] [PubMed]

75. Rogers, I.; Emmett, P.; Ness, A.; Golding, J. Maternal fish intake in late pregnancy and the frequency of low birth weight and intrauterine growth retardation in a cohort of British infants. *J. Epidemiol. Community Health* **2004**, *58*, 486–492. [CrossRef] [PubMed]

76. Carlson, S.E.; Colombo, J.; Gajewski, B.J.; Gustafson, K.M.; Mundy, D.; Yeast, J.; Georgieff, M.K.; Markley, L.A.; Kerling, E.H.; Shaddy, D.J. DHA supplementation and pregnancy outcomes. *Am. J. Clin. Nutr.* **2013**, *97*, 808–815. [CrossRef] [PubMed]

77. Makrides, M.; Gibson, R.A.; McPhee, A.J.; Yelland, L.; Quinlivan, J.; Ryan, P. Effect of DHA supplementation during pregnancy on maternal depression and neurodevelopment of young children: A randomized controlled trial. *JAMA* **2010**, *304*, 1675–1683. [CrossRef] [PubMed]

78. Ramakrishnan, U.; Stein, A.D.; Parra-Cabrera, S.; Wang, M.; Imhoff-Kunsch, B.; Juarez-Marquez, S.; Rivera, J.; Martorell, R. Effects of docosahexaenoic acid supplementation during pregnancy on gestational age and size at birth: Randomized, double-blind, placebo-controlled trial in Mexico. *Food Nutr. Bull.* **2010**, *31*, S108–S116. [CrossRef]

79. Helland, I.B.; Saugstad, O.D.; Smith, L.; Saarem, K.; Solvoll, K.; Ganes, T.; Drevon, C.A. Similar Effects on Infants of n-3 and n-6 Fatty Acids Supplementation to Pregnant and Lactating Women. *Pediatrics* **2001**, *108*, e82. [CrossRef]

80. Olsen, S.F.; Secher, N.J.; Tabor, A.; Weber, T.; Walker, J.J.; Gluud, C. Randomised clinical trials of fish oil supplementation in high risk pregnancies. Fish Oil Trials in Pregnancy (FOTIP) Team. *BJOG Int. J. Obstet. Gynaecol.* **2000**, *107*, 382–395. [CrossRef]
81. Onwude, J.L.; Lilford, R.J.; Hjartardottir, H.; Staines, A.; Tuffnell, D. A randomised double blind placebo controlled trial of fish oil in high risk pregnancy. *BJOG: Int. J. Obstet. Gynaecol.* **1995**, *102*, 95–100. [CrossRef] [PubMed]
82. Huisjes, H.J.; Visser, G.H.A.; Bulstra-Ramakers, M.T.E.W.; Bulstra-Ramakers, M.T.E.W. The effects of 3g eicosapentaenoic acid daily on recurrence of intrauterine growth retardation and pregnancy induced hypertension. *BJOG: Int. J. Obstet. Gynaecol.* **1995**, *102*, 123–126.
83. Olsen, S.; Sorensen, J.; Secher, N.; Hedegaard, M.; Henriksen, T.; Hansen, H.; Grant, A. Randomised controlled trial of effect of fish-oil supplementation on pregnancy duration. *Int. J. Gynecol. Obstet.* **1992**, *39*, 365–366. [CrossRef]
84. Mardones, F.; Urrutia, M.T.; Villarroel, L.; Rioseco, A.; Castillo, O.; Rozowski, J.; Tapia, J.L.; Bastias, G.; Bacallao, J.; Rojas, I. Effects of a dairy product fortified with multiple micronutrients and omega-3 fatty acids on birth weight and gestation duration in pregnant Chilean women. *Public Health Nutr.* **2008**, *11*, 30–40. [CrossRef] [PubMed]
85. Smuts, C.M.; Huang, M.; Mundy, D.; Plasse, T.; Major, S.; Carlson, S.E. A randomized trial of docosahexaenoic acid supplementation during the third trimester of pregnancy. *Obstet. Gynecol.* **2003**, *101*, 469–479. [PubMed]
86. Glaser, C.; Heinrich, J.; Koletzko, B. Role of FADS1 and FADS2 polymorphisms in polyunsaturated fatty acid metabolism. *Metabolism* **2010**, *59*, 993–999. [CrossRef] [PubMed]
87. Moltó-Puigmartí, C.; Van Dongen, M.C.J.M.; Dagnelie, P.C.; Plat, J.; Mensink, R.P.; Tan, F.E.S.; Heinrich, J.; Thijs, C. Maternal but Not Fetal FADS Gene Variants Modify the Association between Maternal Long-Chain PUFA Intake in Pregnancy and Birth Weight. *J. Nutr.* **2014**, *144*, 1430–1437. [CrossRef] [PubMed]
88. Carlson, S.E.; Gajewski, B.J.; Valentine, C.J.; Rogers, L.K.; Weiner, C.P.; DeFranco, E.A.; Buhimschi, C.S. Assessment of DHA on reducing early preterm birth: The ADORE randomized controlled trial protocol. *BMC Pregnancy Childbirth* **2017**, *17*, 62. [CrossRef]
89. Zhou, S.J.; Best, K.; Gibson, R.; McPhee, A.; Yelland, L.; Quinlivan, J.; Makrides, M. Study protocol for a randomised controlled trial evaluating the effect of prenatal omega-3 LCPUFA supplementation to reduce the incidence of preterm birth: The ORIP trial. *BMJ Open* **2017**, *7*, e018360. [CrossRef]
90. Briggs, V.; Goldenberg, T.; Ramakrishnan, U.; Imhoff-Kunsch, B.; Imhoff-Kunsch, B. Effect of n-3 Long-chain Polyunsaturated Fatty Acid Intake during Pregnancy on Maternal, Infant, and Child Health Outcomes: A Systematic Review. *Paediatr. Périnat. Epidemiol.* **2012**, *26*, 91–107.
91. Szajewska, H.; Horvath, A.; Koletzko, B. Effect of n-3 long-chain polyunsaturated fatty acid supplementation of women with low-risk pregnancies on pregnancy outcomes and growth measures at birth: A meta-analysis of randomized controlled trials. *Am. J. Clin. Nutr.* **2006**, *83*, 1337–1344. [CrossRef] [PubMed]
92. Makrides, M.; Duley, L.; Olsen, S.F. Marine oil, and other prostaglandin precursor, supplementation for pregnancy uncomplicated by pre-eclampsia or intrauterine growth restriction. *Cochrane Database Syst. Rev.* **2006**, *3*, CD003402. [CrossRef] [PubMed]
93. Horvath, A.; Koletzko, B.; Szajewska, H. Effect of supplementation of women in high-risk pregnancies with long-chain polyunsaturated fatty acids on pregnancy outcomes and growth measures at birth: A meta-analysis of randomized controlled trials. *Br. J. Nutr.* **2007**, *98*, 253–259. [CrossRef] [PubMed]
94. Kar, S.; Wong, M.; Rogozinska, E.; Thangaratinam, S. Effects of omega-3 fatty acids in prevention of early preterm delivery: A systematic review and meta-analysis of randomized studies. *Eur. J. Obstet. Gynecol. Reprod. Biol.* **2016**, *198*, 40–46. [CrossRef] [PubMed]
95. Middleton, P.; Gomersall, J.C.; Gould, J.F.; Shepherd, E.; Olsen, S.F.; Makrides, M. Omega-3 fatty acid addition during pregnancy. *Cochrane Database Syst. Rev.* **2018**, *11*, CD003402. [CrossRef] [PubMed]
96. Park, H.G.; Lawrence, P.; Engel, M.G.; Kothapalli, K.; Brenna, J.T. Metabolic fate of docosahexaenoic acid (DHA; 22:6n-3) in human cells: Direct retroconversion of DHA to eicosapentaenoic acid (20:5n-3) dominates over elongation to tetracosahexaenoic acid (24:6n-3). *FEBS Lett.* **2016**, *590*, 3188–3194. [CrossRef] [PubMed]
97. Olsen, S.F.; Secher, N.J.; Bjornsson, S.; Weber, T.; Atke, A. The potential benefits of using fish oil in relation to preterm labor: The case for a randomized controlled trial? *Acta Obstet. Gynecol. Scand.* **2003**, *82*, 978–982. [CrossRef] [PubMed]

98. Calder, P.C. The role of marine omega-3 (n-3) fatty acids in inflammatory processes, atherosclerosis and plaque stability. *Mol. Nutr. Food Res.* **2012**, *56*, 1073–1080. [CrossRef] [PubMed]
99. MacDonald, R.S. The role of zinc in growth and cell proliferation. *J. Nutr.* **2000**, *130*, 1500s–1508s. [CrossRef]
100. Black, R.E.; Allen, L.H.A.; Bhutta, Z.; Caulfield, L.E.; De Onis, M.; Ezzati, M.; Mathers, C.; Rivera, J. Maternal and child undernutrition: Global and regional exposures and health consequences. *Lancet* **2008**, *371*, 243–260. [CrossRef]
101. Keen, C.L.; Uriu-Adams, J.Y.; Uriu-Adams, J.Y. Zinc and reproduction: Effects of zinc deficiency on prenatal and early postnatal development. *Birth Defects Res. Part B Dev. Reprod. Toxicol.* **2010**, *89*, 313–325.
102. Chaffee, B.W.; King, J.C. Effect of Zinc Supplementation on Pregnancy and Infant Outcomes: A Systematic Review. *Paediatr. Périnat. Epidemiol.* **2012**, *26*, 118–137. [CrossRef] [PubMed]
103. Ota, E.; Mori, R.; Middleton, P.; Tobe-Gai, R.; Mahomed, K.; Miyazaki, C.A.; Bhutta, Z. Zinc supplementation for improving pregnancy and infant outcome. *Cochrane Database Syst. Rev.* **2015**, *2*, CD000230. [CrossRef] [PubMed]
104. Wilson, R.L.; Grieger, J.A.; Bianco-Miotto, T.; Roberts, C.T. Association between Maternal Zinc Status, Dietary Zinc Intake and Pregnancy Complications: A Systematic Review. *Nutrients* **2016**, *8*, 641. [CrossRef] [PubMed]
105. DeLuca, H.F. Overview of general physiologic features and functions of vitamin D. *Am. J. Clin. Nutr.* **2004**, *80*, 1689s–1696s. [CrossRef] [PubMed]
106. Mithal, A.; Wahl, D.A.; Bonjour, J.P.; Burckhardt, P.; Dawson-Hughes, B.; Eisman, J.A.; El-Hajj Fuleihan, G.; Josse, R.G.; Lips, P.; Morales-Torres, J. Global vitamin D status and determinants of hypovitaminosis D. *Osteoporos. Int.* **2009**, *20*, 1807–1820. [CrossRef] [PubMed]
107. Liu, N.Q.; Hewison, M. Vitamin D, the placenta and pregnancy. *Arch. Biochem. Biophys.* **2012**, *523*, 37–47. [CrossRef] [PubMed]
108. Liu, N.Q.; Kaplan, A.T.; Lagishetty, V.; Ouyang, Y.B.; Ouyang, Y.; Simmons, C.F.; Equils, O.; Hewison, M. Vitamin D and the Regulation of Placental Inflammation. *J. Immunol.* **2011**, *186*, 5968–5974. [CrossRef]
109. Zhou, S.; Tao, Y.; Huang, K.; Zhu, B. Vitamin D and risk of preterm birth: Up-to-date meta-analysis of randomized controlled trials and observational studies. *J. Obstet. Gynaecol. Res.* **2017**, *43*, 247–256. [CrossRef] [PubMed]
110. Qin, L.L.; Lu, F.G.; Yang, S.H.; Xu, H.L.; Luo, B.A. Does Maternal Vitamin D Deficiency Increase the Risk of Preterm Birth: A Meta-Analysis of Observational Studies. *Nutrients* **2016**, *8*, 301. [CrossRef] [PubMed]
111. Thorne-Lyman, A.; Fawzi, W.W. Vitamin D during pregnancy and maternal, neonatal and infant health outcomes: A systematic review and meta-analysis. *Paediatr. Périnat. Epidemiol.* **2012**, *26*, 75–90. [CrossRef] [PubMed]
112. De-Regil, L.M.; Palacios, C.; Lombardo, L.K.; Peña-Rosas, J.P. Vitamin D supplementation for women during pregnancy. *Cochrane Database Syst. Rev.* **2016**, *1*, CD008873.
113. Cooper, C.; Harvey, N.C.; Bishop, N.J.; Kennedy, S.; Papageorghiou, A.T.; Schoenmakers, I.; Fraser, R.; Gandhi, S.V.; Carr, A.; D'Angelo, S.; et al. Maternal gestational vitamin D supplementation and offspring bone health (MAVIDOS): A multicentre, double-blind, randomised placebo-controlled trial. *Lancet Diabetes Endocrinol.* **2016**, *4*, 393–402. [CrossRef]
114. Arikan, G.M.; Panzitt, T.; Gücer, F.; Scholz, H.S.; Reinisch, S.; Haas, J.; Weiss, P.A. Course of Maternal Serum Magnesium Levels in Low-Risk Gestations and in Preterm Labor and Delivery. *Fetal Diagn. Ther.* **1999**, *14*, 332–336. [CrossRef] [PubMed]
115. King, D.E.; Mainous, A.G., 3rd; Geesey, M.E.; Woolson, R.F. Dietary magnesium and C-reactive protein levels. *J. Am. Coll. Nutr.* **2005**, *24*, 166–171. [CrossRef] [PubMed]
116. Wynn, A.; Wynn, M. Magnesium and Other Nutrient Deficiencies as Possible Causes of Hypertension and Low Birthweight. *Nutr. Health* **1988**, *6*, 69–88. [CrossRef] [PubMed]
117. Lopez Bernal, A. The regulation of uterine relaxation. *Semin. Cell Dev. Biol.* **2007**, *18*, 340–347. [CrossRef] [PubMed]
118. Makrides, M.A.; Crowther, C. Magnesium supplementation in pregnancy. *Cochrane Database Syst. Rev.* **2001**, CD000937. [CrossRef]
119. Crosby, D.D.; Shepherd, E.A.; Crowther, C.; Makrides, M. Magnesium supplementation in pregnancy. *Cochrane Database Syst. Rev.* **2014**, *4*, CD000937.

120. Crowther, C.A.; Brown, J.; McKinlay, C.J.D.; Middleton, P. Magnesium sulphate for preventing preterm birth in threatened preterm labour. *Cochrane Database Syst. Rev.* **2014**, *8*, CD001060. [CrossRef]

121. Alves, J.G.B.; De Araújo, C.A.F.L.; Pontes, I.E.; Guimarães, A.C.; Ray, J.G. The BRAzil MAGnesium (BRAMAG) trial: A randomized clinical trial of oral magnesium supplementation in pregnancy for the prevention of preterm birth and perinatal and maternal morbidity. *BMC Pregnancy Childbirth* **2014**, *14*, 222. [CrossRef] [PubMed]

122. Buppasiri, P.; Lumbiganon, P.; Thinkhamrop, J.; Ngamjarus, C.; Laopaiboon, M.; Medley, N. Calcium supplementation (other than for preventing or treating hypertension) for improving pregnancy and infant outcomes. *Cochrane Database Syst. Rev.* **2015**, CD007079. [CrossRef] [PubMed]

123. Villar, J.; Merialdi, M.; Gulmezoglu, A.M.; Abalos, E.; Carroli, G.; Kulier, R.; de Onis, M. Nutritional interventions during pregnancy for the prevention or treatment of maternal morbidity and preterm delivery: An overview of randomized controlled trials. *J. Nutr.* **2003**, *133*, 1606s–1625s. [CrossRef] [PubMed]

124. Peña-Rosas, J.P.; Dowswell, T.; Peña-Rosas, J.P.; De-Regil, L.M.; Garcia-Casal, M.N.; Pena-Rosas, J.P.; De-Regil, L.M.; Garcia-Casal, M.N. Daily oral iron supplementation during pregnancy. *Cochrane Database Syst. Rev.* **2015**, CD004736. [CrossRef] [PubMed]

125. De-Regil, L.M.; Peña-Rosas, J.P.; Fernández-Gaxiola, A.C.; Rayco-Solon, P. Effects and safety of periconceptional oral folate supplementation for preventing birth defects. *Cochrane Database Syst. Rev.* **2015**, CD007950. [CrossRef] [PubMed]

126. Klebanoff, M.; Shiono, P.; Selby, J.; Trachtenberg, A.; Graubard, B. Anemia and spontaneous preterm birth. *Int. J. Gynecol. Obstet.* **1991**, *164*, 59–63.

127. Scholl, T.O.; Hediger, M.L.; Fischer, R.L.; Shearer, J.W. Anemia vs. iron deficiency: Increased risk of preterm delivery in a prospective study. *Am. J. Clin. Nutr.* **1992**, *55*, 985–988. [CrossRef]

128. Lassi, Z.S.; Salam, R.A.; Haider, B.A.; Bhutta, Z. Folic acid supplementation during pregnancy for maternal health and pregnancy outcomes. *Cochrane Database Syst. Rev.* **2013**, *3*, CD006896. [CrossRef]

129. West, K.P., Jr. Extent of vitamin A deficiency among preschool children and women of reproductive age. *J. Nutr.* **2002**, *132*, 2857s–2866s. [CrossRef]

130. Thorne-Lyman, A.L.; Fawzi, W.W. Vitamin A and carotenoids during pregnancy and maternal, neonatal and infant health outcomes: A systematic review and meta-analysis. *Paediatr. Périnat. Epidemiol.* **2012**, *26*, 36–54. [CrossRef]

131. West, K.P., Jr.; Katz, J.; Khatry, S.K.; LeClerq, S.C.; Pradhan, E.K.; Shrestha, S.R.; Connor, P.B.; Dali, S.M.; Christian, P.; Pokhrel, R.P.; et al. Double blind, cluster randomised trial of low dose supplementation with vitamin A or beta carotene on mortality related to pregnancy in Nepal. The NNIPS-2 Study Group. *BMJ* **1999**, *318*, 570–575. [CrossRef]

132. Mistry, H.D.; Williams, P.J. The importance of antioxidant micronutrients in pregnancy. *Oxid. Med. Cell. Longev.* **2011**, *2011*, 841749. [CrossRef] [PubMed]

133. Ray, J.G.; Laskin, C.A. Folic acid and homocyst(e)ine metabolic defects and the risk of placental abruption, pre-eclampsia and spontaneous pregnancy loss: A systematic review. *Placenta* **1999**, *20*, 519–529. [CrossRef] [PubMed]

134. Himes, K.P.; Simhan, H.N. Risk of recurrent preterm birth and placental pathology. *Obstet. Gynecol.* **2008**, *112*, 121–126. [CrossRef] [PubMed]

135. Catov, J.M.; Bodnar, L.M.; Olsen, J.; Olsen, S.A.; Nohr, E. Periconceptional multivitamin use and risk of preterm or small-for-gestational-age births in the Danish National Birth Cohort1234. *Am. J. Clin. Nutr.* **2011**, *94*, 906–912. [CrossRef] [PubMed]

136. Haider, B.A.; Bhutta, Z.A. Multiple-micronutrient supplementation for women during pregnancy. *Cochrane Database Syst. Rev.* **2015**, *11*, CD004905.

137. de Onis, M.; Villar, J.; Gulmezoglu, M. Nutritional interventions to prevent intrauterine growth retardation: Evidence from randomized controlled trials. *Eur. J. Clin. Nutr.* **1998**, *52*, S83–S93.

138. Kramer, M.S.; Kakuma, R. Energy and protein intake in pregnancy. *Cochrane Database Syst. Rev.* **2003**, *4*, CD000032.

139. Hillier, S.L.; Martin, D.H.; Pastorek, J.G.; Rao, A.V.; McNellis, D.; Regan, J.A.; Nugent, R.P.; Eschenbach, D.A.; Krohn, M.A.; Gibbs, R.S.; et al. Association between Bacterial Vaginosis and Preterm Delivery of a Low-Birth-Weight Infant. *N. Engl. J. Med.* **1995**, *333*, 1737–1742. [CrossRef]

140. Brocklehurst, P.; Gordon, A.; Heatley, E.; Milan, S.J. Antibiotics for treating bacterial vaginosis in pregnancy. *Cochrane Database Syst. Rev.* **2013**. [CrossRef]

141. Al-Ghazzewi, F.H.; Tester, R.F. Biotherapeutic agents and vaginal health. *J. Appl. Microbiol.* **2016**, *121*, 18–27. [CrossRef] [PubMed]

142. Hemarajata, P.; Versalovic, J. Effects of probiotics on gut microbiota: Mechanisms of intestinal immunomodulation and neuromodulation. *Ther. Adv. Gastroenterol.* **2013**, *6*, 39–51. [CrossRef] [PubMed]

143. Krauss-Silva, L.; Moreira, M.E.L.; Alves, M.B.; Rezende, M.R.; Braga, A.; Camacho, K.G.; Batista, M.R.R.; Savastano, C.; Almada-Horta, A.; Guerra, F. Randomized controlled trial of probiotics for the prevention of spontaneous preterm delivery associated with intrauterine infection: Study protocol. *Reprod. Health* **2010**, *7*, 14. [CrossRef] [PubMed]

144. Krauss-Silva, L.; Moreira, M.E.L.; Alves, M.B.; Braga, A.; Camacho, K.G.; Batista, M.R.R.; Almada-Horta, A.; Rebello, M.R.; Guerra, F. A randomised controlled trial of probiotics for the prevention of spontaneous preterm delivery associated with bacterial vaginosis: Preliminary results. *Trials* **2011**, *12*, 239. [CrossRef] [PubMed]

145. Gille, C.; Böer, B.; Marschal, M.; Urschitz, M.S.; Heinecke, V.; Hund, V.; Speidel, S.; Tarnow, I.; Mylonas, I.; Franz, A.; et al. Effect of probiotics on vaginal health in pregnancy. EFFPRO, a randomized controlled trial. *Am. J. Obstet. Gynecol.* **2016**, *215*, 608.e1–608.e7. [CrossRef] [PubMed]

146. Luoto, R.; Laitinen, K.; Nermes, M.; Isolauri, E. Impact of maternal probiotic-supplemented dietary counselling on pregnancy outcome and prenatal and postnatal growth: A double-blind, placebo-controlled study. *Br. J. Nutr.* **2010**, *103*, 1792–1799. [CrossRef]

147. Mantaring, J.; Benyacoub, J.; Destura, R.; Pecquet, S.; Vidal, K.; Volger, S.; Guinto, V. Effect of maternal supplement beverage with and without probiotics during pregnancy and lactation on maternal and infant health: A randomized controlled trial in the Philippines. *BMC Pregnancy Childbirth* **2018**, *18*, 193. [CrossRef]

148. Rautava, S.; Collado, M.C.; Salminen, S.; Isolauri, E. Probiotics modulate host-microbe interaction in the placenta and fetal gut: A randomized, double-blind, placebo-controlled trial. *Neonatology* **2012**, *102*, 178–184. [CrossRef]

149. Nordqvist, M.; Jacobsson, B.; Brantsæter, A.-L.; Myhre, R.; Nilsson, S.; Sengpiel, V. Timing of probiotic milk consumption during pregnancy and effects on the incidence of preeclampsia and preterm delivery: A prospective observational cohort study in Norway. *BMJ Open* **2018**, *8*, e018021. [CrossRef]

150. Myhre, R.; Brantsaeter, A.L.; Myking, S.; Gjessing, H.K.; Sengpiel, V.; Meltzer, H.M.; Haugen, M.; Jacobsson, B. Intake of probiotic food and risk of spontaneous preterm delivery. *Am. J. Clin. Nutr.* **2011**, *93*, 151–157. [CrossRef]

151. Othman, M.; Neilson, J.P.; Alfirevic, Z. Probiotics for preventing preterm labour. *Cochrane Database Syst. Rev.* **2007**, *1*, CD005941. [CrossRef] [PubMed]

152. Jarde, A.; Lewis-Mikhael, A.-M.; Moayyedi, P.; Stearns, J.C.; Collins, S.M.; Beyene, J.; McDonald, S.D. Pregnancy outcomes in women taking probiotics or prebiotics: A systematic review and meta-analysis. *BMC Pregnancy Childbirth* **2018**, *18*, 14. [CrossRef] [PubMed]

153. Grev, J.; Berg, M.; Soll, R. Maternal probiotic supplementation for prevention of morbidity and mortality in preterm infants. *Cochrane Database Syst. Rev.* **2018**, *12*, CD012519. [CrossRef] [PubMed]

154. Stojanovic, N.; Plecas, D.; Plesinac, S. Normal vaginal flora, disorders and application of probiotics in pregnancy. *Arch. Gynecol. Obstet.* **2012**, *286*, 325–332. [CrossRef] [PubMed]

155. Jespers, V.; van de Wijgert, J.; Cools, P.; Verhelst, R.; Verstraelen, H.; Delany-Moretlwe, S.; Mwaura, M.; Ndayisaba, G.F.; Mandaliya, K.; Menten, J.; et al. The significance of Lactobacillus crispatus and L. vaginalis for vaginal health and the negative effect of recent sex: A cross-sectional descriptive study across groups of African women. *BMC Infect. Dis.* **2015**, *15*, 115. [CrossRef]

156. Srinivasan, S.; Morgan, M.T.; Fiedler, T.L.; Djukovic, D.; Hoffman, N.G.; Raftery, D.; Marrazzo, J.M.; Fredricks, D.N. Metabolic signatures of bacterial vaginosis. *MBio* **2015**, *6*, e00204–e00215. [CrossRef]

157. Kim, J.Y.; Kwon, J.H.; Ahn, S.H.; Lee, S.I.; Han, Y.S.; Choi, Y.O.; Lee, S.Y.; Ahn, K.M.; Ji, G.E. Effect of probiotic mix (Bifidobacterium bifidum, Bifidobacterium lactis, Lactobacillus acidophilus) in the primary prevention of eczema: A double-blind, randomized, placebo-controlled trial. *Pediatr. Allergy Immunol.* **2010**, *21*, e386–e393. [CrossRef]

158. Ou, C.Y.; Kuo, H.C.; Wang, L.; Hsu, T.Y.; Chuang, H.; Liu, C.A.; Chang, J.C.; Yu, H.R.; Yang, K.D. Prenatal and postnatal probiotics reduces maternal but not childhood allergic diseases: A randomized, double-blind, placebo-controlled trial. *Clin. Exp. Allergy* **2012**, *42*, 1386–1396. [CrossRef]

159. Vitali, B.; Cruciani, F.; Baldassarre, M.E.; Capursi, T.; Spisni, E.; Valerii, M.C.; Candela, M.; Turroni, S.; Brigidi, P. Dietary supplementation with probiotics during late pregnancy: Outcome on vaginal microbiota and cytokine secretion. *BMC Microbiol.* **2012**, *12*, 236. [CrossRef]

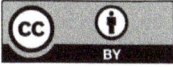

nutrients

MDPI

Article

Associations between the Prenatal Diet and Neonatal Outcomes—A Secondary Analysis of the Cluster-Randomised GeliS Trial

Julia Günther [1], Julia Hoffmann [1], Monika Spies [1], Dorothy Meyer [1], Julia Kunath [1], Lynne Stecher [1], Eva Rosenfeld [2], Luzia Kick [2], Kathrin Rauh [1,2] and Hans Hauner [1,*]

[1]   Else Kröner-Fresenius-Centre for Nutritional Medicine, School of Medicine, Klinikum rechts der Isar, Technical University of Munich, Georg-Brauchle-Ring 62, 80992 Munich, Germany
[2]   Competence Centre for Nutrition (KErn), Am Gereuth 4, 85354 Freising, Germany
*   Correspondence: hans.hauner@tum.de; Tel.: +49-(0)-892-892-4921

Received: 9 July 2019; Accepted: 9 August 2019; Published: 13 August 2019

Abstract: The prenatal lifestyle, including maternal dietary behaviour, is an important determinant of offspring health. This secondary cohort analysis of the GeliS ("healthy living in pregnancy") trial investigated associations between antenatal dietary factors and neonatal weight parameters. The cluster-randomised GeliS trial included 2286 pregnant women. Dietary information was collected with food frequency questionnaires before or in the 12th (T0) and after the 29th week of gestation (T1). Consumption of vegetables (41.28 g per portion at T0, $p = 0.001$; 36.67 g per portion at T1, $p = 0.001$), fruit (15.25 g per portion at T1, $p = 0.010$) and dietary quality, measured with a Healthy Eating Index (39.26 g per 10 points at T0, $p = 0.004$; 42.76 g per 10 points at T1, $p = 0.002$) were positively associated with birth weight. In contrast, sugar-sweetened beverages (10.90 g per portion at T0, $p = 0.003$; 8.19 g per portion at T1, $p = 0.047$), higher sugar consumption at T0 (8.27 g per 10 g, $p = 0.032$) and early pregnancy alcohol intake (15.32 g per g, $p = 0.039$) were inversely associated with birth weight. Most other dietary factors were not associated with neonatal weight. Some components reflecting a healthy maternal diet were associated with a modest increase in offspring birth weight, whereas some unhealthy components slightly reduced neonatal weight.

Keywords: lifestyle intervention; pregnancy; dietary behaviour; neonatal outcomes; birth weight; large for gestational age (LGA); small for gestational age (SGA); obesity prevention

1. Introduction

In recent decades, concern about childhood obesity has grown worldwide. The intrauterine environment has been found to have a profound impact on body weight and health development during childhood and adulthood. Offspring birth weight and weight-related parameters such as a high birth weight and large for gestational age (LGA) at birth have been suggested to modify the risk of future health consequences, including obesity [1] and metabolic diseases such as diabetes mellitus [2].

Maternal over-nutrition can result in excessive gestational weight gain (GWG) and has been found to increase the risk of a high birth weight by its influence on the intrauterine environment [3]. Ultimately, excessive GWG can increase the risk of childhood overweight and obesity [4,5] and may promote health complications in the offspring, including metabolic and cardiovascular diseases [6,7]. Several studies have investigated the specific role of the maternal diet in offspring growth and development [8,9]. While clear associations between the antenatal diet and offspring birth weight have been shown in malnourished women [10], the findings in well-nourished women were less conclusive. Although some components of the maternal diet have been suggested to influence the offspring's birth weight including for instance, milk [11], fruit and vegetables [12] and fish [13], evidence in this field is sparse [8]. Comprehensive data on the impact of the overall antenatal maternal diet on neonatal growth parameters are lacking [14].

The importance of a healthy lifestyle during pregnancy, including adequate GWG, a healthy diet, and regular physical activity, has been increasingly recognised. Different approaches aiming to improve the antenatal maternal lifestyle have been developed. While some of these trials have been effective in reducing excessive GWG, data on diet and physical activity have been less often reported [15]. The large-scale cluster-randomised controlled GeliS study ("Gesund leben in der Schwangerschaft"/healthy living in pregnancy), which primarily aimed to reduce excessive GWG using a routine care approach, extensively reported on pregnancy and obstetric outcomes, as well as behavioural parameters after a lifestyle intervention [16]. Data on the effects of the intervention on GWG, as well as on maternal and infant outcomes, have recently been published [17]. The large GeliS cohort, recruited in the setting of routine prenatal care, collated a large and diverse maternal and offspring data set which provides a valuable opportunity to comprehensively analyse associations between maternal antenatal behaviour and infant growth and health parameters. This secondary analysis aims to investigate associations between the maternal diet during early and late pregnancy and neonatal outcomes in the GeliS cohort. The impact of mean daily intake of food groups, energy and macronutrients as well as dietary quality by means of a Healthy Eating Index (HEI) on offspring weight parameters at birth was elucidated herein.

2. Materials and Methods

2.1. Study Design

The cluster-randomised, controlled GeliS trial was conducted within the German routine care setting in medical practices. In five administrative regions of Bavaria, pairs of ten urban and rural areas were randomised into one intervention and one control area per pair. The randomisation process and study procedures have been described in detail in the published study protocol [16].

Study procedures were conducted in accordance with the declaration of Helsinki as well as with local regulatory requirements and laws. The study protocol was approved by the ethics committee of the Technical University of Munich and is registered at the ClinicalTrials.gov Protocol Registration System (NCT01958307).

2.2. Study Participants

Pregnant women were recruited before or in the 12th week of gestation in gynaecological and midwifery practices. Inclusion criteria were fulfilled if women were aged between 18 and 43 years, had a body mass index (BMI) between 18.5 and 40.0 kg/m^2, had a singleton pregnancy, sufficient German language skills and provided written informed consent for participation in the trial. Women were excluded in case of a multiple or complicated pregnancy and if severe illnesses were diagnosed [16].

2.3. The Lifestyle Intervention Program

In the intervention group (IV), women attended a structured lifestyle intervention programme attached to routine prenatal care visits. They participated in three individual antenatal and one postpartum counselling sessions. Counselling included standardised information about an adequate GWG, a balanced diet and regular physical activity during pregnancy, and was conducted according to German recommendations [18]. Lifestyle counselling was performed by specifically trained midwives, gynaecologists and medical assistants in their practices.

Women in the control group (C) received routine prenatal care, complemented by a leaflet with general recommendations on a healthy antenatal lifestyle.

2.4. Study Outcomes

The primary outcome of the trial was the proportion of women showing excessive GWG as defined by the American Institute of Medicine (IOM) [19]. Data on the effect of the intervention on excessive GWG and some secondary outcomes have been published recently [17]. Despite a slight difference in offspring birth weight and length, no considerable between-group differences in maternal and neonatal outcomes were found [17]. Data from IV and C were thus pooled to form one cohort for the investigation of potential associations between the maternal diet and neonatal weight parameters.

2.5. Data Collection and Processing

Baseline characteristics of study participants were recorded by means of a screening questionnaire at study entry (≤12th week of gestation).

Maternal diet was assessed in both groups in early (≤12th week of gestation, T0) and late pregnancy (>29th week of gestation, T1) with food frequency questionnaires (FFQ). The self-administered FFQ was developed and validated by the Robert Koch Institute, Berlin, Germany for the "German Health Examination Survey for Adults" (DEGS) study [20] and was slightly modified for use in the GeliS trial. In the modified version, mean consumption frequency over the last four weeks was ranked by study participants from "never" to "more than five times per day" for 54 food items. Mean portion size was reported in standard measures such as cups, glasses, plates or bowls, and daily intake was calculated by combining frequency and portion size. If more than 20 out of the 54 food item questions were not answered, questionnaires were excluded from dietary analyses. Further, data of women reporting implausibly high daily intakes (either liquids >15 kg, or solid foods >10 kg, or both liquids >4 kg and solid foods >6 kg) were discarded due to over-reporting of food intake (according to personal communication by Dr. Gert Mensink, Robert Koch Institute, Berlin, Germany, 2018).

Recorded food items were summarised in food groups. Estimations of energy and macronutrient intake were made on the basis of information retrieved from the German food composition database ("Bundeslebensmittelschlüssel", version 3.02, Max Rubner Institute (MRI), Karlsruhe, Germany) using OptiDiet PLUS software (version 6.0, GOE mbH, Linden, Germany). Some questions in the FFQ referred to food groups in sum and not to single food items. For these food groups, data of the German National Consumption Survey II (NVS II) assessing typical patterns in the consumption of food items within food groups were considered (personal communication from MRI, Federal Research Institute of Nutrition and Food, "Verzehrsmengen ausgewählter Lebensmittel aus der Nationalen Verzehrsstudie II" (NVS II), Karlsruhe, Germany, July 2018). Data of women were excluded from analyses of energy and macronutrient consumption if their estimated mean energy intake was below 4500 kJ or exceeded 20,000 kJ per day [21].

Dietary quality was rated by means of a Healthy Eating Index (HEI) specifically developed for the applied DEGS-FFQ from the Robert Koch Institute [22]. Intake of 14 food groups assessed with the FFQ was compared with the German Nutrition Society (DGE) recommendations for a healthy diet and scored from 0 (no adherence to recommendations) to 100 (high adherence to recommendations) points. Correspondingly, a HEI-score was calculated as mean from the group scores [22].

Information on birth weight and length was retrieved from birth records collected from medical practices. Neonatal weight below the 10th percentile for gestational age was defined as "small for gestational age" (SGA), weight above the 90th percentile for gestational age as "large for gestational age" (LGA). Offspring were considered to have a low birth weight if they weighed less than 2500 g and to have a high birth weight if they weighed more than 4000 g.

2.6. Statistical Analysis

Women were included in the analyses if dietary data on at least one assessment point as well as neonatal data (body weight and length) were available. Women dropping out of the study due to a miscarriage or pregnancy termination, severe pregnancy complications or maternal death were excluded from the analyses. IV and C were pooled to form one cohort. Baseline characteristics are presented as mean ± standard deviation or proportion if appropriate.

For the analysis of associations between dietary variables (as mean daily portion or percent of energy if appropriate) and continuous offspring outcomes (birth weight, BMI), linear regression models were applied. Portions sizes were defined according to the FFQ for the different food items. For the analysis of dichotomous outcomes (SGA, LGA, low birth weight, high birth weight), binary logistic regression models were applied. Regression models were adjusted for group assignment, maternal pre-pregnancy age, BMI category and parity. Results are presented as effect sizes or odds ratios with 95% confidence intervals. *p*-values below 0.05 were considered as statistically significant. All analyses were conducted using SPSS software (IBM SPSS Statistics for Windows, version 24.0, IBM Corp, Armonk, NY, USA).

3. Results

3.1. Study Participants and Baseline Characteristics

Altogether, 2286 women were recruited for participation in the GeliS trial. A total of 112 women dropped out during the course of pregnancy (Figure 1). Women were further excluded from cohort analyses if they did not provide the relevant infant parameters (*n* = 156), resulting in a total of 2018 eligible participants. The maternal and neonatal characteristics of this sample are shown in Table 1. Dietary intake data were provided by 1995 of the 2018 women. After exclusion of invalid questionnaires and over-reporters, dietary data of 1902 (T0) and 1861 (T1) women were analysed in relation to neonatal weight parameters.

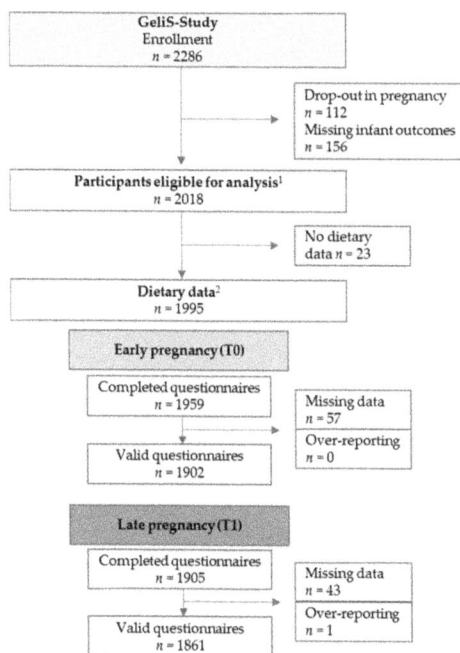

Figure 1. Participant flow. [1] Women without miscarriages, late loss of pregnancy, terminations, pregnancy complications that interfered with the intervention, maternal deaths and/or lack of infant outcomes (birth weight, birth length). [2] Women who provided dietary data at T0 or T1. T0: Dietary assessment before or in the 12th week of gestation; T1: Dietary assessment after the 29th week of gestation.

Table 1. Characteristics of study participants eligible for cohort analyses.

Maternal and Neonatal Characteristics	Total (n = 2018)
Maternal characteristics	
Pre-pregnancy age, years	30.3 ± 4.4 [a]
Pre-pregnancy weight, kg	68.2 ± 13.4 [a]
Pre-pregnancy BMI, kg/m^2	24.4 ± 4.5 [a]
Pre-pregnancy BMI category	
BMI 18.5–24.9 kg/m^2	1311/2018 (65.0%)
BMI 25.0–29.9 kg/m^2	464/2018 (23.0%)
BMI 30.0–40.0 kg/m^2	243/2018 (12.0%)
Educational level	
General secondary school	320/2014 (15.9%)
Intermediate secondary school	856/2014 (42.5%)
(Technical) High school	838/2014 (41.6%)
Country of birth	
Germany	1790/2014 (88.9%)
Others	224/2014 (11.1%)
Further maternal characteristics	
Nulliparous	1162/2018 (57.6%)
Living with a partner	1939/2011 (96.4%)
Full-time employed	1056/1996 (52.9%)
Gestational diabetes mellitus [b]	209/1940 (10.8%)
Pregnancy hypertension [c]	161/2015 (8.0%)
Preterm delivery [d]	131/2016 (6.5%)
Neonatal characteristics	
Birth weight, g	3337.6 ± 517.8 [a]
Birth length, cm	51.3 ± 2.6 [a]
Head circumference, cm	34.7 ± 1.6 [a]
BMI, kg/m^2	12.7 ± 1.3 [a]
SGA	172/2016 (8.5%)
LGA	148/2016 (7.3%)
Low birth weight	101/2018 (5.0%)
High birth weight	169/2018 (8.4%)

[a] mean ± SD. [b] diagnosed with a 2-h oral glucose tolerance test at weeks 24–28 of gestation according to national and international standards [23,24]. [c] Systolic blood pressure > 140 mmHg or diastolic blood pressure > 90 mmHg at at least two time points. [d] < 37 weeks of gestation. BMI: body mass index; SGA: Small for gestational age; LGA: Large for gestational age.

3.2. Associations between the Maternal Diet and Infant Weight and Weight-Related Parameters

Associations between antenatal food intake and neonatal birth weight and BMI are shown in Table 2. Associations with BMI z-scores are shown in Supplementary Table S1. There was evidence for a positive association between maternal fruit and vegetable consumption and infant birth weight (Table 2). An increase in offspring weight at birth by 41.28 g (95% CI 17.87 to 64.70 g, $p = 0.001$) was observed per portion of vegetables (150 g) in early pregnancy, and by 36.67 g/portion in late pregnancy (95% CI 15.95 to 57.39 g, $p = 0.001$). These observations were also reflected in the BMI of the neonates (T0: $p = 0.017$, T1: $p = 0.002$). A significant association between fruit intake and birth weight and BMI was found for the late pregnancy dietary assessment (birth weight: 15.25 g increase per portion of fruit (95% CI 3.67 to 26.83 g, $p = 0.010$), BMI: 0.04 kg/m^2 increase per portion (95% CI 0.01 to 0.07, $p = 0.009$)), but not for early pregnancy (birth weight: $p = 0.322$, BMI: $p = 0.172$). In contrast, maternal consumption of sugar-containing beverages was significantly inversely associated with weight at birth. In early pregnancy, one glass of soft drinks (200 mL) consumed by the mother reduced offspring birth weight by 10.90 g (95% CI −18.17 to −3.64 g, p = 0.003). In late pregnancy, there was evidence of a reduction by 8.19 g (95% CI −16.26 to −0.11 g, p = 0.047) per consumed glass of soft drinks. The association between soft drink intake and weight was not reflected in the BMI of the neonates (T0: p = 0.076, T1: p = 0.437). For the other food groups, such as dairy products, fast food and meat, no significant association between the consumed amount and offspring weight and BMI could be shown, either in early or in late pregnancy (Table 2).

Table 2. Associations between maternal food intake and offspring birth weight and body mass index.

Food Groups	Birth Weight (g)		BMI (kg/m^2)	
	Adjusted Effect Size [a] (95% CI)	Adjusted p Value [a]	Adjusted Effect Size [a] (95% CI)	Adjusted p Value [a]
Soft drinks [b] (200 mL/day)				
T0	−10.90 (−18.17, −3.64)	0.003	−0.02 (−0.03,0.00)	0.076
T1	−8.19 (−16.26, −0.11)	0.047	−0.01 (−0.03,0.01)	0.437
Light drinks [c] (200 mL/day)				
T0	−5.70 (−17.59,6.19)	0.347	−0.00 (−0.03,0.03)	0.919
T1	−5.89 (−18.34,6.55)	0.353	0.01 (−0.02,0.04)	0.577
Vegetables (150 g/day)				
T0	41.28 (17.87,64.70	0.001	0.07 (0.01,0.13)	0.017
T1	36.67 (15.95,57.39)	0.001	0.09 (0.03,0.14)	0.002
Fruit (150 g/day)				
T0	5.55 (−5.44,16.55)	0.322	0.02 (−0.01,0.05)	0.172
T1	15.25 (3.67,26.83)	0.010	0.04 (0.01,0.07)	0.009
Dairy products (200 g/day)				
T0	8.41 (−5.60,22.41)	0.239	0.00 (−0.03,0.04)	0.838
T1	3.13 (−9.37,15.62)	0.624	0.02 (−0.01,0.05)	0.233
Meat and meat products (150 g/day)				
T0	6.79 (−54.36,67.94)	0.828	0.00 (−0.15,0.15)	0.993
T1	3.35 (−60.86,67.55)	0.919	0.00 (−0.16,0.17)	0.966
Sweets and snacks (50 g/day)				
T0	11.69 (−8.07,31.44)	0.246	0.00 (−0.05,0.05)	0.895
T1	−4.97 (−21.12,11.18)	0.547	0.00 (−0.04,0.05)	0.855
Fast food (250 g/day)				
T0	9.08 (−153.36,171.52)	0.913	0.08 (−0.32,0.48)	0.702
T1	−95.15 (−273.51,83.22)	0.296	−0.17 (−0.63,0.29)	0.470

Estimated is the regression coefficient describing the association between the intake of a portion of a food item or food group and infant weight and BMI. Portion sizes are defined according to the applied food frequency questionnaire. [a] linear regression models adjusted for pre-pregnancy BMI, age, parity and group assignment. [b] sugar-containing sweetened beverages. [c] low or non-caloric sweetened beverages. BMI: body mass index; T0: assessment before or in the 12th week of gestation; T1: assessment after the 29th week of gestation.

Table 3 shows associations between antenatal food intake and infant weight-related outcomes. Fruit consumption in early pregnancy was significantly associated with increased odds of having a LGA neonate (OR 1.08 per portion, 95% CI 1.02 to 1.15, p = 0.016). Moreover, fast food consumption in early pregnancy but not in late pregnancy increased the odds of the offspring weighing > 4000 g at birth (T0: OR 3.14 per 250 g portion, 95% CI 1.26 to 7.84, p = 0.014).

Table 3. Associations between maternal food intake and neonatal weight-related parameters.

Food Groups	Low Birth Weight		High Birth Weight		SGA		LGA	
	Adjusted Odds Ratio [a] (95% CI)	Adjusted p Value [a]	Adjusted Odds Ratio [a] (95% CI)	Adjusted p Value [a]	Adjusted Odds Ratio [a] (95% CI)	Adjusted p Value [a]	Adjusted Odds Ratio [a] (95% CI)	Adjusted p Value [a]
Soft drinks [b] (200 mL/day)								
T0	1.04(0.99,1.09)	0.150	0.95(0.88,1.02)	0.149	1.03(0.99,1.08)	0.123	0.94(0.87,1.02)	0.155
T1	1.01(0.94,1.09)	0.766	0.95(0.88,1.03)	0.221	1.00(0.94,1.07)	0.973	0.95(0.87,1.03)	0.212
Light drinks [c] (200 mL/day)								
T0	0.98(0.87,1.11)	0.778	0.99(0.91,1.08)	0.858	1.01(0.93,1.10)	0.783	1.00(0.92,1.09)	0.971
T1	1.01(0.90,1.14)	0.864	1.01(0.94,1.10)	0.763	1.05(0.98,1.12)	0.213	1.02(0.94,1.10)	0.627
Vegetables (150 g/day)								
T0	0.85(0.67,1.08)	0.184	1.09(0.94,1.27)	0.262	0.98(0.84,1.16)	0.841	1.13(0.96,1.32)	0.138
T1	0.81(0.63,1.05)	0.113	1.14(1.00,1.31)	0.058	0.88(0.74,1.05)	0.146	1.14(0.98,1.32)	0.081
Fruit (150 g/day)								
T0	1.05(0.96,1.14)	0.284	1.06(0.99,1.13)	0.094	0.97(0.89,1.05)	0.460	1.08(1.02,1.15)	0.016
T1	1.07(0.96,1.18)	0.224	1.05(0.97,1.14)	0.197	0.90(0.81,1.01)	0.063	1.06(0.97,1.14)	0.187
Dairy products (200 g/day)								
T0	0.95(0.82,1.10)	0.458	1.04(0.95,1.14)	0.387	1.05(0.96,1.14)	0.294	1.06(0.97,1.16)	0.177
T1	0.98(0.85,1.13)	0.772	0.95(0.85,1.06)	0.321	0.95(0.84,1.06)	0.343	0.99(0.90,1.10)	0.903
Meat and meat products (150 g/day)								
T0	1.40(0.87,2.25)	0.172	1.20(0.82,1.76)	0.349	0.85(0.54,1.33)	0.474	1.16(0.77,1.72)	0.481
T1	1.52(0.82,2.82)	0.183	1.25(0.79,1.98)	0.347	1.00(0.61,1.63)	0.998	1.19(0.73,1.94)	0.486
Sweets and snacks (50 g/day)								
T0	1.07(0.91,1.25)	0.423	1.02(0.90,1.17)	0.722	0.97(0.84,1.12)	0.683	1.06(0.93,1.20)	0.424
T1	1.14(0.99,1.30)	0.066	0.96(0.84,1.09)	0.496	1.00(0.88,1.13)	0.963	0.93(0.81,1.07)	0.308
Fast food (250 g/day)								
T0	1.35(0.36,5.09)	0.655	3.14(1.26,7.84)	0.014	1.10(0.37,3.25)	0.862	2.31(0.85,6.33)	0.103
T1	1.87(0.34,10.36)	0.473	2.21(0.64,7.61)	0.210	1.68(0.47,5.97)	0.427	1.04(0.26,4.16)	0.955

Estimated is the regression coefficient describing the association between the intake of a portion of a food item or food group and infant weight-related parameters. Portion sizes are defined according to the applied food frequency questionnaire. [a] linear regression models adjusted for pre-pregnancy BMI, age, parity and group assignment; [b] sugar-containing sweetened beverages; [c] low or non-caloric sweetened beverages. BMI: body mass index; LGA: large for gestational age; SGA: small for gestational age; T0: assessment before or in the 12th week of gestation; T1: assessment after the 29th week of gestation.

There was no evidence for an association between energy or macronutrient intake as percent of energy and offspring birth weight and BMI (Table 4). With increasing saccharose intake (per 10 g of sugar) in early pregnancy, a slight reduction in birth weight by 8.27 g (95% CI −15.83 to −0.70 g, $p = 0.032$) was observed. There was no statistical evidence for such an association in late pregnancy ($p = 0.074$). Similarly, alcohol consumption in early but not late pregnancy was related to a reduction in offspring weight at birth by 15.32 g per g (95% CI −29.83 to −0.80 g, $p = 0.039$).

Table 4. Associations between maternal energy, macronutrient intake and dietary quality and offspring birth weight and body mass index.

Energy and Macronutrient Intake	Birth Weight (g)		BMI (kg/m^2)	
	Adjusted Effect Size [a] (95% CI)	Adjusted *p* Value [a]	Adjusted Effect Size [a] (95% CI)	Adjusted *p* Value [a]
Energy [100 kcal/day]				
T0	−0.04 (−3.89,3.80)	0.984	−0.01 (−0.02,0.00)	0.224
T1	3.15 (−0.45,6.76)	0.087	0.01 (−0.00,0.02)	0.218
Carbohydrates [10 E%]				
T0	−8.69 (−39.35,21.97)	0.579	0.01 (−0.06,0.09)	0.769
T1	9.16 (−22.26,40.58)	0.568	0.01 (−0.07,0.09)	0.764
Saccharose [10 g/day]				
T0	−8.27 (−15.83,−0.70)	0.032	−0.02 (−0.04,0.00)	0.074
T1	3.72 (−3.90,11.34)	0.339	0.01 (−0.01,0.03)	0.271
Protein [10 E%]				
T0	48.88 (−28.19,125.95)	0.214	0.08 (−0.12,0.27)	0.439
T1	14.36 (−60.91,89.64)	0.708	0.08 (−0.11,0.27)	0.425
Fat [10 E%]				
T0	5.35 (−33.39,44.08)	0.787	−0.03 (−0.13,0.06)	0.489
T1	−17.00 (−55.49,21.50)	0.387	−0.04 (−0.14,0.06)	0.458
Alcohol [g]				
T0	−15.32 (−29.83,−0.80)	0.039	−0.01 (−0.05,0.02)	0.439
T1	−40.67 (−105.97,24.63)	0.222	−0.11 (−0.28,0.05)	0.182
Caffeine [100 mg]				
T0	−6.57 (−32.54,19.41)	0.620	−0.03 (−0.10,0.03)	0.313
T1	−12.20 (−40.04,15.64)	0.390	−0.05 (−0.13,0.02)	0.139
HEI [10 points]				
T0	39.26 (12.29,66.22)	0.004	0.06 (−0.01,0.13)	0.081
T1	42.76 (15.98,69.55)	0.002	0.10 (0.03,0.16)	0.006

Estimated is the regression coefficient describing the association between the intake of a certain amount or percentage and infant weight and BMI. [a] linear regression models adjusted for pre-pregnancy BMI, age, parity and group assignment. BMI: body mass index; HEI: Healthy Eating Index; T0: assessment before or in the 12th week of gestation; T1: assessment after the 29th week of gestation.

3.3. Diet Quality and Infant Weight Outcomes

Maternal dietary quality, measured with a HEI, was positively associated with birth weight in both early (39.26 g per 10 points (95% CI 12.29 to 66.22 g, *p* = 0.004)) and late pregnancy (42.76 g per 10 points (95% CI 15.98 to 69.55 g, *p* = 0.002)). Additionally, late pregnancy HEI was positively associated with the neonatal BMI (*p* = 0.006), whereas there was no evidence for such an association with early HEI (*p* = 0.081). These observations did not translate into increased odds of the offspring being LGA or having a birth weight above 4000 g (Table 5). Per 10 g maternal sugar consumption in early pregnancy, the odds of the offspring being born with a low birth weight were increased by 1.07 (95% CI 1.01 to 1.13, *p* = 0.026). Maternal energy intake, as well as macronutrient intake as percent of energy, did not show any further associations with the offspring's risk of being born with low or high birth weight, SGA or LGA (Table 5).

Table 5. Associations between maternal energy, macronutrient intake and dietary quality and neonatal weight-related parameters.

Energy and Macronutrient Intake	Low Birth Weight		High Birth Weight		SGA		LGA	
	Adjusted Odds Ratio [a] (95% CI)	Adjusted *p* Value [a]	Adjusted Odds Ratio [a] (95% CI)	Adjusted *p* Value [a]	Adjusted Odds Ratio [a] (95% CI)	Adjusted *p* Value [a]	Adjusted Odds Ratio [a] (95% CI)	Adjusted *p* Value [a]
Energy [100 kcal/day]								
T0	1.01 (0.98,1.05)	0.560	1.01 (0.98,1.04)	0.509	1.00 (0.97,1.03)	0.854	1.01 (0.98,1.04)	0.630
T1	0.99 (0.95,1.03)	0.594	1.01 (0.98,1.03)	0.659	0.98 (0.96,1.01)	0.267	0.99 (0.96,1.02)	0.604
Carbohydrates [10 E%]								
T0	0.96 (0.73,1.26)	0.761	0.94 (0.76,1.17)	0.587	0.92 (0.74,1.13)	0.408	1.03 (0.83,1.29)	0.780
T1	1.05 (0.76,1.45)	0.786	1.01 (0.79,1.27)	0.966	0.83 (0.65,1.06)	0.131	1.09 (0.85,1.39)	0.501
Saccharose [10 g/day]								
T0	1.07 (1.01,1.13)	0.026	0.97 (0.92,1.03)	0.358	1.01 (0.96,1.07)	0.627	0.99 (0.94,1.05)	0.702
T1	0.98 (0.90,1.07)	0.664	0.98 (0.92,1.04)	0.513	0.96 (0.90,1.02)	0.210	0.96 (0.90,1.03)	0.244
Protein [10 E%]								
T0	0.77 (0.38,1.55)	0.457	1.31 (0.76,2.23)	0.331	0.95 (0.56,1.61)	0.852	1.02 (0.58,1.81)	0.940
T1	1.11 (0.51,2.40)	0.802	1.32 (0.76,2.30)	0.329	0.98 (0.55,1.75)	0.948	1.49 (0.84,2.66)	0.173
Fat [10 E%]								
T0	1.14 (0.80,1.61)	0.467	1.05 (0.80,1.38)	0.735	1.14 (0.88,1.49)	0.329	0.94 (0.71,1.25)	0.673
T1	0.91 (0.61,1.36)	0.647	0.92 (0.69,1.23)	0.584	1.33 (0.99,1.79)	0.057	0.79 (0.58,1.07)	0.131
Alcohol [g]								
T0	1.01 (0.88,1.15)	0.905	0.77 (0.55,1.07)	0.115	1.05 (0.98,1.13)	0.181	1.03 (0.94,1.12)	0.555
T1	1.05 (0.53,2.07)	0.887	0.85 (0.46,1.58)	0.616	0.74 (0.35,1.58)	0.442	0.81 (0.42,1.59)	0.544
Caffeine [100 mg]								
T0	1.09 (0.88,1.34)	0.431	0.94 (0.77,1.14)	0.494	1.03 (0.86,1.24)	0.739	1.03 (0.87,1.22)	0.718
T1	0.93 (0.68,1.27)	0.638	0.84 (0.66,1.07)	0.154	1.13 (0.93,1.37)	0.210	0.87 (0.68,1.10)	0.245
HEI [10 points]								
T0	0.86 (0.68,1.09)	0.220	1.11(0.92,1.34)	0.290	0.84(0.70,1.02)	0.076	1.10(0.90,1.35)	0.363
T1	0.80 (0.61,1.06)	0.117	1.15(0.94,1.41)	0.171	0.85(0.69,1.04)	0.104	1.15(0.93,1.43)	0.188

Estimated is the regression coefficient describing the association between the intake of a certain amount or percentage and infant weight-related parameters. [a] linear regression models adjusted for pre-pregnancy BMI, age, parity and group assignment. BMI: body mass index; HEI: Healthy Eating Index; LGA: large for gestational age; SGA: small for gestational age; T0: assessment before or in the 12th week of gestation; T1: assessment after the 29th week of gestation.

4. Discussion

This secondary analysis of the GeliS trial shows associations between the maternal diet in early and late pregnancy and offspring weight parameters. Although no consistent associations between energy intake and macronutrient composition and neonatal birth weight and weight-derived parameters were shown, several aspects of maternal dietary behaviour were related to neonatal weight parameters.

Our analysis provides evidence that a healthy balanced antenatal diet, indicated by higher scores on the HEI, promotes birth weight within an adequate range and does not increase the risk of high birth weight or LGA. An increase in neonatal body weight with an increasing HEI has also been reported by others [25]. We could not confirm findings by investigators who observed that women with a healthier dietary pattern bore offspring with a reduced risk for low birth weight [26]. However, the latter study was performed in Ghana where the risk of low birth weight is much higher compared to developed countries [27]. Moreover, fruit and vegetable consumption were identified as factors that are positively associated with infant weight and BMI at birth. This observation is in line with findings of other studies reporting an increase in birth weight with increasing intake of fruits and vegetables [12,28]. While maternal vegetable intake did not modify the risk of being born SGA or LGA in our study, a high fruit intake in early pregnancy seemed to slightly increase the risk of LGA.

Our data did not indicate a beneficial association between the consumption of fruits and vegetables and the odds of being born SGA. In general, the data showing a protective effect of vegetable and fruit consumption on infants being born SGA is conflicting [12]. This may result from the heterogeneity in methods used for dietary assessment in the few studies. Moreover, effects may differ between high-

and low-income countries [12]. The observed effects of fruit and vegetable intake in our cohort may be a surrogate reflecting healthier dietary choices, as similar associations were observed regarding the HEI.

For instance, factors related to a lower neonatal body weight in the GeliS cohort included food parameters reflecting a rather unhealthy diet, such as soft drinks, sugar and alcohol intake. Soft drink and saccharose consumption were inversely associated with birth weight. An increase in sugar consumption in early pregnancy was additionally found to increase the risk of being born with a low birth weight. Both soft drinks and saccharose are energy-providing components of the diet that do not deliver any further nutrients of specific value. A high consumption may be accompanied by a lower consumption of nutritious foods and this could explain the negative association with birth weight. A negative effect of the intake of sugar and sugar-rich products on offspring birth weight has also been reported in other studies [28,29], whereas the role of soft drinks needs to be further elucidated. In the literature, the consumption of sugar-containing beverages has been suggested to have both an increasing [14] and a decreasing effect [30] on neonatal birth weight. Another factor, which we found to be negatively associated with birth weight, was alcohol consumption. This is consistent with evidence from a recent review and meta-analysis suggesting a relationship between low amounts of alcohol intake and the prevalence of children born SGA [31]. Although alcohol intake was found to be associated with a reduction in birth weight in the GeliS trial, there was no evidence for a modification of the SGA risk. However, reported alcohol consumption was generally low among our study population [32] and intake may be underreported, thus limiting the validity of our observations as well as those from others.

Fast food consumption was associated with an increased risk of the offspring being born with a high birth weight. This may be related to the high energy density of fast food which can generally increase overall energy intake [33]. A higher risk for delivering macrosomic infants in women eating a diet rich in energy-dense fast food has been suggested [34], but evidence is sparse. In our cohort, we found no evidence for an effect of energy and fat intake itself on birth weight and weight-related parameters. Likewise, although other maternal dietary factors, such as the intake of dairy products [11] or fish [13], have previously been shown to modify infant birth weight, we were not able to confirm these observations.

The presented cohort data have some limitations. Due to the high number of recruited pregnant women, maternal diet was assessed by means of a self-administered FFQ and energy and macronutrient intake were estimated based on the FFQ. More precise methods for the assessment of the maternal diet, such as weighted dietary records, were not feasible in the context of the large-scale GeliS study. However, they may have a greater potential to reveal significant effects of the maternal diet on neonatal weight and weight-related characteristics. In addition, maternal antenatal physical activity was not considered as a covariate in exploring associations between food intake and offspring weight data. We acknowledge that physical activity may be an additional modifying factor for food and energy intake and may likewise influence neonatal outcomes [35]. Due to the nature of the trial designed as a routine care study, offspring data were limited to reported body weight and weight-derived parameters. An additional assessment of infant body composition may provide a more comprehensive picture of the observed associations, as suggested for instance in the INFAT trial [36]. Moreover, infant weight was measured at different clinics, and it is possible that measurements may not have been conducted completely standardised.

The reported effects of the maternal diet on infant weight and weight-related parameters at birth were only modest and clinical relevance of the observed associations is thus questionable. Nonetheless, this secondary analysis of the GeliS cohort has some strengths that merit particular attention. A wide spectrum of dietary data was analysed with regard to offspring weight and weight-related data, including the consumption of particular foods and food groups, energy and macronutrient intake, as well as dietary quality measured with an HEI that was specifically developed for the FFQ used in this study [20,22]. Within the large-scale GeliS trial, we collected dietary and infant data directly in the setting of routine prenatal care. We were able to follow participants from early pregnancy through the postpartum period. In contrast to many other studies, dietary data were collected twice during pregnancy in the GeliS cohort, enabling separate analyses of potential effects of the antenatal diet on offspring outcomes in early and late pregnancy. Our cohort included both primi- and multiparous women from different BMI categories with varying educational levels. This offered a view on the impact of the maternal diet on offspring weight in a diverse target population which is, in many characteristics, representative for German women of childbearing age.

5. Conclusions

In conclusion, a healthy maternal diet characterised by a high intake of fruit and vegetables, as well as a high HEI, was shown to modestly increase birth weight within the adequate range without augmenting the risk for high birth weight or LGA. In contrast, intake of soft-drinks, saccharose and alcohol represented factors associated with a decrease in birth weight. Maternal intake of fast food in early pregnancy was related to a higher risk for infants to have a high birth weight. In the on-going follow-up of the GeliS cohort, the long-term effects of the maternal diet on offspring weight development during infancy will be evaluated.

Supplementary Materials: The following are available online at http://www.mdpi.com/2072-6643/11/8/1889/s1, Table S1: Associations between dietary parameters and offspring body mass index z-score at birth.

Author Contributions: Conceptualization, H.H., K.R., J.G. and J.H.; methodology, H.H., K.R., J.G., J.H. and L.S.; formal analysis, J.G. and L.S.; investigation, J.G. and J.K.; resources, K.R., E.R., L.K., J.K. and J.G.; data curation, J.G. and L.S.; writing—original draft preparation, J.G.; writing—review and editing, J.H., K.R., L.S., J.K., M.S., D.M., E.R., L.K. and H.H.; visualization, J.G.; supervision, H.H.; project administration, H.H. and K.R.; funding acquisition, H.H.

Funding: The study was funded by the Else Kröner-Fresenius Centre for Nutritional Medicine at the Technical University of Munich, the Competence Centre for Nutrition (KErn) in Bavaria, the Bavarian State Ministry of Food, Agriculture and Forestry, the Bavarian State Ministry of Health and Care (Health Initiative "Gesund.Leben.Bayern."), the AOK Bayern, the largest statutory health insurance in Bavaria, as well as the DEDIPAC consortium by the Joint Programming Initiative (JPI) "A Healthy Diet for a Healthy Life". Data collection, analysis, interpretation of data and manuscript preparation were independent from the funding bodies.

Acknowledgments: We gratefully acknowledge the valuable contribution from the Munich Study Centre at the Technical University of Munich and project managers at the expert centres for nutrition/community catering at the regional offices (AELF) of the Bavarian State Ministry of Food, Agriculture and Forestry (StMELF) which have been coordinating the study on the regional level. We gratefully acknowledge the support of our colleague Christina Holzapfel, Institute for Nutritional Medicine. The support from Martin Wabitsch and Stefanie Brandt, Pediatric Endocrinology and Diabetes, Department of Pediatrics and Adolescent Medicine, University Medical Center Ulm, Kurt Ulm and Victoria Kehl, Institute of Medical Informatics, Statistics and Epidemiology, Klinikum rechts der Isar of the Technical University of Munich, the network "Healthy Start - Young Family Network", Federal Center for Nutrition (BZfE), Federal Office for Agriculture and Food (BLE), belonging to the national IN FORM initiative (Maria Flothkötter, Katharina Krüger), Bonn, Uta Engels, Sports Centre, University of Regensburg, Karl-Heinz Ladwig, Head of Research Group Mental Health at the Institute of Epidemiology, Helmholtz Centre Munich, K.T.M. Schneider, Division of Obstetrics and Perinatal Medicine, Technical University of Munich, Rüdiger von Kries, Institute of Social Paediatrics and Adolescent Medicine, Ludwig-Maximilians-University Munich, Regina Ensenauer, von Hauner Children's Hospital, Ludwig-Maximilians-University Munich and Heinrich Heine University Düsseldorf, Rolf Holle, Institute of Health Economics and Health Care Management, Institute of Epidemiology, Helmholtz Centre Munich, Gabi Pfeifer, Educational Center Nuremberg, and Eveline Rieg, Competence Centre for Nutrition, Freising/Kulmbach, are gratefully acknowledged. We gratefully acknowledge Gert Mensink, Robert Koch Institute, Berlin for guidance in the analysis of the FFQ including the Healthy Eating Index and the Max Rubner Institute, Karlsruhe for provision of reference data from the German National Consumption Survey II (NVS II). Finally, we would like to thank our colleagues Annie Naujoks, Kristina Geyer and Roxana Raab, Institute for Nutritional Medicine, for their support and all participating practices, gynecologists, medical personnel, midwives, participants and their families for their involvement.

Conflicts of Interest: The authors declare no conflict of interest. The funders had no role in the design of the study; in the collection, analyses, or interpretation of data; in the writing of the manuscript, or in the decision to publish the results.

References

1. Schellong, K.; Schulz, S.; Harder, T.; Plagemann, A. Birth weight and long-term overweight risk: Systematic review and a meta-analysis including 643,902 persons from 66 studies and 26 countries globally. *PLoS ONE* **2012**, *7*, e47776. [CrossRef]
2. Harder, T.; Rodekamp, E.; Schellong, K.; Dudenhausen, J.W.; Plagemann, A. Birth weight and subsequent risk of type 2 diabetes: A meta-analysis. *Am. J. Epidemiol.* **2007**, *165*, 849–857. [CrossRef]
3. Kim, S.Y.; Sharma, A.J.; Sappenfield, W.; Wilson, H.G.; Salihu, H.M. Association of maternal body mass index, excessive weight gain, and gestational diabetes mellitus with large-for-gestational-age births. *Obstet. Gynecol.* **2014**, *123*, 737–744. [CrossRef] [PubMed]
4. Lau, E.Y.; Liu, J.; Archer, E.; McDonald, S.M.; Liu, J. Maternal weight gain in pregnancy and risk of obesity among offspring: A systematic review. *J. Obes.* **2014**, *2014*, 524939. [CrossRef] [PubMed]
5. Mamun, A.A.; Mannan, M.; Doi, S.A.R. Gestational weight gain in relation to offspring obesity over the life course: A systematic review and bias-adjusted meta-analysis. *Obes. Rev.* **2014**, *15*, 338–347. [CrossRef] [PubMed]
6. Fraser, A.; Tilling, K.; Macdonald-Wallis, C.; Sattar, N.; Brion, M.-J.; Benfield, L.; Ness, A.; Deanfield, J.; Hingorani, A.; Nelson, S.M.; et al. Association of maternal weight gain in pregnancy with offspring obesity and metabolic and vascular traits in childhood. *Circulation* **2010**, *121*, 2557–2564. [CrossRef] [PubMed]
7. Pérez-Morales, M.E.; Bacardi-Gascon, M.; Jimenez-Cruz, A. Association of excessive GWG with adiposity indicators and metabolic diseases of their offspring: Systematic review. *Nutr. Hosp.* **2015**, *31*, 1473–1480. [CrossRef]
8. Grieger, J.A.; Clifton, V.L. A review of the impact of dietary intakes in human pregnancy on infant birthweight. *Nutrients* **2014**, *7*, 153–178. [CrossRef]
9. Abu-Saad, K.; Fraser, D. Maternal nutrition and birth outcomes. *Epidemiol. Rev.* **2010**, *32*, 5–25. [CrossRef]
10. Imdad, A.; Bhutta, Z.A. Effect of balanced protein energy supplementation during pregnancy on birth outcomes. *BMC Public Health* **2011**, *11* (Suppl. 3), S17. [CrossRef]
11. Brantsæter, A.L.; Olafsdottir, A.S.; Forsum, E.; Olsen, S.F.; Thorsdottir, I. Does milk and dairy consumption during pregnancy influence fetal growth and infant birthweight? A systematic literature review. *Food Nutr. Res.* **2012**, *56*. [CrossRef] [PubMed]
12. Murphy, M.M.; Stettler, N.; Smith, K.M.; Reiss, R. Associations of consumption of fruits and vegetables during pregnancy with infant birth weight or small for gestational age births: A systematic review of the literature. *Int. J. Womens Health* **2014**, *6*, 899–912. [CrossRef] [PubMed]
13. Leventakou, V.; Roumeliotaki, T.; Martinez, D.; Barros, H.; Brantsaeter, A.-L.; Casas, M.; Charles, M.-A.; Cordier, S.; Eggesbø, M.; van Eijsden, M.; et al. Fish intake during pregnancy, fetal growth, and gestational length in 19 European birth cohort studies. *Am. J. Clin. Nutr.* **2014**, *99*, 506–516. [CrossRef] [PubMed]
14. Phelan, S.; Hart, C.; Phipps, M.; Abrams, B.; Schaffner, A.; Adams, A.; Wing, R. Maternal behaviors during pregnancy impact offspring obesity risk. *Exp. Diabetes Res.* **2011**, *2011*, 985139. [CrossRef] [PubMed]
15. International Weight Management in Pregnancy (i-WIP) Collaborative Group. Effect of diet and physical activity based interventions in pregnancy on gestational weight gain and pregnancy outcomes: Meta-analysis of individual participant data from randomised trials. *BMJ* **2017**, *358*, j3119. [CrossRef]
16. Rauh, K.; Kunath, J.; Rosenfeld, E.; Kick, L.; Ulm, K.; Hauner, H. Healthy living in pregnancy: A cluster-randomized controlled trial to prevent excessive gestational weight gain—Rationale and design of the GeliS study. *BMC Pregnancy Childbirth* **2014**, *14*, 119. [CrossRef]
17. Kunath, J.; Günther, J.; Rauh, K.; Hoffmann, J.; Stecher, L.; Rosenfeld, E.; Kick, L.; Ulm, K.; Hauner, H. Effects of a lifestyle intervention during pregnancy to prevent excessive gestational weight gain in routine care—The cluster-randomised GeliS trial. *BMC Med.* **2019**, *17*, 5. [CrossRef] [PubMed]
18. Koletzko, B.; Bauer, C.-P.; Bung, P.; Cremer, M.; Flothkötter, M.; Hellmers, C.; Kersting, M.; Krawinkel, M.; Przyrembel, H.; Rasenack, R.; et al. Ernährung in der Schwangerschaft—Teil 2. Handlungsempfehlungen des Netzwerks "Gesund ins Leben—Netzwerk Junge Familie". *Deutsche Medizinische Wochenschrift* **2012**, *137*, 1366–1372. [CrossRef]
19. National Research Council. *Weight Gain during Pregnancy. Reexamining the Guidelines*; Rasmussen, K.M., Yaktine, A.L., Eds.; National Academies Press: Washington, DC, USA, 2009; ISBN 9780309131131.

20. Haftenberger, M.; Heuer, T.; Heidemann, C.; Kube, F.; Krems, C.; Mensink, G.B.M. Relative validation of a food frequency questionnaire for national health and nutrition monitoring. *Nutr. J.* **2010**, *9*, 36. [CrossRef]

21. Meltzer, H.M.; Brantsaeter, A.L.; Ydersbond, T.A.; Alexander, J.; Haugen, M. Methodological challenges when monitoring the diet of pregnant women in a large study: Experiences from the Norwegian Mother and Child Cohort Study (MoBa). *Matern. Child Nutr.* **2008**, *4*, 14–27. [CrossRef]

22. Kuhn, D.-A. Entwicklung eines Index zur Bewertung der Ernährungsqualität in der Studie zur Gesundheit Erwachsener in Deutschland (DEGS1), German ("Development of a dietary quality index in the German Health Examination Survey for Adults"). Master's Thesis, Robert Koch Institute, Berlin, Germany, 2017.

23. Kleinwechter, H.; Schäfer-Graf, U.; Bührer, C.; Hoesli, I.; Kainer, F.; Kautzky-Willer, A.; Pawlowski, B.; Schunck, K.; Somville, T.; Sorger, M. Gestationsdiabetes mellitus (GDM)—Diagnostik, Therapie und Nachsorge. *Diabetologie und Stoffwechsel* **2016**, *11*, S182–S194. [CrossRef]

24. Metzger, B.E.; Gabbe, S.G.; Persson, B.; Buchanan, T.A.; Catalano, P.A.; Damm, P.; Dyer, A.R.; de Leiva, A.; Hod, M.; Kitzmiler, J.L.; et al. International association of diabetes and pregnancy study groups recommendations on the diagnosis and classification of hyperglycemia in pregnancy. *Diabetes Care* **2010**, *33*, 676–682. [CrossRef] [PubMed]

25. Rodríguez-Bernal, C.L.; Rebagliato, M.; Iñiguez, C.; Vioque, J.; Navarrete-Muñoz, E.M.; Murcia, M.; Bolumar, F.; Marco, A.; Ballester, F. Diet quality in early pregnancy and its effects on fetal growth outcomes: The Infancia y Medio Ambiente (Childhood and Environment) Mother and Child Cohort Study in Spain. *Am. J. Clin. Nutr.* **2010**, *91*, 1659–1666. [CrossRef] [PubMed]

26. Abubakari, A.; Jahn, A. Maternal Dietary Patterns and Practices and Birth Weight in Northern Ghana. *PLoS ONE* **2016**, *11*, e0162285. [CrossRef] [PubMed]

27. He, Z.; Bishwajit, G.; Yaya, S.; Cheng, Z.; Zou, D.; Zhou, Y. Prevalence of low birth weight and its association with maternal body weight status in selected countries in Africa: A cross-sectional study. *BMJ Open* **2018**, *8*, e020410. [CrossRef] [PubMed]

28. Kjøllesdal, M.K.R.; Holmboe-Ottesen, G. Dietary Patterns and Birth Weight-a Review. *AIMS Public Health* **2014**, *1*, 211–225. [CrossRef] [PubMed]

29. Lenders, C.M.; Hediger, M.L.; Scholl, T.O.; Khoo, C.S.; Slap, G.B.; Stallings, V.A. Gestational age and infant size at birth are associated with dietary sugar intake among pregnant adolescents. *J. Nutr.* **1997**, *127*, 1113–1117. [CrossRef]

30. Grundt, J.H.; Eide, G.E.; Brantsaeter, A.-L.; Haugen, M.; Markestad, T. Is consumption of sugar-sweetened soft drinks during pregnancy associated with birth weight? *Matern. Child Nutr.* **2017**, *13*. [CrossRef]

31. Mamluk, L.; Edwards, H.B.; Savović, J.; Leach, V.; Jones, T.; Moore, T.H.M.; Ijaz, S.; Lewis, S.J.; Donovan, J.L.; Lawlor, D.; et al. Low alcohol consumption and pregnancy and childhood outcomes: Time to change guidelines indicating apparently 'safe' levels of alcohol during pregnancy? A systematic review and meta-analyses. *BMJ Open* **2017**, *7*, e015410. [CrossRef]

32. Günther, J.; Hoffmann, J.; Kunath, J.; Spies, M.; Meyer, D.; Stecher, L.; Rosenfeld, E.; Kick, L.; Rauh, K.; Hauner, H. Effects of a Lifestyle Intervention in Routine Care on Prenatal Dietary Behavior—Findings from the Cluster-Randomized GeliS Trial. *JCM* **2019**, *8*, 960. [CrossRef]

33. Ledikwe, J.H.; Blanck, H.M.; Kettel Khan, L.; Serdula, M.K.; Seymour, J.D.; Tohill, B.C.; Rolls, B.J. Dietary energy density is associated with energy intake and weight status in US adults. *Am. J. Clin. Nutr.* **2006**, *83*, 1362–1368. [CrossRef] [PubMed]

34. Wen, L.M.; Simpson, J.M.; Rissel, C.; Baur, L.A. Maternal "junk food" diet during pregnancy as a predictor of high birthweight: Findings from the healthy beginnings trial. *Birth* **2013**, *40*, 46–51. [CrossRef] [PubMed]

35. Hoffmann, J.; Günther, J.; Geyer, K.; Stecher, L.; Kunath, J.; Meyer, D.; Spies, M.; Rosenfeld, E.; Kick, L.; Rauh, K.; et al. Effects of prenatal physical activity on neonatal and obstetric outcomes—Findings from the cluster-randomised GeliS trial. *BMC Pregnancy Childbirth* **2019**, under review.

36. Brei, C.; Stecher, L.; Meyer, D.M.; Young, V.; Much, D.; Brunner, S.; Hauner, H. Impact of Dietary Macronutrient Intake during Early and Late Gestation on Offspring Body Composition at Birth, 1, 3, and 5 Years of Age. *Nutrients* **2018**, *10*, 579. [CrossRef] [PubMed]

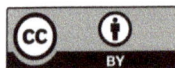

nutrients

MDPI

Article

Maternal Fatty Fish Intake Prior to and during Pregnancy and Risks of Adverse Birth Outcomes: Findings from a British Cohort

Camilla Nykjaer [1,2,*], Charlotte Higgs [3], Darren C. Greenwood [4], Nigel A.B. Simpson [3], Janet E. Cade [1] and Nisreen A. Alwan [5,6]

[1] Nutritional Epidemiology Group, School of Food Science and Nutrition, University of Leeds, Leeds LS2 9JT, UK; J.E.Cade@leeds.ac.uk
[2] School of Biomedical Sciences, Faculty of Biological Sciences, University of Leeds, Leeds LS2 9JT, UK
[3] Department of Obstetrics and Gynaecology, University of Leeds, Leeds LS2 9JT, UK; charlotte.higgs@nhs.net (C.H.); N.A.B.Simpson@leeds.ac.uk (N.A.B.S.)
[4] Division of Biostatistics, Centre for Epidemiology and Biostatistics, University of Leeds, Leeds LS2 9JT, UK; D.C.Greenwood@leeds.ac.uk
[5] School of Primary Care and Population Sciences, Faculty of Medicine, University of Southampton, Southampton General Hospital, Southampton SO16 6YD, UK; N.A.Alwan@soton.ac.uk
[6] NIHR Southampton Biomedical Research Centre, University of Southampton and University Hospital Southampton NHS Foundation Trust, Southampton SO16 6YD, UK
*   Correspondence: c.nykjaer@leeds.ac.uk

Received: 1 February 2019; Accepted: 13 March 2019; Published: 16 March 2019

Abstract: Fish is an important source of the essential fatty acids contributing to foetal growth and development, but the evidence linking maternal fatty fish consumption with birth outcomes is inconsistent. In the UK, pregnant women are recommended to consume no more than two 140 g portions of fatty fish per week. This study aimed to investigate the association between fatty fish consumption before and during pregnancy with preterm birth and size at birth in a prospective birth cohort. Dietary intake data were acquired from a cohort of 1208 pregnant women in Leeds, UK (CARE Study) to assess preconception and trimester-specific fatty fish consumption using questionnaires. Multiple 24-h recalls during pregnancy were used to estimate an average fatty fish portion size. Intake was classified as ≤ 2, > 2 portions/week and no fish categories. Following the exclusion of women taking cod liver oil and/or omega-3 supplements, the associations between fatty fish intake with size at birth and preterm delivery (<37 weeks gestation) were examined in multivariable regression models adjusting for confounders including salivary cotinine as a biomarker of smoking status. The proportion of women reporting any fatty fish intake decreased throughout pregnancy, with the lowest proportion observed in trimester 3 (43%). Mean intakes amongst consumers were considerably lower than that recommended, with the lowest intake amongst consumers observed in the 1st trimester (106 g/week, 95% CI: 99, 113). This was partly due to small portion sizes when consumed, with the mean portion size of fatty fish being 101 g. After adjusting for confounders, no association was observed between fatty fish intake before or during pregnancy with size at birth and preterm delivery.

Keywords: fatty fish; essential fatty acids; omega-3; pregnancy; birth weight; foetal growth; preterm birth

---

1. Introduction

Preterm birth (<37 weeks gestation) and low birth weight (LBW) are important determinants of neonatal mortality and morbidity. They are also linked with higher risks of metabolic, neurological and cardiovascular disease in adult life [1–3]. Maternal nutrition during pregnancy has been postulated to play a role in the prevention of these adverse birth outcomes [4,5].

Recent research has focused on the role of fatty acids, in particular the omega-6 and omega-3 long chain polyunsaturated fatty acids (LCPUFA), which are derived from their respective precursors, linoleic (LA) and linolenic (LNA) acids. These are vital for the development of cell membranes and new tissues [6–8] and are classified as essential fatty acids (EFA) as they can only be derived from the maternal diet. During pregnancy the most biologically active LCPUFAs, docosahexaenoic acid (DHA) and arachidonic acid (AA) have been shown to have beneficial effects [9], particularly on the development of the foetal brain and retina [8]. These EFA cannot be synthesised in the human body [6,7,10] and the conversion rate of precursor to LCPUFA derivative within the foetus is limited [11]. Consequently, the foetus is heavily dependent on the maternal diet for EFA through transport across the placenta [11–13]. Additionally, as the EFA status of the mother has been found to decline during pregnancy [6,14], a dietary source is paramount for meeting the demand for maternal-foetal exchange.

Fish are an important source of essential LCPUFAs, particularly the n-3 PUFAs. However, the extent to which fish intake plays a role in shaping pregnancy outcomes is unclear, as evidence regarding maternal consumption and birth outcomes is inconclusive. Findings from some birth cohorts suggest a positive association between total fish intake and birth weight [15–19], with women with a high total fish intake being less likely to have low birthweight (LBW) babies [16,19] as well as preterm birth [20,21]. However, negative associations have also been found [15,18,22–24] and in some cases no association with preterm birth [15,17,23–25] nor size at birth [15,24–27] has been evident.

It has been hypothesised that adverse associations may be due to contaminants in fish including mercury and persistent organic pollutants (POPs). Fatty fish is a known source of these contaminants, particularly in larger fish species [22]. However, studies that have focused on differentiating between types of fish consumed including lean, fatty and shellfish in relation to birth outcomes have been inconclusive [15,18,19,24,27] although there may be a trend toward a negative association between fatty fish and foetal growth [18,22].

The current advice in the UK is to consume at least two portions of fish/week (~140 g/portion), one of which should be fatty fish [28]. This recommendation also applies to pregnant women and women trying to conceive but with an upper limit of maximum two portions of fatty fish/week. Pregnant women and women trying to conceive are also advised to avoid consumption of larger species such as marlin, swordfish and shark [28]. Despite the guideline stating that intake of up to two portions of fatty fish/week does not present any harm, many Western pregnant women consume limited amounts of fish [10,29,30] resulting in low intakes of LCPUFA which could be potentially detrimental to foetal development.

Using data from a prospective UK-based birth cohort (the Caffeine and Reproductive Health study (CARE)) [31], this paper aimed to estimate maternal fatty fish intake frequency and portion size before and during pregnancy, and investigate the association between maternal fatty fish intake before and during pregnancy with both preterm birth and size at birth.

2. Materials and Methods

2.1. Participants and Study Design

The CARE study is a British prospective birth cohort with the primary aim of investigating the associations between caffeine in the maternal diet and pregnancy outcomes [31]. Between 2003 and 2006, low risk pregnant women aged 18–45 years were recruited from Leeds Teaching Maternity Hospitals at 8–12 weeks gestation. A total of 5959 women were considered, of whom 4571 met the inclusion criteria. Eligible women were sent detailed information about the study and 1374 consented to participate. All participants gave written, informed consent and the study was conducted in accordance with the Declaration of Helsinki and approved by the Leeds West Local Research Ethics Committee (reference number 03/054).

2.2. Assessment of Maternal Fatty Fish Intake

2.2.1. Recall Data

Rather than using the Scientific Advisory Committee on Nutrition (SACN) estimate of 140 grams (g) per portion of fatty fish [28], which is based on data from a non-pregnant population (the National Diet and Nutrition Survey) we derived an estimate of the average portion size of fatty fish from 24 h dietary recalls administered by research midwives at 14–16 and 28 weeks gestation. To get a better picture of usual consumption throughout pregnancy an average portion size of fatty fish was derived for women who consumed fatty fish at both recalls. Participants were asked to record all food and drink consumed in a 24 h period (12 midnight to 12 midnight), including portion size and drink amounts. An example recall was provided as guidance. Reported canned tuna intake was removed from the analysis as it is not considered a fatty fish due the majority of the fat content being removed during the canning process [28].

2.2.2. Self-Reported Questionnaires

Fatty fish consumption was ascertained prior to and throughout pregnancy using a frequency type self-reported questionnaire adapted from the UK Women's Cohort Study [32] and administered at enrolment (12–18 weeks gestation), assessing consumption in the 4 weeks leading up to pregnancy and trimester 1; week 28, assessing trimester 2 consumption and postpartum (weeks 46–50) assessing trimester 3 consumption. Participants were asked how often (never; less than once/month; 1–3 times/month; once/week; 2–4 times/week; 5–6 times/week; once/day; 2–3 times/day; 4–5 times/day and >6 times/day) they consumed fatty fish (examples given were: salmon, tuna (fresh only), herring, kipper, mackerel, pilchards, sprats and swordfish). No examples of what constitutes a portion were given in the questionnaire. Frequency of fish consumption derived from the questionnaires was converted to times per week, which was then multiplied by the portion estimate of fish obtained from the recall data (see above) in order to get weekly consumption in grams for each of the trimesters.

2.3. Assessment of Pregnancy Outcomes

Information regarding pregnancy outcomes was collected from hospital maternity records. The two primary outcomes assessed were preterm birth (defined as <37 weeks gestation) and small for gestational age (SGA), defined as <10th individualised birth centile taking into account gestational age, maternal height, weight, ethnicity, parity, child sex and birth weight [33]. Actual birth weight was also analysed as a secondary measurement and expressed as a continuous variable in grams and a binary variable LBW defined as <2500 g. Duration of gestation was calculated from the date of the last menstrual period, and confirmed by ultrasound scans dating at around 12 and 20 weeks gestation.

2.4. Assessment of Participant Characteristics

Maternal characteristics including age, ethnicity, pre-pregnancy weight, height, parity, education (university degree versus no degree) were self-reported in the preliminary administered questionnaire. Caffeine intake (mg/day) and alcohol consumption (units/day) were assessed throughout pregnancy using the same frequency type questionnaire used to assess fatty fish intake. Smoking status was objectively measured using salivary cotinine levels at enrolment. Participants were classified based on cotinine concentrations as active smokers (>5 ng/mL), passive smokers (1–5 ng/mL) or non-smokers (<1 ng/mL). Daily total energy intake was derived from the 1st 24 h of food recall data.

2.5. Statistical Power Calculation

Comparing mothers consuming > 2 portions/week to non-consumers, the study had 80% power to detect an odds ratio of approximately 0.4 for SGA. The equivalent test for linear trend including the intermediate category half way between these extremes would have 90% power. Similarly, comparing the birth weight of babies born to mothers consuming > 2 portions of fish/week with non-consumers, assuming the SD to be approximately 500 g, this study had 85% power to detect a difference of 150 g in birth weight at $p < 0.05$.

2.6. Statistical Analysis

Analysis was conducted using the continuous weekly fish variable assigned into three categories of intake based on the current UK guidelines of no more than 2 portions of fatty fish per week [28] with the addition of a "no fish" category which was used as the referent group: no fish, ≤2 portions/week and >2 portions/week.

Univariable analyses were performed using one-way ANOVA for normally distributed variables, Kruskal-Wallis for non-parametric variables and chi-squared test for categorical outcomes. Multivariable linear and logistic regression models were used to assess the association between maternal fatty fish intake and continuous and dichotomous birth outcomes respectively. Maternal pre-pregnancy weight, height, ethnicity, parity, gestation and neonatal sex were accounted for when calculating the SGA variable and were adjusted for in the preterm delivery (omitting gestation) and birth weight models. Covariates adjusted for in all models were selected based on *a priori* knowledge from the literature and included maternal age, salivary cotinine levels, self-reported caffeine intake and alcohol consumption and university degree status as a marker for socioeconomic status.

In order to separate the effect of fatty fish from supplements as opposed to dietary sources on birth outcomes, women taking any cod liver oil and/or omega-3 supplements were removed from the analysis. Women with extreme values for energy intake (highest 1% and lowest 1%), obtained from the 24 h recall data, were excluded due to possible bias with self-reported dietary intake, as proposed by Meltzer et al. [34].

Sensitivity analyses were conducted taking into account previous high-risk pregnancies (including a previous LBW baby, previous gestational diabetes (GDM) and previous gestational hypertension (GHT)) and total energy intake during pregnancy. Sensitivity analyses were also done by excluding women who developed GHT and GDM during their current pregnancy (3rd trimester only). All analyses were performed using the Stata 14 software (Stata, College Station, TX, USA).

3. Results

Of the 1374 mothers who consented, 1303 agreed to participate and were enrolled into the CARE study. Of these, nine were lost to follow-up, five terminated pregnancies and others were excluded due to stillbirth (n = 6), neonatal death (n = 3) and late miscarriage (n = 10). Following exclusions of women taking cod liver oil and/or omega-3 supplements (n = 37) as well as those with extreme energy intakes (n = 25) left 1208 mothers with data available on birth outcomes.

3.1. Estimation of Portion Size and Types of Fatty Fish Consumed (24-h Recall)

A total of 1276 women reported dietary information by recall at weeks 14–16, and 601 women at week 28. Of these women, 162/1276 (13%) and 70/601 (12%) reported intakes of any fatty fish at the 1st and 2nd recall respectively. Combining both sets of recall data together, a total of 106 women reported fatty fish intake during the 1st and 2nd recall. The amount of fish consumed in grams at each meal was used to obtain an average portion size of 101 g (min: 10 g, max: 300 g).

Of the 106 women consuming fatty fish in the 24 h recall data (14–28 weeks gestation), 52 (49%) women ate salmon, 25 (24%) ate raw tuna and 14 (13%) ate mackerel. Other types of fatty fish included anchovies (5%), sardines (7%), trout (6%) and orange roughy (0.9%). Fatty fish consumption accounted for 4.8% of the total energy intake.

3.2. Frequency of Fatty Fish Consumption (Questionnaire)

Of the 1208 women with birth outcome data, 1116 (92%) women had information available on frequency of fatty fish intake before pregnancy, 1114 (92%) in the 1st trimester, 812 (67.2%) in the 2nd trimester and 409 (34%) in the 3rd trimester (Table 1). For those women who reported consuming any fatty fish, intake before pregnancy (123.5 g/week) was significantly higher ($p < 0.0001$) than trimester 1 & 2 (106.4 and 107.4 g/week respectively) but slightly lower than the mean intake in the 3rd trimester (136.5 g/week). The proportion of women reporting any fatty fish intake, however, decreased throughout pregnancy with the lowest proportion observed in trimester 3 (43%).The prevalence of women consuming within the recommended guidelines of no more than 2 portions of fatty fish per week was highest in trimester 1 (47%) and in the 2nd trimester (49%), with mean intakes for women reaching 64.3 g (95% CI 61.0 to 67.7) and 71.3 g (95% CI 66.6 to 75.7) per week, respectively.

Table 1. Self-reported fatty fish intake across pregnancy.

	n (%)	Mean (g)	95% CI
Fish intake (g/week) (consumers only):			
4 weeks before pregnancy (*n* = 1116)	648 (58.1)	123.5	115.1, 131.9
First trimester (*n* = 1114)	652 (58.5)	106.4	98.9, 112.9
Second trimester (*n* = 812)	466 (57.4)	107.4	98.2, 116.6
Third trimester (*n* = 409)	177 (43.3)	136.5	118.8, 154.1
Categories of intake 4 weeks before pregnancy *			
No fish	468 (41.9)	0	0
≤2 portions/week	491 (44.0)	67.6	64.8, 70.5
>2 portions/week	157(14.1)	298.1	286.7, 309.6
Categories of intake trimester 1			
No fish	462 (41.47)	0	0
≤2 portions/week	524 (47.0)	64.3	61.0, 67.7
>2 portions/week	128 (11.5)	278.9	267.1, 290.7
Categories of intake trimester 2			
No fish	346 (42.6)	0	0
≤2 portions/week	396 (48.8)	71.3	66.6, 75.7
>2 portions/week	70 (8.6)	311.8	291.9, 331.7
Categories of intake trimester 3			
No fish	232 (56.7)	0	0
≤2 portions/week	131 (32.0)	75.4	70.4, 80.4
>2 portions/week	46 (11.3)	310.5	279.0, 341.9

* Categories based on the UK recommendations of no more than 2 portions of fatty fish/week [28]. One portion of fish is 101 g.

3.3. Maternal Characteristics According to Categories of Fish Intake

Table 2 shows characteristics of participants according to maternal fatty fish intake in trimester 1. Women who consumed fatty fish during pregnancy were more likely to be older, have a university degree, to consume alcohol, were less likely to smoke and less likely to live in an area within the most deprived Index of Multiple Deprivation (IMD) quartile. These characteristics were consistent across all trimesters and the four weeks leading up to pregnancy. Women consuming fish in trimester 1 & 2 were also more likely to have a lower BMI, and those consuming fish in trimester 1 were shown to have a lower caffeine intake than non-fish consumers.

Table 2. Characteristics of mothers by fatty fish intake in the 1st trimester of pregnancy (*n* = 1114).

	No Fatty Fish	≤2 Portions/Week	>2 Portions/Week	*p* *
	(*n* = 462)	(*n* = 524)	(*n* = 128)	
Age (years) mean (SD)	28.5 (5.6)	30.8 (4.4)	31.7 (4.6)	0.0001
Pre-pregnancy BMI (kg/m^2) mean (SD)	25.1 (5.3)	24.4 (4.3)	23.9 (5.3)	0.01
Total energy intake (kcal) mean (SD)	2109.4 (595.6)	2111.5 (614.3)	2183.5 (670.8)	0.8
Caffeine intake (mg/day) mean (SD)	223.3 (225.4)	159.9 (151.3)	190.6 (177.6)	0.0001
Alcohol intake: % non-drinkers (*n*)	28.3 (127)	16.4 (84)	20.0 (24)	0.0001
Smoker at 12 weeks % (*n*) **	26.8 (117)	9.1 (461)	10.6 (13)	0.0001
IMD most deprived quartile % (*n*)	41.1 (182)	21.7 (109)	19.1 (24)	0.0001
University degree % (*n*)	24.5 (113)	50.4 (264)	56.3 (72)	<0.0001
European origin % (*n*)	94.8 (437)	93.5 (489)	94.5 (121)	0.7
Primigravida % (*n*)	45.3 (209)	51.1 (267)	40.9 (52)	0.06
Baby's gender: % male (*n*)	52.6 (243)	49.1 (257)	43.8 (56)	0.2
Gestational hypertension % (*n*)	1.1 (5)	1.9 (10)	1.6 (2)	0.6
Gestational diabetes % (*n*)	0.2 (1)	0.4 (2)	0 (0)	0.7
Past history of miscarriage % (*n*)	22.4 (102)	22.9 (119)	27.8 (35)	0.4

* *p*-Value using one-way ANOVA and Kruskal-Wallis for normally and non-normally distributed continuous variables respectively, and χ^2-test & Fisher's exact test for categorical variables. Significant difference at *p* < 0.05. ** Smoking status based on salivary cotinine concentrations: non-smoker < 1 ng/mL, passive smoker 1–5 ng/mL, current smoker > 5 ng/mL. Where numbers do not add up it is due to a small proportion of missing data. SD, standard deviation; BMI, body mass index; IMD, Index of Multiple Deprivation.

3.4. Pregnancy Outcomes

Of the 1208 women with information on birth outcomes, 44 babies (4%) were delivered preterm (<37 weeks gestation) with a mean gestational age of 34.29 weeks (SD = 2.99). A further 153 (13%) babies were born SGA (<10th centile) and 46 (4%) were LBW (<2500 g); the latter of which 27 (56%) were born preterm. The mean birth weight of the total sample was 3446 g (SD = 537 g).

3.5. Relationship between Fish Intake before Pregnancy and Birth Outcomes

There was no evidence of an association between fatty fish intake before pregnancy and preterm birth nor size at birth (Table 3).

3.6. Relationship between Fish Intake during Pregnancy and Preterm Birth

Compared to mothers consuming no fish in trimester 1, in unadjusted analysis mothers consuming up to 2 portions and >2 portions of fatty fish/week were less likely to have babies born preterm (OR: 0.5, 95% CI: 0.3, 1.0 & OR: 0.3, 95% CI: 0.1, 1.1 respectively; p_{trend} = 0.05) (Table 4). After adjustment for potential confounders, these estimates were largely unchanged, though no longer statistically significant (OR: 0.6, 95% CI: 0.3, 1.3 & OR: 0.3, 95% CI: 0.1, 1.3 respectively, p_{trend} = 0.2). A similar trend could be observed in trimester 2 for mothers consuming ≤2 portions of fatty fish/week compared to non-consumers (OR: 0.4, 95% CI: 0.2, 0.9; p_{trend} = 0.06), becoming non-significant after adjustment (OR: 0.5, 95% CI: 0.2, 1.2, p_{trend} = 0.2). There was no association between fatty fish intake in the 3rd trimester and preterm birth.

Table 3. The relationship between maternal fatty fish intake 4 weeks before pregnancy and size at birth & preterm delivery.

Birth weight (g)	*n*	Unadjusted Change (95% CI)	*p* *	*n*	Adjusted Change ** (95% CI)	*p* *
No fatty fish	468	0	0.3	426	0	0.7
≤2 portions/week	491	45.8 (−23.3, 115.0)		459	−17.9 (−75.3, 39.5)	
>2 portions/week	157	71.6 (−27.1, 170.3)		144	−35.7 (−115.6, 44.1)	

		Unadjusted OR (95% CI)	*p* *		Adjusted OR ** (95% CI)	*p* *
SGA (<10th centile) ***	cases/*n*			cases/*n*		
No fatty fish	70/468	1	0.3	67/444	1	0.6
≤2 portions/week	57/491	0.7 (0.5, 1.1)		55/473	1.0 (0.6, 1.5)	
>2 portions/week	23/157	1.0 (0.6, 1.6)		23/150	1.3 (0.8, 2.3)	
Low birth weight (≤2500 g)						
No fatty fish	21/468	1	0.8	19/426	1	0.3
≤2 portions/week	20/491	0.9 (0.5, 1.7)		19/459	1.9 (0.7, 5.3)	
>2 portions/week	5/157	0.7 (0.3, 1.9)		5/144	3.1 (0.8, 12.7)	
Preterm birth (<37 weeks gestation)						
No fatty fish	24/468	1	0.2	23/426	1	0.4
≤2 portions/week	17/491	0.7 (0.4, 1.3)		17/459	0.8 (0.4, 1.6)	
>2 portions/week	3/157	0.4 (0.1, 1.2)		3/144	0.4 (0.1, 1.5)	

* p for trend for categories of fish intake ** Adjusted for maternal pre-pregnancy weight, height, age, parity, ethnicity, salivary cotinine levels, caffeine intake, alcohol intake, education, gestation and baby's sex in multivariable linear regression for continuous outcome and multivariable logistic regression for categorical outcomes. *** Takes into account maternal pre-pregnancy weight, height, parity, ethnicity, gestation and baby's sex.

3.7. Relationship between Fish Intake during Pregnancy and Size at Birth

When comparing babies born to mothers consuming no fatty fish in trimester 1, mothers consuming up to two portions of fatty fish/week had babies weighing 58.4 g less (95% CI: −115.1, −1.5) although there was no linear trend ($p_{trend} = 0.1$). There was no evidence of any relationship between fish intake in the second or third trimester and size at birth expressed as birth weight (g), SGA (<10th centile) or low birth weight (Table 4).

3.8. Sensitivity Analysis

Adding total energy intake to the regression models did not affect the results. Similarly, including an indicator for high risk pregnancies as a possible moderator ($n = 175$) did not significantly alter findings nor did excluding women who developed GDM ($n = 3$) or GHT ($n = 19$).

Table 4. The relationship between maternal fatty fish intake during pregnancy and size at birth & preterm delivery.

	Trimester 1						Trimester 2						Trimester 3					
	n	Unadjusted Change (95% CI)	p*	n	Adjusted Change ** (95% CI)	p*	n	Unadjusted Change (95% CI)	p*	n	Adjusted Change ** (95% CI)	p*	n	Unadjusted Change (95% CI)	p*	n	Adjusted Change ** (95% CI)	p*
Birth weight (g)																		
No fatty fish	462	0	0.3	422	0	0.1	346	0	0.2	316	0	0.3	232	0	0.3	218	0	0.8
≤2 portions/week	524	30.4 (−37.9, 98.7)		488	−58.4 (−115.1, −1.7)		396	75.3 (−6.5, 157.1)		371	−47.3 (−113.0, 18.4)		131	109.6 (−25.4, 244.6)		126	−35.6 (−139.9, 68.7)	
>2 portions/week	128	87.7 (−19.2, 194.6)		118	−64.0 (−151.1, 23.1)		70	42.3 (−103.4, 188.1)		64	−71.4 (−185.8, 43.13)		46	52.6 (−146.8, 251.9)		43	−21.8 (−169.0, 125.4)	
	cases/n	Unadjusted OR (95% CI)	p*	cases/n	Adjusted OR ** (95% CI)	p*	cases/n	Unadjusted OR (95% CI)	p*	cases/n	Adjusted OR ** (95% CI)	p*	cases/n	Unadjusted OR (95% CI)	p*	cases/n	Adjusted OR ** (95% CI)	p*
SGA (<10th centile) * **																		
No fatty fish	69/462	1	0.2	65/436	1	0.3	60/346	1	0.6	56/328	1	0.6	74/232	1	0.9	69/220	1	0.8
≤2 portions/week	69/524	0.9 (0.6, 1.2)		68/506	1.2 (0.8, 1.8)		58/396	0.8 (0.6, 1.2)		58/385	1.1 (0.4, 1.7)		40/131	0.9 (0.6, 1.5)		40/129	1.1 (0.7, 1.9)	
>2 portions/week	11/128	0.5 (0.3, 1.0)		11/123	0.7 (0.4, 1.5)		12/70	1.0 (0.5, 1.9)		12/67	1.5 (0.7, 3.0)		5/46	1.0 (0.5, 2.0)		5/43	1.2 (0.6, 2.5)	
Low birth weight (≤2500 g)																		
No fatty fish	23/462	1	0.3	21/422	1	0.4	23/346	1	0.3	21/316	1	0.2	26/232	1	0.5	24/218	1	0.2
≤2 portions/week	21/524	0.8 (0.4, 1.5)		20/488	2.0 (0.7, 5.6)		17/396	0.6 (0.3, 1.2)		17/371	3.0 (0.9, 9.7)		10/131	0.7 (0.3, 1.4)		10/126	2.4 (0.6, 9.7)	
>2 portions/week	2/128	0.3 (0.1, 1.3)		2/118	1.2 (0.2, 7.4)		3/70	0.6 (0.2, 2.2)		3/64	1.5 (0.3, 8.1)		5/46	1.0 (0.4, 2.7)		5/43	5.5 (0.9, 31.9)	
Preterm birth (<37 weeks gestation)																		
No fatty fish	26/462	1	0.05	25/422	1	0.2	21/346	1	0.06	21/316	1	0.2	18/232	1	0.3	18/218	1	0.6
≤2 portions/week	16/524	0.5 (0.3, 1.0)		16/488	0.6 (0.3, 1.3)		10/396	0.4 (0.2, 0.9)		10/371	0.5 (0.2, 1.2)		5/131	0.5 (0.2, 1.3)		5/126	0.6 (0.2, 1.7)	
>2 portions/week	2/128	0.3 (0.1, 1.1)		2/118	0.3 (0.1, 1.3)		4/70	0.9 (0.3, 2.8)		4/64	1.1 (0.4, 3.6)		3/46	0.8 (0.2, 2.9)		3/43	0.7 (0.2, 2.8)	

* p for trend for categories of maternal fish intake in linear and logistic regression models for continuous and dichotomous outcomes respectively. ** Adjusted for maternal pre-pregnancy weight, height, age, parity, ethnicity, salivary cotinine levels, caffeine intake, alcohol intake, education, gestation and baby's sex in multivariable linear regression for continuous outcome and multivariable logistic regression for categorical outcomes. *** Takes into account maternal pre-pregnancy weight, height, parity, ethnicity, gestation and baby's sex. LBW, low birth weight; n, number; OR, odds ratio; SGA, small for gestation age.

4. Discussion

As far as we are aware this is the only British prospective birth cohort study assessing maternal fatty fish intake prior to and throughout each of the trimesters separately in relation to pregnancy outcomes.

The results showed the majority of pregnant women were consuming considerably less than two portions of fatty fish per week prior to and throughout pregnancy and a trend towards a decreased fatty fish consumption with the progression of pregnancy. Within this study there was no evidence of a statistically significant association between maternal fatty fish intake and gestational length and size at birth, when taking known confounders into account.

4.1. Fish Intake and Maternal Characteristics

The proportion of mothers reporting any fatty fish consumption decreased as pregnancy progressed. Among consumers, mean weekly intakes were highest for the period leading up to pregnancy and the 3rd trimester (124 g and 137 g/week respectively) but still considerably lower than the mean of 190 g of fatty fish/week reported in a UK national survey of women (non-pregnant women aged 19–64) carried out around the same time [35] and noticeably lower than the UK guidelines of up to two portions of 140 g fatty fish/week.

The proportion of women in our study not consuming any fatty fish in the 3rd trimester (56.7%) was slightly higher compared to results from the Avon Longitudinal Study of Parents and Children (ALSPAC) which showed in their study of fish intake in pregnancy and birth weight that 42.6% of pregnant women (*n* = 11,511) reported never or rarely consumed any fatty fish in the 3rd trimester [17]. Compared to other non UK studies assessing fatty fish intakes in Western pregnant women, the proportion not consuming any fatty fish were 33% during the 1st trimester in a Dutch birth cohort (*n* = 3380) [25], 11% during the 2nd trimester in a large Norwegian birth cohort (*n* = 62,099) [19] and 24% reported consuming <0.2 portions of fatty fish/month before pregnancy in a US cohort [27], all lower than that observed in our cohort. Results from the Danish National Birth Cohort (DNBC) however (*n* = 44,824) reported a similar proportion of 54% of non-consumers from their assessment of fatty fish intake in the 2nd trimester [22]. Similarly, results from a Spanish cohort of pregnant women (INMA) showed 41% of women reporting consuming <1 portion of fatty fish/month [18]. Results from a meta-analysis by Leventakou et al., (2014) of 19 European cohorts (some of which are mentioned above) showed a considerable variation in fatty fish intake between countries; with Italian, Spanish and Portuguese mothers consuming fatty fish more than twice as often as Irish & French mothers. It is however impossible to tell how much more fatty fish the Spanish mothers ate than the Irish mothers, for instance, because the researchers had data only on frequency, not quantity [36].

Although it is probable that some women simply do not like fish, reasons for low consumption are likely to include perceptions about cost, access to stores that sell fish, and uncertainty about preparation and cooking methods. Furthermore, some women may abstain from eating fish out of a worry that they and their babies will be harmed by contaminants present in some types of fish, a concern which is highlighted in the current UK guidelines but may actually result in a lack of consumption rather than a lowered intake of fatty fish. The characteristics of the mothers in our study across categories of increased fatty fish consumption are consistent with those observed in other studies where slightly older women, those consuming alcohol and women of higher socioeconomic status and higher education tended to consume higher levels of fish and were less likely to be smokers [16,17,19,22,23,25,26].

4.2. Interpretation of Main Findings

We did not find any evidence of an association between maternal fatty fish intake before and during pregnancy with gestational age or size at birth.

In another British birth cohort (ALSPAC), Rogers et al., (2004) used n-3 fatty acids as a marker of fish consumption and found no association with preterm birth, LBW or intrauterine growth retardation once they adjusted for confounders [17]. Despite having data on type of fish consumed they did not relate this to birth outcomes but focused instead on n-3 fatty acid intake from fish as well as frequency of total fish consumption making it impossible to make direct comparisons to our study. Other studies have reported a similar lack of association between maternal fatty fish intake and birth outcomes [18,19,24,27]. In their meta-analysis Leventakou et al. (2014) in addition to assessing total fish intake, also assessed types of fish (fatty, lean and seafood) in relation to birth outcomes and similarly to our results, they found no association between fatty fish and gestational age or LBW. Where lean fish and shellfish had no significant associations with any birth outcomes, they did observe a positive association between fatty fish and birth weight, albeit a small one at 2.38 g (95% CI: 0.51, 4.25) for every 1 unit (times/week) increment. The authors stipulated that the n-3 LCPUFA content in fatty fish could be the contributing factor behind the overall positive association they found between total fish intake and birth weight [36]. Contrary to this, Halldorson et al. (2007) reported a reduction of 27.5 g in birthweight of babies born to mothers consuming fatty fish more than four times/month compared to non-consumers as well as an increased risk of having babies born SGA [22].

Differences in findings are partly due to heterogeneity between studies. In particular what constitutes a portion of fish varies from study to study and has been shown to range from 85 g to 200 g depending on the type of fish as well as the country of the study [15,27,36]. In addition, categories of intake differ from study to study with some choosing very high or low categories of intake. We chose to assess intake from a more public health relevant context, but this resulted in very small numbers in the high consumption category (>2 portions/week), which limited the power to detect a true association. Furthermore, it is unclear whether the timing of exposure has any effect on outcomes and to our knowledge; no study to date has looked at all trimester specific fatty fish intakes in relation to birth outcomes. Of the studies which have assessed intake in more than one trimester and/or prior to pregnancy [16,20,23,26], one found a positive association with size at birth in overweight women for intakes before pregnancy but not in the final period of pregnancy [26]. Another found an increased risk of LBW babies in women reporting no fish consumption in the 3rd trimester, but not in trimester 1 [16]. Results from a Danish study showed a decreased risk of preterm birth with increasing total fish consumption in both trimester 1 and 2 [20]. Finally one study found a negative association with size at birth and fish intake reported in the 1st trimester but not in the 2nd trimester [23]. None of these studies however looked at types of fish consumed. Moreover, the choice of confounders tends to be inconsistent across studies and since not only in the present study, but also in other studies, high fish consumption has been shown to be strongly related to a higher education level and more healthy lifestyle habits, any positive associations between fish consumption and birth outcomes may be partly due to residual confounding by lifestyle-related characteristics if studies have failed to take these into account in their analysis. Additionally, discrepancies in findings between countries may be a reflection of differences in dietary patterns. This heterogeneity makes it hard to compare results.

4.3. Strengths

As a unique feature of this study we had two sources of dietary intake available which allowed us to derive a study specific estimation of a portion of fatty fish rather than using the SACN estimation of 140 g/portion [28]. This may have given a truer picture of actual intake of fatty fish within a cohort of British pregnant women. Fatty fish intake was averaged to weekly consumption and then divided into categories. This was done so as to better reflect the current UK guidelines on fatty fish consumption for pregnant women and women trying to conceive, and to make the results more applicable in a public health context.

We assessed maternal fish intake at three time points covering a wide window of exposure and taking into account variations across trimesters. Furthermore, only self-reported fatty fish intake was accounted for in the questionnaire. Therefore, the relationship with fatty fish could be assessed, as previous studies have combined type of fish such as lean fish, shellfish and molluscs in their overall analysis, biasing the true effect. Halldorsson et al. (2007) found a negative association with size at birth [22] and Ramon et al. (2009) found that consumption of larger fatty fish ≥ twice/week (such as swordfish) compared to <once/month was associated with a higher risk of SGA, however the P for trend across categories of intake was not significant [18]. Other studies have not specifically identified fatty fish within their analysis and therefore findings cannot be explicitly compared.

In our study information was available for a wide range of confounders. The objective measurement of salivary cotinine samples meant that smoking, a significant confounder in relation to maternal fish intake and birth outcomes, was assessed accurately with a biomarker.

4.4. Limitations

The questionnaires used in this study were originally designed to assess caffeine intake in pregnancy and not dietary fatty fish consumption. However, the questionnaire was validated with reference to caffeine intake in pregnant women [37]; and other food related questions were comparable to other methods used in the assessment of fish. Despite intakes being self-reported and thus presenting the issue of possible under-reporting, fatty fish consumption was assessed prospectively in trimesters 1 and 2, reducing the potential for differential measurement (recall) bias.

An explanation for non-statistically significant findings with fatty fish intake and birth outcomes could be due to the number of women included in the analysis (n = 1208) compared to other large well known cohorts [15,17,20,22,23] as well as the low consumption of fatty fish reported in our cohort. We had limited power to detect small associations due to the low numbers in the high consumption category, especially in trimester 3 (n = 409). The original study of caffeine and birth outcomes planned to follow up women several weeks after delivery to investigate whether their caffeine metabolism had returned to normal, using a caffeine challenge. This proposed data collection was expensive. To reduce costs without introducing selection bias, all cases (SGA and LBW infants) were recruited for postpartum follow-up, but only a sample of controls were taken to be the next two births that were not SGA or LBW. However, previous studies with smaller cohorts have detected associations in relation to fatty fish intake [18,24], although these women consumed high intakes of fish due to their Mediterranean diets.

In this analysis, fresh tuna was considered a fatty fish and was therefore included in the estimation of fatty fish intake and portion size. UK guidance has recently changed to exclude fresh tuna from being considered a type of fatty fish [38,39]. However, our analysis included fresh tuna as a fatty fish, to facilitate comparison with previous studies. With the low intake of fatty fish within this cohort and the relatively low proportion of consumers reporting fresh tuna intake (n = 25) this is unlikely to have influenced results. Canned tuna was excluded in the estimation of fatty fish intake as it is not considered a fatty fish in the UK. However, it is important to acknowledge that canned tuna still contains levels of EPA and DHA, and with tuna being the second most consumed type of fish in our cohort, it could still be a contributor to total EPA and DHA intake. Nevertheless, the few studies that have looked at fish subtypes such as canned tuna in relation to birth outcomes have been inconclusive making it hard to elucidate the potential impact excluding it could have on our findings. Mendez et al. (2010) found in their Spanish cohort of 657 pregnant women that maternal consumption of canned tuna (more than 1 portion per week) was associated with a significantly increased risk of SGA (adjusted OR: 2.49, 95% CI: 1.04 to 5.97). However, another Spanish study [18] similar in size found that mothers consuming more than or equal to 2 portions per week of canned tuna had a lower risk of having infants who were SGA (adjusted OR: 0.3, 95% CI: 0.1, 0.8) compared to mothers in the lower consumption categories.

Finally, a major weakness within this cohort was the lack of objective measurement of self-reported fish consumption. This could have been validated using a biomarker, such as erythrocytes concentrations of n-3 fatty acids, to indicate accurate fish intake during pregnancy, which has been addressed in previous studies [18,19,22–24].

5. Conclusions

Within this UK cohort of low risk pregnant women there was a low prevalence of fatty fish consumption and no evidence of an association between fatty fish intake prior to or throughout pregnancy with size at birth or preterm birth after adjusting for confounding.

Ideally, large cohort studies focusing on types of fish as well as timing of exposure, with a particular focus on the preconception period, are needed to help improve the understanding of the relationship between maternal fish intake during pregnancy and birth outcomes.

Author Contributions: The CARE study was designed by and carried out under the leadership of J.E.C. and N.A.B.S. N.A.A., N.A.B.S. and C.H. conceptualised the research questions. C.N. & C.H. conducted the statistical analysis with guidance from D.C.G. and N.A.A. and led the drafting of the manuscript. All authors contributed to subsequent drafts of the manuscript and have read and approved the final manuscript.

Funding: The CARE study was supported by a grant from the Food Standard Agency, UK (T01033). Camilla Nykjaer's PhD studentship is jointly funded by the Medical Research Council (MR/K500914/1) and the Rank Prize Foundation.

Acknowledgments: We would like to acknowledge the women participating in this study and the research midwives for their invaluable contribution, Sinead Boylan for recruitment and data collection, Susan Shires, Alastair Kay & Kay White for laboratory analysis of cotinine and caffeine levels and James Thomas & Neil Hancock for database management.

Conflicts of Interest: The authors declare no conflicts of interests.

References

1. Barker, D. Fetal origins of coronary heart disease. *BMJ* **1995**, *311*, 171–174. [CrossRef] [PubMed]
2. Osmond, C.; Barker, D.J. Fetal, infant and childhood growth are predictors of coronary heart disease, diabetes, and hypertension in adult men and women. *Environ. Health Perspect.* **2000**, *108*, 545–553. [PubMed]
3. NICE. *Scope Guideline—Preterm Labour and Birth*; National Collaborating Centre for Women's and Children's Health: London, UK, 2013.
4. Wu, G.; Bazer, F.W.; Cudd, T.A.; Meininger, C.J.; Spencer, T.E. Maternal nutrition and fetal development. *J. Nutr.* **2004**, *134*, 2169–2172. [CrossRef] [PubMed]
5. Burdge, G.C.; Hanson, M.A.; Slater-Jefferies, J.L.; Lillycrop, K.A. Epigenetic regulation of transciption: A mechanism of inducing variations in phenotype (fetal programming) by differences in nutrition during early life? *Br. J. Nutr.* **2007**, *97*, 1036–1046. [CrossRef] [PubMed]
6. Hornstra, G. Essential fatty acids in mothers and their neonates. *Am. J. Clin. Nutr.* **2000**, *71*, 1262–1269. [CrossRef] [PubMed]
7. McGregor, J.A.; Allen, K.G.; Harris, M.A.; Reece, M.; Wheeler, M.; French, J.I.; Morrison, J. The omega-3 story: Nutritional prevention of preterm birth and other adverse pregnancy outcomes. *Obstet. Gynecol. Surv.* **2001**, *56*, S1–S13. [CrossRef]
8. Simopoulos, A.P.; Leaf, A.; Salem, N., Jr. Essentiality of and recommended dietary intakes for omega-6 and omega-3 fatty acids. *Ann. Nutr. Metab.* **1999**, *43*, 127–130. [CrossRef]
9. Coletta, J.M.; Bell, S.J.; Roman, A.S. Omega-3 fatty acids and pregnancy. *Rev. Obstetrics Gynaecol.* **2010**, *3*, 163–171.
10. Oken, E.; Belfort, M.B. Fish, fish oil, and pregnancy. *JAMA J. Am. Med. Assoc.* **2010**, *304*, 1717–1718. [CrossRef]
11. Makrides, M.; Neumann, M.; Simmer, K.; Gibson, R.; Pater, J. Are long-chain polyunsaturated fatty acids essential nutrients in infancy? *Lancet* **1995**, *345*, 1463–1468. [CrossRef]
12. Williamson, C. Nutrition in pregnancy. *Br. Nutr. Found. Nutr. Bull.* **2006**, *31*, 28–59. [CrossRef]
13. Hanebutt, F.L.; Demmelmair, H.; Schiessl, B.; Larqué, E.; Koletzko, B. Long-chain polyunsaturated fatty acid (lc-pufa) transfer across the placenta. *Clin. Nutr.* **2008**, *27*, 685–693. [CrossRef] [PubMed]
14. Makrides, M.; Gibson, R.A. Long-chain polyunsaturated fatty acid requirements during pregnancy and lactation. *Am. J. Clin. Nutr.* **2000**, *71*, S307–S311. [CrossRef] [PubMed]
15. Guldner, L.; Monfort, C.; Rouget, F.; Garlantezec, R.; Cordier, S. Maternal fish and shellfish intake and pregnancy outcomes: A prospective cohort study in brittany, france. *Environ. Health* **2007**, *6*, 33. [CrossRef] [PubMed]

16. Muthayya, S.; Dwarkanath, P.; Thomas, T.; Ramprakash, S.; Mehra, R.; Mhaskar, A.; Mhaskar, R.; Thomas, A.; Bhat, S.; Vaz, M.; et al. The effect of fish and n-3 lcpufa intake on low birth weight in indian pregnancy women. *Eur. J. Clin. Nutr.* **2009**, *63*, 340–346. [CrossRef]

17. Rogers, I.; Emmett, P.; Ness, A.; Golding, J. ALSPAC Study Team. Maternal fish intake in late pregnancy and the frequency of low birth weight and intrauterine growth retardation in a cohort of british infants. *J. Epidemiol. Community Health* **2004**, *58*, 486–492. [CrossRef] [PubMed]

18. Ramon, R.; Ballester, F.; Aguinagalde, X.; Amurrio, A.; Vioque, J.; Lacasana, M.; Rebagliato, M.; Murcia, M.; Iniguez, C. Fish consumption during pregnancy, prenatal mercury exposure, and anthropometric measures at birth in a prospective mother-infant cohort in spain. *Am. J. Clin. Nutr.* **2009**, *90*, 1047–1055. [CrossRef] [PubMed]

19. Brantsaeter, A.L.; Birgisdottir, B.E.; Meltzer, H.M.; Kvalem, H.E.; Alexander, J.; Magnus, P.; Haugen, M. Maternal seafood consumption and infant birth weight, length and head circumference in the norwegian mother and child cohort study. *Br. J. Nutr.* **2012**, *107*, 436–444. [CrossRef]

20. Olsen, S.F.; Østerdal, M.L.; Salvig, J.D.; Kesmodel, U.; Henriksen, T.B.; Hedegaard, M.; Secher, N.J. Duration of pregnancy in relation to seafood intake during early and mid pregnancy: Prospective cohort. *Perinat. Epidemol.* **2006**, *21*, 749–758. [CrossRef] [PubMed]

21. Haugen, M.; Margrete Meltzer, H.; Lise Brantsæter, A.; Mikkelsen, T.; Louise Østerdal, M.; Alexander, J.; Olsen, S.F.; Bakketeig, L. Mediterranean-type diet and risk of preterm birth among women in the norwegian mother and child cohort study (moba): A prospective cohort study. *Acta Obstet. Gynecol. Scand.* **2008**, *87*, 319–324. [CrossRef] [PubMed]

22. Halldorsson, T.I.; Meltzer, H.M.; Thorsdottir, I.; Knudsen, V.; Olsen, S.F. Is high consumption of fatty fish during pregnancy a risk factor for fetal growth retardation? A study of 44824 danish pregnant women. *Am. J. Epidemiol.* **2007**, *166*, 687–696. [CrossRef]

23. Oken, E.; Kleinman, K.P.; Olsen, S.F.; Rich-Edwards, J.W.; Gillman, M.W. Associations of seafood and elongated n-3 fatty acid intake with fetal growth and length of gestation: Results from a us pregnancy cohort. *Am. J. Epidemiol.* **2004**, *160*, 774–783. [CrossRef] [PubMed]

24. Mendez, M.A.; Plana, E.; Guxens, M.; Morillo, C.M.F.; Albareda, R.M.; Garcia-Esteban, R.; Goñi, F.; Kogevinas, M.; Sunyer, J. Seafood consumption in pregnancy and infant size at birthl results from a prospective spanish cohort. *J. Epidemiol. Community Health* **2010**, *64*, 216–222. [CrossRef]

25. Heppe, D.H.; Steegers, E.A.; Timmermans, S.; Breeijen, H.; Tiemeier, H.; Hofman, A.; Jaddoe, V.W. Maternal fish consumption, fetal growth and the risks of neonatal complications: The generation r study. *Br. J. Nutr.* **2011**, *105*, 938–949. [CrossRef]

26. Drouillet, P.; Kaminski, M.; De Lauzon-Guillain, B.; Forhan, A.; Ducimetiere, P.; Schweitzer, M.; Magnin, G.; Goua, V.; Thiebaugeorges, O.; Charles, M.A. Association between maternal seafood consumption before pregnancy and fetal growth: Evidence for an association in overweight women. The eden mother-child cohort. *Paediatr. Perinat. Epidemiol.* **2009**, *23*, 76–86. [CrossRef] [PubMed]

27. Mohanty, A.F.; Thompson, M.L.; Burbacher, T.M.; Siscovick, D.S.; Williams, M.A.; Enquobahrie, D.A. Periconceptional seafood intake and fetal growth. *Paediatr. Perinat. Epidemiol.* **2015**, *29*, 376–387. [CrossRef]

28. SACN. *Advice on Fish Consumption: Benefits & Risks*; SACN: London, UK, 2004.

29. Cetin, I.; Koletzko, B. Long-chain omega-3 fatty acid supply in pregnancy and lactation. *Curr. Opin. Clin. Nutr. Metab. Care* **2008**, *11*, 297–302. [CrossRef] [PubMed]

30. Bloomingdale, A.; Guthrie, L.B.; Price, S.; Wright, R.O.; Platek, D.; Haines, J.; Oken, E. A qualitative study of fish consumption during pregnancy. *Am. J. Clin. Nutr.* **2010**, *92*, 1234–1240. [CrossRef]

31. CARE Study Group. Maternal caffeine intake during pregnancy and risk of fetal growth restriction: A large prospective observational study. *BMJ* **2008**, *337*, a2332. [CrossRef]

32. Cade, J.E.; Burley, V.J.; Greenwood, D.C.; UK Women's Cohort Study Steering Group. The UK women's cohort study: Comparison of vegetarians, fish-eaters and meat-eaters. *Public Health Nutr.* **2004**, *7*, 871–878. [CrossRef]

33. Gardosi, J. New definition of small for gestational age based on fetal growth potential. *Horm. Res.* **2006**, *65*, 15–18. [CrossRef] [PubMed]

34. Meltzer, H.M.; Brantsæter, A.L.; Ydersbond, T.A.; Alexander, J.; Haugen, M.; MoBa Dietary Support Group. Methodological challenges when monitoring the diet of pregnant women in a large study: Experiences from the norwegian mother and child cohort study (MoBa). *Matern. Child Nutr.* **2008**, *4*, 14–27. [CrossRef] [PubMed]

35. Henderson, L.; Gregory, J.; Swan, G. *The National Diet and Nutrition Survey: Adults Aged 19 to 64 Years. Volume 1: Types and Quantities of Foods Consumed*; The Stationery Office: London, UK, 2002.

36. Leventakou, V.; Roumeliotaki, T.; Martinez, D.; Barros, H.; Brantsaeter, A.L.; Casas, M.; Charles, M.A.; Cordier, S.; Eggesbo, M.; van Eijsden, M.; et al. Fish intake during pregnancy, fetal growth, and gestational length in 19 european birth cohort studies. *Am. J. Clin. Nutr.* **2014**, *99*, 506–516. [CrossRef]

37. Boylan, S.M.; Cade, J.E.; Kirk, S.F.; Greenwood, D.C.; White, K.L.; Shires, S.; Simpson, N.A.; Wild, C.P.; Hay, A.W. Assessing caffeine exposure in pregnant women. *Br. J. Nutr.* **2008**, *100*, 875–882. [CrossRef] [PubMed]

38. Roe, M.; Pinchen, H.; Finglas, P. *Nutrient Analysis of Fish and Fish Products*; Department of Health: London, UK, 2018.

39. Clark, R. In the News: Fresh Tuna no Longer Counts as an Oily Fish. Available online: https://www.wcrf-uk.org/informed/articles/news-fresh-tuna-no-longer-counts-oily-fish (accessed on 21 January 2019).

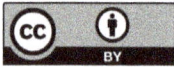

nutrients

MDPI

Review

Effects of Vitamin D Supplementation During Pregnancy on Birth Size: A Systematic Review and Meta-Analysis of Randomized Controlled Trials

Andrea Maugeri, Martina Barchitta, Isabella Blanco and Antonella Agodi *

Department of Medical and Surgical Sciences and Advanced Technologies "GF Ingrassia", University of Catania, Via S. Sofia 87, 95123 Catania, Italy; andreamaugeri88@gmail.com (A.M.); martina.barchitta@unict.it (M.B.); dott.ssa.blanco.isabella@gmail.com (I.B.)
* Correspondence: agodia@unict.it

Received: 23 January 2019; Accepted: 15 February 2019; Published: 20 February 2019

Abstract: During pregnancy, vitamin D supplementation may be a feasible strategy to help prevent low birthweight (LBW) and small for gestational age (SGA) births. However, evidence from randomized controlled trials (RCTs) is inconclusive, probably due to heterogeneity in study design and type of intervention. A systematic literature search in the PubMed-Medline, EMBASE, and Cochrane Central Register of Controlled Trials databases was carried out to evaluate the effects of oral vitamin D supplementation during pregnancy on birthweight, birth length, head circumference, LBW, and SGA. The fixed-effects or random-effects models were used to calculate mean difference (MD), risk ratio (RR), and 95% Confidence Interval (CI). On a total of 13 RCTs, maternal vitamin D supplementation had a positive effect on birthweight (12 RCTs; MD = 103.17 g, 95% CI 62.29–144.04 g), length (6 RCTs; MD = 0.22 cm, 95% CI 0.11–0.33 cm), and head circumference (6 RCTs; MD:0.19 cm, 95% CI 0.13–0.24 cm). In line with these findings, we also demonstrated that maternal vitamin D supplementation reduced the risk of LBW (3 RCTs; RR = 0.40, 95% CI 0.22–0.74) and SGA (5 RCTS; RR = 0.69, 95% CI 0.51–0.92). The present systematic review and meta-analysis confirmed the well-established effect of maternal vitamin D supplementation on birth size. However, further research is required to better define risks and benefits associated with such interventions and the potential implications for public health.

Keywords: nutrition; diet; vitamin D; birthweight; birth length; head circumference; gestational age; pregnancy outcomes

1. Introduction

Nutrition in women of childbearing age has a critical role on their health as well as on infant outcomes. A balanced supply of maternal nutrients, before conception, during pregnancy, and during breastfeeding, promotes optimal growth and development both in fetus and offspring [1,2]. During pregnancy, the fetus is entirely dependent on maternal sources of vitamin D, which also regulates placental function [3]. Several observational studies have shown that pregnancy is a crucial period in which vitamin D deficiency may affect mother and neonatal outcomes, thereby influencing the risk of recurrent pregnancy losses, preeclampsia, gestational diabetes, maternal infections, preterm birth, low birthweight (LBW), small for gestational age (SGA), and poor offspring health [4]. Thus, hypovitaminosis D in pregnancy requires an adequate treatment, and vitamin D supplementation represents a valid strategy for preventing and controlling vitamin D deficiency [5]. The Food and Nutrition Board at the Institute of Medicine of the National Academies suggests that a proper integration of vitamin D in pregnancy and in lactation is 15 micrograms (600 IU) per day [6]. Recently, many randomized controlled trials (RCTs) have been conducted to evaluate the benefits of vitamin D supplementation in pregnancy. Although vitamin D supplementation may increase serum 25(OH)D levels in both mothers and infants [7], it remains unclear whether vitamin D supplementation is protective for LBW, SGA or intrauterine growth restriction, and generally for long-term offspring health. To our knowledge, the meta-analysis by Thorne-Lyman et al. was the first to summarize the effect of vitamin D on birthweight and LBW incidence [8]. Pooled estimates of observational studies showed a positive relationship between vitamin D status and birthweight [8]. However, pooled analysis of interventional studies suggested, on one hand, no significant effect on mean birthweight, but on the other hand a lower risk of LBW newborns in women supplemented with vitamin D [8]. A recent systematic review by Harvey et al. [4] partially confirmed these results: out of seven studies, three trials showed that maternal vitamin D supplementation significantly increased birthweight in infants [4]. Although this evidence was also corroborated by Perez-Lopez et al. in a meta-analysis of 8 RCTs, the authors did not demonstrate the influence on the risk of LBW and SGA (3 RCTs, respectively) [5]. In contrast, four trials included in the most recent systematic review by De-Regil et al. reported that maternal vitamin D supplementation significantly reduced the risk of LBW [7]. However, no difference was reported in the mean birthweight of infants [7]. Therefore, evidence is currently inconclusive to drawn convincing assumptions on the usefulness of maternal vitamin D supplementation against LBW and SGA births. Moreover, previous mentioned reviews [4,5,7,8] showed heterogeneity in dose, duration and timing of supplementation, and study design (i.e., observational studies, quasi-RCTs, and RCTs). Herein, we provide a systematic review and a meta-analysis of data from RCTs, to evaluate the effects of oral vitamin D supplementation during pregnancy on fetal growth as indicated by neonatal anthropometric measures and incidence of LBW and SGA births. Moreover, we also performed subgroup analyses to demonstrate whether alternative formulations and regimens had different effect on birth size.

2. Materials and Methods

2.1. Literature Search

A systematic literature search in the PubMed-Medline, EMBASE, and Cochrane Central Register of Controlled Trials databases was carried out for RCTs investigating the role of oral vitamin D supplementation during pregnancy on neonatal anthropometric measures and incidence of LBW and SGA. Literature search was conducted independently by two authors (A.M. and I.B.) using the following keywords: (vitamin d OR ergocalciferol OR cholecalciferol OR calcifediol OR vitamin d supplementation OR 25-hydroxyvitamin D) AND (birth size OR birth weight OR birth length OR head circumference OR low birth weight OR SGA OR neonatal anthropometric measures). Full details of literature search terms are included in Supplementary Materials. The databases were searched from inception to May 2017 without language restriction; abstracts and unpublished studies were not included. Moreover, the reference lists from selected articles, including relevant review papers, were searched to identify all relevant studies. The preferred reporting items for systematic reviews and meta-analysis (PRISMA) guidelines were followed [9].

2.2. Inclusion and Exclusion Criteria

Studies were selected only if they satisfied the following criteria: (1) RCTs, with randomization at either individual or cluster level, (2) of pregnant women of any gestational age (3) without pregnancy complications, (4) that assessed the effect of oral vitamin D supplementation, irrespective of dose, duration or time of commencement, on birthweight, birth length, head circumference, and incidence of LBW, and/or SGA. Eligible intervention groups included daily or single-intermitted vitamin D supplementation (vitamin D2 or D3), alone or in combination with calcium and/or other micronutrients. For studies with more than two intervention groups, we combined disaggregated data into subgroup category to create a single pair-wise group comparison [10]. Control groups included no treatment or placebo. Exclusion criteria were as follows: (1) systematic reviews or meta-analyses;

(2) observational studies, cross-over trials, or quasi-RCTs; (3) no appropriate treatment group (pregnant women with pre-existing pregnancy complications); (4) no appropriate control group (i.e., vitamin D supplementation); (5) not available data on birth size and/or incidence of LBW and SGA.

2.3. Study Selection and Data Extraction

Two of the authors (A.M. and I.B.) independently assessed for inclusion all the references identified through the literature search. From all the eligible studies, two authors (A.M. and I.B.) independently extracted the following information in a standard format: first author's last name, year of publication, country, and latitude where the study was performed, season when the study was performed, number of participants, age and information about vitamin D intervention (i.e., Formulation, regimen, method of administration, and treatment duration). Primary outcomes were birthweight (g), birth length (cm), head circumference (cm), low birthweight (LBW; <2500 g) and SGA, defined as birthweight below the 10th percentile of a reference distribution of weights specific for sex and gestational age. Other outcomes were: maternal serum 25-OHD levels at baseline and at the end of the intervention, cord 25-OHD levels, gestational age, caesarean delivery, pregnancy complications (i.e., preterm birth, gestational diabetes, pre-eclampsia), and Apgar score. Cross-checked data were entered into Review Manager software (RevMan, version 5.3, Copenhagen, Denmark)) by A.M., and checked for accuracy by M.B. During study selection and data extraction, any disagreements between A.M. and M.B. were resolved by discussion and consensus with a third Author (A.A.).

2.4. Risk-of-Bias and Quality Assessment

The risk of bias from each eligible RCT was evaluated using the Cochrane's Collaboration tool for assessing risk of bias in randomized trials [10]. This tool includes the following items, which were assigned as either 'low risk of bias', 'unclear risk of bias' or 'high risk of bias': random sequence generation (selection bias); concealment of the allocation sequence (selection bias); blinding of participants and personnel (performance bias); blinding of outcome assessment (detection bias); incomplete outcome data (attrition bias); selective outcome reporting (reporting bias); and other biases [8]. Risk of bias was assessed by two of the authors (A.M. and M.B.) using the Review Manager software (RevMan, version 5.3), and presented as a risk-of-bias summary figure. Disagreements were resolved by consensus or discussion with a third Author (A.A.). For each outcome, two of the authors (A.M. and M.B.) independently assessed the quality of the evidence using the Grading of Recommendations Assessment, Development and Evaluation (GRADE) approach [11]. The GRADE system considers eight criteria for assessing the quality of evidence: risk of bias, inconsistency, indirectness, imprecision, publication bias, and other (large magnitude of effect, dose response, and no plausible confounding). Based on these criteria, the quality of evidence was classified as high, moderate, low, or very low. Disagreements were resolved by consensus or discussion with a third Author (A.A.).

2.5. Statistical Analysis

Data on dichotomous outcomes were combined and effect sizes were presented as RR with 95% confidence intervals (CIs). For continuous outcomes, we estimated mean differences (MDs) with 95% CI. Forest plots were generated to illustrate the study-specific effect sizes along with a 95% CI. The significance of pooled effect size was determined using the Z test, and $p < 0.05$ was considered significant. Heterogeneity across studies was assessed using the Q-test based on the χ2 statistic ($p < 0.1$ was considered statistically significant). To quantify heterogeneity, the I2 value was calculated and interpreted as follows: an I2 value of 0% indicates "no heterogeneity," whereas 25% is "low," 50% is "moderate," and 75% is "high" heterogeneity. We considered heterogeneity as significant if $p < 0.1$ for Q-test based on the χ2 statistic and I^2 was greater than 30% [12]. To calculate pooled effect estimates, the fixed-effects model (Mantel-Haenszel method) was used in absence of significant heterogeneity, otherwise the random-effects model (Der Simonian-Laird method). In the random effect model, the between-study variance was estimated using the tau-squared ($\tau2$) statistic [10]. The leave-one-out sensitivity analysis was performed by the omission of a single study at a time, to assess whether a particular omission could affect effect sizes and heterogeneity across studies. Sensitivity analysis by the omission of studies with daily vitamin D dose of 200 IU [13,14] was also performed to assess whether they affected the pooled effect sizes. We also performed subgroup analyses by formulation (vitamin D alone vs. vitamin D in combination with calcium and/or other micronutrients) and supplementation regimen (daily vs. single/intermitted high dose). Since vitamin D might have a dose-dependent effect on birth sizes, we performed a meta-regression using the Comprehensive Meta-analysis software (Version 2.0; Biostat Inc., Englewood, NJ, USA). Particularly, meta-regression analyses were performed on those outcomes with at least three studies evaluating daily vitamin D supplementation alone [15]. Heterogeneity in formulation, dose, duration, and timing of supplementation, did not allow us to perform meta-regression of studies with single supplementation and/or combination of supplements. In those outcomes with at least two group comparisons for subgroup, we assessed subgroup differences by the $\chi2$ statistic, and the interaction test I^2 value. In those outcomes with 10 or more group comparisons, the presence of publication bias was investigated by visually assessment of funnel plot asymmetry, followed by Begg's test and Egger's regression asymmetry test [16,17]. Except for the Q-test, $p < 0.05$ was considered statistically significant, and all tests were 2-sided. All statistical analyses were performed using the Review Manager software (RevMan, version 5.3).

3. Results

3.1. Study Selection

The detailed steps of the study selection are given as a PRISMA flow diagram in Figure 1. A total of 669 abstracts were retrieved from the databases; 542 were excluded after reading titles and/or abstracts, and 127 articles were subjected to a full-text review. From these, 114 studies were excluded according to selection criteria, whereas 13 RCTs, published between 1980 and 2016, were included in the meta-analysis [13,14,18–28]. However, since four articles showed more eligible intervention groups [19–21,28], the meta-analysis reported data on 17 group comparisons between eligible intervention ($n = 17$) and control groups ($n = 13$) (Table 1).

PRISMA 2009 Flow Diagram

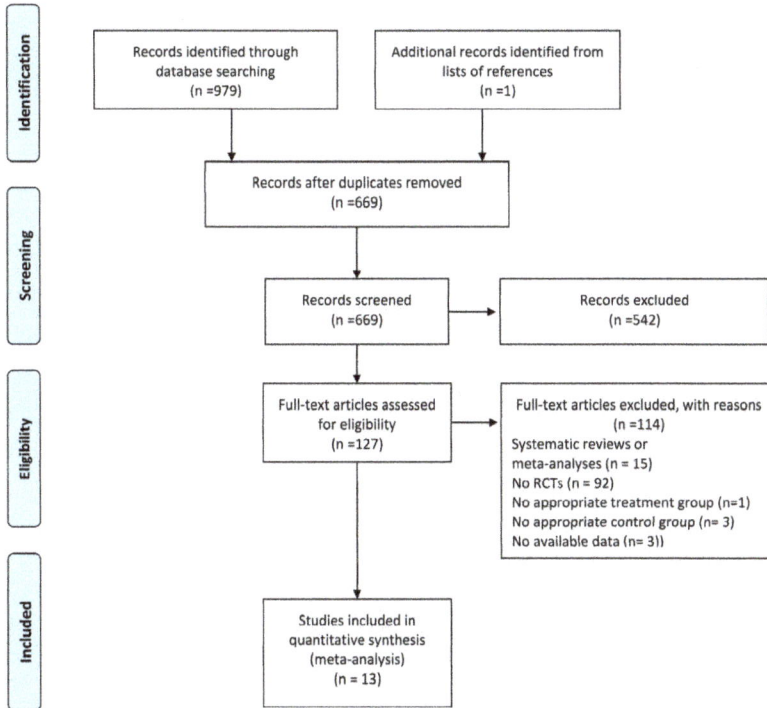

Figure 1. PRISMA flow diagram of study selection.

Table 1. Characteristics of randomized controlled trials included in the meta-analysis.

First Author, Year	Country	Treatment (Vitamin D Dosage)	CONTROL GROUP	Size of Intervention/ Control Groups	Treatment Duration (Week)	Outcomes
Asemi, 2016 [13]	Iran	Vit D3 + Ca (200 IU/day)	Placebo	21/21	9	Birthweight, birth length, head circumference
Brooke, 1980 [18]	UK	Vit D2 (1000 IU/day)	Placebo	59/67	8–12	Birthweight, birth length, head circumference, LBW, SGA
Brough, 2010 [14]	UK	Vit D3 + micronutrients (200 IU/day)	Placebo	88/61	NA	Birthweight, head circumference, LBW, SGA
Charandabi, 2015 [19]	Iran	Vit D + Ca (1000 IU/day) Vit D (1000 IU/day)	Placebo	40/42 42/42	9	Birthweight, birth length, head circumference
Goldring, 2013 [20]	UK	Vit D2 (800 IU/day) Vit D3 (single dose of 200000 IU)	No intervention	56/50	12	Birthweight
Hollis, 2011 [21]	USA	Vit D3 + micronutrients (1600 IU/day) Vit D3 + micronutrients (3600 IU/day)	Placebo	122/111 117/111	24–28	Birthweight

Table 1. *Cont.*

First Author, Year	Country	Treatment (Vitamin D Dosage)	CONTROL GROUP	Size of Intervention/ Control Groups	Treatment Duration (Week)	Outcomes
Hossain, 2014 [22]	Pakistan	Vit D3 (4000 IU/day)	No intervention	86/89	16	Birthweight, birth length, head circumference, SGA
Marya, 1988 [23]	India	Vit D3 (two doses of 600000 IU)	No intervention	100/100	12	Birthweight, birth length
Naghshineh, 2016 [24]	Iran	Vit D (600 IU/day)	No intervention	68/70	20	Birthweight
Roth, 2013 [25]	Bangladesh	Vit D3 (35,000 IU/week)	Placebo	80/80	12	Birthweight, birth length, head circumference
Sabet, 2012 [26]	Iran	Vit D3 (100000 IU/mol)	Placebo	25/25	12	Birthweight, birth length
Sablok, 2015 [27]	India	Vit D3 (single-intermitted dose depending upon the serum 25OHD levels)	No intervention	108/57	16	Birthweight, SGA
Yu, 2009 [28]	UK	Vit D2 (800 IU/d) Vit D2 (single dose of 200000 IU)	No intervention	60/59 60/59	13	LBW, SGA

Abbreviations: Ca, Calcium; IU, International Unit; 25-OHD, 25-hydroxyvitamin D; LBW, low birth weight; SGA, small for gestational age; NA, not available.

3.2. Systematic Review

A total of 8 studies were from Asian countries, 4 from European countries, and 1 from USA. Accordingly, the latitude of the setting was the Northern tropic in all the included studies. To avoid confounding due to seasonal variation in sunlight exposure, 6 RCTs were carried out in different seasons [14,18,22,24,26,27]. Otherwise, the seasons varied from winter [19] to spring-summer period [13,20,25,28]; this information was not available for 2 RCTs [21,23]. Overall, sample sizes ranged between 40 and 400 pregnant women, and neonatal outcomes of 2016 newborns were reported: 1184 from mothers in the intervention groups and 832 from controls. All the eligible studies were carried out using an individual randomization. Intervention groups were characterized by vitamin D2 (n = 4) or D3 (n = 10) supplementation alone (n = 12) or in combination with calcium (n = 2) or other micronutrients (n = 3). Two trials did not report the vitamin D form used in 3 intervention groups [19,24]. The duration of vitamin D intervention was 6–28 weeks of gestation. Women in 11 intervention groups were supplemented with daily dose of vitamin D, whereas subjects in the remaining 6 intervention groups were supplemented with single-intermitted high dose. The daily dose ranged from 200 IU to 4000 IU; among single-intermitted interventions, the high dose varied from 35000 IU to 600000 IU. Control groups included patients who received placebo (n = 8) or no treatment (n = 5). In those studies evaluating the effect of vitamin D supplementation on 25-hydroxyvitamin D levels, the intervention significantly increased 25-OHD concentration in both mothers [13,14,18,21–23,25–28] and infants [21,22,25–28]. Although 3 RCTs suggested that women who received vitamin D supplementation during pregnancy had a lower risk of preterm birth than controls [13,24,27], in other trials the intervention did not affect gestational age [13,14,20–22,24] and preterm birth risk [14,19,22].

3.3. Meta-Analysis

3.3.1. Birthweight

The effect of vitamin D supplementation on birthweight was assessed by 12 RCTs [13,14,18–27] and 15 group comparisons. Compared to controls, birthweight was significantly higher in the intervention groups (MD: 103.17 g, 95% CI 62.29–144.04 g; p < 0.001). Q-test and I2 statistics showed no significant heterogeneity across studies (p > 0.1; I2 = 7.0%). Particularly, vitamin D supplementation alone, but not in combination with other micronutrients, significantly increased birthweight (MD: 118.46 g,

95% CI 70.47–166.45 g, $p < 0.001$; MD: 62.76 g, 95% CI −15.24–140.77 g, $p = 0.520$, respectively) (Figure 2). The effect of vitamin D in combination with other micronutrients remained no significant also after the omission of studies with daily vitamin D dose of 200 IU [13,14] (MD: 49.30 g, 95% CI −43.52–142.11 g, $p = 0.300$). Particularly, meta-regression did not reveal a dose-dependent effect of vitamin D supplementation alone on birthweight ($p = 0.773$). Subgroup analysis by regimen showed that both daily and single-intermitted high dose supplementation significantly increased birthweight (MD: 74.66 g, 95% CI 18.80–130.52 g, $p < 0.001$; MD: 136.02 g, 95% CI 76.05–195.98 g, $p < 0.001$, respectively).

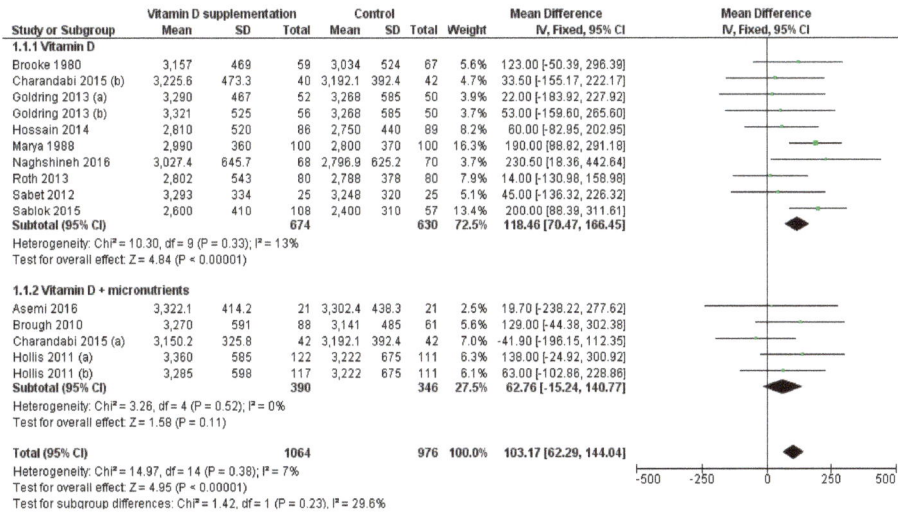

Study or Subgroup	Vitamin D supplementation Mean	SD	Total	Control Mean	SD	Total	Weight	Mean Difference IV, Fixed, 95% CI
1.1.1 Vitamin D								
Brooke 1980	3,157	469	59	3,034	524	67	5.6%	123.00 [−50.39, 296.39]
Charandabi 2015 (b)	3,225.6	473.3	40	3,192.1	392.4	42	4.7%	33.50 [−155.17, 222.17]
Goldring 2013 (a)	3,290	467	52	3,268	585	50	3.9%	22.00 [−183.92, 227.92]
Goldring 2013 (b)	3,321	525	56	3,268	585	50	3.7%	53.00 [−159.60, 265.60]
Hossain 2014	2,810	520	86	2,750	440	89	8.2%	60.00 [−82.95, 202.95]
Marya 1988	2,990	360	100	2,800	370	100	16.3%	190.00 [88.82, 291.18]
Naghshineh 2016	3,027.4	645.7	68	2,796.9	625.2	70	3.7%	230.50 [18.36, 442.64]
Roth 2013	2,802	543	80	2,788	378	80	7.9%	14.00 [−130.98, 158.98]
Sabet 2012	3,293	334	25	3,248	320	25	5.1%	45.00 [−136.32, 226.32]
Sablok 2015	2,600	410	108	2,400	310	57	13.4%	200.00 [88.39, 311.61]
Subtotal (95% CI)			674			630	72.5%	118.46 [70.47, 166.45]
Heterogeneity: Chi² = 10.30, df = 9 (P = 0.33); I² = 13%								
Test for overall effect: Z = 4.84 (P < 0.00001)								
1.1.2 Vitamin D + micronutrients								
Asemi 2016	3,322.1	414.2	21	3,302.4	438.3	21	2.5%	19.70 [−238.22, 277.62]
Brough 2010	3,270	591	88	3,141	485	61	5.6%	129.00 [−44.38, 302.38]
Charandabi 2015 (a)	3,150.2	325.8	42	3,192.1	392.4	42	7.0%	−41.90 [−196.15, 112.35]
Hollis 2011 (a)	3,360	585	122	3,222	675	111	6.3%	138.00 [−24.92, 300.92]
Hollis 2011 (b)	3,285	598	117	3,222	675	111	6.1%	63.00 [−102.86, 228.86]
Subtotal (95% CI)			390			346	27.5%	62.76 [−15.24, 140.77]
Heterogeneity: Chi² = 3.26, df = 4 (P = 0.52); I² = 0%								
Test for overall effect: Z = 1.58 (P = 0.11)								
Total (95% CI)			1064			976	100.0%	103.17 [62.29, 144.04]
Heterogeneity: Chi² = 14.97, df = 14 (P = 0.38); I² = 7%								
Test for overall effect: Z = 4.95 (P < 0.00001)								
Test for subgroup differences: Chi² = 1.42, df = 1 (P = 0.23). I² = 29.6%								

Figure 2. Forest plot of the effect of vitamin D intervention alone or in combination with micronutrients on birthweight (g), based on the fixed-effects model. Charandabi 2015 (**a**): Vit D + Ca (1000 IU/day); Charandabi 2015 (**b**): Vit D (1000 IU/day); Goldring 2013 (**a**): Vit D2 (800 IU/day); Goldring 2013 (**b**): Vit D3 (single dose of 200000 IU); Hollis 2011 (**a**): Vit D3 + micronutrients (1600 IU/day); Hollis 2011 (**b**): Vit D3 + micronutrients (3600 IU/day).

3.3.2. Birth Length

The effect of vitamin D supplementation on birth length was assessed by 7 RCTs [13,18,19,22,23,25,26] and 8 group comparisons. The Q-test and I2 statistics showed significant heterogeneity across studies ($p < 0.001$; I2 = 75.2%). Based on the random effect model, birth length was significantly higher in the intervention groups than in controls (MD: 0.50 cm, 95% CI 0.08–0.92 cm; $p = 0.020$). Moreover, we performed a leave-one-out sensitivity analysis to investigate the sources of heterogeneity across studies. The sensitivity analysis found that the study by Marya et al. [23] affected the heterogeneity across studies. When this study was omitted, the between-studies heterogeneity decreased ($p > 0.1$; I2 = 0.0%) and birth length remained significantly higher in the intervention groups than in controls (MD: 0.22 cm, 95% CI 0.10–0.34 cm; $p < 0.001$). Meta-regression did not reveal a dose-dependent effect of vitamin D supplementation alone on birth length ($p = 0.895$). Subgroup analysis by formulation showed that vitamin D supplementation alone, but not in combination with other micronutrients, significantly increased birth length (MD: 0.22 cm, 95% CI 0.10–0.34 cm, $p < 0.001$; MD: 0.21 cm, 95% CI −0.49–0.92 cm, $p = 0.700$, respectively) (Figure 3). Subgroup analysis by regimen showed that both daily and single-intermitted high dose supplementation significantly increased birth length (MD: 0.20 cm, 95% CI 0.08–0.32 cm; $p = 0.001$; MD: 0.50 cm, 95% CI 0.02–0.97 cm; $p = 0.041$, respectively).

Study or Subgroup	Vitamin D supplementation			Control			Weight	Mean Difference IV, Fixed, 95% CI	Mean Difference IV, Fixed, 95% CI
	Mean	SD	Total	Mean	SD	Total			
1.2.1 Vitamin D									
Brooke 1980	49.7	0.3	59	49.5	0.4	67	87.7%	0.20 [0.08, 0.32]	
Charandabi 2015 (a)	50	2.2	40	49.5	2	42	1.6%	0.50 [-0.41, 1.41]	
Hossain 2014	48.9	2.76	86	48.8	2.37	89	2.3%	0.10 [-0.66, 0.86]	
Roth 2013	48.2	2.5	80	48	2	80	2.7%	0.20 [-0.50, 0.90]	
Sabet 2012	50.75	0.74	25	50	1.48	25	3.1%	0.75 [0.10, 1.40]	
Subtotal (95% CI)			**290**			**303**	**97.3%**	**0.22 [0.10, 0.34]**	
Heterogeneity: Chi² = 3.13, df = 4 (P = 0.54); I² = 0%									
Test for overall effect: Z = 3.71 (P = 0.0002)									
1.2.2 Vitamin D + micronutrients									
Asemi 2016	50.6	2.3	21	50.6	2	21	0.8%	0.00 [-1.30, 1.30]	
Charandabi 2015 (b)	49.8	1.9	42	49.5	2	42	1.9%	0.30 [-0.53, 1.13]	
Subtotal (95% CI)			**63**			**63**	**2.7%**	**0.21 [-0.49, 0.92]**	
Heterogeneity: Chi² = 0.14, df = 1 (P = 0.70); I² = 0%									
Test for overall effect: Z = 0.59 (P = 0.55)									
Total (95% CI)			**353**			**366**	**100.0%**	**0.22 [0.11, 0.33]**	
Heterogeneity: Chi² = 3.27, df = 6 (P = 0.77); I² = 0%									
Test for overall effect: Z = 3.76 (P = 0.0002)									
Test for subgroup differences: Chi² = 0.00, df = 1 (P = 0.98), I² = 0%									

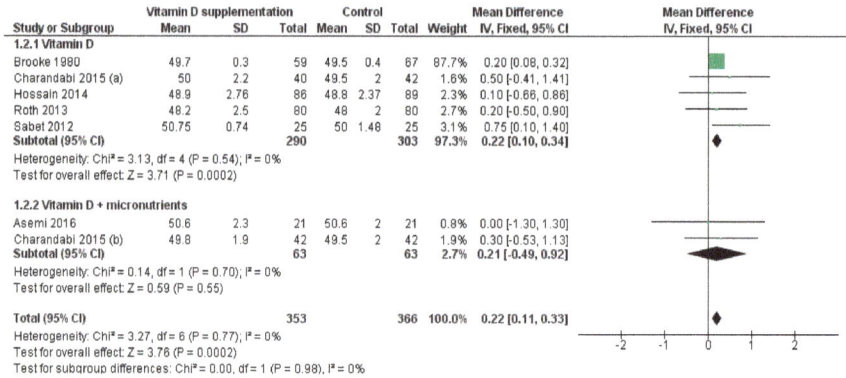

Figure 3. Forest plot of the effect of vitamin D intervention alone or in combination with micronutrients on birth length (cm), based on the fixed-effects model. Charandabi 2015 (**a**): Vit D + Ca (1000 IU/day); Charandabi 2015 (**b**): Vit D (1000 IU/day).

3.3.3. Head Circumference

The effect of vitamin D supplementation on head circumference was assessed by 6 RCTs [13,14,18,19,22,25] and 7 group comparisons. Compared to controls, head circumference was significantly greater in the intervention groups (MD: 0.19 cm, 95% CI 0.13–0.24 cm; $p < 0.001$). Q-test and I2 statistics showed no significant heterogeneity across studies ($p > 0.1$; I2 = 2.0%). Particularly, vitamin D supplementation alone, but not in combination with other micronutrients, significantly increased head circumference (MD: 0.19 cm, 95% CI 0.14–0.25 cm, $p < 0.001$; MD: −0.06 cm, 95% CI −0.41–0.28 cm, $p = 0.720$, respectively; Figure 4). Meta-regression did not reveal a dose-dependent effect of vitamin D supplementation alone on head circumference ($p = 0.746$). Subgroup analysis by regimen showed that daily maternal vitamin D supplementation significantly increased head circumference (MD: 0.19 cm, 95% CI 0.14–0.24 cm; $p < 0.001$). Regarding single-intermitted intervention, Roth et al. reported no significant effect [25].

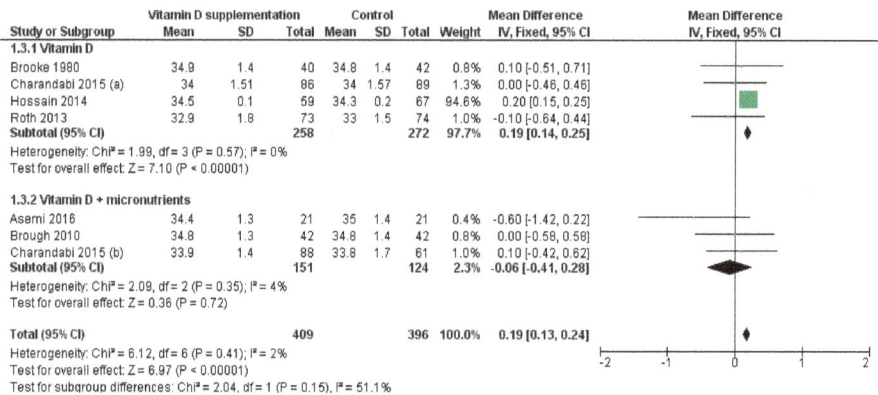

Study or Subgroup	Vitamin D supplementation			Control			Weight	Mean Difference IV, Fixed, 95% CI	Mean Difference IV, Fixed, 95% CI
	Mean	SD	Total	Mean	SD	Total			
1.3.1 Vitamin D									
Brooke 1980	34.9	1.4	40	34.8	1.4	42	0.8%	0.10 [-0.51, 0.71]	
Charandabi 2015 (a)	34	1.51	86	34	1.57	89	1.3%	0.00 [-0.46, 0.46]	
Hossain 2014	34.5	0.1	59	34.3	0.2	67	94.6%	0.20 [0.15, 0.25]	
Roth 2013	32.9	1.8	73	33	1.5	74	1.0%	-0.10 [-0.64, 0.44]	
Subtotal (95% CI)			**258**			**272**	**97.7%**	**0.19 [0.14, 0.25]**	
Heterogeneity: Chi² = 1.99, df = 3 (P = 0.57); I² = 0%									
Test for overall effect: Z = 7.10 (P < 0.00001)									
1.3.2 Vitamin D + micronutrients									
Asemi 2016	34.4	1.3	21	35	1.4	21	0.4%	-0.60 [-1.42, 0.22]	
Brough 2010	34.8	1.3	42	34.8	1.4	42	0.8%	0.00 [-0.58, 0.58]	
Charandabi 2015 (b)	33.9	1.4	88	33.8	1.7	61	1.0%	0.10 [-0.42, 0.62]	
Subtotal (95% CI)			**151**			**124**	**2.3%**	**-0.06 [-0.41, 0.28]**	
Heterogeneity: Chi² = 2.09, df = 2 (P = 0.35); I² = 4%									
Test for overall effect: Z = 0.36 (P = 0.72)									
Total (95% CI)			**409**			**396**	**100.0%**	**0.19 [0.13, 0.24]**	
Heterogeneity: Chi² = 6.12, df = 6 (P = 0.41); I² = 2%									
Test for overall effect: Z = 6.97 (P < 0.00001)									
Test for subgroup differences: Chi² = 2.04, df = 1 (P = 0.15), I² = 51.1%									

Figure 4. Forest plot of the effect of vitamin D intervention alone or in combination with micronutrients on head circumference (cm), based on the fixed-effects model. Charandabi 2015 (**a**): Vit D + Ca (1000 IU/day); Charandabi 2015 (**b**): Vit D (1000 IU/day).

3.3.4. Low Birthweight

The effect of vitamin D supplementation on incidence of LBW was assessed by 3 RCTs [14,18,28] and 4 group comparisons. Compared to control groups, the risk of LBW newborns was lower in the intervention groups (RR = 0.40, 95% CI 0.22–0.74; *p* = 0.003) (Figure 5). Interestingly, the omission of the study by Brough [14], showed that women supplemented with vitamin D alone had a lower risk of LBW than controls (RR = 0.47, 95% CI 0.23–0.97; *p* = 0.040). In contrast, Brough et al. reported no significant effect of vitamin D supplementation with micronutrients [14]. Q-test and I2 statistics showed no significant heterogeneity across studies (*p* > 0.1; I2 = 0%). Subgroup analysis by regimen showed that daily maternal vitamin D supplementation significantly reduced the risk of LBW (RR = 0.40, 95% CI 0.21–0.78; *p* = 0.007). Regarding single-intermitted intervention, Yu et al. reported no significant effect [28].

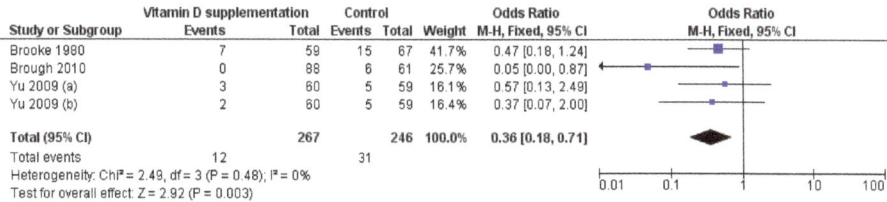

Study or Subgroup	Vitamin D supplementation Events	Total	Control Events	Total	Weight	Odds Ratio M-H, Fixed, 95% CI	Odds Ratio M-H, Fixed, 95% CI
Brooke 1980	7	59	15	67	41.7%	0.47 [0.18, 1.24]	
Brough 2010	0	88	6	61	25.7%	0.05 [0.00, 0.87]	
Yu 2009 (a)	3	60	5	59	16.1%	0.57 [0.13, 2.49]	
Yu 2009 (b)	2	60	5	59	16.4%	0.37 [0.07, 2.00]	
Total (95% CI)		267		246	100.0%	0.36 [0.18, 0.71]	
Total events	12		31				
Heterogeneity: Chi² = 2.49, df = 3 (P = 0.48); I² = 0%							
Test for overall effect: Z = 2.92 (P = 0.003)							

Figure 5. Forest plot of the effect of vitamin D intervention on the risk of low birthweight, based on the fixed-effects model. Yu 2009 (a): Vit D2 (800 IU/day); Yu 2009 (b): Vit D2 (single dose of 200000 IU).

3.3.5. Small for Gestational Age

The effect of vitamin D supplementation on incidence of SGA was assessed by 5 RCTs [14,18,22,27,28] and 6 group comparisons. Compared to control groups, the risk of SGA was lower in the intervention groups (RR = 0.69, 95% CI 0.51–0.92; *p* = 0.018) (Figure 6). Interestingly, the omission of the study by Brough [14], showed that women supplemented with vitamin D alone had a lower risk of SGA than controls (RR = 0.70, 95% CI 0.47–0.97; *p* = 0.047). In contrast, Brough et al. reported no significant effect of vitamin D supplementation with micronutrients [14]. Q-test and I2 statistics showed no significant heterogeneity across studies (*p* > 0.1; I2 = 16.2%). Meta-regression did not reveal a dose-dependent effect of vitamin D supplementation alone on SGA (*p* = 0.903). Subgroup analysis by regimen demonstrated that both daily and single-intermitted dose significantly reduced the risk of SGA (RR = 0.73, 95% CI 0.51–0.98; *p* = 0.042; RR = 0.58, 95% CI 0.32–0.99; *p* = 0.048).

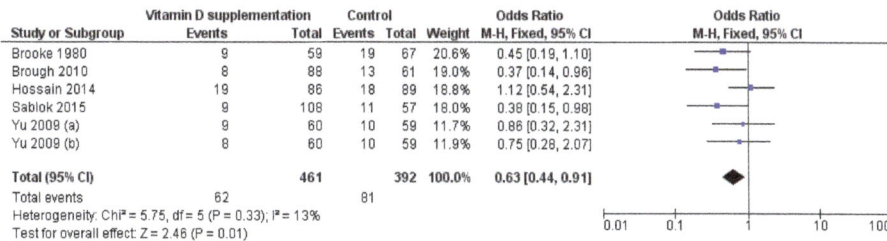

Study or Subgroup	Vitamin D supplementation Events	Total	Control Events	Total	Weight	Odds Ratio M-H, Fixed, 95% CI	Odds Ratio M-H, Fixed, 95% CI
Brooke 1980	9	59	19	67	20.6%	0.45 [0.19, 1.10]	
Brough 2010	8	88	13	61	19.0%	0.37 [0.14, 0.96]	
Hossain 2014	19	86	18	89	18.8%	1.12 [0.54, 2.31]	
Sablok 2015	9	108	11	57	18.0%	0.38 [0.15, 0.98]	
Yu 2009 (a)	9	60	10	59	11.7%	0.86 [0.32, 2.31]	
Yu 2009 (b)	8	60	10	59	11.9%	0.75 [0.28, 2.07]	
Total (95% CI)		461		392	100.0%	0.63 [0.44, 0.91]	
Total events	62		81				
Heterogeneity: Chi² = 5.75, df = 5 (P = 0.33); I² = 13%							
Test for overall effect: Z = 2.46 (P = 0.01)							

Figure 6. Forest plot of the effect of vitamin D intervention on the risk of small for gestational age, based on the fixed-effects model. Yu 2009 (a): Vit D2 (800 IU/day); Yu 2009 (b): Vit D2 (single dose of 200000 IU).

3.4. Risk-of-Bias and Quality Assessment

Risk-of-bias assessment was shown in Figure 7. Overall, we identified low risk of attrition and other biases; however, unclear and/or high risk of selection, performance, detection, and reporting biases cannot be excluded. Overall, the quality of evidence varied from very low (head circumference) to moderate (birthweight, birth length, LBW, and SGA). The main reasons for downgrading the quality of evidence were the risk of bias of RCTs (i.e., high risk of bias for blinding) and the imprecision (i.e., low sample size and/or number of events which resulted in wide 95% CI). Full details of risk-of-bias and quality assessment are included in Supplementary Materials.

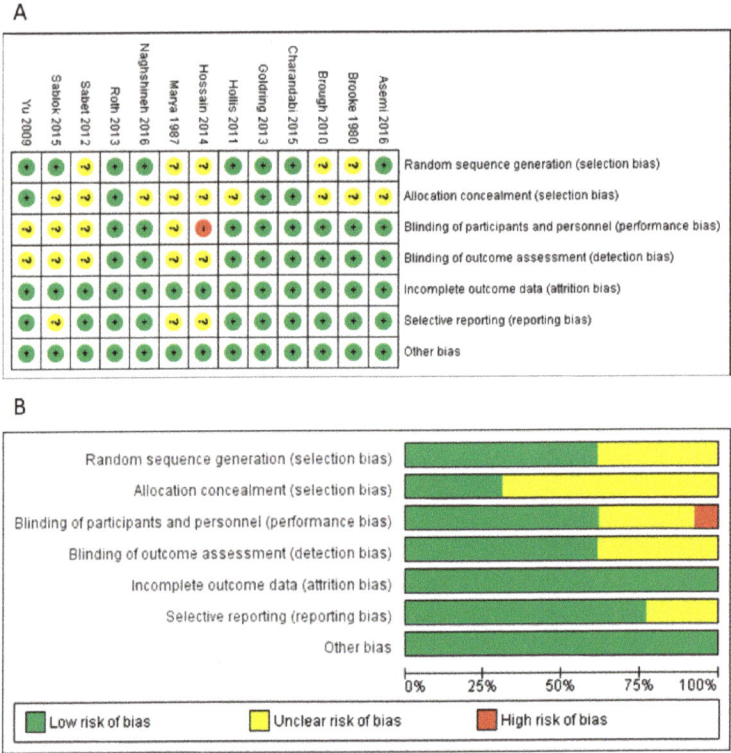

Figure 7. Risk-of-bias assessment of randomized controlled trials included in the meta-analysis. Risk-of-bias summary (**A**) and graph (**B**), according to the Cochrane's Collaboration tool for assessing risk of bias in randomized trials.

3.5. Publication Bias

The funnel plot of the effect of vitamin D supplementation on birthweight appeared symmetric (Figure 8). Accordingly, Begg's rank correlation method and Egger's weighted regression method showed no sources of publication bias (*p*-values > 0.05). Regarding other outcomes, due to the limited number of studies, the extent of publication biases cannot be excluded because the power of the tests for funnel plot asymmetry was too low to identify a real asymmetry [10].

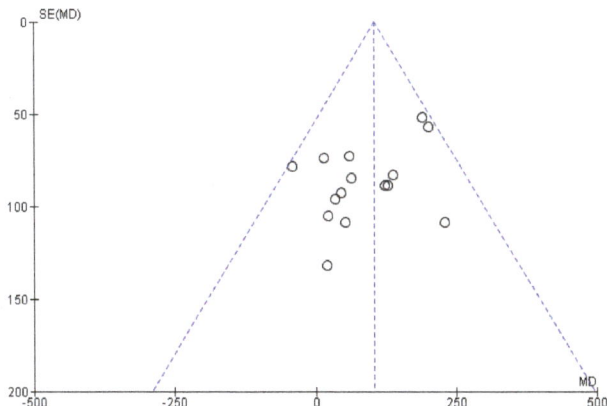

Figure 8. Funnel plot with estimated 95% confidence intervals for meta-analysis of the effect of vitamin D intervention on birthweight.

4. Discussion

When interpreting findings about the effect of maternal vitamin D supplementation on birth size, differences in study design and type of intervention should be considered. To reduce heterogeneity, we limited our analysis to RCTs of pregnant women without pregnancy complications, with randomization at either individual or cluster level. We excluded observational studies, cross-over trials, or quasi-RCTs. Moreover, to demonstrate whether alternative formulations and/or regimens had different effect on birth size, we performed subgroup analyses. Overall, we compared the effect of oral vitamin D (D2 or D3 form) supplementation, alone or in combination with other micronutrients, with placebo or no treatment. Most of the interventions provided daily vitamin supplementation, and to a lesser extent intermitted or single high doses. To date, the recommended dose of vitamin D supplementation, during pregnancy and lactation, is 600 IU per day [6]. This recommendation, based on outcomes related to skeletal health, was proposed as the amount of vitamin D to maintain blood levels of 25(OH)D above 50 nmol/L [29]. However, several lines of evidence argued that deficiency should be defined at thresholds of 75 nmol/L or higher [30–34]. The majority of RCTs included in our work evaluated the benefits of a supplementation greater than 600 IU per day. The daily doses ranged from 200 IU to 4000 IU while, among high single-intermitted interventions, the doses varied from 35000 IU to 600000 IU. During pregnancy, the tolerable upper intake level of vitamin D is now set at 4000 IU/day, although the adverse effects of higher levels are uncertain [30]. As suggested by several RCTs included in the present systematic review, interventions which reached or exceed the tolerable upper intake level did not manifest adverse effects [20,22,23,25,26,28]. However, due to inconclusive evidence, monitoring of toxicity and potential adverse effects of high intermittent dosages should be an important consideration in RCTs design [30].

Our findings add to the growing body of evidence about the effect of vitamin D supplementation on neonatal anthropometric measures and incidence of LBW and SGA births. Compared to previous meta-analyses [5,8], our work summarized data from 13 RCTs, published until May 2017, providing a larger number of group comparisons for each outcome of interest. We confirmed that vitamin D supplementation alone, but not in combination with other micronutrients, significantly increased birthweight, birth length, and head circumference. Compared to the most recent meta-analysis of RCTs by Perez-Lopez et al. [5], we also showed that newborns from women supplemented with vitamin D alone had a lower risk of LBW. This evidence was consistent with four trials included in the recent systematic review by De-Regil et al. [7] and pooled results by Thorne-Lyman et al. [8]. Although birthweight and length are the most used indicators for the assessment of intrauterine growth, the evaluation of weight distribution at birth is more adequate when it is adjusted for gestational age. Accordingly, the reduction of LBW is not the best goal of intervention of RCTs, because it does not distinguish between suboptimal fetal growth and shortened gestation [35]. Evidence about the effect of vitamin D supplementation on gestational age and preterm birth is controversial; De-Regil et al. reported that vitamin D supplementation alone may reduce the risk of preterm birth, while the combined supplementation with calcium increased the risk [7]. Findings from RCTs included in the present study suggested that women who received vitamin D supplementation alone [24,27] or in combination with calcium [13] had a lower risk of preterm birth. However, in other RCTs the intervention did not affect gestational age [13,14,20–22,24] and preterm birth incidence [14,19,22]. To our knowledge, the present study is the first demonstrating that maternal vitamin D supplementation alone significantly reduced the risk of SGA births, defined as birthweight below the 10th percentile for sex and gestational age. SGA newborns show a higher risk of neonatal and infant mortality, childhood malnutrition, neurocognitive disorders, and adulthood metabolic diseases [36]. Subgroup analysis by regimen showed that both daily and high single-intermitted dose significantly increased birthweight and length, reducing the risk of SGA births. In fact, the fat-soluble properties of vitamin D allow the single-intermitted dosage during pregnancy, which may be a feasible strategy against adverse neonatal outcomes in low income countries with poor health infrastructures [8].

Since we included studies with different interventions, we assessed the dose-dependent effect of vitamin D supplementation on birth size. For this purpose, we performed meta-regression analyses of those outcomes with at least three studies evaluating daily vitamin D supplementation alone. By contrast, heterogeneity in formulation, dose, duration, and timing of supplementation, did not allow us to perform meta-regression of studies with single supplementation and/or combination of supplements. However, our analysis did not reveal a dose-dependent effect of vitamin D on birth sizes, probably due to the limited number of studies. Moreover, very few studies investigated the effect of vitamin D supplementation with other micronutrients, and hence we were not able to understand whether the combination with other supplements might affect the efficacy of intervention. Although single and combination interventions were based on similar vitamin D doses, we cannot exclude an antagonistic effect of other micronutrients. Given these limitations, further research is needed to assess the dose-dependent effect of vitamin D alone or in combination with other micronutrients.

The positive effect of maternal vitamin D supplementation on birth size and risk of LBW and SGA might be mediated by changes in fetal cell mass and function, skeletal mineralization, and metabolism [37]. Moreover, maternal serum vitamin D insufficiency is associated with an increased risk of preterm birth [38–40]. The main role of vitamin D in the human body is to maintain adequate levels of calcium and phosphate, enabling the critical processes of bone mineralization and development during fetal life [37]. In many fetal tissues, the active form of vitamin D binds to the vitamin D receptors, regulating genes responsible for the proper implantation of the placenta [41], which is important for fetal growth. Moreover, vitamin D could influence the maternal immune response to the placenta [42] and the expression of human chorionic gonadotropin and sex steroids [43]. Some experimental studies have also proposed the role of vitamin D in glucose and insulin metabolism, affecting availability of energy to the fetus [44], as well as its influence on musculoskeletal growth [45].

Potential weaknesses of our work include the limited number of databases searched. According to selection criteria, some data, such as conference abstracts and/or unpublished reports, were excluded. Our reluctance to include unpublished results is based on: (i) the absence of peer-review of unpublished literature; (ii) the studies that can be located may be an unrepresentative sample of all unpublished studies; (iii) unpublished studies may be of lower methodological quality than published studies [10]. To address publication biases, we visually assessed funnel plot asymmetry followed by Begg's test and Egger's regression asymmetry test. However, in those outcomes with less than 10 intervention groups, the extent of publication bias cannot be completely excluded. Beyond potential reporting and publication biases, we assessed an unclear risk of bias for random sequence generation, allocation concealment, selective reporting and blinding (i.e., absence of blinding should be considered when interpreting results by Hossain et al. [22]). Accordingly, the quality of evidence varied from very low to moderate. The main reasons for downgrading the quality of evidence were the high risk of bias for blinding and the low sample size, which resulted in wide 95% CI. We also recognize that including more group comparisons could have the potential of overestimating or underestimating the effect of vitamin D supplementation. To solve this issue, where possible, we performed subgroup analyses that classified group comparison into different subgroups, whenever possible. Another weakness is the potential effect of confounders. To control for factors that could contribute to the effect of vitamin D supplementation on birth size, RCTs should be based on more standardized protocols [46]: dosage for vitamin D supplementation should be chosen upon the maternal serum 25OHD levels at baseline [8], as performed by Sablok et al. [27], and such trials should take into account risk factors for vitamin D deficiency (i.e., genetic factors, latitude, lifestyles, dietary intake and seasonality) [47–49]. To avoid confounding due to seasonal variation in sunlight exposure, several RCTs were carried out in different seasons [14,18,22,24,26,27]. Taking into account the abovementioned limitations, further research and large multicenter RCTs, evaluating the effect of genetic, environmental, sociodemographic, and life-style factors, is needed.

5. Conclusions

Despite growing interest in the relationship between vitamin D supplementation and pregnancy outcomes, previous evidence about the effect on birth size remained weak. Findings from these systematic review and meta-analysis confirm vitamin D as an essential nutrient for fetal growth and development, with well-established effects on birth size. Moreover, to our knowledge, this work represents the first meta-analysis of RCTs which demonstrates a significant positive effect of maternal vitamin D supplementation on the risk of SGA births. However, further RCTs of vitamin D supplementation during pregnancy are required to better define risks and benefits associated with such interventions and the potential implication as a feasible strategy to prevent adverse pregnancy outcomes.

Supplementary Materials: The following are available online at http://www.mdpi.com/2072-6643/11/2/442/s1, S1: Prisma 2009 Checklist, S2: Search strategy used for PubMed and Cochrane Central Register of Controlled Trials databases, S3: Search strategy used for EMBASE database, S4: Full details of risk of bias assessment, S4: Assessment of the quality of the evidence using the GRADE approach.

Author Contributions: Conceptualization, A.A.; methodology, A.M., M.B., and I.B.; formal analysis, A.M., M.B., and I.B.; data curation, A.M., M.B., and I.B.; writing—original draft preparation, A.M., M.B., I.B., and A.A.; writing—review and editing, A.M., M.B., I.B., and A.A.; supervision, A.A.

Funding: A.M., M.B., and A.A were partially funded by the Department of Medical and Surgical Sciences and Advanced Technologies "GF Ingrassia", University of Catania (Piano Triennale di Sviluppo delle Attività di Ricerca Scientifica del Dipartimento–2016–2018).

Conflicts of Interest: The authors declare no conflict of interest.

References

1. Ramakrishnan, U.; Grant, F.; Goldenberg, T.; Zongrone, A.; Martorell, R. Effect of women's nutrition before and during early pregnancy on maternal and infant outcomes: A systematic review. *Paediatr. Perinat. Epidemiol.* **2012**, *26* (Suppl. 1), 285–301. [CrossRef] [PubMed]
2. Agodi, A.; Barchitta, M.; Valenti, G.; Marzagalli, R.; Frontini, V.; Marchese, A.E. Increase in the prevalence of the MTHFR 677 TT polymorphism in women born since 1959: Potential implications for folate requirements. *Eur. J. Clin. Nutr.* **2011**, *65*, 1302–1308. [CrossRef] [PubMed]
3. Holick, M.F. Vitamin D: A d-lightful solution for health. *J. Investig. Med.* **2011**, *59*, 872–880. [CrossRef] [PubMed]
4. Harvey, N.C.; Holroyd, C.; Ntani, G.; Javaid, K.; Cooper, P.; Moon, R.; Cole, Z.; Tinati, T.; Godfrey, K.; Dennison, E.; et al. Vitamin D supplementation in pregnancy: A systematic review. *Health Technol. Assess.* **2014**, *18*, 1–190. [CrossRef] [PubMed]

5. Pérez-López, F.R.; Pasupuleti, V.; Mezones-Holguin, E.; Benites-Zapata, V.A.; Thota, P.; Deshpande, A.; Hernandez, A.V. Effect of vitamin D supplementation during pregnancy on maternal and neonatal outcomes: A systematic review and meta-analysis of randomized controlled trials. *Fertil. Steril.* **2015**, *103*, 1278–1288. [CrossRef] [PubMed]

6. Ross, A.C. The 2011 report on dietary reference intakes for calcium and vitamin D. *Public Health Nutr.* **2011**, *14*, 938–939. [CrossRef] [PubMed]

7. De-Regil, L.M.; Palacios, C.; Lombardo, L.K.; Peña-Rosas, J.P. Vitamin D supplementation for women during pregnancy. *Sao Paulo Med. J.* **2016**, *134*, 274–275. [CrossRef] [PubMed]

8. Thorne-Lyman, A.; Fawzi, W.W. Vitamin D during pregnancy and maternal, neonatal and infant health outcomes: A systematic review and meta-analysis. *Paediatr. Perinat. Epidemiol.* **2012**, *26* (Suppl. 1), 75–90. [CrossRef] [PubMed]

9. Moher, D.; Shamseer, L.; Clarke, M.; Ghersi, D.; Liberati, A.; Petticrew, M.; Shekelle, P.; Stewart, L.A.; Group, P.-P. Preferred reporting items for systematic review and meta-analysis protocols (PRISMA-P) 2015 statement. *Syst. Rev.* **2015**, *4*, 1. [CrossRef] [PubMed]

10. Higgins, J.; Green, S. *Cochrane Handbook for Systematic Reviews of Interventions*, Version 5.1.0 ed.; The Cochrane Collaboration: London, UK, 2008.

11. Guyatt, G.; Oxman, A.D.; Akl, E.A.; Kunz, R.; Vist, G.; Brozek, J.; Norris, S.; Falck-Ytter, Y.; Glasziou, P.; DeBeer, H.; et al. GRADE guidelines: 1. Introduction-GRADE evidence profiles and summary of findings tables. *J. Clin. Epidemiol.* **2011**, *64*, 383–394. [CrossRef] [PubMed]

12. Higgins, J.P.; Thompson, S.G. Quantifying heterogeneity in a meta-analysis. *Stat. Med.* **2002**, *21*, 1539–1558. [CrossRef] [PubMed]

13. Asemi, Z.; Samimi, M.; Siavashani, M.A.; Mazloomi, M.; Tabassi, Z.; Karamali, M.; Jamilian, M.; Esmaillzadeh, A. Calcium-Vitamin D Co-supplementation Affects Metabolic Profiles, but not Pregnancy Outcomes, in Healthy Pregnant Women. *Int. J. Prev. Med.* **2016**, *7*, 49. [CrossRef] [PubMed]

14. Brough, L.; Rees, G.A.; Crawford, M.A.; Morton, R.H.; Dorman, E.K. Effect of multiple-micronutrient supplementation on maternal nutrient status, infant birth weight and gestational age at birth in a low-income, multi-ethnic population. *Br. J. Nutr.* **2010**, *104*, 437–445. [CrossRef] [PubMed]

15. Thompson, S.G.; Sharp, S.J. Explaining heterogeneity in meta-analysis: A comparison of methods. *Stat. Med.* **1999**, *18*, 2693–2708. [CrossRef]

16. Begg, C.B.; Mazumdar, M. Operating characteristics of a rank correlation test for publication bias. *Biometrics* **1994**, *50*, 1088–1101. [CrossRef] [PubMed]

17. Egger, M.; Davey Smith, G.; Schneider, M.; Minder, C. Bias in meta-analysis detected by a simple, graphical test. *BMJ* **1997**, *315*, 629–634. [CrossRef]

18. Brooke, O.G.; Brown, I.R.; Bone, C.D.; Carter, N.D.; Cleeve, H.J.; Maxwell, J.D.; Robinson, V.P.; Winder, S.M. Vitamin D supplements in pregnant Asian women: Effects on calcium status and fetal growth. *Br. Med. J.* **1980**, *280*, 751–754. [CrossRef]

19. Mohammad-Alizadeh-Charandabi, S.; Mirghafourvand, M.; Mansouri, A.; Najafi, M.; Khodabande, F. The Effect of Vitamin D and Calcium plus Vitamin D during Pregnancy on Pregnancy and Birth Outcomes: A Randomized Controlled Trial. *J. Caring Sci.* **2015**, *4*, 35–44. [CrossRef]

20. Goldring, S.T.; Griffiths, C.J.; Martineau, A.R.; Robinson, S.; Yu, C.; Poulton, S.; Kirkby, J.C.; Stocks, J.; Hooper, R.; Shaheen, S.O.; et al. Prenatal vitamin d supplementation and child respiratory health: A randomised controlled trial. *PLoS ONE* **2013**, *8*, e66627. [CrossRef]

21. Hollis, B.W.; Johnson, D.; Hulsey, T.C.; Ebeling, M.; Wagner, C.L. Vitamin D supplementation during pregnancy: Double-blind, randomized clinical trial of safety and effectiveness. *J. Bone Miner. Res.* **2011**, *26*, 2341–2357. [CrossRef]

22. Hossain, N.; Kanani, F.H.; Ramzan, S.; Kausar, R.; Ayaz, S.; Khanani, R.; Pal, L. Obstetric and neonatal outcomes of maternal vitamin D supplementation: Results of an open-label, randomized controlled trial of antenatal vitamin D supplementation in Pakistani women. *J. Clin. Endocrinol. Metab.* **2014**, *99*, 2448–2455. [CrossRef] [PubMed]

23. Marya, R.K.; Rathee, S.; Dua, V.; Sangwan, K. Effect of vitamin D supplementation during pregnancy on foetal growth. *Indian J. Med. Res.* **1988**, *88*, 488–492. [PubMed]

24. Naghshineh, E.; Sheikhaliyan, S. Effect of vitamin D supplementation in the reduce risk of preeclampsia in nulliparous women. *Adv. Biomed. Res.* **2016**, *5*, 7. [CrossRef] [PubMed]

25. Roth, D.E.; Al Mahmud, A.; Raqib, R.; Akhtar, E.; Perumal, N.; Pezzack, B.; Baqui, A.H. Randomized placebo-controlled trial of high-dose prenatal third-trimester vitamin D3 supplementation in Bangladesh: The AViDD trial. *Nutr. J.* **2013**, *12*, 47. [CrossRef]

26. Sabet, Z.; Ghazi, A.; Tohidi, M.; Oladi, B. Vitamin D supplementation in pregnant Iranian women: Effects on maternal and neonatal vitamin D and parathyroid hormone status. *Acta Endo* **2012**, *8*, 59–66. [CrossRef]

27. Sablok, A.; Batra, A.; Thariani, K.; Bharti, R.; Aggarwal, A.R.; Kabi, B.C.; Chellani, H. Supplementation of vitamin D in pregnancy and its correlation with feto-maternal outcome. *Clin. Endocrinol.* **2015**, *83*, 536–541. [CrossRef] [PubMed]

28. Yu, C.K.; Sykes, L.; Sethi, M.; Teoh, T.G.; Robinson, S. Vitamin D deficiency and supplementation during pregnancy. *Clin. Endocrinol.* **2009**, *70*, 685–690. [CrossRef] [PubMed]

29. Institute of Medicine. *Dietary Reference Intakes for Calcium and Vitamin D*; National Academies Press: Washington, DC, USA, 2011.

30. Heaney, R.P.; Davies, K.M.; Chen, T.C.; Holick, M.F.; Barger-Lux, M.J. Human serum 25-hydroxycholecalciferol response to extended oral dosing with cholecalciferol. *Am. J. Clin. Nutr.* **2003**, *77*, 204–210. [CrossRef] [PubMed]

31. Bischoff-Ferrari, H.A.; Giovannucci, E.; Willett, W.C.; Dietrich, T.; Dawson-Hughes, B. Estimation of optimal serum concentrations of 25-hydroxyvitamin D for multiple health outcomes. *Am. J. Clin. Nutr.* **2006**, *84*, 18–28. [CrossRef] [PubMed]

32. Visser, M.; Deeg, D.J.; Puts, M.T.; Seidell, J.C.; Lips, P. Low serum concentrations of 25-hydroxyvitamin D in older persons and the risk of nursing home admission. *Am. J. Clin. Nutr.* **2006**, *84*, 616–622. [CrossRef]

33. Norman, A.W.; Bouillon, R.; Whiting, S.J.; Vieth, R.; Lips, P. 13th Workshop consensus for vitamin D nutritional guidelines. *J. Steroid Biochem. Mol. Biol.* **2007**, *103*, 204–205. [CrossRef] [PubMed]

34. Henry, H.L.; Bouillon, R.; Norman, A.W.; Gallagher, J.C.; Lips, P.; Heaney, R.P.; Vieth, R.; Pettifor, J.M.; Dawson-Hughes, B.; Lamberg-Allardt, C.J.; et al. 14th Vitamin D Workshop consensus on vitamin D nutritional guidelines. *J. Steroid Biochem. Mol. Biol.* **2010**, *121*, 4–6. [CrossRef] [PubMed]

35. Steer, P. Small for Gestational Age: Causes and Consequences. *J. Anat.* **2009**, *215*, 224. [CrossRef]

36. Institute of Medicine (US) Committee on Improving Birth Outcomes. *Improving Birth Outcomes: Meeting the Challenge in the Developing World*; Bale, J.R., Stoll, B.J., Lucas, A.O., Eds.; National Academies Press: Washington, DC, USA, 2003.

37. Kovacs, C.S. Bone metabolism in the fetus and neonate. *Pediatr. Nephrol.* **2014**, *29*, 793–803. [CrossRef] [PubMed]

38. Qin, L.L.; Lu, F.G.; Yang, S.H.; Xu, H.L.; Luo, B.A. Does Maternal Vitamin D Deficiency Increase the Risk of Preterm Birth: A Meta-Analysis of Observational Studies. *Nutrients* **2016**, *8*, 301. [CrossRef]

39. McDonnell, S.L.; Baggerly, K.A.; Baggerly, C.A.; Aliano, J.L.; French, C.B.; Baggerly, L.L.; Ebeling, M.D.; Rittenberg, C.S.; Goodier, C.G.; Mateus Niño, J.F.; et al. Maternal 25(OH)D concentrations ≥40 ng/mL associated with 60% lower preterm birth risk among general obstetrical patients at an urban medical center. *PLoS ONE* **2017**, *12*, e0180483. [CrossRef]

40. Zhou, S.S.; Tao, Y.H.; Huang, K.; Zhu, B.B.; Tao, F.B. Vitamin D and risk of preterm birth: Up-to-date meta-analysis of randomized controlled trials and observational studies. *J. Obstet. Gynaecol. Res.* **2017**, *43*, 247–256. [CrossRef]

41. Evans, K.N.; Bulmer, J.N.; Kilby, M.D.; Hewison, M. Vitamin D and placental-decidual function. *J. Soc. Gynecol. Investig.* **2004**, *11*, 263–271. [CrossRef]

42. Bodnar, L.M.; Krohn, M.A.; Simhan, H.N. Maternal vitamin D deficiency is associated with bacterial vaginosis in the first trimester of pregnancy. *J. Nutr.* **2009**, *139*, 1157–1161. [CrossRef]

43. Barrera, D.; Avila, E.; Hernández, G.; Méndez, I.; González, L.; Halhali, A.; Larrea, F.; Morales, A.; Díaz, L. Calcitriol affects hCG gene transcription in cultured human syncytiotrophoblasts. *Reprod. Biol. Endocrinol.* **2008**, *6*, 3. [CrossRef]

44. Pittas, A.G.; Lau, J.; Hu, F.B.; Dawson-Hughes, B. The role of vitamin D and calcium in type 2 diabetes. A systematic review and meta-analysis. *J. Clin. Endocrinol. Metab.* **2007**, *92*, 2017–2029. [CrossRef] [PubMed]

45. Giuliani, D.L.; Boland, R.L. Effects of vitamin D3 metabolites on calcium fluxes in intact chicken skeletal muscle and myoblasts cultured in vitro. *Calcif. Tissue Int.* **1984**, *36*, 200–205. [CrossRef] [PubMed]

46. Papageorghiou, A.T.; Ohuma, E.O.; Altman, D.G.; Todros, T.; Cheikh Ismail, L.; Lambert, A.; Jaffer, Y.A.; Bertino, E.; Gravett, M.G.; Purwar, M.; et al. International standards for fetal growth based on serial ultrasound measurements: The Fetal Growth Longitudinal Study of the INTERGROWTH-21st Project. *Lancet* **2014**, *384*, 869–879. [CrossRef]

47. Karras, S.; Paschou, S.A.; Kandaraki, E.; Anagnostis, P.; Annweiler, C.; Tarlatzis, B.C.; Hollis, B.W.; Grant, W.B.; Goulis, D.G. Hypovitaminosis D in pregnancy in the Mediterranean region: A systematic review. *Eur. J. Clin. Nutr.* **2016**, *70*, 979–986. [CrossRef] [PubMed]

48. Wang, T.J.; Zhang, F.; Richards, J.B.; Kestenbaum, B.; van Meurs, J.B.; Berry, D.; Kiel, D.P.; Streeten, E.A.; Ohlsson, C.; Koller, D.L.; et al. Common genetic determinants of vitamin D insufficiency: A genome-wide association study. *Lancet* **2010**, *376*, 180–188. [CrossRef]

49. Barchitta, M.; Maugeri, A.; La Rosa, M.C.; Magnano San Lio, R.; Favara, G.; Panella, M.; Cianci, A.; Agodi, A. Single Nucleotide Polymorphisms in Vitamin D Receptor Gene Affect Birth Weight and the Risk of Preterm Birth: Results From the "Mamma & Bambino" Cohort and A Meta-Analysis. *Nutrients* **2018**, *10*, 1172. [CrossRef]

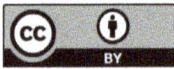

nutrients

MDPI

Article

Maternal Iodine Status and Associations with Birth Outcomes in Three Major Cities in the United Kingdom

Charles J. P. Snart [1,†], **Claire Keeble** [2,†], **Elizabeth Taylor** [1], **Janet E. Cade** [3], **Paul M. Stewart** [4], **Michael Zimmermann** [5], **Stephen Reid** [6], **Diane E. Threapleton** [1], **Lucilla Poston** [7], **Jenny E. Myers** [8], **Nigel A. B. Simpson** [9,‡], **Darren C. Greenwood** [1,2,‡] and **Laura J. Hardie** [1,*,‡]

[1] Department of Clinical and Population Science, Leeds Institute of Cardiovascular and Metabolic Medicine, School of Medicine, University of Leeds, Leeds LS2 9JT, UK; medcjps@leeds.ac.uk (C.J.P.S.); E.Taylor@leeds.ac.uk (E.T.); D.E.Threapleton@leeds.ac.uk (D.E.T.); D.C.Greenwood@leeds.ac.uk (D.C.G.)
[2] Leeds Institute for Data Analytics, University of Leeds, Leeds LS2 9JT, UK; C.M.Owen@leeds.ac.uk
[3] Nutritional Epidemiology Group, School of Food Science & Nutrition, University of Leeds, Leeds LS2 9JT, UK; J.E.Cade@leeds.ac.uk
[4] Faculty of Medicine and Health, University of Leeds, Leeds LS2 9JT, UK; P.M.Stewart@leeds.ac.uk
[5] Laboratory for Human Nutrition, Institute of Food, Nutrition and Health, Swiss Federal Institute of Technology (ETH), 8092 Zürich, Switzerland; michael.zimmermann@hest.ethz.ch
[6] Earth Surface Science Institute, School of Earth and Environment, University of Leeds, Leeds LS2 9JT, UK; S.Reid@leeds.ac.uk
[7] Division of Women's Health, Women's Health Academic Centre, King's College London, London SE1 7EH, UK; lucilla.poston@kcl.ac.uk
[8] Maternal and Fetal Health Research Centre, Institute of Human Development, University of Manchester, Manchester M13 0JH, UK; Jenny.Myers@manchester.ac.uk
[9] Division of Women's and Children's Health, School of Medicine, University of Leeds, Leeds LS2 9JT, UK; N.A.B.Simpson@leeds.ac.uk
* Correspondence: L.J.Hardie@leeds.ac.uk; Tel.: +44(0)-113-343-7769
† These two authors joint first authors.
‡ These three authors joint senior authors.

Received: 28 January 2019; Accepted: 8 February 2019; Published: 20 February 2019

Abstract: Severe iodine deficiency in mothers is known to impair foetal development. Pregnant women in the UK may be iodine insufficient, but recent assessments of iodine status are limited. This study assessed maternal urinary iodine concentrations (UIC) and birth outcomes in three UK cities. Spot urines were collected from 541 women in London, Manchester and Leeds from 2004–2008 as part of the Screening for Pregnancy End points (SCOPE) study. UIC at 15 and 20 weeks' gestation was estimated using inductively coupled plasma-mass spectrometry (ICP-MS). Associations were estimated between iodine status (UIC and iodine-to-creatinine ratio) and birth weight, birth weight centile (primary outcome), small for gestational age (SGA) and spontaneous preterm birth. Median UIC was highest in Manchester (139 µg/L, 95% confidence intervals (CI): 126, 158) and London (130 µg/L, 95% CI: 114, 177) and lowest in Leeds (116 µg/L, 95% CI: 99, 135), but the proportion with UIC <50 µg/L was <20% in all three cities. No evidence of an association was observed between UIC and birth weight centile (−0.2% per 50 µg/L increase in UIC, 95% CI: −1.3, 0.8), nor with odds of spontaneous preterm birth (odds ratio = 1.00, 95% CI: 0.84, 1.20). Given the finding of iodine concentrations being insufficient according to World Health Organization (WHO) guidelines amongst pregnant women across all three cities, further studies may be needed to explore implications for maternal thyroid function and longer-term child health outcomes.

Keywords: Iodine; pregnancy; birth weight; Insufficiency; SGA; preterm Birth

1. Introduction

Iodine is essential for the synthesis of the thyroid hormones triiodothyronine (T3) and thyroxine (T4) which regulate growth and metabolism [1]. Maternal iodine requirements are increased throughout pregnancy to support the thyroid hormone demands of the developing foetus [2]. The foetus is initially reliant on maternal thyroid hormones, but as the foetal thyroid begins functioning from 15–17 weeks gestation, it depends on the maternal iodine supply to maintain thyroid hormone production throughout the remainder of pregnancy [2]. Iodine requirements increase throughout gestation, and iodine deficiency during pregnancy is associated with a number of adverse outcomes for the child, including increased mortality, decreased cognitive performance and delayed physical development [1,3]. Severe deficiency during pregnancy can result in cretinism, a condition characterised by severe mental impairment, motor spasticity and deaf-mutism [1,3].

The introduction of iodine into livestock feed and the widespread adoption of iodophors in the dairy industry after the 1930s resulted in the reduction of overt signs of iodine deficiency in the United Kingdom (UK) population by the 1960s [4–6]. To date, the UK has not implemented an iodine fortification programme for commercial bread or salt production unlike countries such as Denmark and Australia [7,8]. Some authors have suggested that the use of iodophors in the dairy and bread industries in the UK has declined and been superseded by non-iodine alternatives, potentially reducing these sources of dietary iodine [1,9]. In addition, wider changes in dietary practice such as reduced milk and fish intake, the increased availability of dairy substitutes and an increase in vegetarianism may also be affecting iodine status in the UK population [9].

Although the UK adult population is considered iodine sufficient [10], recent studies have suggested that women may become deficient during pregnancy [11–16]. Few studies have provided an up-to-date measure of iodine status during pregnancy, nor have they attempted to link insufficiency with birth outcomes [12–15]. Additionally, these studies have been geographically limited, with many being set in single cities or regions in southern England [12–16]. Recent nationally-representative data have suggested that women of child-bearing age in the UK may be iodine insufficient, though this study specifically excluded pregnant and lactating women and did not assess birth outcomes [10].

We therefore aimed to assess iodine status in the three UK sites of the Screening for Pregnancy Endpoints (SCOPE) international birth cohort, and assess associations between maternal iodine status and birth outcomes, including birth weight, birth centile, small for gestational age (SGA) and spontaneous preterm birth.

2. Materials and Methods

2.1. Study Design and Participants

We analysed samples from three English centres from the Screening for Pregnancy Endpoints (SCOPE) birth cohort. The SCOPE study was previously reported in detail elsewhere [17]. In brief, the SCOPE study recruited 5690 nulliparous women with singleton pregnancies before 15 weeks' gestation, between November 2004 and January 2011 in New Zealand, Australia, UK and Ireland. The UK women were recruited in the cities of Leeds, Manchester and London between November 2004 and August 2008. Women were excluded if they presented a high risk of SGA, pre-eclampsia or spontaneous preterm birth [17]. The original SCOPE study protocol has been registered at clinicaltrials. gov NCT02357667.

Participants were interviewed during antenatal clinic visits at 15 ($\pm$ 1) and 20 ($\pm$ 1) weeks' gestation. Participant characteristics were recorded including age, ethnicity, diet, body mass index (BMI), smoking, marital status, employment and socioeconomic status. Participant socioeconomic index was scored using the New Zealand Socio-economic Index 1996. Spot urines were collected for 643 women at the three UK cities; 619 samples were collected at 15 weeks and 585 at 20 weeks, with 547 providing samples at both time points.

2.2. Urinary Iodine Measurement

Urinary iodine concentration (UIC) was measured in all samples taken at 15 and 20 weeks of gestation. Assessment of individual iodine status typically requires a series of 24 hour urine collections, however spot urines are considered an acceptable tool for assessing iodine status on a population basis [3]. It is additionally possible to eliminate some inter-individual variation from spot-urine samples by correcting UIC by urinary creatinine concentration (g/L) [18]. We report iodine status results both as the raw iodine concentration (μg/L) and the iodine-creatinine ratio (I:Cr) (μg/g).

Urinary ^{127}iodine concentration was measured at the University of Leeds using inductively coupled plasma-mass spectrometry (ICP-MS) (Thermo iCAP Q, Hemel Hempstead, UK), accredited by the Centers for Disease Control and Prevention (CDC) Ensuring the Quality of Urinary Iodine Procedures (EQUIP) standardisation programme. Test samples, calibration standards, and quality control samples were diluted 1:10 prior to analysis. Individual samples consisted of 500 μL of participant urine, 4000 μL of diluent (1% tetramethylammonium hydroxide (Sigma Aldrich), 0.01% Triton X-100 (Sigma Aldrich)) and 500 μL high purity H_2O (>18.2 MΩ.cm). Tellurium (10 μg/L) (Sigma Aldrich) was included as an internal standard for the ICP-MS analysis. Sample concentration was determined against a urine matrix matched calibration curve spiked with 0, 5, 10, 40, 70, 100, 400 and 800 μg/L iodide (Sigma Aldrich). The accuracy of the results was further validated through the inclusion of internal quality control urines: A (target iodine value: 59.9 μg/L, range: 47.2–72.5), B (98.1 μg/L, 88.3–107.9) and C (158.9 μg/L, 140.2–177.5). External validation of our results was provided by inclusion of the certified reference material Seronorm Trace Metal Urine Level 1 (target value: 105 μg/L, certified iodine range: 84–126), and through participation in the CDC EQUIP programme. Observed values were 63.3 μg/L (*n* = 99), 98.6 μg/L (*n* = 99) and 157.9 μg/L (*n* = 99) for quality control urines A, B and C respectively. The observed value for certified reference material was 102.7 μg/L (*n* = 33). Assessment of intra-run precision gave coefficients of variation (CV) of 1.42% at 60 μg/L, 1.67% at 98 μg/L and 2.34% at 159 μg/L. Inter-run precision gave a CV of 2.4% at 60 μg/L, 4.7% at 98 μg/L and 6.0% at 159 μg/L. The method limit of quantification was 1.46 μg/L.

Urinary creatinine concentrations were assessed through a standard microplate assay utilising the Jaffe reaction. Assessment of creatinine intra-assay precision gave a CV of 2% at 10 mg/L, 1% at 70 mg/L and 1.1% at 120 mg/L. Assessment of inter-assay precision gave a CV of 14.5% at 10 mg/L, 9.7% at 70 mg/L and 5.5% at 120 mg/L.

2.3. Outcomes

The primary and a priori outcome for the analysis was birth weight centile. Secondary outcomes were birth weight, SGA, and spontaneous preterm birth. SGA was defined as a birth weight centile <10th on a customised centile chart that accounts for maternal height, weight, parity, ethnicity, neonatal gestation at delivery and sex [19]. This definition was selected due to its standard use in obstetrics and applicability to the UK population, and as it is likely to identify foetal growth restriction. Spontaneous preterm birth was defined as spontaneous preterm labour or preterm premature rupture of the membranes resulting in preterm birth at less than 37 weeks' gestation. These birth outcomes were selected due to the key role of dietary iodine and thyroid hormones in regulating neonatal growth, and the existence of prior studies identifying links between birth weight and preterm birth [20–23].

2.4. Statistical Analysis

Prior to analysis, a set of exclusion parameters were applied. Analysis was limited to participants with urine samples at both time points, using the mean UIC per participant [24]. Exploratory data analysis was then conducted to ensure all values were plausible and all combinations of values were possible. Two participants had duplicate measures at the same time point removed and an additional four participants were excluded due to possessing UIC values more than 3 standard deviations outside of the mean UIC on a log scale. Participant characteristics were described, stratified by location.

Geometric mean and median UIC and I:Cr are presented with 95% confidence intervals (CIs), alongside the proportion of participants with estimated UIC < 50 μg/L. All analyses were completed using Stata version 15.1 (StataCorp. Stata statistical software: Release 15.1. College Station, TX: Stata Corporation, Texas, USA, 2017).

Linear regression was used to quantify associations between UIC and I:Cr for continuous birth outcomes (birth weight and birth weight centile) and logistic regression was used for binary outcomes (SGA and spontaneous preterm birth < 37 weeks). Estimates (with 95% CI) are presented based on the arithmetic mean across the two time points for both UIC and I:Cr for mothers providing both samples (primary analysis) and stratified by time point (secondary analyses). All results are presented as unadjusted and adjusted for known confounders. Directed acyclic graphs were used to inform which variables should be included as covariates, and to prevent over-adjustment [25]. Ethnicity, age, geographic location and socioeconomic index were adjusted for by inclusion in the regression model, except where ethnicity was already accounted for in the birth weight centile and SGA outcomes. Maternal height, weight, parity, neonatal gestation at delivery and sex were also taken into account in the definition of birth weight centile and SGA. The robustness of birthweight and spontaneous preterm birth results to additional adjustment for maternal BMI was assessed.

2.5. Ethics Statement

Ethical approval was gained from local research ethics committees for each SCOPE recruitment site (South East Multi-centre Research Ethics Committee/St Thomas Hospital Research Ethics Committee, 2005082; South East Multi-Centre Research Ethics Committee/Central Manchester Research Ethics Committee, 06/MRE01/98). All participants provided written informed consent.

3. Results

3.1. Participant Characteristics

Table 1 shows participant characteristic summary statistics, including but not limited to maternal age, ethnicity, socioeconomic index, marital status, smoking status, alcohol consumption, height, weight and BMI. The mean maternal age at recruitment was 29 years, 457 (84%) were White Caucasian and 397 (73%) non-smokers (see Table 1). Data were available for 541 participants (151 from London, 260 from Manchester, and 130 from Leeds) after exclusions, with a urine sample available from each participant at both 15 and 20 weeks' gestation. A total of 1082 urine samples were analysed for iodine, with the overall geometric mean of 130 μg/L and a median of 134 μg/L.

3.2. Iodine Status

Geometric mean UIC varied by marital status, geographical location, neonatal gestational age at delivery and gestational time point (Table 2). UIC also varied across time points, with the 20 week concentrations being on average lower than the 15-week concentrations. Participants from Leeds had lower mean UIC (110 μg/L, 95% CI: 99, 121) than participants from Manchester (132 μg/L, 95% CI: 123, 143) or London (145 μg/L, 95% CI: 126, 168). Participants delivering preterm (<37 weeks) generally had similar UIC to those who delivered at term. Consistent with UIC, I:Cr was associated with geographical location and marital status, but not time point or gestational age at delivery. Additionally, I:Cr differed by maternal age category, ethnicity, socioeconomic index and maternal smoking status in the first trimester. Of the three sites, participants at Leeds and Manchester had lower geometric mean I:Cr when compared to London, with Leeds having the lowest. Individuals with UIC (<50 μg/L) constituted 9% (95% CI: 7, 12) across all three sites, with these individuals constituting 9%, 7% and 13% of the Leeds, Manchester and London sites respectively.

Table 1. Participant characteristics by location.

Participant Characteristics	Overall (N = 541)	London (N = 151)	Manchester (N = 260)	Leeds (N = 130)
	n (%)	n (%)	n (%)	n (%)
Mean maternal age (years)				
18–24	121 (22)	12 (8)	62 (24)	47 (36)
25–29	160 (30)	37 (25)	84 (32)	39 (30)
30–34	189 (35)	71 (47)	79 (30)	39 (30)
35+	71 (13)	31 (21)	35 (13)	5 (4)
Maternal ethnicity				
White Caucasian	457 (84)	123 (81)	217 (83)	117 (90)
Other	84 (16)	28 (19)	43 (17)	13 (10)
Maternal socioeconomic index (quartiles)				
Q1 (more deprived)	126 (23)	12 (8)	66 (25)	48 (37)
Q2	133 (25)	31 (21)	68 (26)	34 (26)
Q3	145 (27)	52 (34)	62 (24)	31 (24)
Q4 (less deprived)	137 (25)	56 (37)	64 (25)	17 (13)
Marital status				
Single	84 (16)	14 (9)	38 (15)	32 (25)
Married	258 (48	95 (63)	114 (44)	49 (38)
Living as married	199 (37)	42 (28)	108 (42)	49 (38)
Maternal smoking status in 1st trimester				
Non-smoker	397 (73)	128 (85)	186 (72)	83 (64)
Smoker	144 (27)	23 (15)	74 (28)	47 (36)
Maternal alcohol consumption in 1st trimester (units/week)				
0	153 (28)	34 (23)	85 (33)	34 (26)
<2	94 (17)	38 (25)	38 (15)	18 (14)
2–7	160 (30)	41 (27)	79 (30)	40 (31)
>7	134 (25)	38 (25)	58 (22)	38 (29)
Gravidity				
1	385 (71)	105 (70)	184 (71)	96 (74)
2	119 (22)	35 (23)	61 (23)	23 (18)
3+	37 (7)	11 (7)	15 (6)	11 (8)
Maternal height (cm)				
<160	103 (19)	31 (21)	53 (20)	19 (15)
160–169	300 (55)	85 (56)	148 (57)	67 (52)
170+	138 (26)	35 (23)	59 (23)	44 (34)
Maternal weight at 1st visit (kg)				
<60	154 (28)	44 (29)	77 (30)	33 (25)
60–69	190 (35)	60 (40)	89 (34)	41 (32)
70–79	107 (20)	34 (23	48 (18)	25 (19)
80+	90 (17)	13 (9)	46 (18)	31 (24)
Maternal body mass index at 1st visit (kg/m^2)				
<20	38 (7)	12 (8)	13 (5)	13 (10)
20–25	289 (53)	84 (56)	143 (55)	62 (48)
25–30	148 (27)	42 (28	69 (27)	37 (28)
30+	66 (12)	13 (9)	35 (13)	18 (14)
Spontaneous preterm delivery (<37 weeks)				
No	523 (97)	144 (95)	252 (97)	127 (98)
Yes	18 (3)	7 (5)	8 (3)	3 (2)
Neonatal sex				
Male	277 (51)	78 (52)	140 (54)	59 (45)
Female	264 (49)	73 (48)	120 (46)	71 (55)

Numbers represent the number of individuals in each category, with the percentage in brackets.

Table 2. Urinary iodine concentration and iodine-to-creatinine ratio by participant characteristics.

Participant Characteristics	Mean Urinary Iodine Concentration (μg/L)			Mean Iodine-to-Creatinine ratio (μg/g)	
	Geometric mean (95% CI)	Median (95% CI)	Percent < 50μg/L (95% CI)	Geometric mean (95% CI)	Median (95% CI)
Overall	130 (122, 138)	134 (124, 145)	9 (7, 12)	193 (182, 205)	186 (175, 201)
Maternal age (years)					
18–24	127 (114, 141)	135 (117, 154)	9 (5, 16)	137 (123, 153)	145 (126, 157)
25–29	116 (104, 129)	122 (100, 135)	9 (5, 14)	190 (171, 211)	186 (162, 222)
30–34	138 (124, 154)	140 (119, 164)	11 (7, 16)	228 (208, 251)	219 (201, 254)
35+	147 (122, 176)	144 (122, 191)	6 (2, 14)	232 (197, 272)	210 (175, 249)
Maternal ethnicity					
White Caucasian	130 (122, 139)	134 (124, 147)	10 (7, 13)	201 (189, 214)	190 (176, 209)
Other	127 (112, 143)	124 (103, 147)	4 (1, 10)	155 (135, 178)	160 (142, 193)
Maternal socioeconomic index (quartiles)					
Q1 (More deprived)	125 (112, 139)	128 (109, 163)	6 (2, 11)	157 (141, 174)	153 (144, 182)
Q2	132 (117, 149)	135 (114, 150)	9 (5, 15)	199 (177, 223)	199 (161, 225)
Q3	133 (118, 151)	135 (113, 162)	10 (6, 16)	209 (186, 235)	202 (172, 224)
Q4 (Less deprived)	129 (114, 146)	132 (119, 149)	11 (6, 17)	209 (186, 236)	200 (177, 228)
Marital status					
Single	112 (98, 128)	114 (99, 135)	13 (7, 22)	140 (123, 159)	150 (127, 175)
Married	128 (117, 141)	130 (119, 146)	10 (7, 15)	216 (199, 234)	211 (186, 230)
Living as married	140 (128, 154)	147 (126, 162)	6 (3, 10)	192 (174, 211)	184 (163, 211)
Maternal smoking status in 1st trimester					
Non-smoker	134 (124, 144)	135 (124, 151)	9 (7, 13)	207 (193, 221)	200 (180, 217)
Smoker	119 (108, 132)	126 (111, 143)	8 (4, 14)	160 (145, 177)	154 (143, 180)
Maternal alcohol consumption in 1st trimester (units/week)					
0	133 (120, 148)	135 (117, 161)	7 (4, 12)	183 (166, 202)	184 (163, 212)
<2	124 (107, 143)	125 (99, 153)	11 (5, 19)	193 (168, 222)	186 (161, 206)
2–7	135 (121, 151)	132 (119, 155)	6 (3, 11)	205 (183, 230)	201 (169, 225)
>7	124 (108, 141)	134 (108, 158)	13 (8, 20)	191 (169, 216)	178 (158, 203)
Gravidity					
1	129 (120, 139)	134 (124, 149)	10 (7, 13)	198 (185, 211)	188 (174, 209)
2	131 (117, 147)	131 (115, 151)	7 (3, 13)	183 (161, 209)	183 (147, 210)
3+	130 (104, 163)	120 (102, 174)	8 (2, 22)	179 (148, 218)	188 (154, 217)

Table 2. *Cont.*

Participant Characteristics	Mean Urinary Iodine Concentration (µg/L)			Mean Iodine-to-Creatinine ratio (µg/g)	
	Geometric mean (95% CI)	Median (95% CI)	Percent < 50µg/L (95% CI)	Geometric mean (95% CI)	Median (95% CI)
Maternal height (cm)					
<160	129 (112, 148)	126 (104, 159)	8 (3, 15)	202 (175, 234)	175 (157, 212)
160–169	134 (123, 145)	134 (123, 152)	10 (7, 14)	196 (182, 212)	197 (176, 212)
170+	122 (110, 137)	131 (115, 152)	9 (5, 15)	180 (161, 202)	170 (152, 206)
Maternal weight at 1st visit (kg)					
<60	131 (116, 146)	126 (112, 152)	9 (5, 15)	207 (185, 231)	201 (175, 234)
60–69	124 (112, 137)	125 (111, 141)	8 (5, 13)	195 (177, 214)	190 (170, 209)
70–79	130 (112, 149)	135 (114, 172)	12 (7, 20)	202 (177, 231)	177 (159, 209)
80+	143 (125, 163)	157 (127, 173)	8 (3, 15)	160 (140, 184)	159 (128, 210)
Maternal body mass index at 1st visit (kg/m^2)					
<20	131 (106, 163)	130 (98, 175)	5 (1, 18)	178 (138, 229)	157 (121, 253)
20–25	127 (116, 138)	127 (117, 146)	10 (7, 14)	207 (192, 224)	200 (181, 221)
25–30	128 (115, 143)	134 (115, 151)	9 (5, 15)	186 (167, 209)	177 (161, 205)
30+	149 (128, 174)	164 (126, 182)	8 (3, 17)	162 (139, 190)	161 (132, 210)
Geographical location					
London	145 (126, 168)	130 (114, 177)	13 (8, 20)	242 (210, 279)	228 (181, 273)
Manchester	132 (123, 143)	139 (126, 158)	7 (4, 10)	183 (171, 196)	183 (165, 202)
Leeds	110 (99, 121)	116 (99, 135)	9 (5, 16)	165 (149, 183)	168 (149, 193)
Spontaneous preterm delivery (<37 weeks)					
No	130 (122, 138)	134 (124, 144)	9 (7, 12)	194 (183, 206)	188 (175, 202)
Yes	132 (89, 196)	147 (75, 254)	11 (1, 35)	171 (129, 226)	155 (140, 246)
Neonatal sex					
Male	128 (118, 139)	134 (119, 147)	10 (7, 14)	199 (184, 215)	186 (174, 210)
Female	132 (121, 143)	134 (122, 151)	8 (5, 12)	187 (172, 204)	184 (163, 206)
Appointment					
15 weeks gestation	134 (125, 143)	135 (127, 152)	12 (10, 15)	176 (165, 188)	172 (159, 189)
20 weeks gestation	101 (94, 109)	107 (95, 115)	23 (19, 27)	188 (177, 200)	183 (170, 200)

3.3. Birth Outcomes

Table 3 shows the associations between mean UIC per participant and continuous birth outcomes. There was little evidence of any association between UIC and birth weight (−14 g per 50 μg/L increase in mean UIC, 95% CI: −35, +6). Results were similar when iodine was corrected for creatinine, with no evidence of any association with birth weight (−8 g per 50 μg/g increase in mean I:Cr, 95% CI: −20, +4). When birth weight was considered further as a customised birth centile, again no evidence of an association was found between mean UIC or mean I:Cr. Birth outcome associations with UIC were largely consistent when iodine levels were assessed at individual time points.

Table 3. Change in continuous birth outcomes associated with a 50 μg/L increment in mean urinary iodine concentration or 50 μg/g increment in iodine-to-creatinine ratio. 95% confidence intervals are included in brackets.

		Change in Outcome per 50 μg/L Increment in Urinary Iodine Concentration		Change in Outcome per 50 μg/g Increment in Iodine-to-Creatinine Ratio	
	Appointment	Unadjusted	Adjusted *	Unadjusted	Adjusted *
Birth weight (g)	15 weeks	−6 g (21, +10)	−7 g (−23, +8)	0 g (−9, +9)	−4 g (−14, +5)
	20 weeks	−9 g (−27, +9)	−13 g (−31, +5)	−3 g (−14, +7)	−8 g (−19, +4)
	Mean	−10 g (−30, +10)	−14 g (−35, +6)	−2 g (−14, +9)	−8 g (−20, +4)
Birth weight centile **	15 weeks	0.0% (−0.8, +0.8)	−0.2% (−0.9, +0.6)	+0.1% (−0.3, +0.6)	0.0% (−0.5, +0.4)
	20 weeks	+0.1% (−0.8, +1.0)	−0.2% (−1.1, +0.7)	0.0% (−0.5, +0.5)	−0.2% (−0.7, +0.4)
	Mean	0.0% (−0.9, +1.0)	−0.2% (−1.3, +0.8)	+0.1% (−0.5, +0.6)	−0.1% (−0.7, +0.5)

* Adjusted for maternal age, city, ethnicity and socioeconomic index. ** Additionally, gestation at delivery, maternal height and weight, parity and child's sex were taken into account in the definition of birth weight centile.

Table 4 shows associations between mean UIC per participant and binary birth outcomes. No evidence of an association was observed between SGA and mean UIC or mean I:Cr. There was no evidence that spontaneous preterm birth was associated with mean iodine concentration, with a 50 μg/L increase in mean UIC associated with 0% increase in the odds of spontaneous preterm birth (95% CI: −16%, +20%), nor was there any evidence found of an association between mean urinary I:Cr and spontaneous preterm birth (odds ratio: 0.91, 95% CI: 0.78, 1.07).

Table 4. Relative increase in odds of binary birth outcomes (odds ratios) associated with a 50 μg/L increment in mean urinary iodine concentration or 50 μg/g increment in iodine-to-creatinine ratio. 95% confidence intervals are included in brackets.

		Odds Ratio per 50 μg/L Increment in Urinary Iodine Concentration		Odds Ratio per 50 μg/g Increment in Iodine-to-Creatinine Ratio	
	Visit	Unadjusted	Adjusted *	Unadjusted	Adjusted *
Small for gestational age **	15 weeks	1.03 (0.96, 1.10)	1.05 (0.97, 1.13)	1.00 (0.95, 1.04)	1.01 (0.97, 1.06)
	20 weeks	1.05 (0.97, 1.13)	1.08 (0.99, 1.16)	1.00 (0.95, 1.05)	1.02 (0.97, 1.07)
	Mean	1.05 (0.97, 1.14)	1.09 (1.00, 1.20)	1.00 (0.94, 1.05)	1.02 (0.96, 1.09)
Spontaneous preterm birth (<37 weeks)	15 weeks	1.03 (0.90, 1.18)	1.02 (0.89, 1.17)	0.96 (0.85, 1.09)	0.96 (0.85, 1.08)
	20 weeks	0.98 (0.82, 1.17)	0.97 (0.81, 1.17)	0.89 (0.75, 1.07)	0.89 (0.76, 1.06)
	Mean	1.02 (0.85, 1.22)	1.00 (0.84, 1.20)	0.91 (0.77, 1.08)	0.91 (0.78, 1.07)

* Adjusted for maternal age, city, ethnicity and socioeconomic index. ** Additionally, gestation at delivery, maternal height and weight, parity and child's sex were taken into account in the definition of small-for-gestational-age.

Estimates for birth weight and spontaneous preterm birth outcomes were not substantially changed on adjustment for maternal BMI (data not shown).

4. Discussion

World Health Organization (WHO) guidelines are commonly applied for assessing iodine deficiency disorders [3]. These guidelines define a median population UIC > 100 µg/L as iodine sufficient for school-age children and non-pregnant adults. In addition the proportion of participants with a UIC < 50 µg/L must not exceed 20% of the population to be considered iodine sufficient. Currently, WHO guidelines define iodine status during pregnancy as either sufficient (median UIC 150–249 µg/L) or insufficient (<150 µg/L). Each of the three cities we have assessed in the SCOPE birth cohort would be classed as iodine insufficient under these pregnancy guidelines. Median UIC varied between each city with London and Manchester cohorts giving the highest median UIC, whilst Leeds gave the lowest. On average, UIC decreased between 15 and 20 weeks of pregnancy, though no such decrease was observed when assessing I:Cr.

Despite the presence of iodine insufficiency in the cohort, there was no evidence of any association between UIC or I:Cr and birth outcomes. Only a small number of studies have assessed potential links between UIC in pregnancy and neonatal outcomes [13,20–23], all of which involved populations that were either sufficient [20,23] or borderline sufficient in iodine [13,21,22]. The majority of studies have found no association between UIC and birth weight [13,20,22]. Two studies found positive associations between UIC and birth weight [21,23], but these associations were inconsistent across trimesters.

Charoenratana et al. [20] found that lower UIC was associated with increased odds of preterm birth in Thai women and studies examining links between thyroid hormone concentrations and birth outcomes suggest that pregnant women with hypothyroidism are at greater risk of preterm birth than euthyroid women [26,27]. Whilst these results appear to contradict ours, it should be noted that our study examined gestational time points in the second trimester of pregnancy, whereas Charoenratana et al. measured UIC across all three trimesters and. In addition, a number of other studies have found no evidence of an association between UIC and preterm birth [13,21,22]. Mild iodine deficiency is known to be linked to maternal hypothyroxinemia, a condition characterized by low free T4 levels despite normal free T3 concentrations [28], which in turn has been related to adverse neurodevelopmental outcomes [29]. Conversely, the association between hyperthyroidism and preterm birth is well documented, with the majority of these cases being associated with increased levels of anti-thyroid autoantibodies [27]. However this study was unable to measure thyroid hormone levels, nor examined a hyperthyroid population. We suggest that further studies are warranted in order to clarify the relationship between iodine status and thyroid hormone concentrations with birth outcomes during pregnancy.

Whilst London and Manchester participants had higher UIC values, they also had smaller proportions of participants in the lowest category of socioeconomic status, with London having the smallest. In contrast, Leeds had the highest proportion. As our study found that lower socioeconomic status was associated with lower UIC, our results may suggest that regions of the UK with a greater proportion of citizens with a lower socioeconomic index may be at greater risk of iodine insufficiency. Additionally, participants in the 25–29 age category generally had lower UIC values than participants in other age categories, whilst active smokers generally had lower mean UIC values than non-smokers. Whilst the proportion of participants in each cohort with UIC values <50 µg/L was adequate under WHO guidelines for the general population (<20% of all participants), our observed proportions still constitute a large number of pregnant women who may be at risk for inadequate iodine intakes, if these samples are representative of the UK population as a whole [3].

This study also found that UIC decreased on average between the two time points. A number of changes occur in foetal physiology during the second trimester of pregnancy, with the most notable being the activation of the foetal thyroid between weeks 16–18 of pregnancy [30]. An increase in free T4 allocation to the foetal cerebral cortex also occurs from the mid-point of the first trimester, peaking in weeks 13–20 of pregnancy [30]. These increases in foetal thyroid hormone demand, along with increased iodine trapping and hormone production by the maternal thyroid to meet these demands, could account for the decrease in UIC seen at week 20, compared with week 15. Changes in renal physiology during pregnancy may also have contributed to the observed decrease in UIC [30,31]. Renal iodine clearance via urine increases by roughly 35–50% throughout pregnancy, a change that results in a shortfall in available serum iodine and a compensatory increase of iodine uptake by the thyroid [31]. Previous studies have suggested that the maternal thyroid responds to low iodine status by upregulating thyroid stimulating hormone (TSH) to stimulate increased iodine capture [31]. The decrease in UIC we observe between weeks 15 and 20 may translate into altered TSH, free T3 or T4, but unfortunately this could not be assessed in the present study. A further possibility is that these observed differences were due to differing urine dilutions of participants at these time points. Notably the difference in UIC observed between time points was not observed when using the I:Cr, a correction aimed at reducing inter-individual variability in UIC [22]. This result suggests that iodine excretion may actually remain relatively constant between 15 and 20 weeks.

Our study was limited by a number of factors. Sample collection was restricted to the second trimester of pregnancy, and used spot rather than 24 h urine samples, which are limited in their applicability for assessing iodine status to the population level, rather than providing information on individual chronic iodine intakes. In addition, recruitment was restricted to a small number of UK cities and as a result, the study may have been limited in its assessment of iodine status in surrounding suburban and rural areas. Our study also has a number of strengths. These include the large number of participants available for each of our three geographical sites compared with many prior UK iodine studies, the collection of demographic details through face-to-face interviews with participants, the use of robust analytical procedures for assessing biomarkers of iodine status, and controlling for a number of potentially confounding variables in the statistical modelling. To the best of our knowledge, this is the first study to compare iodine status between geographically separate UK populations.

5. Conclusions

In conclusion, we have demonstrated that the iodine status of pregnant women in our study cohort is generally insufficient by WHO guidelines, with variations in iodine concentrations occurring across different cities in the UK. This finding broadly supports conclusions made by prior UK studies that pregnant women in the UK are insufficient in dietary iodine [10–16]. However, we have not found evidence that this is adversely associated with the birth outcomes assessed in this study. More detailed follow-up of maternal thyroid function, foetal and childhood growth, plus cognitive development are required to assess the long-term implications of this level of iodine insufficiency.

Author Contributions: Conceptualization, D.C.G. and L.J.H.; Methodology, D.C.G., L.J.H., C.J.P.S., E.T., C.K. and D.E.T.; Validation, C.J.P.S., E.T., D.C.G. and C.K.; Formal Analysis, D.C.G., C.K. and D.E.T.; Investigation, C.J.P.S., E.T. and S.R.; Resources, L.J.H., D.C.G., N.A.B.S., L.P. and J.E.M.; Data Curation, D.C.G., C.K. and D.E.T.; Writing—Original Draft Preparation, C.J.P.S. and C.K.; Writing—Review and Editing, C.J.P.S., C.K., E.T., J.E.T., P.M.S., M.Z., S.R., L.P., J.E.M., N.A.B.S., D.E.T., D.C.G. and L.J.H.; Visualization, D.C.G., C.K. and D.E.T.; Supervision, D.C.G. and L.J.H.; Project Administration, L.J.H. and D.C.G.; Funding Acquisition, L.J.H., D.C.G., J.E.C., P.S. and N.A.B.S.

Funding: The report is based on independent research commissioned and funded by the NIHR Policy Research Programme (Assessing iodine status and associated health effects in British women during pregnancy and lactation, PR-R10-0514-11004). The views expressed in the publication are those of the author(s) and not necessarily those of the NHS, the NIHR, the Department of Health, arm's length bodies or other government departments. The SCOPE study sponsors had no role in the study design, data analysis or writing this report.

Acknowledgments: We thank the Iodine in Pregnancy Steering Group for input and advice during study conception, funding acquisition and the wider study timeframe. We thank Amanda McKillion and Sarah Meadows at the Elsie Widdowson Laboratory, University of Cambridge, for additional advice on ICP-MS method development and quality control procedures.

Conflicts of Interest: J.E.C. is director of spin out company Dietary Assessment Ltd, which aims to develop the myfood24 online dietary assessment system for use in research, teaching and for health. The remaining authors have nothing to declare.

References

1. Zimmermann, M.B.; Jooste, P.L.; Pandav, C.S. Iodine-deficiency disorders. *Lancet* **2008**, *372*, 1251–1262. [CrossRef]
2. Delange, F. Iodine requirements during pregnancy, lactation and the neonatal period and indicators of optimal iodine nutrition. *Public Health Nutr.* **2007**, *10*, 1571–1580. [CrossRef] [PubMed]
3. WHO; UNICEF; ICCIDD. *Assessment of Iodine Deficiency Disorders and Monitoring their Elimination*; WHO: Geneva, Switzerland, 2007.
4. Underwood, E.J. Iodine. In *The Mineral Nutrition of Livestock*; Commonwealth Agriculture Bureau: Slough, UK, 1984; pp. 84–85.
5. Wenlock, R.W. Changing patterns of dietary iodine intake in Britain. In *Dietary Iodine and Other Aetiological Factors in Hyperthyroidism*; MRC Conference Report: Southampton, UK, 1987; pp. 1–6.
6. Philips, D.I.W. Iodine, milk, and the elimination of endemic goitre in Britain: The story of an accidental public health triumph. *J. Epidemiol. Community Health* **1997**, *51*, 391–393. [CrossRef]
7. Rasmussen, L.B.; Ovesen, L.; Christensen, T.; Knuthsen, P.; Larsen, E.H.; Lyhnne, N.; Okholm, B.; Saxholt, E. Iodine content in bread and salt in Denmark after iodization and the influence on iodine intake. *Int. J. Food Sci. Nutr.* **2007**, *58*, 231–239. [CrossRef]
8. Seal, J.A.; Doyle, Z.; Burgess, J.R.; Taylor, R.; Cameron, A.R. Iodine status of Tasmanians following voluntary fortification of bread with iodine. *Med. J. Aust.* **2007**, *186*, 69–71.
9. Pearce, N.E. Iodine nutrition in the UK: What went wrong? *Lancet* **2011**, *377*, 1979–1980. [CrossRef]
10. National Diet and Nutrition Survey. NDNS: Results from Years 7 and 8. Public Health England, 2018. Available online: https://www.gov.uk/government/uploads/system/uploads/attachment_data/file/690475/NDNS_survey_results_from_years_7_and_8_of_the_rolling_programme.pdf (accessed on 21 March 2018).
11. Kibirige, M.S.; Hutchison, S.; Owen, C.J.; Delves, H.T. Prevalence of maternal dietary iodine insufficiency in the north east of England: Implications for the fetus. *Arch. Dis. Child. Fetal. Neonatal Ed.* **2004**, *89*, 436–439. [CrossRef]
12. Rayman, M.; Sleeth, M.; Walter, A.; Taylor, A. Iodine deficiency in UK women of child-bearing age. *Proc. Nutr. Soc.* **2008**, *67*, E399. [CrossRef]
13. Bath, S.C.; Steer, C.D.; Golding, J.; Rayman, M.P. Effect of inadequate iodine status in UK pregnant women on cognitive outcomes in their children: Results from the Avon Longitudinal Study of Parents and Children (ALSPAC). *Lancet* **2013**, *382*, 331–337. [CrossRef]
14. Bath, S.C.; Walter, A.; Taylor, A.; Wright, J.; Rayman, M.P. Iodine deficiency in pregnant women living in the South-East of the UK: The influence of diet and nutritional supplements on iodine status. *Br. J. Nutr.* **2014**, *111*, 162–1631. [CrossRef]
15. Bath, S.C.; Furmidge-Owen, V.; Redman, C.W.G.; Rayman, M.P. Gestational changes in iodine status in a cohort study of pregnant women from the United Kingdom: Season as an effect modifier. *Am. J. Clin. Nutr.* **2015**, *101*, 1180–1187. [CrossRef] [PubMed]
16. Knight, B.A.; Shields, B.M.; He, X.; Pearce, E.N.; Braverman, L.E.; Sturley, R.; Vaidya, B. Iodine deficiency amongst pregnant women in South-West England. *Clin. Endocrinol. (Oxf.)* **2017**, *86*, 451–455. [CrossRef] [PubMed]
17. McCowan, L.M.E.; North, R.A.; Taylor, R. ACTRN12607000551493. Australian New Zealand Clinical Trials Registry 2007. Available online: www.anzctr.org.au/trialSearch.aspx (accessed on 12 February 2019).
18. Knudsen, N.; Christiansen, E.; Brandt-Christensen, M.; Nygaard, B.; Perrild, H. Age- and sex-adjusted iodine/creatinine ratio. A new standard in epidemiological surveys? Evaluation of three different estimates of iodine excretion based on casual urine samples and comparison to 24 h values. *Eur. J. Clin. Nutr.* **2000**, *54*, 361–363. [CrossRef] [PubMed]
19. Gardosi, J. Customised fetal growth standards: Rationale and clinical application. *Semin. Perinatol.* **2004**, *28*, 33–40. [CrossRef] [PubMed]
20. Charoenratana, C.; Leelapat, P.; Traisrisilp, K.; Tongsong, T. Maternal iodine insufficiency and adverse pregnancy outcomes. *Matern Child Nutr.* **2016**, *12*, 680–687. [CrossRef] [PubMed]

21. Álvarez-Pedrerol, M.; Guxens, M.; Mendez, M.; Canet, Y.; Martorell, R.; Espada, M.; Plana, E.; Rebagliato, M.; Sunyer, J. Iodine levels and thyroid hormones in healthy pregnant women and birth weight of their offspring. *Eur. J. Endocrinol.* **2009**, *160*, 423–429. [CrossRef] [PubMed]

22. Leon, G.; Murcia, M.; Rebagliato, M.; Álvarez-Pedrerol, M.; Castilla, A.M.; Basterrechea, M.; Iñiguez, C.; Fernández-Somoano, A.; Blarduni, E.; Foradada, C.M.; et al. Maternal thyroid dysfunction during gestation, preterm delivery, and birth weight. The Infancia y Medio Ambiente Cohort, Spain. *Paediatr Perinat Epidemiol.* **2015**, *29*, 113–122. [CrossRef] [PubMed]

23. Casey, B.M.; Dashe, J.S.; Wells, C.E.; McIntire, D.D.; Byrd, W.; Leveno, K.J.; Cunningham, F.G. Subclinical hypothyroidism and pregnancy outcomes. *Obstet Gynecol.* **2005**, *105*, 239–245. [CrossRef] [PubMed]

24. Hynes, K.L.; Otahal, P.; Hay, I.; Burgess, J.R. Mild iodine deficiency during pregnancy is associated with reduced educational outcomes in the offspring: 9-year follow-up of the Gestational Iodine Cohort. *J. Clin. Endocrinol. Metab.* **2013**, *98*, 1954–1962. [CrossRef]

25. Textor, J.; Hardt, J.; Knüppel, S. DAGitty: A graphical tool for analyzing causal diagrams. *Epidemiology* **2011**, *22*, 745. [CrossRef]

26. Stagnaro-Green, A.; Chen, X.; Bogden, J.D.; Davies, T.F.; Scholl, T.O. The thyroid and pregnancy: A novel risk factor for very preterm delivery. *Thyroid* **2005**, *15*, 351–357. [CrossRef]

27. Sheehan, P.M.; Nankervis, A.; Júnior, E.A.; da Silva Costa, F. Maternal thyroid disease and preterm birth: Systematic review and meta-analysis. *J. Clin. Endocrinol. Metab.* **2015**, *100*, 4325–4331. [CrossRef] [PubMed]

28. Glinoer, D. The importance of iodine nutrition during pregnancy. *Public Health Nutr.* **2007**, *10*, 1542–1546. [CrossRef] [PubMed]

29. Henrichs, J.; Bongers-Schokking, J.J.; Schenk, J.J.; Ghassabian, A.; Schmidt, H.G.; Visser, T.J.; Hooijkaas, H.; de Muinck Keizer-Schrama, S.M.; Hofman, A.; Jaddoe, V.V.; et al. Maternal thyroid function during early pregnancy and cognitive functioning in early childhood: The generation R study. *J. Clin. Endocrinol. Metab.* **2010**, *95*, 4227–4234. [CrossRef] [PubMed]

30. Pop, V.J.; Brouwers, E.P.; Vader, H.L.; Vulsma, T.; van Baar, A.L.; de Vijlder, J.J. Maternal hypothyroxinaemia during early pregnancy and subsequent child development: A 3-year follow-up study. *Clin. Endocrinol.* **2003**, *59*, 282–288. [CrossRef]

31. Patel, J.; Landers, K.; Li, H.; Mortimer, R.H.; Richard, K. Thyroid hormones and fetal neurological development. *J. Endocrinol.* **2011**, *209*, 1–8. [CrossRef] [PubMed]

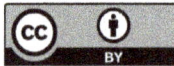

nutrients

MDPI

Review

Preconception and Prenatal Nutrition and Neurodevelopmental Disorders: A Systematic Review and Meta-Analysis

Mengying Li, Ellen Francis, Stefanie N. Hinkle, Aparna S. Ajjarapu and Cuilin Zhang *

Division of Intramural Population Health Research, *Eunice Kennedy Shriver* National Institute of Child Health and Human Development, National Institutes of Health, Bethesda, MD 20817, USA
* Correspondence: zhangcu@mail.nih.gov; Tel.: +1-(301)-435-6917

Received: 17 June 2019; Accepted: 12 July 2019; Published: 17 July 2019

Abstract: Preconception and prenatal nutrition is critical for fetal brain development. However, its associations with offspring neurodevelopmental disorders are not well understood. This study aims to systematically review the associations of preconception and prenatal nutrition with offspring risk of neurodevelopmental disorders. We searched the PubMed and Embase for articles published through March 2019. Nutritional exposures included nutrient intake or status, food intake, or dietary patterns. Neurodevelopmental outcomes included autism spectrum disorders (ASD), attention deficit disorder-hyperactivity (ADHD) and intellectual disabilities. A total of 2169 articles were screened, and 20 articles on ASD and 17 on ADHD were eventually reviewed. We found an overall inverse association between maternal folic acid or multivitamin supplementation and children's risk of ASD; a meta-analysis including six prospective cohort studies estimated an RR of ASD of 0.64 (95% CI: 0.46, 0.90). Data on associations of other dietary factors and ASD, ADHD and related outcomes were inconclusive and warrant future investigation. Future studies should integrate comprehensive and more objective methods to quantify the nutritional exposures and explore alternative study design such as Mendelian randomization to evaluate potential causal effects.

Keywords: pregnancy nutrition; neurodevelopmental disorders; autism spectrum disorder; attention deficit disorder with hyperactivity; developmental origins of health and disease; systematic review; meta-analysis

---

1. Introduction

Maternal nutrition is critical for fetal brain development. Maternal diet prior to pregnancy is important for optimizing nutritional status which plays a vital role in maintaining a healthy pregnancy and supporting the developing fetus [1]. Nutrition around the time of conception is important for gamete function and placental development [2]. Starting 2–3 weeks after fertilization, the embryo undergoes orchestrated processes of neuronal proliferation and migration, synapse formation, myelination, and apoptosis to develop the fetal brain [3]. In this period of rapid development, the brain has heightened sensitivity to the environment, where perturbation may predispose the fetus to postnatal neurodevelopmental disorders [4,5]. Overall, supply of nutrients during the preconception and prenatal periods not only provides the basic building blocks for the brain [6], but may also "program" the brain through epigenetic mechanisms to confer risk or resilience to neurological conditions later in life [7]. The modifiable nature of maternal nutrition during sensitive periods potentially offers opportunities for intervention.

Several nutrients have previously been identified to have a critical role in prenatal neurodevelopment. For example, folate is an essential co-factor in one-carbon metabolism responsible for DNA and RNA synthesis and DNA methylation—processes that are particularly important during periods of rapid growth and development. Inadequate folate intake has been linked to altered DNA methylation [8,9] and compromised fetal brain development [10,11], particularly in animal studies. Preconception and early pregnancy supplementation of folic acid—the synthetic form of folate—was found effective in preventing neural tube defects [12]. In addition to folate, polyunsaturated fatty acids (PUFAs), particularly arachidonic acid (AA) of the omega-6 (n-6) family and docosahexaenoic acid (DHA) of the omega-3 (n-3) family, are structural components of neuronal membrane phospholipids and the myelin sheath insulating the neuronal axons [13]. PUFAs accumulate rapidly in the brain starting in the third trimester and continuing into early postnatal life [14], and the membrane PUFA composition is mainly dependent on maternal dietary supply of DHA [15]. Restriction of DHA and its precursors in the perinatal period negatively impact cognitive and behavioral outcomes in animal studies [16,17].

Some minerals are also known to play important roles in prenatal neurodevelopment. For example, iron is essential for the regulation of neuronal energy metabolism during development; deficiency affects the structure and function of fetal hippocampus, compromising learning and memory [18]. Similarly, iodine is necessary to produce thyroid hormones which regulate brain growth and development; deficiency during the prenatal period results in cognitive deficit [19]. While not a nutrient, caffeine, a psychoactive substance widely consumed through coffee and tea, improves alertness by blocking adenosine receptors in the brain. Prenatal and early postnatal exposure to caffeine alters brain neurochemistry and behavior in animal studies [20]. In addition to individual nutrients and substance, foods and dietary patterns may capture the combined and interactive effects of nutrients in prenatal neurodevelopment.

In the past decade, accumulating evidence from human epidemiological studies support the link between maternal nutrition and offspring cognitive and behavioral abilities [21–25]. Yet, it is unclear whether maternal nutrition is relevant to the risk of clinically defined neurodevelopmental disorders, which are characterized by deficits that produce impairments in daily functioning. A comprehensive and critical review of the evidence may shed light on the question. Limited studies previously reviewed evidence on maternal folic acid intake and offspring autism spectrum disorder (ASD) risk [26,27]; however, an updated review with a comprehensive critique of the evidence is needed. Furthermore, much of the evidence on maternal nutrition and offspring attention-deficit/hyperactivity disorder (ADHD) risk has not been reviewed. Lastly, critical questions regarding the most sensitive time windows (i.e., before vs. during pregnancy) for nutritional exposures remain unanswered. To address these critical knowledge gaps, we conducted a systematic review of epidemiologic studies examining the association of maternal nutrition before and during pregnancy with the risk of offspring neurodevelopmental disorders; we focused on dietary factors including supplements to inform potential public health interventions specific to maternal diet. To provide quantitative syntheses of evidence, we also performed meta-analyses whenever the data were available. A summary of proposed mechanisms in which preconception and prenatal nutrition affects risks of ASD and ADHD and relevant sensitive windows are presented in a schematic figure (Figure 1).

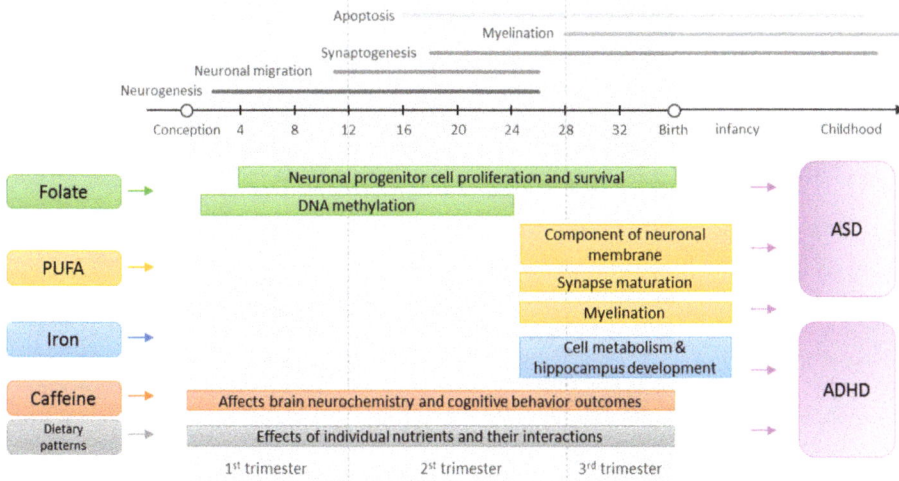

Figure 1. Proposed mechanisms in which preconception and prenatal nutrition affects the risk of autism spectrum disorder (ASD) and attention-deficit/hyperactivity disorder (ADHD). The neurodevelopmental timelines were adapted from the previous publications [3,28]. PUFA, polyunsaturated fatty acids.

2. Materials and Methods

2.1. Eligibility Criteria

The systematic review included studies investigating associations of nutrition before or during pregnancy with offspring major neurodevelopmental disorders, including ASD, ADHD, and intellectual disability (ID). Maternal nutrition was evaluated at multiple levels: nutrient intake, food intake, or dietary patterns. Clinical diagnosis, a positive screening outcome, or a continuous measure of the traits or symptoms of the disorder were considered as outcomes. The studies were conducted in human populations, of case-control, cohort, or experimental design, and published in the English language. Studies were excluded if the exposures were not reflective of maternal dietary intake, such as teratogens (e.g., alcohol), chemicals, certain circulating biomarkers that are not directly reflective of maternal intake (e.g., 25-hydroxyvitamin D and ferritin), biomarkers in umbilical cord blood, or dietary counseling without quantification of actual maternal diet. We also excluded studies where outcomes were not reflective of neurodevelopmental disorders (continuous measures of Intelligence quotient (IQ), or suboptimal IQ defined by a non-clinical cutoff), outcomes were secondary to structural birth defects (e.g., neural tube defect) or chromosomal disorders (e.g., Down Syndrome), relevant associations were not reported, or full-texts were not available. Other neurodevelopmental disorders (i.e., communication disorders, motor disorders, and specific learning disorders) were not covered in this review, as a pilot search found very few epidemiologic studies investigating these disorders in association with maternal nutrition.

2.2. Literature Search, Screening and Abstraction

We searched PubMed and Embase on 27 March 2019. Search strategies were developed a priori for each database with assistance from a librarian. The search targeted title, abstract, and subject headings. Search terms consisted of neurodevelopmental disorders (either the general term or specific terms for ASD, ID, or ADHD), nutrition (nutrients, foods, or dietary patterns), prenatal or preconception periods, and observational or experimental design, combined using the Boolean Operator "AND";

additional search terms were used to exclude animal studies. The search strategy and search history are presented in Table S1.

After the systematic search, we screened the title and abstract of the records for eligibility, and then assessed the full-text of the retained records for final inclusion decisions. We also examined the bibliographies of existing literature reviews on maternal nutrition and neurodevelopmental disorders to identify additional articles not covered in the systematic search. We abstracted relevant data in the included articles using a standardized form.

2.3. Meta-Analysis

We conducted meta-analyses of associations between specific nutritional exposures and neurodevelopmental outcomes whenever three or more relevant independent estimates were available. The analysis pooled relative risks (RRs) and odds ratios (ORs) estimated from cohort studies; OR is a reasonable approximation of RR in these studies as both ASD (prevalence 1–5%) [29] and ADHD (prevalence 5–10%) [30] are relatively rare. Estimates from case-control studies were not pooled with those from cohort studies due to differences in study design and retrospective recall of the nutritional exposures in these studies (all the case-control studies are retrospective); sensitivity analysis including estimates from the case-control studies did not change the findings substantively. Estimates of hazard ratio were not pooled with the RRs, as it is a conceptually different measure [31]. Pooled effect sizes were estimated using DerSimonian and Laird random-effects model. Studies reporting the diagnosis and the screening outcomes of neurodevelopmental disorders were meta-analyzed separately. Attempts were made to separate the effects of specific nutrients from multivitamins, and between exposures at different time periods (e.g., before pregnancy and during pregnancy), whenever possible. The meta-analysis was performed in Stata version 14 (StataCorp LLC, College Station, TX, USA) [32].

2.4. Quality Assessment

While generic tools to evaluate the quality of observational studies exists, these tools may not sufficiently address the methodological concerns important for the topic of interest and the type of studies included. As such, we critiqued the methodological quality of the included studies throughout the narrative review whenever relevant. We also discussed common issues across exposures and outcomes in a separate section following the reviews, with an emphasis for future directions.

3. Results and Commentary

A total of 2167 unique records were obtained from the systematic literature search. After screening the titles and abstracts, 102 relevant records remained. After the full-text review, 36 articles were included. Two additional articles were identified from the bibliographies of existing literature reviews, resulting in a total of 38 studies. Overall, 20 studies reported outcomes related to ASD, 17 ADHD, and 1 ID (Figure 2). The following review focuses on ASD and ADHD. Exposures in these studies included vitamins and minerals (i.e., folate, iron, calcium, and iodine), fatty acids (i.e., PUFA), foods (i.e., fish, fruits), supplements (i.e., multivitamins), and dietary patterns. Nutrients intake or status were grouped together with relevant food sources (e.g., folate with multivitamins, PUFA with seafood) to facilitate the interpretation of the findings. Nutrients or foods reported only in a single study were not reviewed below.

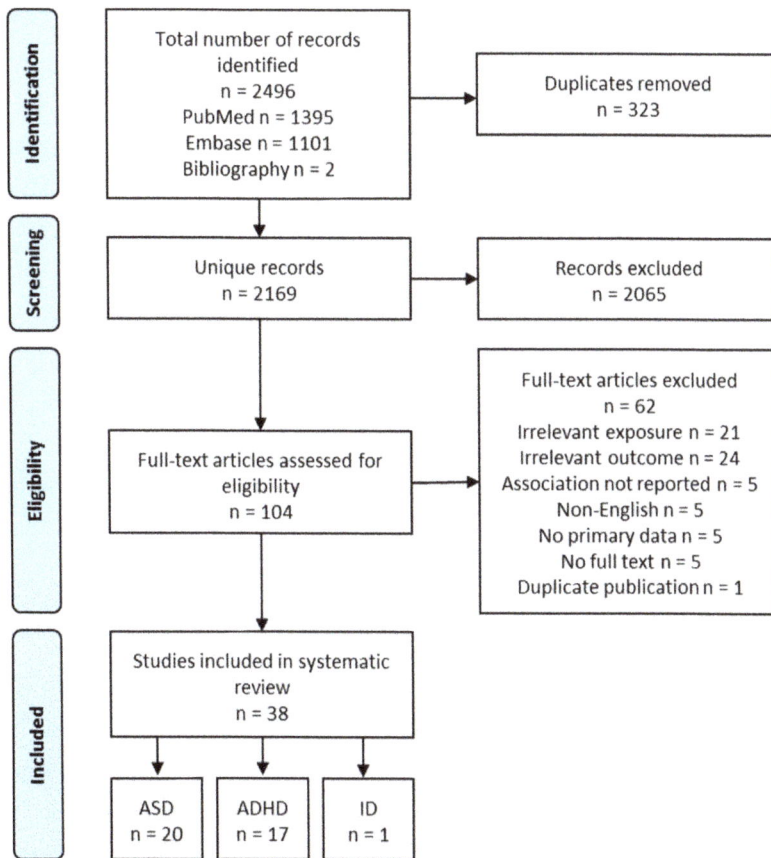

Figure 2. Flow diagram of study selection process, intellectual disability (ID).

3.1. Maternal Nutrition and ASD Risk

The characteristics and main findings of the studies on the associations between maternal nutrition and ASD are presented in Table 1. Of the 20 studies, 14 are prospective study and 6 are retrospective studies. These studies were conducted in the USA, Denmark, Norway, Sweden, The Netherlands, Spain, Israel, and China.

Table 1. Studies on maternal nutrition and offspring ASD risk or traits.

Source (Country)	Design & Sample	Maternal Exposures	Offspring Outcomes	Findings	Covariates
		Vitamins and Minerals			
		Folate and Multivitamin-ASD Diagnosis or Cutoff			
Schmidt et al. 2019 (USA) [33]	Prospective cohort; 332 children who were younger sibling of children with ASD in the MARBLES study	Vitamin and supplement use for the 6 months preconception and each month during the pregnancy assessed in interviews in the first and second halves of pregnancy and after birth	ASD assessed by ADOS at 3 years of age	Prenatal vitamin in the first month of pregnancy was associated with lower ASD risk (RR = 0.50, 95% CI: 0.30 to 0.81) *. Folic acid supplement ≥600 mcg/day in the first month of pregnancy was associated with lower ASD risk (RR = 0.38, 95% CI: 0.16, 0.90) *	Maternal education. The folic acid model further adjusted for iron intake
Levine et al. 2018 (Israel) [34]	Prospective cohort; 45,300 children	Intake of folic acid and multivitamin supplements before and during pregnancy was coded using ATC from the prescription registry	ASD diagnosis identified from health care registers from the Meuhedet health care organization; children were 10 years old	Folic acid and/or multivitamin both before (RR = 0.39, 95% CI: 0.30, 0.50) * and during (RR = 0.27, 95% CI: 0.22, 0.33) * pregnancy were associated with lower risk of ASD. Results on folic acid supplements and multivitamin as two separate exposures were consistent with the main findings	sex, birth year, socioeconomic status, a maternal and paternal psychiatric diagnosis by childbirth, maternal and paternal age at childbirth, and parity
Li et al. 2018 (China) [35]	Retrospective case-control; 374 ASD and 354 TD in the ACED	Food preference and supplement use preconception and during pregnancy assessed 3–6 years after delivery	ASD identified from special education schools; TD identified from ordinary schools; children were 3–6 years of age	Maternal folic acid supplementation before pregnancy was not associated with ASD risk (OR = 0.95, 95% CI: 0.61, 1.50); Maternal folic acid supplementation during pregnancy was associated with lower ASD risk (OR = 0.64, 95% CI: 0.41, 1.00) *	Child's and parental age, child's gender, parental education, maternal BMI before conception and delivery, premature delivery, and intake of other supplements

Table 1. *Cont.*

Source (Country)	Design & Sample	Maternal Exposures	Offspring Outcomes	Findings	Covariates
Raghavan et al. 2018 (USA) [36]	Prospective cohort; 1257 children in the Boston Birth Cohort	Multivitamin supplement intake before pregnancy and in each trimester assessed 1–3 days after delivery; plasma folate and vitamin B12 levels measured 1–3 days after delivery	ASD identified from electronic medical records in Boston Medical Center	Before pregnancy, multivitamin supplement was not associated with ASD risk (HR = 0.5, 95% CI: 0.1, 2.1). In the first trimester, ≤2 (HR = 3.4, 95% CI: 1.6, 7.2) * and >5 (HR = 2.3, 95% CI: 1.2, 3.6) * times/week of multivitamin supplement were both associated with higher risk of ASD compared to 3–5 times/day. Findings are similar at second and third trimester. Very high serum folate (HRs [95% CI] for decile 1 and 10 vs. the rest were 1.2 [0.5, 2.8] and 2.5 [1.3, 4.6]) * and vitamin B12 (HRs [95% CI] for decile 1 and 10 vs. the rest were 0.7 [0.3, 1.7] and 2.5 [1.4, 4.5]) * concentrations were both associate with higher ASD risk.	Maternal age, education, parity, BMI, smoking status, diabetes status, race, and *MTHFR* genotype, offspring gestational age, sex, and year of birth
Strom et al. 2018 (Denmark) [37]	Prospective cohort; 92,676 children in the DNBC	Folic acid supplementation and folate intake from food in the previous 4 weeks assessed by FFQ at GW 25	ASD cases identified in Danish Central Psychiatric Research Registry and the Danish National Patients Registry	Folic acid supplement at GW −4 to 8 was not associated with ASD risk (HR = 1.04, 95% CI: 0.94, 1.19). Folic acid supplement in mid pregnancy was not associated with ASD risk (HRs [95% CI] for <400 and ≥400 mcg/day vs. no intake was 1.01 [0.76, 1.34] and 0.98 [0.75, 1.29]). Folate from food was not associated with SD risk (HRs [95% CI] for quintile 2–5 were 0.82 [0.67, 1.01], 0.96 [0.78, 1.17], 0.85 [0.69, 1.04] and 0.94 [0.77, 1.16])	Maternal age, paternal age, parity, maternal smoking during pregnancy, maternal education, family socioeconomic status, whether the pregnancy was planned, maternal prepregnancy BMI and sex of the child

Table 1. *Cont.*

Source (Country)	Design & Sample	Maternal Exposures	Offspring Outcomes	Findings	Covariates
DeVilbiss et al. 2017 (Sweden) [38]	Prospective cohort; 273,107 children in the Stockholm youth cohort	Supplement use at the first antenatal visit coded in AIC from medical birth registry	ASD identified from computerized registers covering all pathways of ASD diagnosis and care in Stockholm County; children were 4–15 years old	Multivitamin supplement was associated with lower risk of ASD compared to no vitamin/mineral supplement (OR = 0.89, 95% CI: 0.82, 0.97) *. Folic acid supplement alone (OR = 1.27, 95% CI: 1.01, 1.60), iron supplement alone (0.96, 95% CI: 0.90, 1.03) and combined folic acid and iron supplement (OR = 0.92, 0.83 to 1.02) were not associated with ASD risk	Child characteristics (sex, birth year, and years resided in Stockholm County), socioeconomic indicators (education, family income, and maternal birth country), maternal characteristics (age, BMI, parity, smoking status), medication use during pregnancy (antidepressants or antiepileptics), and maternal neuropsychiatric conditions (anxiety disorders, autism, bipolar disorder, depression, epilepsy, intellectual disability, non-affective psychotic disorders, and stress disorders)
Virk et al. 2016 (Denmark) [39]	Prospective cohort; 35,059 children in the DNBC	Folic acid and multivitamin supplementations from 4 weeks preconception to GW 8 assessed by questionnaire at GW 12	ASD identified from National Hospital Register; children were 10 years of age	Folic acid supplement at GW –4 to 8 was not associated with ASD risk (RR = 1.06, 95% CI: 0.82, 1.36). Multivitamin supplement was not associated with ASD risk (RR = 1.00, 95% CI: 0.82, 1.22)	Maternal age; maternal smoking and alcohol consumption during pregnancy; household socioeconomic status-examined more but none changed estimates more than 5%
Braun et al. 2014 (USA) [40]	Prospective cohort; 209 children in the HOMA study	Current vitamin supplementation assessed by interviews at GW 14–39; whole blood folate concentrations measured at GW 11–21	Autistic-behaviors assessed by SRS at 4–5 years of age; scores >60 were defined as abnormal	Vitamin supplementation was associated with lower risk of failed SRS test (weekly/daily vs. never/rare intake: OR = 0.26, 95% CI: 0.08, 0.89) *. Whole blood folate concentrations were not associated with ASD risk (OR per SD = 1.42, 95% CI: 0.81, 2.49)	Whole blood folate concentration, maternal age, race, education, household income, marital status, employment during pregnancy, insurance status, depressive symptoms, serum cotinine concentrations, food security, and fresh fruit/vegetable intake
Nilsen et al. 2013 (Norway) [41]	Prospective cohort; 89,836 children in the MoBa	Folic acid intake before and/or during pregnancy recorded in Medical Birth Registry of Norway	ASD identified in Norwegian Patient Registry; all children were 3 years of older	Folic acid supplement was associated with lower ASD risk (OR = 0.86, 95% CI: 0.78, 0.95) *	Year of birth, maternal age, paternal age, marital status, and parity, hospital size

Table 1. Cont.

Source (Country)	Design & Sample	Maternal Exposures	Offspring Outcomes	Findings	Covariates
Suren et al. 2013 (Norway) [42]	Prospective cohort; 85,176 children in the MoBa	Folic acid and other supplementations from 4 weeks preconception to GW 8 assessed by questionnaire at GW 12	ASD identified through questionnaire screening at 3, 5 and 7 years, professional and parental referral, and the Norwegian Patient Registry when children were 3–10 years of age	Folic acid supplement was associated with lower ASD risk (OR = 0.61, 95% CI: 0.41, 0.90) *. Supplements with folic acid were associated with lower ASD risk, supplements without folic acid were not	Adjusted for year of birth, maternal education level, and parity
DeSoto et al. 2012 (USA) [43]	Retrospective case-control; 256 ASD and 752 TD in the Vaccine Safety Datalink project	Folic acid intake from prenatal vitamins	ASD identified based on medical record	Folic acid supplement/prenatal multivitamin was associated with higher ASD risk (OR = 2.34, 95% CI: 1.14, 4.82) *	Child and family characteristics (e.g., maternal age, birth weight, poverty ratio, birth order, breast feeding duration), maternal prenatal health care/seeking behavior (e.g., adequacy of prenatal care, cholesterol screen, pap smear, prenatal alcohol use, prenatal viral infections), and child medical conditions (e.g., anemia, pica)
Schmidt et al. 2012 (USA) [44]	Retrospective case-control; 429 ASD and 278 TD in CHARGE study	Folic acid intake from supplements and fortified cereals in each month from 3 months before conception to delivery assessed by interviews at 2–5 years after delivery	ASD identified from the California Regional Center System; matched TD identified from state birth files; children were 2 to 5 years old	Higher folic acid intake in the first trimester was associated with lower ASD risk (ORs [95% CI] for <500, 500–799, 800–1000 and >1000 mcg/day vs. no intake were 0.35 [0.10 1.24], 0.27 [0.06 1.36], 0.25 [0.05 1.22] and 0.18 [0.04 0.94]) *	Adjusted for maternal educational level, child's birth year, and log-transformed total iron and vitamin E from supplements and cereals; estimates were not substantially different when further adjusted for log-transformed vitamin B-12, vitamin B-6, vitamin C, vitamin D, or calcium from supplements and cereals or when adjusted for prenatal vitamin use in the first month of pregnancy
Schmidt et al. 2011 (USA) [45]	Retrospective case-control; 288 Autism and 278 TD in CHARGE study	Vitamin use in each month from 3 months before conception to delivery assessed by interviews at 2–5 years after delivery	Autism identified from the California Regional Center System; matched TD identified from state birth files; children were 2 to 5 years old	Prenatal vitamin supplement was associated with lower autism risk (OR [95% CI] for any use was 0.61 [0.39, 0.97]; ORs [95% CI] for irregular or <4 days/week, 4 days/week-daily, and > daily vs. no use were 0.96 [0.18–5.0], 0.61 [0.38–0.98] and 0.51 [0.19–1.4], p-trend = 0.002) * Multivitamin supplement was not associated with ASD risk [OR 1.2, 95% CI [0.51, 2.60]).	Maternal education and the child's year of birth

Table 1. *Cont.*

Source (Country)	Design & Sample	Maternal Exposures	Offspring Outcomes	Findings	Covariates
		Folate and multivitamin–ASD traits			
Steenweg-de Graaff et al. 2015 (The Netherlands) [46]	Prospective cohort; 3893 children in the Generation R study	Plasma folate concentrations at GW 10–17; folic acid supplementation from preconception to early pregnancy assessed by questionnaire early in pregnancy	Autistic traits using the SRS short form at 6 years of age; scores >95th percentile defined as abnormality	Folic acid supplement starting before pregnancy (beta per SD = −0.042, 95% CI: −0.068, −0.017) *, before GW 10 (beta per SD = −0.041, 95% CI: −0.066, −0.016) *, and after GW 10 (beta per SD = −0.057, 95% CI: −0.089, −0.025) * in pregnancy were all associated with fewer autistic traits. Higher serum folate concentration was not associated with fewer autistic traits (beta per SD = −0.007, 95% CI: −0.016, 0.001), nor the risk of being a probable ASD case (OR per SD = 1.03, 95% CI: 0.76, 1.39).	Gestational age at venipuncture, gender and age of the child, maternal psychopathology, education and family income
		Iron–ASD diagnosis or cutoff			
Schmidt et al. 2019 (USA) [33]	Prospective cohort; 332 children who were younger sibling of children with ASD in the MARBLES	Vitamin and supplement use for the 6 months preconception and each month during the pregnancy assessed in interviews in the first and second halves of pregnancy and after birth	ASD assessed by ADOS at 3 years of age	Iron supplement in the first month of pregnancy was not associated with ASD risk (RR = 1.47, 95% CI: 0.61, 3.55)	Maternal education and folic acid supplement
DeVilbiss et al. 2017 (Sweden) [38]	Prospective cohort; 273,107 children in the Stockholm Youth Cohort	Supplement use at the first antenatal visit coded in ATC from medical birth registry	ASD identified from computerized registers covering all pathways of ASD diagnosis and care in Stockholm County; children were 4–15 years old	Folic acid supplement alone (OR = 1.27, 95% CI: 1.01, 1.60), iron supplement alone (OR = 0.96, 95% CI: 0.90 to 1.03) and combined folic acid and iron supplement (OR = 0.92, 95% CI: 0.83, 1.02) were not associated with ASD risk	Child characteristics (sex, birth year, and years resided in Stockholm County), socioeconomic indicators (education, family income, and maternal birth country), maternal characteristics (age, body mass index, parity, smoking status), medication use during pregnancy (antidepressants or antiepileptics), and maternal neuropsychiatric conditions (anxiety disorders, autism, bipolar disorder, depression, epilepsy, intellectual disability, non-affective psychotic disorders, and stress disorders)

Table 1. Cont.

Source (Country)	Design & Sample	Maternal Exposures	Offspring Outcomes	Findings	Covariates
Schmidt et al. 2014 (USA) [47]	Retrospective case-control; 520 ASD and 346 TD in CHARGE study	Iron supplementation in each month from 3 months before conception to delivery assessed by interviews at 2–5 years after delivery	ASD identified from the California Regional Center System; matched TD identified from state birth files; children were 2 to 5 years old	Iron-specific supplement before and during pregnancy was not associated with ASD risk (ORs [95% CI] for gestational months –3 to 9 were 0.89 [0.19, 4.13], 0.89 [0.19, 4.13], and 0.78 [0.21, 2.84], 0.67 [0.29, 1.55], 0.72 [0.37, 1.39], 0.71 [0.40, 1.27], 0.64 [0.39, 1.04], 0.65 [0.41, 1.04], 0.66 [0.43, 1.02], 0.73 [0.48, 1.13], 0.77 [0.49, 1.20] and 0.64 [0.39, 1.03]). Total iron supplement before and during pregnancy were not associated with ASD risk	Maternal folic acid intake, home ownership, child's birth year. The model on total iron supplement was adjusted for folic acid
Calcium-ASD diagnosis or cutoff					
Li et al. 2018 (China) [35]	Retrospective case-control; 374 ASD and 354 TD in the ACED	food preference and supplement use preconception and during pregnancy assessed 3–6 years after delivery	ASD identified from special education schools; TD identified from ordinary schools; children were 3–6 years of age	Maternal calcium supplementation before pregnancy was associated with lower ASD risk (OR = 0.48, 95% CI: 0.28, 0.84) *; during pregnancy, it was not associated with ASD risk (OR = 1.11, 95% CI: 0.70, 1.75)	Child's and parental age, child's gender, parental education, maternal BMI before conception and delivery, premature delivery, and intake of other supplement
PUFA and seafood					
PUFA-ASD diagnosis or cutoff					
Lyall et al. 2013 (USA) [48]	Prospective cohort; 18,045 children in NHSII	Fat intake before pregnancy reported in the year assessed by FFQ after delivery	Autism, Asperger Syndrome, or PDD diagnosis reported by mothers at 4 years of age	Higher total PUFA from food (RRs [95% CI] for quartile 2-4 were 0.74 [0.55, 1.00], 0.73 [0.54, 0.99] and 0.77 [0.47, 1.26], p-trend = 0.05) * was associated with lower ASD risk. Total n-3 PUFA (0.98 [0.73, 1.32], 0.78 [0.57, 1.06] and 0.90 [0.66, 1.22], p-trend = 0.12), ALA (0.91 [0.67, 1.23], 0.86 [0.64, 1.16] and 0.80 [0.58, 1.08], p-trend = 0.14), EPA (1.11 [0.80, 1.54], 1.13 [0.79, 1.61] and 1.07 [0.76, 1.51], p-trend = 0.97), and DHA (1.05 [0.78, 1.42], 0.95 [0.69, 1.31] and 1.07 [0.79, 1.45], p-trend = 0.74) from food were not associated with ASD risk. Total n-6 PUFA (1.01 [0.75, 1.36], 1.01 [0.75, 1.36] and 0.66 [0.47, 0.92], p-trend = 0.01) * and LA (1.01 [0.76, 1.35], 0.86 [0.64, 1.16], 0.86 [0.64, 1.16] and 0.66 [0.48, 0.92], p-trend = 0.008) * from food were associated with lower ASD risk; AA (0.98 [0.73, 1.32], 0.78 [0.57, 1.06] and 0.79 [0.58, 1.09], p-trend = 0.09) were not associated with ASD risk	Adjusted for total energy intake, maternal age, child's year of birth, income level, race, body mass index, and prepregnancy smoking status. Removal of adjustment for smoking did not affect results. Additional adjustment for intake of protein, whole grains, alcohol, fruit, and vegetables, as well as for multivitamin use, physical activity, child birth order, and maternal pregnancy complications did not materially alter the results

Table 1. *Cont.*

Source (Country)	Design & Sample	Maternal Exposures	Offspring Outcomes	Findings	Covariates
PUFA-ASD traits					
Steenweg-De Graaff et al. 2016 (The Netherlands) [49]	Prospective cohort; 4624 children in the Generation R study	Plasma fatty acid profiles measured before GW 25	Autistic traits assessed by SRS at 4 years of age	N-3 PUFA percentage was not associated with autistic trait (beta per SD = −0.002, 95% CI: −0.011, 0.006). Higher n-6 PUFA percentage was associated with fewer autistic traits (beta per SD = 0.011, 95% CI: 0.002, 0.020) *. Higher n-3 to n-6 ratio was associated with fewer autistic traits (beta per SD = −0.009, 95% CI: −0.017, −0.001) *	Gestational age at venipuncture, sex, and age of the child at assessment, maternal IQ, prepregnancy body mass index, educational level, national origin, age at enrollment, psychopathology score in mid-pregnancy, smoking, alcohol consumption, and folic acid supplement use during pregnancy, family income, child day-care attendance, and paternal educational level, national origin, and psychopathology score
Seafood-ASD diagnosis or cutoff					
Gao et al. 2016 (China) [50]	Retrospective case-control; 108 ASD and 108 TD	Fish intake 6 months before pregnancy untill delivery, assessed by FFQ 4-17 years after delivery	ASD identified from the registry of special education schools; matched TD identified from ordinary schools; children were 4-17 years old	Maternal no habit of eating grass carp was associated with higher risk of ASD (OR = 3.59, 95% CI: 1.22, 10.51) *	Maternal habit of eating grass carp, parental habit of eating hairtail, income level at childbirth, current income level. Paternal education, maternal education; matched on child age and sex
Lyall et al. 2013 (USA) [48]	Prospective cohort; 18,045 children in NHSII	Fish intake before pregnancy reported in the year assessed by FFQ after delivery	Autism, Asperger Syndrome, or PDD diagnosis reported by mothers at 4 years of age	Fish intake was not associated with ASD risk (RR [95% CI] for <1, 1 and >1 time/week were 1.10 [0.73, 1.66], 0.99 [0.65, 1.50] and 1.02 [0.59, 1.75])	Adjusted for total energy intake, maternal age, child's year of birth, income level, race, body mass index, and prepregnancy smoking status. Removal of adjustment for smoking did not affect results. Additional adjustment for intake of protein, whole grains, alcohol, fruit, and vegetables, as well as for multivitamin use, physical activity, child birth order, and maternal pregnancy complications did not materially alter the results

Table 1. *Cont.*

Source (Country)	Design & Sample	Maternal Exposures	Offspring Outcomes	Findings	Covariates
			Seafood-ASD traits		
Julvez et al. 2016 (Spain) [51]	Prospective cohort; 1589 children in the INMA study	Seafood intake in the first trimester assessed by interviews with FFQ at GW 10–13	Autism spectrum traits assessed by the Childhood Asperger Syndrome Test based on parent report at 5 years of age	Higher total seafood intake was associated with fewer autistic traits (beta [95% CI] for quintile 2–5 vs. 1 were −0.42 [−0.90, 0.07], −0.45 [−0.95, 0.05], −0.61 [−1.12, −0.11], and −0.55 [−1.06, −0.04], p-trend = 0.04)*. Large fatty fish and lean fish were both associated with fewer autistic traits, whereas small fatty fish and shellfish were not associated	Sex of the child, age during testing, cohort, quality of the test, and maternal energy intake during pregnancy, child's birth weight, gestational age, duration of breastfeeding, maternal age, educational level, social class, prepregnancy body mass index, parity, and country of origin/birth
Steenweg-De Graaff et al. 2016 (The Netherlands) [49]	Prospective cohort; 4624 children in the Generation R study	Fish intake in the past 3 months assessed by FFQ in early pregnancy	Autistic traits assessed by SRS at 6 years of age	Fish intake was not associated with autistic trait (beta = −0.022, 95% CI: −0.055, 0.010)	Gestational age at venipuncture, sex, and age of the child at assessment, maternal IQ, prepregnancy body mass index, educational level, national origin, age at enrollment, psychopathology score in mid-pregnancy, smoking, alcohol consumption, and folic acid supplement use during pregnancy, family income, child day-care attendance, and paternal educational level, national origin, and psychopathology score
			Fish oil-ASD diagnosis or cutoff		
Suren et al. 2013 (Norway) [42]	Prospective cohort; 85,176 children in the MoBa	Folic acid and other supplementations from GW −4 to 8 weeks assessed by questionnaire at GW 12	ASD identified through questionnaire screening at 3, 5 and 7 years, professional and parental referral, and the Norwegian Patient Registry when children were 3–10 years of age	Fish oil supplement at GW −4 to 8 was not associated with ASD risk (OR = 1.29, 95% CI: 0.88, 1.89)	Adjusted for year of birth, maternal education level, and parity

Table 1. *Cont.*

Source (Country)	Design & Sample	Maternal Exposures	Offspring Outcomes	Findings	Covariates
			Fruit-ASD diagnosis or cutoff		
			Fruit		
Gao et al. 2016 (China) [50]	Retrospective case-control; 108 ASD and 108 TD	Fruit intake 6 months before pregnancy until delivery, assessed by FFQ 4–17 years after delivery	ASD identified from the registry of special education schools; matched TD identified from ordinary schools; children were 4–17 years old	Maternal no habit of eating fruits was associated with higher risk of ASD (OR = 2.42, 95% CI: 1.24, 4.73) *	maternal habit of eating grass carp, parental habit of eating hairtail, income level at childbirth, current income level. Paternal education, maternal education; frequency matched on child age and sex
			Dietary patterns		
			Dietary patterns-ASD diagnosis or cutoff		
House et al. 2018 (USA) [52]	Prospective cohort; 325 children in the NEST study	adherence to Mediterranean diet periconception assessed by FFQ in the first trimester of pregnancy or at enrollment	ASD index from ITSEA administered by a parent, caregiver or staff at 1–2 years of age	Adherence to Mediterranean diet was associated with lower ASD risk (ORs [95% CI] for tertile 2 and 3 vs. 1 were 0.46 [0.23, 0.90] and 0.35 [0.15, 0.80]) *. However, the trend was not significant after FDA adjustment (p = 0.09)	Breastfeeding at least 3 months, age of child at behavioral assessment, maternal fiber intake, total calories, folate, education, diabetes, obesity, smoking, and age, as well as paternal age and child parity, premature birth, weight, race, and child sex
Li et al. 2018 (China) [35]	Retrospective case-control; 374 ASD and 354 TD in the ACED	"Mostly meat", "mostly vegetable" or "both meat and vegetable" dietary patterns assessed in questionnaires 3–6 years after delivery	ASD identified from special education schools; TD identified from ordinary schools; children were 3–6 years of age	Before pregnancy, maternal mostly meat (OR = 4.01, 95% CI:1.08, 14.89) * and mostly vegetable dietary pattern (OR = 2.23, 95% CI: 1.01, 4.95) * were both associated with higher ASD risk compared to both meat and vegetable dietary pattern. During pregnancy, they were not associated with ASD risk (ORs [95% CI] were 1.36 [0.29, 6.32] and 1.20 [0.53, 2.68])	Child's and parental age, child's gender, parental education, maternal BMI before conception and delivery, premature delivery, and other maternal dietary patterns

* Statistically significant findings (p-Value < 0.05). Abbreviates of research studies: ACED—Autism Clinical and Environmental Database; CHARGE—Childhood Autism Risks from Genetics and the Environment; DNBC—Danish National Birth Cohort; HOME—Health Outcomes and Measures of the Environment; INMA—Infancia y Medio Ambiente; ITSEA—Infant Toddler Social Emotional Assessment; MARBLES—Markers of Autism Risk in Babies—Learning Early Signs; NHSII—Nurses' Health Study II; MoBa—Norwegian Mother and Child Cohort Study. Other abbreviates: ADOS—the Autism Diagnostic Observation Schedule; ASD—autism spectrum disorder; ATC—Anatomical Therapeutic Chemical; BMI—body mass index; CI—confidence interval; FFQ—food frequency questionnaire; GW—gestational week; HR—hazard ratio; MTHFR—methylenetetrahydrofolate reductase; OR—odds ratio; PDD—pervasive developmental disorders; RR—relative risk; SD—standard deviation; SRS—social response scale; TD—typically developing.

3.1.1. Maternal Folate Intake/Status, Multivitamin Intake and Offspring ASD Risk

Fourteen studies examined the association of folic acid supplementation, folate status, or multivitamin intake in relation to offspring ASD risk. Among them, ten are prospective cohort studies [33,34,36–42], and four are retrospective case-control studies [35,43,45,53]. Studies on folate and multivitamins were combined as it is difficult to separate the two exposures. Among the 12 independent studies [33–38,40–43,53] including 594,229 children (8851 ASD cases), nine found a significant inverse association between maternal folic acid or multivitamin intake during pregnancy (with or without pre-pregnancy use) and offspring ASD risk [33–35,37,38,40–42,44–46], one a null association [37], one a significant positive association [43], and one a curve-linear association with modest intake/status associated with lowest ASD risk [36].

Of the nine studies reporting an inverse association between maternal folic acid or multivitamin intake/status during pregnancy and offspring ASD risk [33–35,37,38,40–42,45], four were large prospective cohort studies which identified ASD cases through population-based patient registries [38,41,42] or medical records of large health care organizations [34]; the ASD cases were either confirmed by specialist providers [34,41] or independently validated [38,42]. These studies included very large sample sizes (45,000–270,000 participants) and contributed the greatest weight to the overall evidence. Three were smaller cohort studies which assessed ASD risk within the study using validated instruments for ASD diagnosis [33] or screening [40,46]. Two were retrospective case-control studies where ASD cases were identified from service registries [35,44].

There are two common methodological concerns about these studies. First, there is potential measurement error in folic acid or multivitamin intake, which were generally assessed by self-report [33,35,42] or administrative records [34,38,41]. Of note, two studies with additional data on whole blood/plasma folate levels found the self-reported measure, but not the biomarker measure, to be associated with lower ASD risk [40,46]. The inconsistent findings may be due to measurement error in either measure, or differences in measurement timing. Second, there is potential bias due to residual confounding. Women who took folic acid supplements generally had higher socioeconomic status, healthier lifestyle, and lower BMI [33,37,38,42]; some of these factors, such as a lower BMI, may contribute to lower risk of ASD [54]. These factors were not always adjusted for, making the results subject to residual confounding.

Despite the methodological concerns, additional data support an inverse association between maternal folate status and ASD risk. For example, the *methylenetetrahydrofolate reductase* (MTHFR) gene encodes the methylenetetrahydrofolate reductase, a rate-limiting enzyme responsible for converting folate to its bioactive form for methylation reactions [55]; the minor T allele at loci *MTHFR 677* is known to confer higher susceptibility to inadequate folate status [55]. In one study, maternal folic acid supplementation was associated with a much greater reduction of children's ASD risk when the mother and/or the child had at least one T allele, but the association was null when neither had a T allele [44]. Furthermore, two studies found maternal folic acid supplementation to be specifically associated with a lower risk of ASD, but not associated with the risk of developmental disorders other than ASD [33,44]. If maternal folic acid supplementation was spuriously associated with ASD due to residual confounding, it is likely that it would also show an association with other developmental disorders. Similarly, one study also found the risk of ASD to be specifically associated with folic acid intake, but not fish oil intake [42].

In contrast to the overall finding of an inverse association between folic acid or multivitamin intake/status and ASD risk, a study among 92,676 children in the Danish National Birth Cohort (DNBC) did not find a significant association between folic acid supplementation and ASD risk [37]. Possible explanations include better folate status without supplementation, lower frequency of T alleles at *MTHFR 677*, and insufficient doses of folic acid in the supplements [37,39]. In addition, a study including 1257 children in the Boston Birth Cohort found both low (<2 times/week) and high (>5 times/week) frequencies of multivitamin intake were associated with an elevated risk of ASD, compared to moderate intake (3–5 times/week) [36]. The increased risk associated with high frequencies of folic acid intake may be a result of the above normal level of folate in the study sample [36].

In the meta-analysis including six cohort studies reporting a linear relationship between maternal folic acid/multivitamin intake with offspring ASD diagnosis, maternal folic acid/multivitamin intake was significantly associated with a 36% reduction in offspring ASD risk (Figure 3. RR = 0.64, 95% CI: 0.46, 0.90). The heterogeneity across studies was highly significant (I^2 = 96.1%, p < 0.001). To further explore the effect of timing on the association, we conducted additional meta-analyses including four studies examining folic acid/multivitamin supplementation during pregnancy only [33,34,38,39], and three studies examining supplementation before pregnancy only [34,36,39]. The overall effect estimates had a similar direction and magnitude compared to the main analysis. However, the confidence intervals were wider, and the associations were not significant for either analyses, likely due to fewer included studies (Figure 4). Of note, most studies that investigated folic acid/multivitamin supplementation during pregnancy were specific to early pregnancy [33,38,39]. Furthermore, studies that investigated supplementation at multiple times during pregnancy consistently found that supplementation in the first or second months of pregnancy, but not later in pregnancy, was associated with lower ASD risk [33,42,44]. We also separately performed meta-analyses for multivitamin or prenatal vitamins and folic acid-specific supplements. The overall effect estimates in both groups were similar to the main analysis, but not significant (Figure S1).

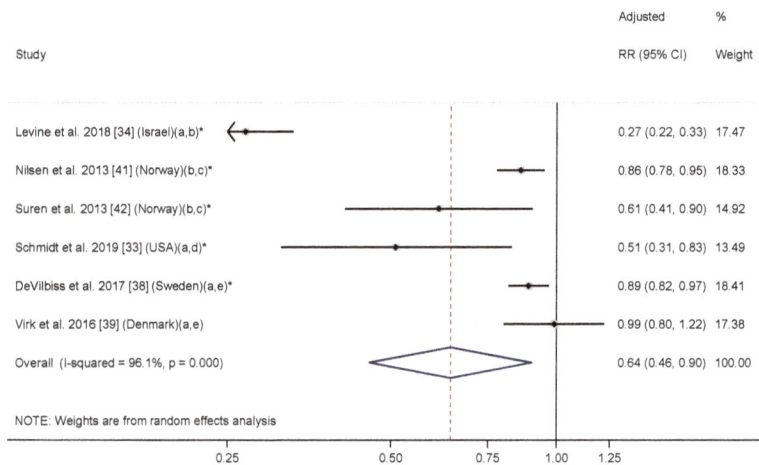

Figure 3. Adjusted relative risk (RRs) of offspring ASD risk associated with maternal intake of supplement containing folic acid, multivitamin or prenatal vitamin during pregnancy (with or without pre-pregnancy use). The overall effect size was estimated using random effects models weighted by inverse variance of each study. One data point was included for each study. Estimates covering any period during pregnancy were included. When estimates for folic acid and multivitamin were both available, the one for folic acid were selected. Notes: (a) Exposure during pregnancy; (b) Intake of supplement containing folic acid vs. no; (c) Exposure before and during pregnancy; (d) Folic acid intake ≥600 mcg/day vs. <600 mcg/day; (e) Intake of multivitamin vs. never/rarely. * p < 0.05.

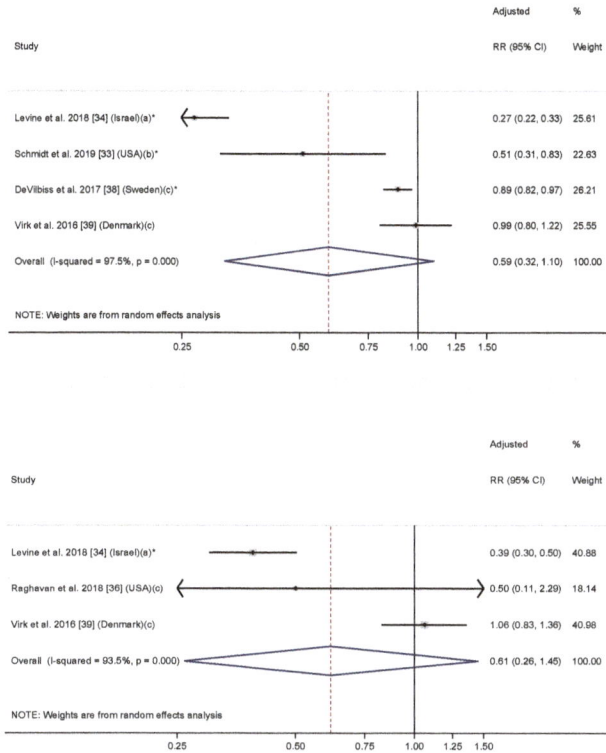

Figure 4. Adjusted relative risk (RRs) of offspring risk of ASD associated with maternal intake of supplement containing folic acid, multivitamin or prenatal vitamin during (top) and before (bottom) pregnancy. The overall effect size was estimated using random effects models weighted by inverse variance of each study. Notes: (a) Intake of supplement containing folic acid vs. no; (b) Folic acid intake ≥600 mcg/day vs. <600 mcg/day; (c) Intake of multivitamin vs. never/rarely. * *p* < 0.05.

Although folic acid is the most widely hypothesized ingredient in multivitamin related to the risk of offspring ASD risk in existing studies, it cannot be explicitly concluded that folic acid was responsible for the observed association yet. Several biological mechanisms support the potential effect of folic acid on reducing offspring ASD risk though. Changes in maternal folate intake result in altered DNA methylation of some genes such as *IGF2* in offspring [8,9], which has been implicated in neurodevelopmental disorders [56,57]. Furthermore, inadequate folate intake affects offspring brain development in animal models through decreasing progenitor cell proliferation [10] and increasing apoptosis [10,11], leading to impaired short-term memory [11]. On the other hand, more than 50 prenatal multivitamins that include folic acid also contain PUFAs [58], for example, and PUFAs are also known to affect prenatal neurodevelopment (see a summary in the introduction section).

In summary, data from the systematic review suggested an overall inverse association between prenatal folic acid/multivitamin supplementation and ASD risk. We also observed large heterogeneity in the association between folic acid/multivitamin intake and ASD risk across studies, which may reflect differences in background nutrient status [59], supplementation dose [39], and genetic polymorphism in nutrient metabolism [60]. Compared with the two earlier reviews [26,27], the present review included six additional recently published articles, thus, providing more conclusive findings. Future studies should simultaneously examine folic acid and other nutrients contained in multivitamins in order to identify the putative nutrients associated with offspring ASD risk; they should also utilize dietary folate intakes in conjunction with folate biomarkers which are more objective.

3.1.2. Maternal Iron Intake and Offspring ASD Risk

Three studies reported maternal iron supplementation and offspring ASD risk—a in large cohort of 273,107 children in Sweden [38], a small cohort of 332 children who had siblings with ASD in the US [33], and 520 ASD cases and 346 typically developing controls in the US [47]. These studies did not find an association between early pregnancy iron supplementation and ASD, regardless of the specific exposure (iron-specific supplementation, any iron supplementation, total iron supplementation). Only the retrospective study in the US examined iron supplementation later in pregnancy, and it found suggestive evidence of an association between total iron supplementation and iron-specific supplementation in the second and third trimester and a lower ASD risk, which did not reach significance. In addition, it also found a significant association between the exposures during breastfeeding and a lower ASD risk. In summary, studies on iron supplementation intakes in pregnancy and offspring ASD risk are limited. Available data do not suggest an association between prenatal iron supplementation and ASD risk.

3.1.3. Maternal PUFA Intake or Status, Seafood Intake and Offspring ASD Risk

Two studies examined maternal PUFA intake or status in relation to offspring ASD risk or traits. Among 18,045 children in the Nurses' Health Study II (NHSII) in the US, total and n-6 PUFA intake before pregnancy were all significantly and inversely associated with children's risk of ASD diagnosis as reported by mothers, whereas n-3 PUFA was not significantly associated with ASD risk [48]. In contrast, among 4624 children in the generation R study in The Netherlands, plasma n-6 PUFA levels in mid-pregnancy were significantly and positively associated with children's ASD traits measured by Social Response Scale (SRS), the ratio of n-3 to n-6 PUFA was inversely associated with the outcome. Similar to NHSII study, plasma n-3 PUFA levels were not associated with the outcome [49]. Both studies controlled for a comprehensive set of potential confounders including other aspects of diet [48] and dietary supplements [48,49]. Both n-3 and n-6 PUFA are necessary for prenatal brain development [13]; however, an elevated n-6 to n-3 PUFA ratio—characteristic of modern western diet [61]—could potentiate inflammatory processes [62]. Discrepant findings from the two studies may be due to the use of absolute versus relative concentrations of n-3 and n-6 PUFA levels, or differences in the timing of the exposure (before pregnancy vs. mid-pregnancy) and outcome measures (clinical diagnosis vs. trait).

Fish is the main dietary source of DHA—the n-3 PUFA most relevant for brain development [15]. In secondary analysis of the above-mentioned studies on PUFA intake/status, maternal fish intake was not associated with ASD diagnosis/traits [48,49]. In contrast, two other studies suggested a potential inverse association between maternal fish intake and offspring ASD risk [42,51]. Among 1589 children in the Spanish INMA study [51], maternal total seafood intake in the first trimester was associated with lower autistic traits measured by Childhood Asperger Syndrome Test; similar associations were observed for large fatty fish and lean fish. Another study of 108 ASD cases and 108 typically developing controls in China [50] found maternal "habit" (>3 times/week) of eating grass carp reported four to 17 years after delivery to be associated with a lower risk of ASD. However, the validity of the food frequency questionnaire in recalling diet after many years was not reported. Lastly, in one study among 85,176 children in the Norwegian Mother and Child Cohort Study (MoBa) [42], fish oil supplementation before and in early pregnancy was not associated with ASD risk.

In conclusion, findings of the associations between maternal PUFA or fish intake and ASD risk are inconclusive. Heterogeneity in the PUFA measurement or assessment (i.e., absolute vs. relative concentrations, intake vs. status) and ASD (i.e., clinical diagnosis vs. traits, intake vs. status) made it difficult to compare findings across studies. Furthermore, recall bias and potential residual confounding are also of concern.

3.1.4. Maternal Dietary Patterns and Offspring risk of ASD

Two studies reported associations between maternal dietary patterns and ASD risk. Among 325 children in the Newborn Epigenetics Study in the US [52], higher periconception Adherence to the Mediterranean diet was associated with a lower risk of ASD assessed by the Infant Toddler Social Emotional Assessment; the association became non-significant after adjusting for multiple comparisons. Among 374 ASD cases and 354 typically developing controls in the Autism Clinical and Environmental Database in China, maternal recall three to six years after delivery of a "mostly meat" and a "mostly vegetable" dietary pattern during pregnancy were both associated with a higher risk of ASD in children compared to a "both meat and vegetable" dietary pattern [35]. However, it appears that the dietary pattern was only assessed using a single question, and a specific definition of each dietary pattern was not given. Thus, it remains inconclusive if maternal dietary patterns are associated with offspring risk of ASD. More studies on this topic are needed in the future.

3.2. Maternal Nutrition and ADHD Risk

Characteristics and main findings of studies assessing the association between maternal nutrition and ADHD are presented in Table 2. Of the 17 studies, 16 are prospective observational study, and one was a randomized controlled trial. These studies were conducted in the UK, France, Spain, The Netherlands, Norway, Denmark, New Zealand, Japan, Brazil, and Mexico.

3.2.1. Maternal Folate Intake/Status, Multivitamin Intake and Offspring ADHD Risk

Three studies examined maternal folic acid supplementation in relation to offspring ADHD risk or symptoms [63–67], with most reporting null findings. Specifically, maternal folic acid-specific supplementation before and in early pregnancy was not associated with clinical diagnosis of hyperkinetic disorders or ADHD medication use in a large study of 35,059 children in the DNBC [65], although it was associated with a lower risk of hyperactivity-inattention problems as measured by the Strength and Difficulties Questionnaire (SDQ) among a subgroup of children followed to age seven. Similarly, maternal intake of any folic acid supplementation before or in early pregnancy was not associated with the risk of the hyperactivity-inattention problem among 6247 children in the Growing Up in New Zealand Study [63] and 420 children in the Menorca cohort in Spain [66].

One study examined maternal folate intake from food in relation to offspring ADHD risk. In the Japanese study including 1199 children in the Kyushu Okinawa Maternal and Child Health Study (KOMCHS) [64], higher intake of folate from food during pregnancy was associated with a non-significant reduction in children's risk of the hyperactivity-inattention problems (p-trend = 0.10), but folic acid supplementation was not accounted for. Lastly, one study examined folate status and total folate intake in relation to ADHD risk. In this small study including 136 children in the UK [67], early pregnancy red blood cell folate concentration and total folate intake from food and supplements, but not late pregnancy intake, were inversely associated with hyperactivity-inattention score. However, unlike the larger studies above, this study only adjusted for a limited set of covariates; residual confounding from maternal lifestyle factors was possible. In summary, no convincing evidence supports an association between folate intake from food or supplements and ADHD risk.

Among the studies previously mentioned, three also assessed the association between maternal multivitamin intake and child ADHD risk [63,65,66]. Overall, the findings are inconsistent. Maternal multivitamin intake was associated with a lower risk of hyperkinetic disorders and ADHD medication in the DNBC [65], but it was not associated with the hyperactivity-inattention problems in the Growing up in New Zealand Study [63]. Maternal intake of multivitamins containing no folic acid was associated with a non-significant reduction in risk of the hyperactivity-inattention problem in the Spanish Menorca cohort (OR = 0.24, 95% CI: 0.05, 1.31) [66]. However, the composition of such multivitamins was not clear. More studies are needed to assess this association further and to examine nutrients other than folate that may be related to ADHD risk.

Table 2. Studies on maternal nutrition and offspring ADHD risk or symptoms.

Source (Country)	Design & Sample	Maternal Exposures	Offspring Outcomes	Findings	Covariates
			Vitamins and Minerals		
			Folate and Multivitamin-ADHD Diagnosis or Cutoff		
D'Souza et al. 2019 (New Zealand) [63]	Prospective cohort; 6246 children in the Growing Up in New Zealand Study	Folic acid and multivitamin supplementation before pregnancy, during the first trimester, and after the first trimester assessed in interviews in late pregnancy	Hyperactivity-inattention symptoms assessed by SDQ using mothers' report at 2 years of age; clinical cutoff was used to define abnormality	Folic acid intake was not associated with ADHD risk (ORs [95% CI] for first trimester only and no intake vs. intake both before pregnancy and at first trimester were 0.98 [0.74, 1.31] and 0.88 [0.57, 1.34]). Multivitamin was not associated with ADHD risk (OR = 0.97, 95% CI: 0.75, 1.24)	Mother's ethnicity, mother's education, mother's age when pregnant, child's gestational age, child's birth weight, child's gender, parity, planned pregnancy, mother in paid employment, area-level deprivation, and rurality
Miyake et al. 2018 (Japan) [64]	Prospective cohort; 1199 children in the KOMCHS	Folate and other B-vitamin intake from food in the past month assessed by FFQ at GW 5 to 39	Hyperactivity-inattention symptoms assessed by SDQ using mothers' report at 5 years of age; clinical cutoff was used to define abnormality	Folate from food was not associated with hyperactivity-inattention problem (ORs [95% CI] for quartile 2–4 were 0.75 [0.46, 1.21], 0.66 [0.40, 1.07], and 0.69 [0.42, 1.12], p-trend = 0.10). Vitamin B12 (ORs [95% CI] for quartile 2–4 were 0.80 [0.49, 1.29], 0.99 [0.61, 1.61] and 0.81 [0.50, 1.32], p-trend = 0.60) and B2 (ORs for quartile 2–4 were 1.09 [0.68, 1.75], 1.03 [0.64, 1.66] and 0.61 [0.36, 1.03], p-trend = 0.08) from food were not associated hyperactivity-inattention problem. Higher vitamin B6 from food was associated with lower risk of hyperactivity-inattention problem (ORs for quartile 2–4 were 0.76 [0.48, 1.21], 0.58 [0.36, 0.94] and 0.57 [0.34, 0.94], p-trend = 0.01) *	Maternal age, gestation at baseline, region of residence at baseline, number of children at baseline, maternal and paternal education, household income, maternal depressive symptoms during pregnancy, maternal alcohol intake during pregnancy, maternal vitamin B complex supplement use during pregnancy, maternal smoking during pregnancy, child's birth weight, child's sex, breastfeeding duration, and smoking in the household during the first year of life.

Table 2. *Cont.*

Source (Country)	Design & Sample	Maternal Exposures	Offspring Outcomes	Findings	Covariates
Virk et al. 2018 (Denmark) [65]	Prospective cohort; 35,059 children in the DNBC	Folic acid and multivitamin supplementations from GW −4 to 8 assessed by questionnaire at GW 12	Hyperkinetic disorder and treatment for ADHD were identified from National Patient Register; children were 7 years of age. Hyperactivity-inattention symptoms assessed by SDQ at age 7 years based on parent reports, and a score ≥7 was defined as abnormal	Folic acid supplement was not associated with risk of hyperkinetic disorder diagnosis (HR = 0.87, 95% CI: 0.54, 1.41) or ADHD medication (HR = 0.96, 95% CI: 0.68, 1.37). Maternal multivitamin use was associated with lower risk of hyperkinetic disorder diagnosis (HR = 0.70, 95% CI: 0.52, 0.96) *, ADHD medication (HR = 0.78, 95% CI: 0.62, 0.98) *	Maternal age, household socio-economic status, maternal smoking and alcohol consumption during pregnancy, maternal prepregnancy body mass index, birth year, and offspring sex
Julvez et al. 2009 (Spain) [66]	Prospective cohort; 420 children in the Menorca cohort	Current folic acid and vitamin supplementations assessed by interviews at GW 12	ADHD assessed by ADHD Rating Scale-IV based on teacher report at 4 years of age; scores >80th percentile was defined abnormal	Folic acid with or without other vitamins compared to no folic acid or vitamins was not associated with ADHD risk (OR = 0.74, 95% CI: 0.38, 1.47). Vitamins without folic acid compared to no folic acid or vitamins was not associated with ADHD risk (OR = 0.26, 95% CI: 0.05, 1.31)	Parental social class and level of education, mother's parity at child's age four, mother's marital status, maternal tobacco smoking during pregnancy, maternal intake of supplementary calcium and iron at the same time as study determinants, gestational age at interview, child's gender, child's duration of breast feeding, child's age and school season during test assessment, evaluator and child's home location at age four
			Folate and multivitamin-ADHD symptoms		
Schlotz et al. 2010 (UK) [67]	Prospective cohort; 139 children	Total folate intake from foods and supplements during early pregnancy assessed by FFQ at GW 14, and during late pregnancy assessed at GW 28	Hyperactivity-inattention symptoms assessed by SDQ based on mothers' report at 8 years	Maternal red cell folate concentration (beta per SD = −1.23, 95% CI: −2.20, −0.26) * and total folate intake from food and supplements (beta per SD = −0.75, 95% CI: −1.39, −0.11) * in early pregnancy were both associated with fewer hyperactivity-inattention symptoms. However, total folate intake from food and supplements in late pregnancy (beta per SD = 0.07, 95% CI: −0.80, 0.93) was not associated with hyperactivity-inattention symptoms	Analysis of red cell folate: child's sex, mother's smoking and drinking alcohol during pregnancy, and mother's educational attainment. Analysis of total folate intake: daily energy, child's sex

Table 2. *Cont.*

Source (Country)	Design & Sample	Maternal Exposures	Offspring Outcomes	Findings	Covariates
		Iodine-ADHD diagnosis or cutoff and ADHD symptoms			
Abel et al. 2017 (Norway) [68]	Prospective cohort; 77,164 children in the MoBa	Iodine intake from foods and supplements assessed by FFQ at GW 22	ADHD identified from Norwegian Patient Registry; ADHD symptom assessed by the ADHD Rating Scale based on mother report at 8 years	Iodine from food was not associated with ADHD diagnosis (p-overall = 0.89). Iodine supplement was not associated with ADHD diagnosis, irrespective of food iodine intake. However, higher iodine from food was associated with fewer ADHD symptoms (beta [95% CI] for 25, 50, 75, 100, 125, 200, 225, 250, 300, 350, 400 vs. 160 mcg/day were 0.05 [−0.02, 0.12], 0.06 [0.01, 0.10], 0.06 [0.03, 0.09], 0.05 [0.02, 0.09], 0.03 [0.01, 0.05], −0.01 [−0.03, −0.00], −0.02 [−0.04, 0.01], −0.01 [−0.05, 0.02], −0.01 [−0.07, 0.05], −0.01 [−0.09, 0.08] and −0.00 [−0.12, 0.11], p-overall = 0.001) *. Higher iodine supplement was associated with higher ADHD score among women with less than 160 mcg/day of food iodine (beta [95% CI] for 1–200 and >200 mcg/day were 0.06 [0.03, 0.10] and 0.06 [−0.03, 0.16]) *, but not among women with more than 160 mcg/day of food iodine	Sibling clusters, total energy intake, maternal age, BMI, parity, education, smoking in pregnancy, and fiber intake

Table 2. *Cont.*

Source (Country)	Design & Sample	Maternal Exposures	Offspring Outcomes	Findings	Covariates
			PUFA and Seafood		
			PUFA-ADHD Diagnosis or Cutoff		
Miyake et al. 2018 (Japan) [69]	Prospective cohort; 1199 children in the KOMCHS	Fat intake from food in the past month assessed by FFQ at GW 5–39	Hyperactivity-inattention symptoms assessed by SDQ using mothers' report at 5 years of age; clinical cutoff was used to define abnormality	Total n-3 PUFA (ORs [95% CI] for quartile 2–4 were 0.82 [0.51, 1.31], 0.75 [0.46, 1.22], and 0.80 [0.49, 1.29], p-trend = 0.31), ALA (0.93 [0.59, 1.49], 0.73 [0.44, 1.20], and 0.72 [0.44, 1.18], p-trend = 0.13), EPA (0.90 [0.55, 1.46], 0.92 [0.56, 1.49], and 0.97 [0.59, 1.59], p-trend = 0.91), and DHA (0.85 [0.52, 1.39], 1.01 [0.62, 1.65], and 1.07 [0.66, 1.73], p-trend = 0.66) were not associated with hyperactivity-inattention problem. Total n-6 PUFA (1.05 [0.66, 1.68], 0.75 [0.45, 1.23], and 0.81 [0.49, 1.33], p-trend = 0.22), LA (1.03 [0.65, 1.64], 0.67 [0.40, 1.11], and 0.81 [0.49, 1.32], p-trend = 0.18), and AA (0.92 [0.56, 1.51], 1.10 [0.69, 1.77], and 0.91 [0.55, 1.50], p-trend = 0.92) were not associated with hyperactivity-inattention problem. Total n-3 to n-6 ratio (1.34 [0.83, 2.18], 1.24 [0.75, 2.04], and 0.97 [0.58, 1.63], p-trend = 0.84) was not associated with hyperactivity-inattention problem	Maternal age, gestation at baseline, region of residence at baseline, number of children at baseline, maternal and paternal education, household income, maternal depressive symptoms during pregnancy, maternal alcohol intake during pregnancy, maternal vitamin B complex supplement use during pregnancy, maternal smoking during pregnancy, child's birth weight, child's sex, breastfeeding duration, and smoking in the household during the first year of life
			PUFA-ADHD symptoms		
Ramakrishnan et al. 2016 (Mexico) [70]	Randomized controlled trial; 797 children in POSGRAD study	Interventions of 400 mg of DHA supplementation or placebo from GW 18–22 to delivery	Hyperactivity-inattention symptoms assessed by K-CPT at 5 years of age. >70th percentile was at clinical risk of suffering from a disorder such as ADHD	DHA supplement of 400 mg/day was not associated with overall K-CPT score >70 (7.2% and 8.1%, p = 0.62)	None

Table 2. *Cont.*

Source (Country)	Design & Sample	Maternal Exposures	Offspring Outcomes	Findings	Covariates
			Seafood-ADHD diagnosis or cutoff		
Gale et al. 2008 (UK) [71]	Prospective cohort; 219 children	Fish intake in the past 3 months assessed by FFQ at GW 15 and 32	Hyperactivity-inattention symptoms assessed by mothers' report at 9 years of age; clinical cutoff was used to define abnormality	More frequent oily fish intake in early pregnancy (ORs [95% CI] for <1 and ≥1 time/week vs. no intake were 0.30 [0.12, 0.76] and 0.41 [0.15, 1.12]) * and late pregnancy (ORs [95% CI] for <1 and ≥1 time/week vs. no intake were 0.40 [0.16, 0.98] and 0.72 [0.26, 1.98]) * were both associated with lower risk of hyperactivity-inattention problem. Frequency of eating all types of fish was not associated with hyperactivity-inattention problem	Maternal social class, educational qualifications, age, IQ, smoking and drinking in pregnancy, duration of breastfeeding and birthweight
Hibbeln et al. 2007 (UK) [72]	Prospective cohort; 8946 children in ALSPAC	Seafood intake during pregnancy assessed by FFQ at GW 32	Hyperactivity-inattention symptoms assessed by mothers' report at 7 years of age; highest quartile was defined as suboptimal outcome	Seafood intake was not associated with hyperactivity-inattention problem (ORs [95% CI] for none and 1–340 g/week vs. ≥340 g/week were 1.13 [0.84, 1.53] and 0.91 [0.73, 1.12], *p*-trend = 0.66)	Maternal education, housing, crowding at home, life events, partner, maternal age, maternal smoking in pregnancy, maternal alcohol use in pregnancy, parity, breastfeeding, gender, ethnic origin, birthweight, preterm delivery, 12 non-fish food groups
			Caffeine, coffee and tea		
			Caffeine-ADHD diagnosis or cutoff		
Miyake et al. 2018 (Japan) [73]	Prospective cohort; 1199 children in the KOMCHS	Caffeine intake from food in the past month assessed by FFQ at GW 5–39	Hyperactivity-inattention symptoms assessed by mothers' report at 5 years of age; clinical cutoff was used to define abnormality	Caffeine was not associated with hyperactivity-inattention problem (ORs [95% CI] for quartile 2–4 were 1.04 [0.64, 1.68], 0.99 [0.61, 1.62], and 0.84 [0.51, 1.38], *p*-trend = 0.49)	Maternal age, gestation at baseline, region of residence at baseline, number of children at baseline, maternal and paternal education, household income, maternal depressive symptoms during pregnancy, maternal alcohol intake during pregnancy, maternal vitamin B complex supplement use during pregnancy, maternal smoking during pregnancy, child's birth weight, child's sex, breastfeeding duration, and smoking in the household during the first year of life

Table 2. Cont.

Source (Country)	Design & Sample	Maternal Exposures	Offspring Outcomes	Findings	Covariates
Del-Ponte et al. 2016 (Brazil) [74]	Prospective cohort; 3485 children	Caffeine intake during each trimester assessed in interviews after delivery	ADHD assessed by DAWBA based on mother's report at 11 years of age; clinical cutoff was used to define abnormality	Caffeine in the entire pregnancy was not associated with ADHD risk (ORs [95% CI] for 100–299 and ≥300 vs. <100 mg/day were 1.12 [0.68 to 1.84] and 0.90 [0.51 to 1.59]). Similar results were found in each of the three trimesters	Maternal mood symptoms during pregnancy, National Economic Index, paternal education level and maternal conjugal situation
Loomans et al. 2012 (The Netherlands) [75]	Prospective cohort; 3439 children in the ABCD study	Caffeine intake from coffee, tea and cola in the past week assessed by questionnaire at GW 16	Hyperactivity-inattention symptoms assessed by SDQ based on mothers' report at 5–6 years of age; clinical cutoff was used to define abnormality	Caffeine was not associated with hyperactivity-inattention problem (ORs [95% CI] for 86–255, 256–425, and >425 vs. 0–85 mg/day were 0.94 [0.68, 1.31], 0.87 [0.57, 1.33], and 1.08 [0.55, 2.12])	Maternal age, ethnicity, maternal education, maternal anxiety, cohabitant status, smoking, alcohol, child's gender, family size
Coffee and tea–ADHD diagnosis or cutoff					
Hvolgaard Mikkelsen et al. 2017 (Denmark) [76]	Prospective cohort; 47,491 children in the DNBC	Current coffee and tea intake assessed by interviews at GW 15 and 30	Hyperactivity-inattention symptoms assessed by SDQ based on children, parents and teachers' report at 11 years of age; computerized algorithms were used to identified ADHD	Higher coffee intake in the first trimester was associated with higher risk of hyperactivity-inattention problem (ORs [95% CI] for 1–3, 4–7 and ≥8 cups/day vs. no intake were 0.97 [0.88, 1.08], 1.09 [0.93, 1.27] and 1.47 [1.18, 1.83], p-trend = 0.03) *. In the third trimester, it was not associated (ORs [95% CI] for 1–3, 4–7 and ≥8 cups/day vs. no intake were 0.94 [0.85, 1.04], 0.96 [0.83, 1.13] and 1.21 [0.95, 1.55], p-trend = 0.88). Tea intake in the first trimester was not associated with hyperactivity-inattention problem (ORs [95% CI] for 1–3, 4–7 and ≥8 cups/day vs. no intake were 0.93 [0.85, 1.03], 0.97 [0.85, 1.12] and 1.21 [0.98, 1.49], p-trend = 0.57). In the third trimester, higher tea intake was associated with lower risk of hyperactivity-inattention problem (ORs [95% CI] for 1–3, 4–7 and ≥8 cups/day vs. no intake were 0.90 [0.81, 1.01], 0.79 [0.66, 0.94] and 0.84 [0.63, 1.11], p-trend = 0.01) *	Sex, birth year, smoking, socioeconomic status, maternal age, parity, maternal BMI, and mutually coffee or tea

Table 2. Cont.

Source (Country)	Design & Sample	Maternal Exposures	Offspring Outcomes	Findings	Covariates
Linnet et al. 2009 (Denmark) [77]	Prospective cohort; 24,068 children in the Aarhus Birth Cohort	Coffee intake during pregnancy assessed by a questionnaire prior to GW 16	Hyperkinetic disorder and ADHD recorded in Danish Psychiatric Central Register; children were 3–12 years of age	Coffee was not associated with ADHD risk (RRs [95% CI] for 1–3, 4–9 and ≥10 cups of coffee were 0.9 [0.5, 1.6], 1.3 [0.7, 2.3] and 2.3 [0.9, 5.9])	Smoking, alcohol, maternal age, gender of the child, parental years of schooling after basic school, employment status, cohabitant status and parental and sibling's psychiatric hospitalizations or contacts as outpatients
			Dietary patterns		
			Dietary patterns-ADHD diagnosis or cutoff		
Galera et al. 2018 (France) [78]	Prospective cohort; 1242 children in the EDEN mother-child cohort	Dietary patterns in the third trimester assessed by FFQ after delivery and derived using principle component analysis	Hyperactivity-inattention symptoms assessed by SDQ based on mother's report at 3, 5, and 8 years of age; clinical cutoff was used to define abnormality; longitudinal trajectories were derived based on mixture models	Lower scores of healthy dietary pattern (OR [95% CI] for quartile 1 vs. the rest was 1.61 [1.09, 2.37]) * and higher scores of Western dietary pattern (OR for quartile 4 vs. the rest was 1.67 [1.13, 2.47]) * were both associated with higher risk of high hyperactivity-inattention trajectory	Centre, child gender, maternal age, prepregnancy BMI, maternal smoking, maternal alcohol-drinking, gestational diabetes, multiparity, gestational length, birth weight, breastfeeding, prenatal maternal depressive symptoms, prenatal maternal anxiety, postnatal maternal depressive symptoms, parental separation, family income, maternal education, child dietary patterns at age 2, and mutual adjusted for healthy and Western dietary patterns
			Dietary patterns-ADHD symptoms		
Rijlaarsdam et al. 2017 (UK) [56]	Prospective cohort; 83 youths with early-onset persistent conduct problems and 81 youths with low conduct problem in ALSPAC	Dietary patterns during pregnancy assessed by FFQ at GW 32 and derived using confirmatory factor analysis	ADHD symptoms assessed by DAWBA based on parent reports at 7 years of age	Unhealthy dietary pattern was indirectly associated with more ADHD symptoms through IGF2 DNA methylation at birth among youths with early-onset persistent conduct problems (beta per SD = 0.069, 95% CI: 0.003, 0.206) *, but not among youths with low conduct problem (beta per SD = −0.015, 95% CI: −0.086, 0.019)	Cumulative risk index during pregnancy and in childhood, including life events, contextual risks, parental risks, interpersonal risks, direct victimization

* Statistically significant findings (p-value < 0.05). Abbreviates of research studies: ABCD—Amsterdam Born Children and their Development; ALSPAC—Avon Longitudinal Study of Parents and Children; DNBC—Danish National Birth Cohort; EDEN—Étude des Déterminants pré et postnatals du développement et de la santé de l'ENfant; KOMCHS—Kyushu Okinawa Maternal and Child Health Study; MoBa—Norwegian Mother and Child Cohort Study; POSGRAD—Prenatal Omega-3 Fatty Acid Supplementation and Child Growth and Development. Other abbreviations: ADHD—attention–deficit/hyperactivity disorder; BMI—body mass index; CI—confidence interval; DAWBA—Development and Well–Being Assessment; DHA—docosahexaenoic acid; FFQ—food frequency questionnaire; GW—gestational week; HR—hazard risk; K-CPT—Conner's Kiddie Continuous Performance Test; OR—odds ratio; RR—relative risk; SD—standard deviation; SDQ—Strengths and Difficulties Questionnaire.

3.2.2. Maternal PUFA and Seafood Intake and Offspring ADHD Risk

Two studies examined maternal PUFA intake in relation to children's ADHD risk and findings did not support a significant association. More specifically, among the 1,199 children in the KOMCHS [69], neither maternal intake of total or specific n-3 and n-6 PUFA from food were associated with children's risk of the hyperactivity-inattention problems. In a randomized controlled trial among 797 children in Mexico [70], maternal DHA supplementation of 400 mg/day from mid-pregnancy to delivery was not associated with clinical risk of ADHD measured by the Conner's Kiddie Continuous Performance Test (K-CPT) core indicating (>70th percentile). Of note, the ability of the K-CPT to accurately identify children at risk for ADHD has been questioned [79].

Two studies examined maternal seafood intake in relation to children's risk of hyperactivity-inattention problems. Among 219 children in the UK [71], more frequent intake of oily fish during pregnancy was associated with lower risk of the hyperactivity-inattention problem, whereas intake of all types of fish was not. In contrast, among 8946 children in Avon Longitudinal Study of Parents and Children (ALSPAC) study in the UK [72], seafood intake was not associated with ADHD risk. However, results for oily fish intake were not reported. In summary, studies on the association between maternal PUFA or seafood intake and children's ADHD risk are inconsistent and provide little evidence for an association; differences in exposure assessments inhibits a clear interpretation of the findings. Future studies need to have a comprehensive assessment of maternal fish, seafood, and PUFA intake/status in relation to offspring ADHD risk.

3.2.3. Maternal Caffeine, Coffee, and Tea Intake and Offspring ADHD Risk

Three cohort studies, including 3485 children in Brazil [74], 3439 children in The Netherlands [75], and 1199 children in Japan [73], consistently found no association between maternal caffeine intake during pregnancy and hyperactivity-inattention problem in children. Across the three studies, the cutoff for the highest intake category was 300–384 mg/day, which is equivalent to three to four and a half cups of coffee/day (a cup coffee is defined as 8 oz). In the meta-analysis pooling all three studies, the overall effect estimate comparing the highest to the lowest category of caffeine intake was null (OR = 0.91, 95% CI: 0.66, 1.27; I^2 = 0.0%, p for I^2 = 0.84).

On the other hand, two large prospective cohort studies [76,77] found suggestive evidence that extremely high levels of coffee intake in early pregnancy were associated with an increased risk of ADHD. Among 47,491 children in the DNBC [76], ≥8 cups/day of coffee in early pregnancy (OR = 1.47, 95% CI: 1.18, 1.83), but not late pregnancy (OR = 1.21, 95% CI: 0.95, 1.55), was associated with a significantly increased risk of hyperactivity inattention problems. Among 24,068 children in the Aarhus Birth Cohort in Denmark [77], ≥10 cups/day of coffee in early pregnancy was also associated with a substantial but non-significant increase in the risk for hyperkinetic disorders and ADHD diagnosis (OR = 2.3, 95% CI: 0.9, 5.9). Less coffee intake (<8 cups/day in the DNBC and <10 cups/day in the Aarhus Birth Cohort) was not associated with ADHD risk in either study. Of note, only about 3% of women had extremely high intake levels in both studies [76,77], and they appeared to be highly selective group, characterized by lower social class, much higher rate of cigarette smoking, and higher rate of hyperactivity themselves [76]. While the two studies adjusted for selected socioeconomic, lifestyle and psychological characteristic of the women [76,77], residual confounding from unmeasured variables cannot be ruled out. On the other hand, it is possible that only extreme levels of caffeine consumption affect fetal neurodevelopment [20]. The extreme levels of coffee intake were not captured in the studies examining caffeine intake. Taken together, these studies suggest a null association between moderate coffee intake and offspring ADHD risk. Further evaluation of extremely high levels of maternal coffee intake and ADHD risk is needed.

3.2.4. Maternal Dietary Patterns and Offspring ADHD Risk

Two cohort studies [56,78] suggested an association between poor dietary quality during pregnancy and increased risk of ADHD or ADHD symptoms in children. Among 1242 children in the EDEN mother-child cohort in France [56], the lowest quartile of "healthy dietary patterns" (i.e., high intake in fruit, vegetables, fish, and whole grain cereals) and the highest quartile of "western dietary pattern" (i.e., high intake in processed and snacking foods) were both associated with increased risk of hyperactivity-inattention trajectory between age three and eight years. In the ALSPAC [56], an "unhealthy dietary pattern" (i.e., high fat and sugar) score was positively associated with ADHD symptoms among 83 youths with early-onset persistent conduct problems, but not associated with ADHD symptoms among the 81 youths with low conduct problems; the association among youths with early-onset persistent conduct problems was mediated by higher levels of *IGF2* DNA methylation at birth. Of note, *IGF2* gene has important roles in regulating placental and fetal growth; genetic and epigenetic changes in the *IGF2* gene and changes in IGF2 hormonal levels has been linked to altered development in the cerebellum and hippocampus, both of which are relevant to ADHD [56]. The significant association between maternal dietary quality and children's ADHD risk should be further evaluated.

4. Methodological Issues and Future Directions

Two major methodological concerns among studies of maternal nutrition and offspring neurodevelopmental disorders merit further discussion. The first is potential measurement error in the exposure assessment. Studies that comprehensively characterized nutrients from both food and supplements are limited. This is relevant as the effect of the supplementation may depend on baseline nutrient sufficiency status before supplementation, as well as the supplementation dose. Similarly, the effects of a nutrient from food may be overwhelmed by supplementation. Moreover, most studies examined maternal nutritional exposures using questionnaires, including food frequency questionnaires, which are prone to recall bias. To address these concerns, future studies need to prospectively quantify nutrient intakes from both foods and dietary supplements, which may help to establish potential dose-response relations and sufficient dose to prevent offspring neurodevelopmental disorders. Future studies should also consider quantifying nutrient status using biomarkers, which complement dietary information from questionnaires and provide a source of validation.

A second methodological concern with regard to existing studies is potential bias due to residual confounding. Many maternal demographic, lifestyle, and psychosocial factors that contribute to poorer maternal nutritional status may also contribute to the risk of neurodevelopmental disorders in children [4,80]. Smaller studies frequently lack the power to adjust for a comprehensive list of potential confounders. Even in large studies where such adjustments were made, residual confounding from unknown risk factors are still possible, and a causal link cannot be established. Alternative study designs may help to ameliorate this concern and strengthen the evidence. For example, variants in *MTHFR* gene encoding methylenetetrahydrofolate reductase affect vulnerability to low folate intake [55]; variants in *FADS* gene encoding fatty acid desaturase are determinants of long change PUFA status [81]. These genetic variants have been found to modify the association between maternal intake of respective nutrients and offspring neurodevelopmental outcomes [15,44]. Futures studies may use these variants to implement Mendelian randomization in observational studies to further evaluate a potential causal effect of nutrients on offspring outcomes.

Besides these major methodological concerns, several others may merit consideration in designing future studies. First, the effect of a nutrient on neurodevelopmental disorders may vary by fetal developmental period, reflecting the underlying developmental processes affected. Many existing studies did not investigate the timing of the exposure explicitly. Future studies should have explicit hypotheses about the window of sensitivity, and use it inform study design and implementation and the interpretation of results. Longitudinal assessment of the exposures throughout relevant periods would be particularly suitable to identify the most relevant window of sensitivity to the nutrient. Knowledge of the sensitive window of exposure is essential for establishing evidence and designing interventions. Second, epigenetic modification is postulated to be major mechanism by which early life nutrition contributes to risk of health and disease later in life [82], and maternal intake of nutrients such as folate and DHA has been linked to differential DNA methylation patterns [8]. Two studies have reported promising findings where maternal diet has been simultaneously linked to altered methylation of specific genes and neurodevelopmental disorders [52,56]. More studies incorporating epigenetic data are needed to better understand the mechanism.

5. Conclusions

Maternal nutrition is a potentially modifiable factor important for fetal neurodevelopment. In the past decade, a body of research emerged examining the impact of maternal nutritional status and offspring developmental disorders. To our knowledge, this is the first comprehensive and systematic review of maternal nutrition during the preconception and perinatal period and offspring risk of neurodevelopmental disorders. This review included studies on maternal intake (or status) at multiple levels: nutrients (i.e., vitamins, minerals, PUFA, multivitamins), food (i.e., fish), and dietary patterns in relation to children's risk of ASD and ADHD. Findings from the review supported an inverse association between maternal folic acid or multivitamin intake and children's risk of ASD, although large heterogeneity existed across studies. Data on associations of other dietary factors and ASD, ADHD and related outcomes are inconclusive and warrant future investigation. Future studies that comprehensively quantify maternal nutrient intake from both food and supplements and integrate more objective measures of biomarkers reflecting intake and metabolism are warranted. In addition, incorporating genetic variants related to nutrient metabolism shall enable Mendelian randomization analyses to inform causal inferences and a better understanding of gene-diet interactions in relation to neurodevelopmental disorders. Understanding the sensitive window of exposure and gene-diet interactions may help inform precise intervention and prevention.

Supplementary Materials: The following are available online at http://www.mdpi.com/2072-6643/11/7/1628/s1, Table S1: Search strategy and history in PubMed and Embase; Figure S1: Adjusted relative risk (RR) of offspring risk of autism spectrum disorder associated with maternal intake of multivitamin or prenatal vitamin and supplement with folic acid only formulation during pregnancy.

Author Contributions: C.Z., M.L. and S.N.H. conceptualized the study; M.L., S.N.H. and E.F. designed the study; M.L., E.F. and A.S.A. contributed to the acquisition, analysis, and interpretation of the data; M.L. wrote the first draft of the manuscript; all authors substantially revised the manuscript for important intellectual content and approved the submitted version of the manuscript.

Funding: The research and the publication cost were supported by the Intramural Research Program of the Eunice Kennedy Shriver National Institute of Child Health and Human Development, National Institutes of Health.

Conflicts of Interest: The authors declare no conflict of interest. The sponsors had no role in the design, execution, interpretation, or writing of the study.

References

1. King, J.C. A summary of pathways or mechanisms linking preconception maternal nutrition with birth outcomes. *J. Nutr.* **2016**, *146*, 1437s–1444s. [CrossRef] [PubMed]
2. Stephenson, J.; Heslehurst, N.; Hall, J.; Schoenaker, D.; Hutchinson, J.; Cade, J.E.; Poston, L.; Barrett, G.; Crozier, S.R.; Barker, M.; et al. Before the beginning: Nutrition and lifestyle in the preconception period and its importance for future health. *Lancet* **2018**, *391*, 1830–1841. [CrossRef]
3. Tau, G.Z.; Peterson, B.S. Normal development of brain circuits. *Neuropsychopharmacology* **2010**, *35*, 147–168. [CrossRef] [PubMed]
4. Lyall, K.; Schmidt, R.J.; Hertz-Picciotto, I. Maternal lifestyle and environmental risk factors for autism spectrum disorders. *Int. J. Epidemiol.* **2014**, *43*, 443–464. [CrossRef] [PubMed]

5. Linnet, K.M.; Dalsgaard, S.; Obel, C.; Wisborg, K.; Henriksen, T.B.; Rodriguez, A.; Kotimaa, A.; Moilanen, I.; Thomsen, P.H.; Olsen, J.; et al. Maternal lifestyle factors in pregnancy risk of attention deficit hyperactivity disorder and associated behaviors: review of the current evidence. *Am. J. Psychiatry* **2003**, *160*, 1028–1040. [CrossRef] [PubMed]

6. Prado, E.L.; Dewey, K.G. Nutrition and brain development in early life. *Nutr. Rev.* **2014**, *72*, 267–284. [CrossRef] [PubMed]

7. Bale, T.L.; Baram, T.Z.; Brown, A.S.; Goldstein, J.M.; Insel, T.R.; McCarthy, M.M.; Nemeroff, C.B.; Reyes, T.M.; Simerly, R.B.; Susser, E.S.; et al. Early life programming and neurodevelopmental disorders. *Biol. Psychiatry* **2010**, *68*, 314–319. [CrossRef] [PubMed]

8. Lee, H.S. Impact of maternal diet on the epigenome during in utero life and the developmental programming of diseases in childhood and adulthood. *Nutrients* **2015**, *7*, 9492–9507. [CrossRef] [PubMed]

9. Steegers-Theunissen, R.P.; Obermann-Borst, S.A.; Kremer, D.; Lindemans, J.; Siebel, C.; Steegers, E.A.; Slagboom, P.E.; Heijmans, B.T. Periconceptional maternal folic acid use of 400 microg per day is related to increased methylation of the *IGF2* gene in the very young child. *PLoS ONE* **2009**, *4*, e7845. [CrossRef]

10. Craciunescu, C.N.; Brown, E.C.; Mar, M.H.; Albright, C.D.; Nadeau, M.R.; Zeisel, S.H. Folic acid deficiency during late gestation decreases progenitor cell proliferation and increases apoptosis in fetal mouse brain. *J. Nutr.* **2004**, *134*, 162–166. [CrossRef]

11. Jadavji, N.M.; Deng, L.; Malysheva, O.; Caudill, M.A.; Rozen, R. MTHFR deficiency or reduced intake of folate or choline in pregnant mice results in impaired short-term memory and increased apoptosis in the hippocampus of wild-type offspring. *Neuroscience* **2015**, *300*, 1–9. [CrossRef] [PubMed]

12. Pitkin, R.M. Folate and neural tube defects. *Am. J. Clin. Nutr.* **2007**, *85*, 285s–288s. [CrossRef] [PubMed]

13. Yehuda, S.; Rabinovitz, S.; Mostofsky, D.I. Essential fatty acids are mediators of brain biochemistry and cognitive functions. *J. Neurosci. Res.* **1999**, *56*, 565–570. [CrossRef]

14. Martinez, M. Tissue levels of polyunsaturated fatty acids during early human development. *J. Pediatrics* **1992**, *120*, S129–S138. [CrossRef]

15. Lauritzen, L.; Brambilla, P.; Mazzocchi, A.; Harsløf, L.; Ciappolino, V.; Agostoni, C. DHA effects in brain development and function. *Nutrients* **2016**, *8*, 6. [CrossRef]

16. McCann, J.C.; Ames, B.N. Is docosahexaenoic acid, an n-3 long-chain polyunsaturated fatty acid, required for development of normal brain function? An overview of evidence from cognitive and behavioral tests in humans and animals. *Am. J. Clin. Nutr.* **2005**, *82*, 281–295. [CrossRef] [PubMed]

17. Carlson, S.E. Docosahexaenoic acid and arachidonic acid in infant development. *Semin. Neonatol.* **2001**, *6*, 437–449. [CrossRef]

18. Fretham, S.J.; Carlson, E.S.; Georgieff, M.K. The role of iron in learning and memory. *Adv. Nutr.* **2011**, *2*, 112–121. [CrossRef]

19. Skeaff, S.A. Iodine deficiency in pregnancy: The effect on neurodevelopment in the child. *Nutrients* **2011**, *3*, 265–273. [CrossRef]

20. Porciúncula, L.O.; Sallaberry, C.; Mioranzza, S.; Botton, P.H.S.; Rosemberg, D.B. The Janus face of caffeine. *Neurochem. Int.* **2013**, *63*, 594–609. [CrossRef]

21. Bougma, K.; Aboud, F.E.; Harding, K.B.; Marquis, G.S. Iodine and mental development of children 5 years old and under: A systematic review and meta-analysis. *Nutrients* **2013**, *5*, 1384–1416. [CrossRef] [PubMed]

22. Borge, T.C.; Aase, H.; Brantsaeter, A.L.; Biele, G. The importance of maternal diet quality during pregnancy on cognitive and behavioural outcomes in children: A systematic review and meta-analysis. *BMJ Open* **2017**, *7*, e016777. [CrossRef] [PubMed]

23. Freedman, R.; Hunter, S.K.; Hoffman, M.C. Prenatal primary prevention of mental illness by micronutrient supplements in pregnancy. *Am. J. Psychiatry* **2018**, *175*, 607–619. [CrossRef] [PubMed]

24. Starling, P.; Charlton, K.; McMahon, A.T.; Lucas, C. Fish intake during pregnancy and foetal neurodevelopment—A systematic review of the evidence. *Nutrients* **2015**, *7*, 2001–2014. [CrossRef] [PubMed]

25. Gould, J.F.; Smithers, L.G.; Makrides, M. The effect of maternal omega-3 (n-3) LCPUFA supplementation during pregnancy on early childhood cognitive and visual development: A systematic review and meta-analysis of randomized controlled trials. *Am. J. Clin. Nutr.* **2013**, *97*, 531–544. [CrossRef] [PubMed]

26. Wang, M.; Li, K.; Zhao, D.; Li, L. The association between maternal use of folic acid supplements during pregnancy and risk of autism spectrum disorders in children: A meta-analysis. *Mol. Autism* **2017**, *8*, 51. [CrossRef] [PubMed]

27. DeVilbiss, E.A.; Gardner, R.M.; Newschaffer, C.J.; Lee, B.K. Maternal folate status as a risk factor for autism spectrum disorders: A review of existing evidence. *Br. J. Nutr.* **2015**, *114*, 663–672. [CrossRef]

28. Bayer, S.A.; Altman, J.; Russo, R.J.; Zhang, X. Timetables of neurogenesis in the human brain based on experimentally determined patterns in the rat. *Neurotoxicology* **1993**, *14*, 83–144.

29. Centers for Disease Control and Prevention. Data & Statistics on Autism Spectrum Disorder. Available online: https://www.cdc.gov/ncbddd/autism/data.html (accessed on 5 June 2019).

30. Centers for Disease Control and Prevention. Data & Statistics about ADHD. Available online: https://www.cdc.gov/ncbddd/adhd/data.html (accessed on 5 June 2019).

31. Tierney, J.F.; Stewart, L.A.; Ghersi, D.; Burdett, S.; Sydes, M.R. Practical methods for incorporating summary time-to-event data into meta-analysis. *Trials* **2007**, *8*, 16. [CrossRef]

32. StataCorp LP. *Stata Statistical Software: Release 14. (computer program)*; StataCorp LP: College Station, TX, USA, 2015.

33. Schmidt, R.J.; Iosif, A.M.; Angel, E.G.; Ozonoff, S. Association of maternal prenatal vitamin use with risk for autism spectrum disorder recurrence in young siblings. *JAMA Psychiatry* **2019**, *76*, 391–398. [CrossRef]

34. Levine, S.Z.; Kodesh, A.; Viktorin, A.; Smith, L.; Uher, R.; Reichenberg, A.; Sandin, S. Association of maternal use of folic acid and multivitamin supplements in the periods before and during pregnancy with the risk of autism spectrum disorder in offspring. *JAMA Psychiatry* **2018**, *75*, 176–184. [CrossRef] [PubMed]

35. Li, Y.M.; Shen, Y.D.; Li, Y.J.; Xun, G.L.; Liu, H.; Wu, R.R.; Ou, J.J. Maternal dietary patterns, supplements intake and autism spectrum disorders: A preliminary case-control study. *Medicine* **2018**, *97*, e13902. [CrossRef] [PubMed]

36. Raghavan, R.; Riley, A.W.; Volk, H.; Caruso, D.; Hironaka, L.; Sices, L.; Hong, X.; Wang, G.; Ji, Y.; Brucato, M.; et al. Maternal multivitamin intake, plasma folate and vitamin B12 levels and autism spectrum disorder risk in offspring. *Paediatr. Perinat. Epidemiol.* **2018**, *32*, 100–111. [CrossRef]

37. Strom, M.G.C.; Lyall, K.; Ascherio, A.; Olsen, S.F. Research letter: Folic acid supplementation and intake of folate in pregnancy in relation to offspring risk of autism spectrum disorder. *Psychol. Med.* **2018**, *48*, 1048–1054. [CrossRef] [PubMed]

38. DeVilbiss, E.A.; Magnusson, C.; Gardner, R.M.; Rai, D.; Newschaffer, C.J.; Lyall, K.; Dalman, C.; Lee, B.K. Antenatal nutritional supplementation and autism spectrum disorders in the Stockholm youth cohort: Population based cohort study. *BMJ* **2017**, *359*, j4273. [CrossRef] [PubMed]

39. Virk, J.; Liew, Z.; Olsen, J.; Nohr, E.A.; Catov, J.M.; Ritz, B. Preconceptional and prenatal supplementary folic acid and multivitamin intake and autism spectrum disorders. *Autism* **2016**, *20*, 710–718. [CrossRef] [PubMed]

40. Braun, J.M.; Froehlich, T.; Kalkbrenner, A.; Pfeiffer, C.M.; Fazili, Z.; Yolton, K.; Lanphear, B.P. Brief report: Are autistic-behaviors in children related to prenatal vitamin use and maternal whole blood folate concentrations? *J. Autism Dev. Disord.* **2014**, *44*, 2602–2607. [CrossRef]

41. Nilsen, R.M.; Surén, P.; Gunnes, N.; Alsaker, E.R.; Bresnahan, M.; Hirtz, D.; Roth, C. Analysis of self-selection bias in a population-based cohort study of autism spectrum disorders. *Paediatr. Perinat. Epidemiol.* **2013**, *27*, 553–563. [CrossRef]

42. Suren, P.; Roth, C.; Bresnahan, M.; Haugen, M.; Hornig, M.; Hirtz, D.; Lie, K.K.; Lipkin, W.I.; Magnus, P.; Reichborn-Kjennerud, T.; et al. Association between maternal use of folic acid supplements and risk of autism spectrum disorders in children. *Jama* **2013**, *309*, 570–577. [CrossRef]

43. DeSoto, M.C.; Hitlan, R.T. Synthetic folic acid supplementation during pregnancy may increase the risk of developing autism. *J. Pediatric Biochem.* **2012**, *2*, 251–261.

44. Schmidt, R.J.; Tancredi, D.J.; Ozonoff, S.; Hansen, R.L.; Hartiala, J.; Allayee, H.; Schmidt, L.C.; Tassone, F.; Hertz-Picciotto, I. Maternal periconceptional folic acid intake and risk of autism spectrum disorders and developmental delay in the CHARGE (Childhood Autism Risks from Genetics and Environment) case-control study. *Am. J. Clin. Nutr.* **2012**, *96*, 80–89. [CrossRef] [PubMed]

45. Schmidt, R.J.; Hansen, R.L.; Hartiala, J.; Allayee, H.; Schmidt, L.C.; Tancredi, D.J.; Tassone, F.; Hertz-Picciotto, I. Prenatal vitamins, one-carbon metabolism gene variants, and risk for autism. *Epidemiology* **2011**, *22*, 476–485. [CrossRef] [PubMed]

46. Steenweg-de Graaff, J.; Ghassabian, A.; Jaddoe, V.W.; Tiemeier, H.; Roza, S.J. Folate concentrations during pregnancy and autistic traits in the offspring. The Generation R Study. *Eur. J. Public Health* **2015**, *25*, 431–433. [CrossRef] [PubMed]

47. Schmidt, R.J.; Tancredi, D.J.; Krakowiak, P.; Hansen, R.L.; Ozonoff, S. Maternal intake of supplemental iron and risk of autism spectrum disorder. *Am. J. Epidemiol.* **2014**, *180*, 890–900. [CrossRef] [PubMed]

48. Lyall, K.; Munger, K.L.; O'Reilly, E.J.; Santangelo, S.L.; Ascherio, A. Maternal dietary fat intake in association with autism spectrum disorders. *Am. J. Epidemiol.* **2013**, *178*, 209–220. [CrossRef]

49. Steenweg-De Graaff, J.; Tiemeier, H.; Ghassabian, A.; Rijlaarsdam, J.; Jaddoe, V.W.V.; Verhulst, F.C.; Roza, S.J. Maternal fatty acid status during pregnancy and child autistic traits: The Generation R Study. *Am. J. Epidemiol.* **2016**, *183*, 792–799. [CrossRef]

50. Gao, L.; Cui, S.S.; Han, Y.; Dai, W.; Su, Y.Y.; Zhang, X. Does periconceptional fish consumption by parents affect the incidence of autism spectrum disorder and intelligence deficiency? A Case-control study in Tianjin, China. *Biomed. Environ. Sci.* **2016**, *29*, 885–892. [CrossRef]

51. Julvez, J.; Mendez, M.; Fernandez-Barres, S.; Romaguera, D.; Vioque, J.; Llop, S.; Ibarluzea, J.; Guxens, M.; Avella-Garcia, C.; Tardon, A.; et al. Maternal consumption of seafood in pregnancy and child neuropsychological development: A longitudinal study based on a population with high consumption levels. *Am. J. Epidemiol.* **2016**, *183*, 169–182. [CrossRef]

52. House, J.S.; Mendez, M.; Maguire, R.L.; Gonzalez-Nahm, S.; Huang, Z.; Daniels, J.; Murphy, S.K.; Fuemmeler, B.F.; Wright, F.A.; Hoyo, C. Periconceptional maternal mediterranean diet is associated with favorable offspring behaviors and altered CpG methylation of imprinted genes. *Front. Cell Dev. Biol.* **2018**, *6*, 107. [CrossRef]

53. Schmidt, R.J.; Ozonoff, S.; Hansen, R.; Hartiala, J.; Allayee, H.; Schmidt, L.; Tassone, F.; Hertz-Picciotto, I. (old record 6424) Maternal periconceptional folic acid intake and risk for developmental delay and autism spectrum disorder: A case-control study. *Am. J. Epidemiol.* **2012**, *175*, S126. [CrossRef]

54. Li, Y.-M.; Ou, J.-J.; Liu, L.; Zhang, D.; Zhao, J.-P.; Tang, S.-Y. Association between maternal obesity and autism spectrum disorder in offspring: A meta-analysis. *J. Autism Dev. Disord.* **2016**, *46*, 95–102. [CrossRef] [PubMed]

55. Ueland, P.M.; Hustad, S.; Schneede, J.; Refsum, H.; Vollset, S.E. Biological and clinical implications of the *MTHFR* C677T polymorphism. *Trends Pharmacol. Sci.* **2001**, *22*, 195–201. [CrossRef]

56. Rijlaarsdam, J.; Cecil, C.A.; Walton, E.; Mesirow, M.S.; Relton, C.L.; Gaunt, T.R.; McArdle, W.; Barker, E.D. Prenatal unhealthy diet, *insulin-like growth factor 2 gene (IGF2)* methylation, and attention deficit hyperactivity disorder symptoms in youth with early-onset conduct problems. *J. Child Psychol. Psychiatry* **2017**, *58*, 19–27. [CrossRef] [PubMed]

57. Pidsley, R.; Dempster, E.; Troakes, C.; Al-Sarraj, S.; Mill, J. Epigenetic and genetic variation at the *IGF2/H19* imprinting control region on 11p15. 5 is associated with cerebellum weight. *Epigenetics* **2012**, *7*, 155–163. [CrossRef] [PubMed]

58. Office of Dietary Supplements; National Library of Medicine. Dietary Supplement Label Database. Available online: https://www.dsld.nlm.nih.gov/dsld/index.jsp (accessed on 7 February 2019).

59. Stamm, R.; Houghton, L. Nutrient intake values for folate during pregnancy and lactation vary widely around the world. *Nutrients* **2013**, *5*, 3920–3947. [CrossRef] [PubMed]

60. Wilcken, B.; Bamforth, F.; Li, Z.; Zhu, H.; Ritvanen, A.; Redlund, M.; Stoll, C.; Alembik, Y.; Dott, B.; Czeizel, A. Geographical and ethnic variation of the 677C> T allele of 5, 10 *methylenetetrahydrofolate reductase (MTHFR)*: Findings from over 7000 newborns from 16 areas world wide. *J. Med Genet.* **2003**, *40*, 619–625. [CrossRef] [PubMed]

61. Schmitz, G.; Ecker, J. The opposing effects of n-3 and n-6 fatty acids. *Prog. Lipid Res.* **2008**, *47*, 147–155. [CrossRef]

62. Patterson, E.; Wall, R.; Fitzgerald, G.F.; Ross, R.P.; Stanton, C. Health implications of high dietary omega-6 polyunsaturated fatty acids. *J. Nutr. Metab.* **2012**, *2012*, 539426. [CrossRef]

63. D'Souza, S.W.; Waldie, K.E.; Peterson, E.R.; Underwood, L.; Morton, S.M.B. Antenatal and postnatal determinants of behavioural difficulties in early childhood: Evidence from growing up in New Zealand. *Child Psychiatry Hum. Dev.* **2019**, *50*, 45–60. [CrossRef]

64. Miyake, Y.T.K.; Okubo, H.; Sasaki, S.; Arakawa, M. Maternal B vitamin intake during pregnancy and childhood behavioral problems in Japan: The Kyushu Okinawa maternal and child health study. *Nutr. Neurosci.* **2018**, *19*, 1–8. [CrossRef]

65. Virk, J.; Liew, Z.; Olsen, J.; Nohr, E.A.; Catov, J.M.; Ritz, B. Pre-conceptual and prenatal supplementary folic acid and multivitamin intake, behavioral problems, and hyperkinetic disorders: A study based on the Danish National Birth Cohort (DNBC). *Nutr. Neurosci.* **2018**, *21*, 352–360. [CrossRef] [PubMed]

66. Julvez, J.; Fortuny, J.; Mendez, M.; Torrent, M.; Ribas-Fitó, N.; Sunyer, J. Maternal use of folic acid supplements during pregnancy and four-year-old neurodevelopment in a population-based birth cohort. *Paediatr. Perinat. Epidemiol.* **2009**, *23*, 199–206. [CrossRef] [PubMed]

67. Schlotz, W.; Jones, A.; Phillips, D.I.; Gale, C.R.; Robinson, S.M.; Godfrey, K.M. Lower maternal folate status in early pregnancy is associated with childhood hyperactivity and peer problems in offspring. *J. Child Psychol. Psychiatry* **2010**, *51*, 594–602. [CrossRef] [PubMed]

68. Abel, M.H.; Ystrom, E.; Caspersen, I.H.; Meltzer, H.M.; Aase, H.; Torheim, L.E.; Askeland, R.B.; Reichborn-Kjennerud, T.; Brantsaeter, A.L. Maternal iodine intake and offspring attention-deficit/hyperactivity disorder: Results from a large prospective cohort study. *Nutrients* **2017**, *9*, 1239. [CrossRef] [PubMed]

69. Miyake, Y.T.K.; Okubo, H.; Sasaki, S.; Arakawa, M. Maternal fat intake during pregnancy and behavioral problems in 5-y-old Japanese children. *Nutrition* **2018**, *50*, 91–96. [CrossRef]

70. Ramakrishnan, U.; Gonzalez-Casanova, I.; Schnaas, L.; DiGirolamo, A.; Quezada, A.D.; Pallo, B.C.; Hao, W.; Neufeld, L.M.; Rivera, J.A.; Stein, A.D.; et al. Prenatal supplementation with DHA improves attention at 5 years of age: A randomized controlled trial. *Am. J. Clin. Nutr.* **2016**, *104*, 1075–1082. [CrossRef] [PubMed]

71. Gale, C.R.; Robinson, S.M.; Godfrey, K.M.; Law, C.M.; Schlotz, W.; O'Callaghan, F.J. Oily fish intake during pregnancy—Association with lower hyperactivity but not with higher full-scale IQ in offspring. *J. Child Psychol. Psychiatry Allied Discip.* **2008**, *49*, 1061–1068. [CrossRef]

72. Hibbeln, J.R.; Davis, J.M.; Steer, C.; Emmett, P.; Rogers, I.; Williams, C.; Golding, J. Maternal seafood consumption in pregnancy and neurodevelopmental outcomes in childhood (ALSPAC study): An observational cohort study. *Lancet* **2007**, *369*, 578–585. [CrossRef]

73. Miyake, Y.T.K.; Okubo, H.; Sasaki, S.; Arakawa, M. Maternal caffeine intake in pregnancy is inversely related to childhood peer problems in Japan: The Kyushu Okinawa maternal and child health study. *Nutr. Neurosci.* **2018**, *13*, 1–8. [CrossRef]

74. Del-Ponte, B.; Santos, I.S.; Tovo-Rodrigues, L.; Anselmi, L.; Munhoz, T.N.; Matijasevich, A. Caffeine consumption during pregnancy and ADHD at the age of 11 years: A birth cohort study. *BMJ Open* **2016**, *6*, e012749. [CrossRef]

75. Loomans, E.M.; Hofland, L.; van der Stelt, O.; van der Wal, M.F.; Koot, H.M.; Van den Bergh, B.R.; Vrijkotte, T.G. Caffeine intake during pregnancy and risk of problem behavior in 5- to 6-year-old children. *Pediatrics* **2012**, *130*, e305–e313. [CrossRef] [PubMed]

76. Hvolgaard Mikkelsen, S.; Obel, C.; Olsen, J.; Niclasen, J.; Bech, B.H. Maternal caffeine consumption during pregnancy and behavioral disorders in 11-year-old offspring: A Danish National Birth Cohort study. *J. Pediatrics* **2017**, *189*, 120–127.e121. [CrossRef] [PubMed]

77. Linnet, K.M.; Wisborg, K.; Secher, N.J.; Thomsen, P.H.; Obel, C.; Dalsgaard, S.; Henriksen, T.B. Coffee consumption during pregnancy and the risk of hyperkinetic disorder and ADHD: A prospective cohort study. *Acta Paediatr.* **2009**, *98*, 173–179. [CrossRef] [PubMed]

78. Galera, C.; Heude, B.; Forhan, A.; Bernard, J.Y.; Peyre, H.; Van der Waerden, J.; Pryor, L.; Bouvard, M.P.; Melchior, M.; Lioret, S.; et al. Prenatal diet and children's trajectories of hyperactivity-inattention and conduct problems from 3 to 8 years: The EDEN mother-child cohort. *J. Child Psychol. Psychiatry* **2018**, *59*, 1003–1011. [CrossRef] [PubMed]

79. McGee, R.A.; Clark, S.E.; Symons, D.K. Does the conners' continuous performance test aid in ADHD diagnosis? *J. Abnorm. Child Psychol.* **2000**, *28*, 415–424. [CrossRef] [PubMed]

80. Thapar, A.; Cooper, M.; Jefferies, R.; Stergiakouli, E. What causes attention deficit hyperactivity disorder? *Arch. Dis. Child.* **2012**, *97*, 260–265. [CrossRef]
81. Mathias, R.A.; Pani, V.; Chilton, F.H. Genetic Variants in the FADS gene: Implications for dietary recommendations for fatty acid intake. *Curr. Nutr. Rep.* **2014**, *3*, 139–148. [CrossRef]
82. Symonds, M.E.; Sebert, S.P.; Hyatt, M.A.; Budge, H. Nutritional programming of the metabolic syndrome. *Nat. Rev. Endocrinol.* **2009**, *5*, 604–610. [CrossRef]

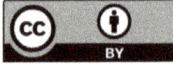

![nutrients logo] *nutrients*

MDPI

Communication

Choline and DHA in Maternal and Infant Nutrition: Synergistic Implications in Brain and Eye Health

Jonathan G. Mun *, LeeCole L. Legette, Chioma J. Ikonte and Susan H. Mitmesser

Science & Technology, Pharmavite LLC, West Hills, CA 91304, USA; llegette@pharmavite.net (L.L.L.); cikonte@pharmavite.net (C.J.I.); smitmesser@pharmavite.net (S.H.M.)
* Correspondence: jmun@pharmavite.net; Tel.: +1-818-221-6365

Received: 29 March 2019; Accepted: 17 May 2019; Published: 21 May 2019

Abstract: The aim of this review is to highlight current insights into the roles of choline and docosahexaenoic acid (DHA) in maternal and infant nutrition, with special emphasis on dietary recommendations, gaps in dietary intake, and synergistic implications of both nutrients in infant brain and eye development. Adequate choline and DHA intakes are not being met by the vast majority of US adults, and even more so by women of child-bearing age. Choline and DHA play a significant role in infant brain and eye development, with inadequate intakes leading to visual and neurocognitive deficits. Emerging findings illustrate synergistic interactions between choline and DHA, indicating that insufficient intakes of one or both could have lifelong deleterious impacts on both maternal and infant health.

Keywords: choline; pregnancy; infant nutrition; brain health; docosahexaenoic acid; DHA; eye function

---

1. Introduction

Pregnancy is an important time for both mother and baby and a long-standing strategy in supporting healthy pregnancies involves adequate prenatal care. Health care during pregnancy is one of the most frequently used wellness services in the US, with more than 18 million prenatal visits in 2015 [1]. Increasing the percentage of pregnant women who receive early and adequate prenatal care is a key objective for the US Healthy People 2020 public health initiative [2]. As part of adequate prenatal health consciousness and self-care, optimal nutrition plays a key role in maternal and infant health, prior to, during, and after pregnancy. Leading health organizations including the American Congress of Obstetricians and Gynecologists (ACOG), American Academy of Pediatrics (AAP), Europe Food Safety Authority (EFSA), and the World Health Organization (WHO) have highlighted several key nutrients as vital during pregnancy, including choline and DHA. The 2018 AAP policy statement emphasized the role of nutrition in the first 1000 days of life. The AAP recognized choline and long-chain polyunsaturated fatty acids (LC-PUFAs) as key nutrients in supporting early neurodevelopment and lifelong mental health [3]. Both docosahexaenoic acid (DHA) and arachidonic acid (ARA) are common LC-PUFAs that accumulate in tissues and are known for their importance in brain function and development [4,5]. Docosahexaenoic acid and ARA are synthesized from precursor essential fatty acids, omega-3 α-linolenic acid (ALA) and omega-6 linoleic acid (LA), respectively [6]. Endogenous synthesis of choline and DHA is insufficient to meet nutrient demands, reinforcing the need for adequate daily intake. While general dietary intake of omega-6s meets daily recommendations, omega-3 intake is low in the American diet [7]. National survey data in the US population indicates inadequate dietary intakes of choline and DHA. Over 90% of the US population does not meet adequate intake for choline (550 mg/day for men, 425 mg/day for women) [8]. Among US adults, pregnant and lactating women are at increased risk for choline insufficiency as their requirements increase to

450 and 550 mg, respectively, during these life stages [9]. Dietary intakes of DHA are also low in American diet, with general recommendations of 7–8 oz of fish and seafood weekly to equate to 250 mg EPA + DHA omega-3 fatty acids daily. However, the majority of US adults fail to consume adequate amounts of seafood, with averages of 0.43 oz seafood (63 mg DHA) daily [10]. Docosahexaenoic acid recommendations for pregnant and lactating women are slightly higher, with the 2015 US Department of Agriculture Dietary Guidelines advising weekly consumption of 8–12 oz of low-mercury content seafood, noting that DHA is associated with improved infant health outcomes [11]. However, nearly all US women of child-bearing age and pregnant women (95%) have low seafood consumption and do not meet recommended daily intakes of 250 mg total of eicosapentaenoic acid (EPA) and DHA [12]. While supplement use has increased DHA and EPA intakes over time, current intakes are still low, suggesting a need for more effective nutrition education programs to address nutrient shortfalls [12], especially during pregnancy and lactation. Choline and DHA, as a LC-PUFA, are essential nutrients for normal brain development as they are integral structural components of neurological systems, and deficits during early life can have long-term impacts on brain function [3]. Both are also utilized in retinal development and lack of adequate amounts could adversely impact eye health. The main objective of this review is to critically evaluate the roles of choline and DHA in infant and maternal nutrition, to elucidate possible synergistic implications of both nutrients in brain and eye health and increase the awareness of this public health concern.

2. Role of Choline in Maternal and Infant Nutrition

2.1. Essential Functions

Discovered as a component of lecithin from heated pig and ox bile in the 1860s, choline was named from the Greek word for bile, "chole" [13]. Lecithin was later characterized as being largely comprised of phosphatidylcholine, a major constituent of biological membranes. As researchers began to study how nerves communicated with each other in the 1920s, a substance secreted from a stimulated vagus nerve was identified (acetylcholine) and found to be the same molecule as a choline-containing molecule derived from fungi that could activate nerves when applied to organs. This discovery was awarded a Nobel Prize to Otto Loewi and Henry Dale in 1936.

For decades following this work, choline was recognized as being a critical component of the two biologically relevant molecules, phosphatidylcholine and acetylcholine, and yet its requirement in the human diet was substantially underappreciated. In animal models, pancreatectomized dogs developed fatty degeneration of the liver, which could be reversed by feeding raw pancreas or lecithin [14], a consequence later understood to be due to the impaired lipid packaging into lipoproteins for export from the liver. Choline deficiencies were documented in a number of other animal species, including perosis in poultry (deforming leg weakness), atherosclerosis in rodents, and related conditions in rabbit, cattle, and baboon. In addition, choline-deficient animals were found to develop liver cancer, which uncovered yet another a role of choline, as a betaine precursor in the methylation process and DNA repair [15]. Supporting these observations in animal species, human patients fed total parenteral nutrition solutions lacking choline had low circulating levels of choline, coupled with impaired liver function and fatty liver [16–18].

Today, choline is recognized by the National Academy of Medicine (formerly the Institute of Medicine) as an essential nutrient that must be acquired from the diet, as de novo biosynthesis is insufficient to meet human requirements [9]. We now know that choline plays a key role in lipid transport (as phosphatidylcholine in lipoprotein assembly and secretion), cell membrane structural support (as phosphatidylcholine and sphingomyelin), neurotransmission (as acetylcholine), and as a source of methyl groups (as a precursor of betaine).

2.2. Choline: Role in Maternal Health

In addition to the role of choline in general physiology, choline is critically important during pregnancy. Lower serum choline levels are associated with increased risk of neural tube defects [19], suggesting that choline intakes should be increased prior to pregnancy, as closing of the neural tube occurs by the fourth week of pregnancy (28 days after conception) [20]. As pregnancy progresses, the demand for choline significantly increases, as membrane biosynthesis is needed for placental development, increased workload by maternal organs, and to support exponential fetal organ growth. The growing need for choline by the developing fetus is facilitated by elevated maternal plasma free choline, placental accumulation (approximately 50 times higher concentration than maternal blood), and elevated plasma free choline levels that are three times higher than adult concentrations. Consequences of low choline status during pregnancy have major implications not only for fetal development, but also for maternal health. Acute fatty liver of pregnancy, while uncommon, is a potentially fatal complication that occurs in the third trimester or early postpartum period and shares symptoms with more common conditions like pre-eclampsia and cholestasis [21]. Furthermore, increased choline supplementation during pregnancy has demonstrated downregulation of antiangiogenic factor and preeclampsia risk marker, fms-like tyrosine kinase-1 (sFLT1) in in human placental tissues [22]. Simulating decreased placental efficiency in preeclampsia and intrauterine growth restriction, the *Dlx3*+/− mouse model has been used to show that dietary choline drives placental betaine concentration, which downregulates inflammatory gene expression [23] and improves fetal growth patterns [24].

Common genetic variants in choline-metabolizing enzymes are known to alter the metabolic fate of dietary choline, thereby increasing choline intake requirements in some individuals [25]. For instance, choline contributes to phosphatidylcholine synthesis by way of two metabolic pathways—through phosphorylation via the cytidine diphosphate-choline (CDP-choline) pathway or sequential methylation of phosphatidylethanolamine by the phosphatidylethanolamine N-methyltransferase (PEMT) pathway. The latter pathway is critically important in that it enables phosphatidylcholine synthesis even in the absence of dietary choline intake. Activity of PEMT is greater in pre-menopausal women, due to its upregulation by estrogen, but is considered inadequate to support endogenous production alone, necessitating a dietary choline requirement to prevent deficiency. Variations in single-base pairs (single-nucleotide polymorphisms or SNPs) in the *Pemt* gene are known to impact endogenous choline production, thereby influencing interindividual choline requirements and risk for choline deficiency [26,27].

Despite choline's importance in maternal health, many do not meet the daily recommendation. Approximately 90–95% of pregnant women are consuming less than the adequate intake (AI) [28]. Experts note that choline is not found in most prenatal supplements [29,30], suggesting that increased awareness of choline's place in infant and maternal health is needed to improve intakes through consumption of choline-rich foods and/or dietary supplementation.

2.3. Choline: Role in Infant Health

In the late 1970s, Steven Zeisel [31], a pediatric resident and graduate student, observed that blood choline concentrations were much higher in human newborns than in adults. Collaborator, Jan Blusztajn [32], observed that endogenous synthesis of phosphatidylcholine was increased in the brain and liver of rodent pups, demonstrating an increased metabolic demand for choline in newborns. In addition, mechanistic studies in rodents also showed that hepatic choline pools are depleted during pregnancy when fed a normal diet [33–35]. Soon after, choline was found to concentrate across the placenta, raising fetal tissue concentrations of choline [36]. Zeisel's research group and colleagues subsequently discovered that mammary glands accumulate and export choline in milk, providing substantial dietary choline to the developing infant postpartum [37]. Adequate intake recommendations (AI) are 125 mg choline/day for infants 0–6 months and 150 mg choline/day for infants 7–12 months; these AIs are based on choline concentrations in human milk (160 mg/L) and mean volume output of human milk (0.78 L/day) for infants 0–6 months with a reference body weight of 7 kg (approximately 18 mg/kg), and extrapolation for reference body weight at ages 7–12 months [9].

The increased availability of choline for the brain led to the hypothesis that acetylcholine concentrations impact neurological processes and cognitive function. Testing this hypothesis, researchers Christina Williams and Warren Meck [38] found that prenatal and postnatal choline supplementation of developing rat pups improved performance as adults on the 12- and 18-arm radial maze task, a test of spatial memory. Several potential roles that maternal dietary choline play on fetal brain biochemistry that impart lifelong behavioral changes have been suggested. Amongst this is the observation that choline alters timing of neuronal differentiation in the septum and the hippocampus, two brain regions known to be involved in learning and memory [39,40]. Others have confirmed these findings, showing that prenatal choline modulated rates of adult hippocampal neurogenesis, increased hippocampal brain-derived neurotrophic factor, improved cognitive performance on memory tasks as adults [41,42], accelerated hippocampal maturation [43], and decreased the threshold for induction of long-term potentiation (an indication of synapse strength) [44,45]. These findings are especially significant, given that rates of hippocampal neurogenesis decline with age and that nutritional intervention produced a marked change in behavioral output. These impacts of dietary choline on neurogenesis extend beyond the hippocampal development, showing increased neurogenesis in the cerebral cortex [46,47] and increased levels of nerve growth factor (NGF) in both the hippocampus and cortical areas [48]. This is further supported by the observation that maternal choline status influences brain gray and white matter development in piglet brains using magnetic resonance spectroscopy neuroimaging, which is consistent with choline's role in myelin components, phospholipids, and sphingomyelin, and emphasizes the role of choline in early brain development [49]. In humans, the role of choline in cognition have also been observed, with higher choline intakes during pregnancy associated with higher performance on memory tasks in their 7-year-old children [50]. As in brain development, emerging research by Zeisel and colleagues [51] suggests that fetal eye development may also be dependent on choline intakes, with low maternal choline intakes resulting in fewer retinal stem cells and worse eyesight in animal models. Together, the accumulating evidence underscores the long-term significance of choline in prenatal nutrition.

Beyond prenatal brain development, choline plays a significant role in continued growth of the brain and in cognitive measures. In animal models, inadequate choline intakes have demonstrated reductions in maternal plasma and milk concentrations of choline metabolites, and therefore nutrient availability for neonatal development [52]. Observational studies have shown that higher choline intakes during pregnancy have been associated with modestly better visual memory in children at age seven [50]. In a sample of 15-year-old children ($n = 324$), the sum of school grades in 17 major subjects were used as an outcome measure for academic achievement. Researchers showed that plasma choline level was significantly and positively associated with academic achievement, independent of socioeconomic status (SES) factors, and folate intake [53]. In randomized, double-blind, controlled feeding studies, maternal choline supplementation did not improve measures of infant memory or language development [54], but did improve infant information processing speed [55], bolstering support for prenatal choline supplementation. Recent evidence suggests that postnatal choline supplementation should also be considered, especially in preterm infants, when a choline deficiency may contribute to impaired lean body mass growth and neurocognitive development, despite adequate macronutrient intake and weight gain [56].

3. Role of DHA in Maternal and Infant Nutrition

3.1. Essential Functions

While proteins and carbohydrates were widely regarded as indispensable dietary constituents by the early 20th century, there were still conflicting views on the role of dietary fats in nutrition with initial findings on essential fatty acids not emerging until the late 1920s and early 1930s [57]. Between

1929 and 1932, George O. Burr and colleagues [57–60] conducted animal studies which demonstrated that exclusion of dietary fat led to a deficiency disease in rats. Results from Burr's work also showed that dietary fat, in particular fatty acids, was required to stimulate growth and prevent disease leading Burr to be the first to propose LA as an essential fatty acid in 1930 [58,59]. In 1931, Wesson and Burr also noted that similarly to LA, ALA is not synthesized by rats and can stimulate weight gain in rats consuming an essential fatty acid-deficient diet, which led them to conclude that ALA is also an essential fatty acid [61]. Animal work continued until 1960s to elucidate physiological actions of ALA and LA, including roles as precursors for ARA and DHA fatty acids. Key findings in 1950s led to purification of DHA and determination of its structure from animal brain phosphatides. In 1960, Klerk et al. [62] determined the metabolic pathway for conversion of DHA from ALA. Subsequent work in the 1960s and 1970s illustrated a functional role of DHA in brain and eye health, as DHA was shown to be abundant in both retinal [63,64] and synaptic membrane [65] phospholipids. Clinical research in the 1970s and 80s provided definitive findings on ALA and LA as essential fatty acids for human nutrition. Case reports and clinical studies of infants with essential fatty acid deficiency showed that it is resolved with administration of LA and/or ALA [66–70]. Presently, the National Academy of Medicine (formerly the Institute of Medicine) recognizes LA and ALA as essential fatty acids, recommends amounts for adequate daily intakes (AI), and state the main role of omega-3 fatty acids as structural membrane lipids, particularly in nerve tissue and retina [6]. After establishment of LA and ALA as essential fatty acids, majority of fatty acid research focused on physiological roles of common omega-3s (DHA and EPA) and omega-6 (ARA) synthesized from ALA and LA precursors, respectively. Specifically, observational findings in the 1980s and 1990s on EPA content in plasma phospholipids as well as fish oil/fish consumption (major EPA and DHA) dietary source and associations with heart health parameters led to greater understanding of the role of omega-3s in vascular biology and heart health [57]. Concurrently, omega-6 research focused on the role of ARA in eicosanoid production and downstream impact on inflammation and immune system, rather than its abundance and role in brain gray matter phospholipids. Beginning in the 1990s, focus shifted from omega-3s and heart health to role of DHA specifically in brain and eye health due to its presence in brain and retinal tissues. It is prevalent in structures that underlie cognitive abilities, including the eyes and brain (cerebellum, frontal, and occipital lobe).

The brain is largely comprised of lipids. The predominant LC-PUFAs in the brain are ARA omega-6 fatty acid and DHA omega-3 fatty acid [5,71,72]. Both ARA and DHA can be provided in diet or synthesized via desaturation and elongation pathways from LA and ALA precursors. Findings show DHA affects brain function by modulating neurogenesis [73,74], influencing neurotransmission [75], and promoting synaptic activity [76]. Additionally, DHA exerts other important actions that affect overall health including playing a key role in cell signaling, lipid metabolism, cell membrane function, and eye development and function. Docosahexaenoic acid (DHA) acts as a precursor for autocoid signaling molecules as well as an activator of several gene transcription factors including peroxisome proliferator activated receptors [77], which modulate metabolic processes, cholesterol homeostasis, and inflammation [78]. It also impacts cell membrane properties by increasing membrane permeability [79–83] and facilitating membrane fluidity [84–87]. Docosahexaenoic acid contributes to eye development and function through its signaling [88] and structural [89] effects on retinal photoreceptor cells. Low levels of plasma DHA have been observed in individuals with genetic retinal disorders such as retinitis pigmentosa leading some to theorize that DHA deficiencies could lead to defects in central retinal cones adversely impacting eye health [90]. In all, the totality of scientific literature strongly suggests a role of dietary DHA in various aspects of health including neonatal neurodevelopment.

3.2. DHA: Role in Maternal Health

Pregnancy is a time when higher nutrient demands can impact maternal health and pregnancy outcomes. Maternal DHA intake, endogenous synthesis, and body stores help meet DHA needs for mother and fetus through pregnancy [86,91]. Various genetic and lifestyle factors can influence maternal DHA stores including nutrition as well as pre-pregnancy health conditions, which may alter DHA utilization. Impaired fatty acid metabolism, due to the various single nucleotide polymorphisms (SNPs), can affect DHA status, and consequently, alter DHA requirements [92]. Researchers assessed several SNPs for genes encoding for key enzymes involved in LC-PUFA production—fatty acid desaturase (FADS) and elongase (ELOVL)—and found that *FADS1* and *FADS2* variants impacted mainly omega-6 fatty acid levels, whereas *ELOVL* genetic variants affected omega-3 fatty acid levels [93]. Investigators also observed normal weight women with *FADS1* SNPs had significantly lower levels of ARA and overweight/obese women with ELOVL2 SNPs had an association with lower DHA levels [93]. Gonzalez-Casanova et al. [94] examined the impact of 15 different FADS SNPs along with prenatal DHA supplementation on birth weight in the Mexican population based on earlier observations of high prevalence of SNPs associated with slow LC-PUFA conversion in Hispanic populations. Results showed differential response to prenatal supplementation due to the FADS genotype. Women with *FADS2* SNP that received supplementation had higher birth weight children than those who received the placebo. This led the authors to propose that mixed findings on DHA supplementation's effects on birth weight could be attributed to differential responses due to genetic variance [94]. Xie and Innis [95] found that genetic variation in *FADS1* and *FADS2* influenced maternal plasma and erythrocyte levels of both omega-3 (DHA) and omega-6 (ARA) fatty acids during pregnancy and lipids levels in breast milk during lactation. Overall maternal health status can also impact the role of DHA during pregnancy. A recent study showed pre-pregnancy obesity is associated with higher inflammation and attenuated response to DHA supplementation [96]. In general, the DHA needs of the fetus rise during pregnancy, peaking towards the end of the third trimester (after week 32), a time of great growth and development as well as significant accretion of DHA in fetal brain tissue [97–100]. Kuipers et al. [100] evaluated DHA fetal content at 25, 35, and 40 weeks of gestation. At term (40 weeks), 21% of DHA was present in skeletal muscle, 23% in brain tissue, and most of the DHA residing in fetal adipose tissue (50%), leading researchers to suggest fetal DHA adipose content serves as a reservoir for DHA that can be utilized in infant development. Higher maternal DHA intakes may be required in the late stage of pregnancy to help meet elevating needs. With advancing gestation, there is increased transfer of DHA to the developing fetus which may lead to depleted maternal DHA levels [101]. Low levels of DHA have been associated with increased incidence of various diseases during perinatal period, including postpartum depression [101]. Maternal DHA supplementation (600 mg daily) starting in the last half of gestation (week 20 to birth) resulted in greater gestational duration and infant birth size [102]. Observational and clinical research shows maternal DHA dietary intakes during pregnancy impact blood DHA status of newborns [103]. Maternal and fetal DHA is associated with several brain and eye health outcomes in infants [77,103,104].

3.3. DHA: Role in Infant Health

Maternal DHA status during fetal development can have lasting impacts on brain and eye health throughout life as evident by key recommendations for DHA intakes during the first 1000 days of life [3]. Docosahexaenoic acid is essential for normal vision and brain development. There is rapid DHA accretion in utero during the last weeks of the third trimester to support growth [77,97–100,105,106] and DHA is a major structural lipid in both the brain and retina. It reaches levels of about 4 g in the brain and represents 50% of the fatty acids present in retinal rod and cone components [106]. During pregnancy, DHA insufficiency was noticed to be associated with lower infant neurodevelopment scores up to 18 months old; however, this finding was not detected at later follow up (5 years of age) [107]. Maternal DHA intake, particularly in the last 5 weeks of pregnancy, influences visual acuity development up towards the end of the first year of life [108].

Recent studies have observed an effect of maternal and fetal DHA status on general health including various brain and eye health outcomes well into early and mid-childhood. Researchers found associations with umbilical cord plasma DHA levels and metabolic measures in early childhood

(3 years of age) [109]. Specifically, higher cord plasma DHA was associated with lower body mass index (BMI) scores, waist circumference, and leptin levels. This association was stronger when infant–mother pairs experienced hyperglycemia during pregnancy [109]. Prenatal DHA status may also contribute to improved sustained attention in preschool children [110]. In contrast, some findings have not shown an impact of maternal DHA on brain health measures in childhood. Crozier et al. [111] found neither maternal ARA or DHA levels during pregnancy were associated with cognitive performance in 4- and 6-year-old children. Investigators speculated that diet quality, which was positively associated with neurodevelopment at four years of age may compensate for maternal DHA insufficiencies during pregnancy [111], indicating an effect of postnatal nutrition on health as well. Daily postnatal DHA supplementation, via DHA enriched solid baby food from 6–12 months old, led to improved visual acuity [112]. Some early communicative development benefits were also observed with DHA supplementation during early infancy [113]. However, other neurodevelopment outcomes were not significantly changed in the study [113]. Current findings indicate various factors affect the overall impact of DHA in infant brain and eye health including both pre-pregnancy maternal health status as well as prenatal and postnatal nutritional status of mother and child.

4. Synergistic Relationship between Choline and DHA

4.1. Proposed Mechanisms: Insights from Preclinical Studies

Choline and DHA are two important lipid-based nutrients needed for growth and development. Findings from in vitro studies highlight potential interactions between both nutrients and effects on metabolism. For example, DHA supplementation significantly increased cellular choline uptake in human retinal cells compared to cultured cells without supplemental DHA [114], which demonstrates how DHA may impact choline status. This finding is consistent with an earlier report demonstrating that the high unsaturated fatty acid content of human retinoblastoma cell membranes facilitated the capacity of the high-affinity choline uptake system to transport low concentrations of choline [114,115]. Docosahexaenoic acid has been shown to stimulate choline acetyltransferase (ChAT) enzymatic activity as well as support growth and function in neural cell culture studies [116,117]. The interaction of DHA and choline status has also been demonstrated in vivo, in the *Pemt*–/– mouse model. Discussed in Section 2.2, the PEMT enzyme facilitates endogenous hepatic synthesis of phosphatidylcholine from phosphatidylethanolamine. Deficiency of PEMT in *Pemt* gene knockout (*Pemt*–/–) mice yields disrupted fetal hippocampal development that can be reversed through maternal dietary DHA supplementation compared to control diets [118]. Maternal DHA supplementation not only increased fetal brain *Pemt*–/– phospholipid-DHA levels to wild-type levels, and eliminated differences in neural progenitor cell proliferation and apoptosis differences, but the DHA supplementation also halved the rate of neural apoptosis in wild type [118], affirming roles of DHA and choline in developmental neurogenesis. This observation is consistent with the specificity of PEMT in synthesizing polyunsaturated-phosphatidylcholine species [119] and highlights the coordinated roles of choline and DHA in neural lipid metabolism. Recent work in evaluating aspects of neural development processes revealed that specific nutrient combinations have a beneficial impact on brain function. Both in vitro and in vivo studies illustrate the role of nutrient combinations in neurodevelopment, particularly the presence of both DHA and choline. van Deijk et al. [120] showed that a medical food with DHA and choline, as well as other micronutrients, positively affected synaptic function in neuronal cells. When assessing aspects of neuroinflammation, investigators observed that administration of a DHA-containing choline phospholipid led to decreased lipopolysaccharide (LPS)-induced neuroinflammation in both cell culture and animal models [121]. Similar to its anti-inflammatory effects, supplementing with choline and DHA also attenuated brain oxidative stress in a perinatal maternal separation stress rodent model [122]. Favorable effects of nutrient combinations were also seen when supplementing during pregnancy. Results from several studies indicate a valuable impact of prenatal choline and DHA supplementation on offspring brain function in rats [123,124], dogs [125], and pigs [126]. In a study of choline, DHA, or saline control supplementation of pregnant rat dams and pups from choline or DHA supplemented groups showed significantly increased numbers of CA1 hippocampal neurons compared to both untreated and saline control group pups ($p < 0.05$). The combined supplementation of choline and DHA during pregnancy further enhanced neurodevelopment of the fetal hippocampus in rats compared to control ($p < 0.001$), with these effects proving better than supplementing with choline ($p < 0.05$) or DHA ($p < 0.05$) alone [124]. These results are supported by work by van Wijk et al. [123], who showed that supplementation of DHA in rats significantly increased DHA levels in plasma and red blood cells compared to control, and supplementation of choline from lecithin significantly increased plasma free choline, but did not affect DHA levels. However, combined supplementation of DHA and lecithin increased DHA to levels significantly greater than DHA supplementation alone ($p < 0.025$), which indicated that the impact of combined choline and DHA supplementation on circulating DHA levels were greater than an additive effect [123]. Advantageous effects of nutrient combinations could be due to the role of choline in placental nutrient transport. Kwan et al. [127] found that maternal choline supplementation modulates placental nutrient metabolism in a late gestational mouse pregnancy model, which may be attributed to its influence on vascular development. Furthermore, maternal choline supplementation increased placental transcript abundance of DHA, choline, and acetylcholine transporters [127]. Collectively, the evidence presented in this section supports the hypothesis that supplementation of choline or DHA alone yield complementary outcomes on choline and DHA metabolism, and that supplementation in combination produce benefits that must be greater than additive effects. Current in vivo and in vitro evidence supports co-supplementation of choline and DHA, particularly during pregnancy to support brain and eye development of offspring, and while the literature to date provides novel leads on how choline and DHA function in synergy, additional work is needed to clarify its mechanism of action.

4.2. Proposed Mechanisms: Insights from Clinical Findings

In this review, we have thus far discussed the roles of choline and DHA independently on infant brain and eye development, and synergistic relationships from preclinical models. From a clinical standpoint, the roles of choline and DHA on infant development may be best observed in premature birth, a circumstance wherein nutrient availability is interrupted, when levels would otherwise remain high *in utero*. Furthermore, human brain and eye development is known to begin *in utero*, and continue postnatally, with choline and LC-PUFAs (DHA, ARA) supplied together postpartum from human milk or supplemental infant formula. Human milk choline content from mothers of preterm infants have also been reported to be lower than from mothers following full-term delivery [128]. Preterm births in the US occurred in about 1 in 10 babies from 2007 to 2014, with an estimated associated cost of $26.2 billion USD annually, equating to approximately $51,600 per infant born preterm [129,130]. More importantly, premature births are associated with increased health problems, longer hospital stays, and learning and behavioral problems through childhood. To highlight the mechanistic synergy of choline and DHA, Bernhard and colleagues [131] demonstrated through a randomized, controlled trial that in preterm infants supplemented with choline, DHA, both, or neither, choline alone did not significantly increase phosphatidylcholine-DHA (PC-DHA), DHA alone increased PC-DHA content by only 35% ($p < 0.05$), but the combined treatment increased PC-DHA by 63% compared to control ($p < 0.001$). Additionally, supplementation with choline increased plasma choline concentrations in preterm infants to near-fetal concentrations and improved DHA status [131]. Since phosphatidylcholine is the major transport form of DHA in plasma, these findings provide strong support for the hypothesis that actions of each nutrient are metabolically linked through phosphatidylcholine and that their actions cannot be mutually exclusive.

To better understand the role(s) choline and DHA play in unison in infant brain and eye health, researchers have studied how choline intakes influence phosphatidylcholine-DHA enrichment [132]. West and colleagues [133] showed that phosphatidylcholine-DHA levels were greater in pregnant women than non-pregnant women, suggesting a greater demand for methyl donors and increased

PEMT activity. Additionally, they showed that when choline and DHA were both supplemented in non-pregnant women, higher choline intakes resulted in greater PC-DHA enrichment, suggesting that higher choline intakes may increase PEMT activity [132,134]. These findings suggest a metabolic synergy between choline and DHA, and are further supported by research that demonstrated consumption of n-3 fatty acid-enriched eggs increased plasma free choline and betaine compared to non-enriched eggs [133]. Consistent with these findings, McNamara et al. [135] showed that low DHA status is associated with lower cortical metabolism of choline using proton magnetic resonance spectroscopy. To explore the relationship between infant nutrition and subsequent cognitive performance, Cheatham et al. [136] collected and analyzed human milk samples at 3–4 months postpartum and tested recognition memory ability in infants at 6-months old. Through this work, Cheatham demonstrated that brain electrical activity expressed as event-related potential latency scores from the frontal, central, and midline areas were predicted by the DHA and choline interaction and that higher choline and DHA content was related to better recognition memory [136]. Together, these clinical findings provide evidence that choline and DHA function is synergistic in infant neurocognitive development.

5. Conclusions and Future Directions

The evidence presented in this review of cell culture, animal model, and human clinical trials provide compelling support for choline and DHA in maternal and infant nutrition. The interactions between choline and DHA support roles in brain and eye health, and the findings that supplementation with one augments the other points to synergy between the two nutrients. Dietary intakes of choline and DHA in the US population are lower than recommended levels, and vulnerable populations may require additional supplementation, particularly women during pregnancy and lactation. Infants receiving nutrition from breastmilk are provided with choline and LC-PUFAs (inclusive of ARA, LA, and DHA) from the maternal intake, but those who are not breastfed will require formula that contains choline and LC-PUFAs for proper growth and development.

Ensuring optimal nutrition during pregnancy requires a multi-faceted approach. Effective strategies are needed to determine nutrient status, address key nutrient gaps, and gain a deeper understanding of nutrient interactions during pregnancy. Prenatal testing for DHA status has been proposed [137] and should also include choline to inform on nutrient adequacy and guide strategy for obtaining optimal intake levels. Moreover, commercial tools for screening of common SNPs may enable personalized tailoring of dietary recommendations. With a greater understanding of maternal nutrient needs and how genetic and lifestyle factors impact metabolism, we are empowered to improve nutritional approaches to prenatal care.

Author Contributions: J.G.M. and L.L.L. conceptualized and drafted the manuscript; C.J.I. and S.H.M. contributed, reviewed, and edited the manuscript. All authors read and approved the final manuscript.

Funding: This research received no external funding.

Conflicts of Interest: J.G.M., L.L.L., C.J.I., and S.H.M. are employed at Pharmavite LLC.

References

1. Rui, O.T.P. National Ambulatory Medical Care Survey: 2015 State and National Summary Tables. Available online: https://www.cdc.gov/nchs/data/ahcd/namcs_summary/2015_namcs_web_tables.pdf (accessed on 20 February 2019).
2. US Department of Health and Human Services. Healthy People 2020: Maternal, Infant, and Child Health Objectives. Available online: https://www.healthypeople.gov/2020/topics-objectives/topic/maternal-infant-and-child-health/objectives (accessed on 20 February 2020).
3. Schwarzenberg, S.J.; Georgieff, M.K.; Committee on Nutrition. Advocacy for Improving Nutrition in the First 1000 Days to Support Childhood Development and Adult Health. *Pediatrics* **2018**, *141*. [CrossRef]
4. Koletzko, B.; Carlson, S.E.; van Goudoever, J.B. Should Infant Formula Provide Both Omega-3 DHA and Omega-6 Arachidonic Acid? *Ann. Nutr. Metab.* **2015**, *66*, 137–138. [CrossRef] [PubMed]

5. Martinez, M. Tissue levels of polyunsaturated fatty acids during early human development. *J. Pediatr.* **1992**, *120*, S129–S138. [CrossRef]

6. Institute of Medicine (US). Dietary Fat: Total Fat and Fatty Acids. In *Dietary References Intakes: The Essential Guide to Nutrient Requirements*; National Academies Press: Washington, DC, USA, 2006.

7. US Department of Agriculture—Agricultural Research Service. Nutrient Intakes from Food: Mean Amounts Consumed per Individual, by Gender and Age. Available online: https://www.ars.usda.gov/ARSUserFiles/80400530/pdf/1516/Table_1_NIN_GEN_15.pdf (accessed on 22 April 2019).

8. Wallace, T.C.; Fulgoni, V.L., 3rd. Assessment of Total Choline Intakes in the United States. *J. Am. Coll. Nutr.* **2016**, *35*, 108–112. [CrossRef] [PubMed]

9. IoM (US). Choline. In *Dietary Reference Intakes for Thiamin, Riboflavin, Niacin, Vitamin B_6, Folate, Vitamin B_{12}, Pantothenic Acid, Biotin, and Choline*; National Academies Press: Washington, DC, USA, 1998. [CrossRef]

10. Papanikolaou, Y.; Brooks, J.; Reider, C.; Fulgoni, V.L. US adults are not meeting recommended levels for fish and omega-3 fatty acid intake: Results of an analysis using observational data from NHANES 2003–2008. *Nutr. J.* **2014**, *13*, 31. [CrossRef]

11. US Department of Health and Human Services. 2015–2020 Dietary Guidelines for Americans. Available online: https://health.gov/dietaryguidelines/2015/resources/2015-2020_Dietary_Guidelines.pdf (accessed on 4 March 2019).

12. Zhang, Z.; Fulgoni, V.L.; Kris-Etherton, P.M.; Mitmesser, S.H. Dietary Intakes of EPA and DHA Omega-3 Fatty Acids among US Childbearing-Age and Pregnant Women: An Analysis of NHANES 2001–2014. *Nutrients* **2018**, *10*, 416. [CrossRef]

13. Zeisel, S.H. A brief history of choline. *Ann. Nutr. Metab.* **2012**, *61*, 254–258. [CrossRef]

14. Hershey, J.M.; Soskin, S. Substitution of "lecithin" for raw pancreas in the diet of the depancreatized dog. *Am. J. Physiol.-Leg. Content* **1931**, *98*, 74–85. [CrossRef]

15. Mehedint, M.G.; Zeisel, S.H. Choline's role in maintaining liver function: New evidence for epigenetic mechanisms. *Curr. Opin. Clin. Nutr. Metab. Care* **2013**, *16*, 339–345. [CrossRef] [PubMed]

16. Chawla, R.K.; Berry, C.J.; Kutner, M.H.; Rudman, D. Plasma concentrations of transsulfuration pathway products during nasoenteral and intravenous hyperalimentation of malnourished patients. *Am. J. Clin. Nutr.* **1985**, *42*, 577–584. [CrossRef]

17. Sheard, N.F.; Tayek, J.A.; Bistrian, B.R.; Blackburn, G.L.; Zeisel, S.H. Plasma choline concentration in humans fed parenterally. *Am. J. Clin. Nutr.* **1986**, *43*, 219–224. [CrossRef]

18. Tayek, J.A.; Bistrian, B.; Sheard, N.F.; Zeisel, S.H.; Blackburn, G.L. Abnormal liver function in malnourished patients receiving total parenteral nutrition: A prospective randomized study. *J. Am. Coll. Nutr.* **1990**, *9*, 76–83. [CrossRef] [PubMed]

19. Shaw, G.M.; Finnell, R.H.; Blom, H.J.; Carmichael, S.L.; Vollset, S.E.; Yang, W.; Ueland, P.M. Choline and risk of neural tube defects in a folate-fortified population. *Epidemiology* **2009**, *20*, 714–719. [CrossRef]

20. Cavalli, P. Prevention of Neural Tube Defects and proper folate periconceptional supplementation. *J. Prenat. Med.* **2008**, *2*, 40–41. [PubMed]

21. Ko, H.; Yoshida, E.M. Acute fatty liver of pregnancy. *Can. J. Gastroenterol. J. Can. Gastroenterol.* **2006**, *20*, 25–30. [CrossRef]

22. Jiang, X.; Bar, H.Y.; Yan, J.; Jones, S.; Brannon, P.M.; West, A.A.; Perry, C.A.; Ganti, A.; Pressman, E.; Devapatla, S.; et al. A higher maternal choline intake among third-trimester pregnant women lowers placental and circulating concentrations of the antiangiogenic factor fms-like tyrosine kinase-1 (sFLT1). *FASEB J.* **2013**, *27*, 1245–1253. [CrossRef]

23. King, J.H.; Kwan, S.T.; Yan, J.; Jiang, X.; Fomin, V.G.; Roberson, M.S.; Caudill, M.A. Maternal Choline Supplementation Modulates Maternal and Fetal Choline Metabolism and Downregulates Inflammatory Gene Expression in a Mouse Model of Placental Insufficiency. *FASEB J.* **2016**, *30*, 272.1. [CrossRef]

24. King, J.H.; Kwan, S.T.C.; Yan, J.; Klatt, K.C.; Jiang, X.; Roberson, M.S.; Caudill, M.A. Maternal Choline Supplementation Alters Fetal Growth Patterns in a Mouse Model of Placental Insufficiency. *Nutrients* **2017**, *9*, 765. [CrossRef] [PubMed]

25. Ganz, A.B.; Cohen, V.V.; Swersky, C.C.; Stover, J.; Vitiello, G.A.; Lovesky, J.; Chuang, J.C.; Shields, K.; Fomin, V.G.; Lopez, Y.S.; et al. Genetic Variation in Choline-Metabolizing Enzymes Alters Choline Metabolism in Young Women Consuming Choline Intakes Meeting Current Recommendations. *Int. J. Mol. Sci.* **2017**, *18*, 252. [CrossRef]

26. da Costa, K.A.; Kozyreva, O.G.; Song, J.; Galanko, J.A.; Fischer, L.M.; Zeisel, S.H. Common genetic polymorphisms affect the human requirement for the nutrient choline. *FASEB J.* **2006**, *20*, 1336–1344. [CrossRef]

27. Resseguie, M.E.; da Costa, K.-A.; Galanko, J.A.; Patel, M.; Davis, I.J.; Zeisel, S.H. Aberrant Estrogen Regulation of PEMT Results in Choline Deficiency-associated Liver Dysfunction. *J. Biol. Chem.* **2011**, *286*, 1649–1658. [CrossRef]

28. Brunst, K.J.; Wright, R.O.; DiGioia, K.; Enlow, M.B.; Fernandez, H.; Wright, R.J.; Kannan, S. Racial/ethnic and sociodemographic factors associated with micronutrient intakes and inadequacies among pregnant women in an urban US population. *Public Health Nutr.* **2014**, *17*, 1960–1970. [CrossRef]

29. Bell, C.; Aujla, J. Prenatal vitamins deficient in recommended Choline intake for pregnant women. *J. Fam. Med. Dis. Prev.* **2016**, *2*, 048. [CrossRef]

30. Caudill, M.A. Pre- and postnatal health: Evidence of increased choline needs. *J. Am. Diet. Assoc.* **2010**, *110*, 1198–1206. [CrossRef]

31. Zeisel, S.H.; Epstein, M.F.; Wurtman, R.J. Elevated choline concentration in neonatal plasma. *Life Sci.* **1980**, *26*, 1827–1831. [CrossRef]

32. Blusztajn, J.K.; Zeisel, S.H.; Wurtman, R.J. Synthesis of lecithin (phosphatidylcholine) from phosphatidylethanolamine in bovine brain. *Brain Res.* **1979**, *179*, 319–327. [CrossRef]

33. Gwee, M.C.; Sim, M.K. Free choline concentration and cephalin-N-methyltransferase activity in the maternal and foetal liver and placenta of pregnant rats. *Clin. Exp. Pharmacol. Physiol.* **1978**, *5*, 649–653. [CrossRef]

34. Gwee, M.C.; Sim, M.K. Changes in the concentration of free choline and cephalin-N-methyltransferase activity of the rat material and foetal liver and placeta during gestation and of the maternal and neonatal liver in the early postpartum period. *Clin. Exp. Pharmacol. Physiol.* **1979**, *6*, 259–265. [CrossRef]

35. Zeisel, S.H.; Mar, M.H.; Zhou, Z.; da Costa, K.A. Pregnancy and lactation are associated with diminished concentrations of choline and its metabolites in rat liver. *J. Nutr.* **1995**, *125*, 3049–3054. [CrossRef]

36. Sweiry, J.H.; Page, K.R.; Dacke, C.G.; Abramovich, D.R.; Yudilevich, D.L. Evidence of saturable uptake mechanisms at maternal and fetal sides of the perfused human placenta by rapid paired-tracer dilution: Studies with calcium and choline. *J. Dev. Physiol.* **1986**, *8*, 435–445.

37. Chao, C.K.; Pomfret, E.A.; Zeisel, S.H. Uptake of choline by rat mammary-gland epithelial cells. *Biochem. J.* **1988**, *254*, 33–38. [CrossRef]

38. Meck, W.H.; Smith, R.A.; Williams, C.L. Pre- and postnatal choline supplementation produces long-term facilitation of spatial memory. *Dev. Psychobiol.* **1988**, *21*, 339–353. [CrossRef]

39. Albright, C.D.; Friedrich, C.B.; Brown, E.C.; Mar, M.H.; Zeisel, S.H. Maternal dietary choline availability alters mitosis, apoptosis and the localization of TOAD-64 protein in the developing fetal rat septum. *Brain Res. Dev. Brain Res.* **1999**, *115*, 123–129. [CrossRef]

40. Craciunescu, C.N.; Albright, C.D.; Mar, M.H.; Song, J.; Zeisel, S.H. Choline availability during embryonic development alters progenitor cell mitosis in developing mouse hippocampus. *J. Nutr.* **2003**, *133*, 3614–3618. [CrossRef]

41. Glenn, M.J.; Gibson, E.M.; Kirby, E.D.; Mellott, T.J.; Blusztajn, J.K.; Williams, C.L. Prenatal choline availability modulates hippocampal neurogenesis and neurogenic responses to enriching experiences in adult female rats. *Eur. J. Neurosci.* **2007**, *25*, 2473–2482. [CrossRef]

42. Tees, R.C.; Mohammadi, E. The effects of neonatal choline dietary supplementation on adult spatial and configural learning and memory in rats. *Dev. Psychobiol.* **1999**, *35*, 226–240. [CrossRef]

43. Mellott, T.J.; Williams, C.L.; Meck, W.H.; Blusztajn, J.K. Prenatal choline supplementation advances hippocampal development and enhances MAPK and CREB activation. *FASEB J.* **2004**, *18*, 545–547. [CrossRef]

44. Pyapali, G.K.; Turner, D.A.; Williams, C.L.; Meck, W.H.; Swartzwelder, H.S. Prenatal dietary choline supplementation decreases the threshold for induction of long-term potentiation in young adult rats. *J. Neurophysiol.* **1998**, *79*, 1790–1796. [CrossRef]

45. Jones, J.P.; Meck, W.H.; Williams, C.L.; Wilson, W.A.; Swartzwelder, H.S. Choline availability to the developing rat fetus alters adult hippocampal long-term potentiation. *Brain Res. Dev. Brain Res.* **1999**, *118*, 159–167. [CrossRef]

46. Trujillo-Gonzalez, I.; Wang, Y.; Friday, W.B.; Vickers, K.C.; Toth, C.L.; Molina-Torres, L.; Surzenko, N.; Zeisel, S.H. microRNA-129-5p is regulated by choline availability and controls EGF receptor synthesis and neurogenesis in the cerebral cortex. *FASEB J.* **2018**. [CrossRef]

47. Wang, Y.; Surzenko, N.; Friday, W.B.; Zeisel, S.H. Maternal dietary intake of choline in mice regulates development of the cerebral cortex in the offspring. *FASEB J.* **2016**, *30*, 1566–1578. [CrossRef]
48. Sandstrom, N.J.; Loy, R.; Williams, C.L. Prenatal choline supplementation increases NGF levels in the hippocampus and frontal cortex of young and adult rats. *Brain Res.* **2002**, *947*, 9–16. [CrossRef]
49. Mudd, A.T.; Getty, C.M.; Dilger, R.N. Maternal Dietary Choline Status Influences Brain Gray and White Matter Development in Young Pigs. *Curr. Dev. Nutr.* **2018**, *2*, nzy015. [CrossRef]
50. Boeke, C.E.; Gillman, M.W.; Hughes, M.D.; Rifas-Shiman, S.L.; Villamor, E.; Oken, E. Choline intake during pregnancy and child cognition at age 7 years. *Am. J. Epidemiol.* **2013**, *177*, 1338–1347. [CrossRef]
51. Surzenko, N.; Trujillo-González, I.; Zeisel, S.H. Low Intake of Choline During Pregnancy Leads to Aberrant Retinal Architecture and Poor Visual Function in the Offspring. *FASEB J.* **2016**, *30*, 679. [CrossRef]
52. Mudd, A.T.; Alexander, L.S.; Johnson, S.K.; Getty, C.M.; Malysheva, O.V.; Caudill, M.A.; Dilger, R.N. Perinatal Dietary Choline Deficiency in Sows Influences Concentrations of Choline Metabolites, Fatty Acids, and Amino Acids in Milk throughout Lactation. *J. Nutr.* **2016**, *146*, 2216–2223. [CrossRef]
53. Nilsson, T.K.; Hurtig-Wennlof, A.; Sjostrom, M.; Herrmann, W.; Obeid, R.; Owen, J.R.; Zeisel, S. Plasma 1-carbon metabolites and academic achievement in 15-yr-old adolescents. *FASEB J.* **2016**, *30*, 1683–1688. [CrossRef]
54. Cheatham, C.L.; Goldman, B.D.; Fischer, L.M.; da Costa, K.A.; Reznick, J.S.; Zeisel, S.H. Phosphatidylcholine supplementation in pregnant women consuming moderate-choline diets does not enhance infant cognitive function: A randomized, double-blind, placebo-controlled trial. *Am. J. Clin. Nutr.* **2012**, *96*, 1465–1472. [CrossRef]
55. Caudill, M.A.; Strupp, B.J.; Muscalu, L.; Nevins, J.E.H.; Canfield, R.L. Maternal choline supplementation during the third trimester of pregnancy improves infant information processing speed: A randomized, double-blind, controlled feeding study. *FASEB J.* **2018**, *32*, 2172–2180. [CrossRef]
56. Bernhard, W.; Poets, C.F.; Franz, A.R. Choline and choline-related nutrients in regular and preterm infant growth. *Eur. J. Nutr.* **2018**. [CrossRef]
57. Spector, A.A.; Kim, H.Y. Discovery of essential fatty acids. *J. Lipid Res.* **2015**, *56*, 11–21. [CrossRef]
58. Burr, G.O.; Burr, M.M. A new deficiency disease produced by the rigid exclusion of fat from the diet. *J. Biol. Chem.* **1929**, *82*, 345–367. [CrossRef]
59. Burr, G.O.; Burr, M.M. On the nature and role of the fatty acids essential in nutrition. *J. Biol. Chem.* **1930**, *86*, 587–621. [CrossRef]
60. Burr, G.O.; Burr, M.M.; Miller, E.S. On the fatty acids essential in nutrition. III. *J. Biol. Chem.* **1932**, *97*, 1–9.
61. Wesson, L.G.; Burr, G.O. The metabolic rate and respiratory quotients of rats on a fat-deficient diet. *J. Biol. Chem.* **1931**, *91*, 525–539.
62. Klenk, E.; Mohrhauer, H. Studies on the metabolism of polyenoic fatty acids in the rat. *Hoppe Seylers Z. Physiol. Chem.* **1960**, *320*, 218–232. [CrossRef] [PubMed]
63. Anderson, R.E.; Benolken, R.M.; Dudley, P.A.; Landis, D.J.; Wheeler, T.G. Proceedings: Polyunsaturated fatty acids of photoreceptor membranes. *Exp. Eye Res.* **1974**, *18*, 205–213. [CrossRef]
64. Benolken, R.M.; Anderson, R.E.; Wheeler, T.G. Membrane fatty acids associated with the electrical response in visual excitation. *Science* **1973**, *182*, 1253–1254. [CrossRef]
65. Cotman, C.; Blank, M.L.; Moehl, A.; Snyder, F. Lipid composition of synaptic plasma membranes isolated from rat brain by zonal centrifugation. *Biochemistry* **1969**, *8*, 4606–4612. [CrossRef]
66. Caldwell, M.D.; Jonsson, H.T.; Othersen, H.B., Jr. Essential fatty acid deficiency in an infant receiving prolonged parenteral alimentation. *J. Pediatr.* **1972**, *81*, 894–898. [CrossRef]
67. Collins, F.D.; Sinclair, A.J.; Royle, J.P.; Coats, D.A.; Maynard, A.T.; Leonard, R.F. Plasma lipids in human linoleic acid deficiency. *Nutr. Metab.* **1971**, *13*, 150–167. [CrossRef]
68. Holman, R.T.; Johnson, S.B.; Hatch, T.F. A case of human linolenic acid deficiency involving neurological abnormalities. *Am. J. Clin. Nutr.* **1982**, *35*, 617–623. [CrossRef]
69. Postuma, R.; Pease, P.W.; Watts, R.; Taylor, S.; McEvoy, F.A. Essential fatty acid deficiency in infants receiving parenteral nutrition. *J. Pediatr. Surg.* **1978**, *13*, 393–398. [CrossRef]
70. Tashiro, T.; Ogata, H.; Yokoyama, H.; Mashima, Y.; Itoh, K. The effect of fat emulsion (Intralipid) on essential fatty acid deficiency in infants receiving intravenous alimentation. *J. Pediatr. Surg.* **1976**, *11*, 505–515. [CrossRef]
71. Carlson, S.E.; Colombo, J. Docosahexaenoic Acid and Arachidonic Acid Nutrition in Early Development. *Adv. Pediatr.* **2016**, *63*, 453–471. [CrossRef]

72. Svennerholm, L.; Vanier, M.T. The distribution of lipids in the human nervous system. 3. Fatty acid composition of phosphoglycerides of human foetal and infant brain. *Brain Res.* **1973**, *50*, 341–351. [CrossRef]

73. Dyall, S.C.; Michael, G.J.; Michael-Titus, A.T. Omega-3 fatty acids reverse age-related decreases in nuclear receptors and increase neurogenesis in old rats. *J. Neurosci. Res.* **2010**, *88*, 2091–2102. [CrossRef]

74. Janssen, C.I.; Zerbi, V.; Mutsaers, M.P.; de Jong, B.S.; Wiesmann, M.; Arnoldussen, I.A.; Geenen, B.; Heerschap, A.; Muskiet, F.A.; Jouni, Z.E.; et al. Impact of dietary n-3 polyunsaturated fatty acids on cognition, motor skills and hippocampal neurogenesis in developing C57BL/6J mice. *J. Nutr. Biochem.* **2015**, *26*, 24–35. [CrossRef]

75. Kodas, E.; Galineau, L.; Bodard, S.; Vancassel, S.; Guilloteau, D.; Besnard, J.C.; Chalon, S. Serotoninergic neurotransmission is affected by n-3 polyunsaturated fatty acids in the rat. *J. Neurochem.* **2004**, *89*, 695–702. [CrossRef]

76. Cao, D.; Kevala, K.; Kim, J.; Moon, H.S.; Jun, S.B.; Lovinger, D.; Kim, H.Y. Docosahexaenoic acid promotes hippocampal neuronal development and synaptic function. *J. Neurochem.* **2009**, *111*, 510–521. [CrossRef]

77. Lauritzen, L.; Brambilla, P.; Mazzocchi, A.; Harslof, L.B.; Ciappolino, V.; Agostoni, C. DHA Effects in Brain Development and Function. *Nutrients* **2016**, *8*, 6. [CrossRef]

78. Muskiet, F.A.; Fokkema, M.R.; Schaafsma, A.; Boersma, E.R.; Crawford, M.A. Is Docosahexaenoic Acid (DHA) Essential? Lessons from DHA Status Regulation, Our Ancient Diet, Epidemiology and Randomized Controlled Trials. *J. Nutr.* **2004**, *134*, 183–186. [CrossRef]

79. Ehringer, W.; Belcher, D.; Wassall, S.R.; Stillwell, W. A comparison of the effects of linolenic (18:3 omega 3) and docosahexaenoic (22:6 omega 3) acids on phospholipid bilayers. *Chem. Phys. Lipids* **1990**, *54*, 79–88. [CrossRef]

80. Jenski, L.J.; Sturdevant, L.K.; Ehringer, W.D.; Stillwell, W. Omega-3 fatty acid modification of membrane structure and function. I. Dietary manipulation of tumor cell susceptibility to cell- and complement-mediated lysis. *Nutr. Cancer* **1993**, *19*, 135–146. [CrossRef]

81. Stillwell, W.; Ehringer, W.; Jenski, L.J. Docosahexaenoic acid increases permeability of lipid vesicles and tumor cells. *Lipids* **1993**, *28*, 103–108. [CrossRef]

82. Stillwell, W.; Jenski, L.J.; Crump, F.T.; Ehringer, W. Effect of docosahexaenoic acid on mouse mitochondrial membrane properties. *Lipids* **1997**, *32*, 497–506. [CrossRef]

83. Stillwell, W.; Wassall, S.R. Docosahexaenoic acid: Membrane properties of a unique fatty acid. *Chem. Phys. Lipids* **2003**, *126*, 1–27. [CrossRef]

84. Lee, A.G.; East, J.M.; Froud, R.J. Are essential fatty acids essential for membrane function? *Prog. Lipid Res.* **1986**, *25*, 41–46. [CrossRef]

85. Stubbs, C.D.; Smith, A.D. The modification of mammalian membrane polyunsaturated fatty acid composition in relation to membrane fluidity and function. *Biochim. Biophys. Acta* **1984**, *779*, 89–137. [CrossRef]

86. Uauy, R.; Mena, P.; Rojas, C. Essential fatty acids in early life: Structural and functional role. *Proc. Nutr. Soc.* **2000**, *59*, 3–15. [CrossRef]

87. Wheeler, T.G.; Benolken, R.M.; Anderson, R.E. Visual membranes: Specificity of fatty acid precursors for the electrical response to illumination. *Science* **1975**, *188*, 1312–1314. [CrossRef]

88. Knott, E.J.; Gordon, W.C.; Jun, B.; Do, K.; Bazan, N.G. Retinal Pigment Epithelium and Photoreceptor Preconditioning Protection Requires Docosanoid Signaling. *Cell. Mol. Neurobiol.* **2018**, *38*, 901–917. [CrossRef]

89. Shindou, H.; Koso, H.; Sasaki, J.; Nakanishi, H.; Sagara, H.; Nakagawa, K.M.; Takahashi, Y.; Hishikawa, D.; Iizuka-Hishikawa, Y.; Tokumasu, F.; et al. Docosahexaenoic acid preserves visual function by maintaining correct disc morphology in retinal photoreceptor cells. *J. Biol. Chem.* **2017**, *292*, 12054–12064. [CrossRef]

90. Gong, J.; Rosner, B.; Rees, D.G.; Berson, E.L.; Weigel-DiFranco, C.A.; Schaefer, E.J. Plasma docosahexaenoic acid levels in various genetic forms of retinitis pigmentosa. *Investig. Ophthalmol. Vis. Sci.* **1992**, *33*, 2596–2602.

91. Singh, M. Essential Fatty Acids, DHA and Human Brain. *Indian J. Pediatr.* **2005**, *72*, 239–242. [CrossRef]

92. Minihane, A.M. Impact of Genotype on EPA and DHA Status and Responsiveness to Increased Intakes. *Nutrients* **2016**, *8*, 123. [CrossRef]

93. de la Garza Puentes, A.; Montes Goyanes, R.; Chisaguano Tonato, A.M.; Torres-Espinola, F.J.; Arias Garcia, M.; de Almeida, L.; Bonilla Aguirre, M.; Guerendiain, M.; Castellote Bargallo, A.I.; Segura Moreno, M.; et al. Association of maternal weight with FADS and ELOVL genetic variants and fatty acid levels- The PREOBE follow-up. *PLoS ONE* **2017**, *12*, e0179135. [CrossRef]

94. Gonzalez-Casanova, I.; Rzehak, P.; Stein, A.D.; Garcia Feregrino, R.; Rivera Dommarco, J.A.; Barraza-Villarreal, A.; Demmelmair, H.; Romieu, I.; Villalpando, S.; Martorell, R.; et al. Maternal single nucleotide polymorphisms in the fatty acid desaturase 1 and 2 coding regions modify the impact of prenatal supplementation with DHA on birth weight. *Am. J. Clin. Nutr.* **2016**, *103*, 1171–1178. [CrossRef]
95. Xie, L.; Innis, S.M. Genetic variants of the FADS1 FADS2 gene cluster are associated with altered (n-6) and (n-3) essential fatty acids in plasma and erythrocyte phospholipids in women during pregnancy and in breast milk during lactation. *J. Nutr.* **2008**, *138*, 2222–2228. [CrossRef]
96. Monthe-Dreze, C.; Penfield-Cyr, A.; Smid, M.C.; Sen, S. Maternal Pre-Pregnancy Obesity Attenuates Response to Omega-3 Fatty Acids Supplementation During Pregnancy. *Nutrients* **2018**, *10*, 1908. [CrossRef]
97. Bernhard, W.; Raith, M.; Koch, V.; Maas, C.; Abele, H.; Poets, C.F.; Franz, A.R. Developmental changes in polyunsaturated fetal plasma phospholipids and feto-maternal plasma phospholipid ratios and their association with bronchopulmonary dysplasia. *Eur. J. Nutr.* **2016**, *55*, 2265–2274. [CrossRef]
98. Clandinin, M.T.; Chappell, J.E.; Leong, S.; Heim, T.; Swyer, P.R.; Chance, G.W. Intrauterine fatty acid accretion rates in human brain: Implications for fatty acid requirements. *Early Hum. Dev.* **1980**, *4*, 121–129. [CrossRef]
99. van Houwelingen, A.C.; Foreman-van Drongelen, M.M.; Nicolini, U.; Nicolaides, K.H.; Al, M.D.; Kester, A.D.; Hornstra, G. Essential fatty acid status of fetal plasma phospholipids: Similar to postnatal values obtained at comparable gestational ages. *Early Hum. Dev.* **1996**, *46*, 141–152. [CrossRef]
100. Kuipers, R.S.; Luxwolda, M.F.; Offringa, P.J.; Boersma, E.R.; Dijck-Brouwer, D.A.; Muskiet, F.A. Fetal intrauterine whole body linoleic, arachidonic and docosahexaenoic acid contents and accretion rates. *Prostaglandins Leukot Essent Fat. Acids* **2012**, *86*, 13–20. [CrossRef]
101. Kuipers, R.S.; Luxwolda, M.F.; Sango, W.S.; Kwesigabo, G.; Dijck-Brouwer, D.A.; Muskiet, F.A. Maternal DHA equilibrium during pregnancy and lactation is reached at an erythrocyte DHA content of 8 g/100 g fatty acids. *J. Nutr.* **2011**, *141*, 418–427. [CrossRef]
102. Carlson, S.E.; Colombo, J.; Gajewski, B.J.; Gustafson, K.M.; Mundy, D.; Yeast, J.; Georgieff, M.K.; Markley, L.A.; Kerling, E.H.; Shaddy, D.J. DHA supplementation and pregnancy outcomes. *Am. J. Clin. Nutr.* **2013**, *97*, 808–815. [CrossRef]
103. Guesnet, P.; Alessandri, J.M. Docosahexaenoic acid (DHA) and the developing central nervous system (CNS)—Implications for dietary recommendations. *Biochimie* **2011**, *93*, 7–12. [CrossRef]
104. Rogers, L.K.; Valentine, C.J.; Keim, S.A. DHA supplementation: Current implications in pregnancy and childhood. *Pharm. Res.* **2013**, *70*, 13–19. [CrossRef]
105. Harris, W.S.; Baack, M.L. Beyond building better brains: Bridging the docosahexaenoic acid (DHA) gap of prematurity. *J. Perinatol.* **2015**, *35*, 1–7. [CrossRef]
106. Koletzko, B.; Lien, E.; Agostoni, C.; Bohles, H.; Campoy, C.; Cetin, I.; Decsi, T.; Dudenhausen, J.W.; Dupont, C.; Forsyth, S.; et al. The roles of long-chain polyunsaturated fatty acids in pregnancy, lactation and infancy: Review of current knowledge and consensus recommendations. *J. Perinat. Med.* **2008**, *36*, 5–14. [CrossRef]
107. Mulder, K.A.; Elango, R.; Innis, S.M. Fetal DHA inadequacy and the impact on child neurodevelopment: A follow-up of a randomised trial of maternal DHA supplementation in pregnancy. *Br. J. Nutr.* **2018**, *119*, 271–279. [CrossRef]
108. Rees, A.; Sirois, S.; Wearden, A. Prenatal maternal docosahexaenoic acid intake and infant information processing at 4.5 mo and 9 mo: A longitudinal study. *PLoS ONE* **2019**, *14*, e0210984. [CrossRef]
109. Maslova, E.; Rifas-Shiman, S.L.; Olsen, S.F.; Gillman, M.W.; Oken, E. Prenatal n-3 long-chain fatty acid status and offspring metabolic health in early and mid-childhood: Results from Project Viva. *Nutr. Diabetes* **2018**, *8*, 29. [CrossRef]
110. Ramakrishnan, U.; Gonzalez-Casanova, I.; Schnaas, L.; DiGirolamo, A.; Quezada, A.D.; Pallo, B.C.; Hao, W.; Neufeld, L.M.; Rivera, J.A.; Stein, A.D.; et al. Prenatal supplementation with DHA improves attention at 5 y of age: A randomized controlled trial. *Am. J. Clin. Nutr.* **2016**, *104*, 1075–1082. [CrossRef]
111. Crozier, S.R.; Sibbons, C.M.; Fisk, H.L.; Godfrey, K.M.; Calder, P.C.; Gale, C.R.; Robinson, S.M.; Inskip, H.M.; Baird, J.; Harvey, N.C.; et al. Arachidonic acid and DHA status in pregnant women is not associated with cognitive performance of their children at 4 or 6–7 years. *Br. J. Nutr.* **2018**, *119*, 1400–1407. [CrossRef]
112. Hoffman, D.R.; Theuer, R.C.; Castañeda, Y.S.; Wheaton, D.H.; Bosworth, R.G.; O'Connor, A.R.; Morale, S.E.; Wiedemann, L.E.; Birch, E.E. Maturation of visual acuity is accelerated in breast-fed term infants fed baby food containing DHA-enriched egg yolk. *J. Nutr.* **2004**, *134*, 2307–2313. [CrossRef]

113. Meldrum, S.J.; D'Vaz, N.; Simmer, K.; Dunstan, J.A.; Hird, K.; Prescott, S.L. Effects of high-dose fish oil supplementation during early infancy on neurodevelopment and language: A randomised controlled trial. *Br. J. Nutr.* **2012**, *108*, 1443–1454. [CrossRef]

114. Treen, M.; Uauy, R.D.; Jameson, D.M.; Thomas, V.L.; Hoffman, D.R. Effect of docosahexaenoic acid on membrane fluidity and function in intact cultured Y-79 retinoblastoma cells. *Arch. Biochem. Biophys.* **1992**, *294*, 564–570. [CrossRef]

115. Hyman, B.T.; Spector, A.A. Choline uptake in cultured human Y79 retinoblastoma cells: Effect of polyunsaturated fatty acid compositional modifications. *J. Neurochem.* **1982**, *38*, 650–656. [CrossRef]

116. Machova, E.; Novakova, J.; Lisa, V.; Dolezal, V. Docosahexaenoic acid supports cell growth and expression of choline acetyltransferase and muscarinic receptors in NG108-15 cell line. *J. Mol. Neurosci.* **2006**, *30*, 25–26. [CrossRef]

117. Machova, E.; Malkova, B.; Lisa, V.; Novakova, J.; Dolezal, V. The increase of choline acetyltransferase activity by docosahexaenoic acid in NG108-15 cells grown in serum-free medium is independent of its effect on cell growth. *Neurochem. Res.* **2006**, *31*, 1239–1246. [CrossRef]

118. da Costa, K.-A.; Rai, K.S.; Craciunescu, C.N.; Parikh, K.; Mehedint, M.G.; Sanders, L.M.; McLean-Pottinger, A.; Zeisel, S.H. Dietary Docosahexaenoic Acid Supplementation Modulates Hippocampal Development in the Pemt−/− Mouse. *J. Biol. Chem.* **2010**, *285*, 1008–1015. [CrossRef]

119. Pynn, C.J.; Henderson, N.G.; Clark, H.; Koster, G.; Bernhard, W.; Postle, A.D. Specificity and rate of human and mouse liver and plasma phosphatidylcholine synthesis analyzed in vivo. *J. Lipid Res.* **2011**, *52*, 399–407. [CrossRef]

120. van Deijk, A.F.; Broersen, L.M.; Verkuyl, J.M.; Smit, A.B.; Verheijen, M.H.G. High Content Analysis of Hippocampal Neuron-Astrocyte Co-cultures Shows a Positive Effect of Fortasyn Connect on Neuronal Survival and Postsynaptic Maturation. *Front. Neurosci.* **2017**, *11*, 440. [CrossRef]

121. Fourrier, C.; Remus-Borel, J.; Greenhalgh, A.D.; Guichardant, M.; Bernoud-Hubac, N.; Lagarde, M.; Joffre, C.; Laye, S. Docosahexaenoic acid-containing choline phospholipid modulates LPS-induced neuroinflammation in vivo and in microglia in vitro. *J. Neuroinflam.* **2017**, *14*, 170. [CrossRef]

122. Almeida, P.M.D.; Kamath, S.U.; Shenoy, P.R.; Bernhardt, L.K.; Kishore, A.; Rai, K.S. Persistent attenuation of brain oxidative stress through aging in perinatal maternal separated rat pups supplemented with choline and docosahexaenoic acid or Clitoria ternatea aqueous root extract. *Folia Neuropathol.* **2018**, *56*, 206–214. [CrossRef]

123. van Wijk, N.; Balvers, M.; Cansev, M.; Maher, T.J.; Sijben, J.W.; Broersen, L.M. Dietary Crude Lecithin Increases Systemic Availability of Dietary Docosahexaenoic Acid with Combined Intake in Rats. *Lipids* **2016**, *51*, 833–846. [CrossRef]

124. Rajarethnem, H.T.; Megur Ramakrishna Bhat, K.; Jc, M.; Kumar Gopalkrishnan, S.; Mugundhu Gopalram, R.B.; Rai, K.S. Combined Supplementation of Choline and Docosahexaenoic Acid during Pregnancy Enhances Neurodevelopment of Fetal Hippocampus. *Neurol Res. Int.* **2017**, *2017*, 8748706. [CrossRef]

125. Zicker, S.C.; Jewell, D.E.; Yamka, R.M.; Milgram, N.W. Evaluation of cognitive learning, memory, psychomotor, immunologic, and retinal functions in healthy puppies fed foods fortified with docosahexaenoic acid-rich fish oil from 8 to 52 weeks of age. *J. Am. Vet. Med. Assoc.* **2012**, *241*, 583–594. [CrossRef]

126. Lima, H.K.; Lin, X.; Jacobi, S.K.; Man, C.; Sommer, J.; Flowers, W.; Blikslager, A.; Gonzalez, L.; Odle, J. Supplementation of Maternal Diets with Docosahexaenoic Acid and Methylating Vitamins Impacts Growth and Development of Fetuses from Malnourished Gilts. *Curr. Dev. Nutr.* **2018**, *2*, nzx006. [CrossRef]

127. Kwan, S.T.C.; King, J.H.; Yan, J.; Wang, Z.; Jiang, X.; Hutzler, J.S.; Klein, H.R.; Brenna, J.T.; Roberson, M.S.; Caudill, M.A. Maternal Choline Supplementation Modulates Placental Nutrient Transport and Metabolism in Late Gestation of Mouse Pregnancy. *J. Nutr.* **2017**, *147*, 2083–2092. [CrossRef]

128. Maas, C.; Franz, A.R.; Shunova, A.; Mathes, M.; Bleeker, C.; Poets, C.F.; Schleicher, E.; Bernhard, W. Choline and polyunsaturated fatty acids in preterm infants' maternal milk. *Eur. J. Nutr.* **2017**, *56*, 1733–1742. [CrossRef]

129. Ferre, C.; Callaghan, W.; Olson, C.; Sharma, A.; Barfield, W. Effects of Maternal Age and Age-Specific Preterm Birth Rates on Overall Preterm Birth Rates—United States, 2007 and 2014. *Mmwr. Morb. Mortal. Wkly. Rep.* **2016**, *65*, 1181–1184. [CrossRef]

130. Institute of Medicine Committee on Understanding Premature Birth; Assuring Healthy Outcomes. The National Academies Collection: Reports funded by National Institutes of Health. In *Preterm Birth: Causes, Consequences, and Prevention*; Behrman, R.E., Butler, A.S., Eds.; National Academies Press (US), National Academy of Sciences: Washington, DC, USA, 2007. [CrossRef]

131. Bernhard, W.; Böckmann, K.; Maas, C.; Mathes, M.; Hovelmann, J.; Shunova, A.; Hund, V.; Schleicher, E.; Poets, C.F.; Franz, A.R. Combined choline and DHA supplementation: A randomized controlled trial. *Eur. J. Nutr.* **2019**. [CrossRef]

132. West, A.A.; Yan, J.; Jiang, X.; Perry, C.A.; Innis, S.M.; Caudill, M.A. Choline intake influences phosphatidylcholine DHA enrichment in nonpregnant women but not in pregnant women in the third trimester. *Am. J. Clin. Nutr.* **2013**, *97*, 718–727. [CrossRef]

133. West, A.A.; Shih, Y.; Wang, W.; Oda, K.; Jaceldo-Siegl, K.; Sabate, J.; Haddad, E.; Rajaram, S.; Caudill, M.A.; Burns-Whitmore, B. Egg n-3 fatty acid composition modulates biomarkers of choline metabolism in free-living lacto-ovo-vegetarian women of reproductive age. *J. Acad. Nutr. Diet.* **2014**, *114*, 1594–1600. [CrossRef]

134. da Costa, K.A.; Sanders, L.M.; Fischer, L.M.; Zeisel, S.H. Docosahexaenoic acid in plasma phosphatidylcholine may be a potential marker for in vivo phosphatidylethanolamine N-methyltransferase activity in humans. *Am. J. Clin. Nutr.* **2011**, *93*, 968–974. [CrossRef]

135. McNamara, R.K.; Jandacek, R.; Tso, P.; Weber, W.; Chu, W.J.; Strakowski, S.M.; Adler, C.M.; Delbello, M.P. Low docosahexaenoic acid status is associated with reduced indices in cortical integrity in the anterior cingulate of healthy male children: A 1H MRS Study. *Nutr. Neurosci.* **2013**, *16*, 183–190. [CrossRef]

136. Cheatham, C.L.; Sheppard, K.W. Synergistic Effects of Human Milk Nutrients in the Support of Infant Recognition Memory: An Observational Study. *Nutrients* **2015**, *7*, 9079–9095. [CrossRef]

137. Jackson, K.H.; Harris, W.S. A Prenatal DHA Test to Help Identify Women at Increased Risk for Early Preterm Birth: A Proposal. *Nutrients* **2018**, *10*, 1933. [CrossRef]

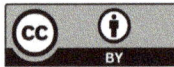

![nutrients logo] *nutrients*

MDPI

Article

Maternal Choline Supplementation Modulates Placental Markers of Inflammation, Angiogenesis, and Apoptosis in a Mouse Model of Placental Insufficiency

Julia H. King [1], Sze Ting (Cecilia) Kwan [1], Jian Yan [1], Xinyin Jiang [1,2], Vladislav G. Fomin [1], Samantha P. Levine [1], Emily Wei [1], Mark S. Roberson [3,*] and Marie A. Caudill [1,*]

[1] Division of Nutritional Sciences, Cornell University, Ithaca, NY 14850, USA; jhk288@cornell.edu (J.H.K.); sk2563@cornell.edu (S.T.K.); jy435@cornell.edu (J.Y.); XinyinJiang@brooklyn.cuny.edu (X.J.); vgf6@cornell.edu (V.G.F.); spl63@cornell.edu (S.P.L.); ew376@cornell.edu (E.W.)
[2] Department of Health and Nutrition Sciences, Brooklyn College, Brooklyn, NY 11210, USA
[3] Department of Biomedical Sciences, Cornell University, Ithaca, NY 14850, USA
* Correspondence: msr14@cornell.edu (M.S.R.); mac379@cornell.edu (M.A.C.); Tel.: +1-607-253-3336 (M.S.R.); +1-607-254-7456 (M.A.C.)

Received: 7 December 2018; Accepted: 5 February 2019; Published: 12 February 2019

Abstract: *Dlx3* (distal-less homeobox 3) haploinsufficiency in mice has been shown to result in restricted fetal growth and placental defects. We previously showed that maternal choline supplementation (4X versus 1X choline) in the *Dlx3*+/− mouse increased fetal and placental growth in mid-gestation. The current study sought to test the hypothesis that prenatal choline would modulate indicators of placenta function and development. Pregnant *Dlx3*+/− mice consuming 1X (control), 2X, or 4X choline from conception were sacrificed at embryonic (E) days E10.5, E12.5, E15.5, and E18.5, and placentas and embryos were harvested. Data were analyzed separately for each gestational day controlling for litter size, fetal genotype (except for models including only +/− pups), and fetal sex (except when data were stratified by this variable). 4X choline tended to increase ($p < 0.1$) placental labyrinth size at E10.5 and decrease ($p < 0.05$) placental apoptosis at E12.5. Choline supplementation decreased ($p < 0.05$) expression of pro-angiogenic genes *Eng* (E10.5, E12.5, and E15.5), and *Vegf* (E12.5, E15.5); and pro-inflammatory genes *Il1b* (at E15.5 and 18.5), *Tnfα* (at E12.5) and *Nfκb* (at E15.5) in a fetal sex-dependent manner. These findings provide support for a modulatory effect of maternal choline supplementation on biomarkers of placental function and development in a mouse model of placental insufficiency.

Keywords: choline; Dlx3; placenta; placental insufficiency; inflammation; angiogenesis; apoptosis

---

1. Introduction

Abnormal placental development underlies many pathologies of pregnancy including preeclampsia, intrauterine growth restriction (IUGR), and spontaneous abortion [1]. These conditions have serious consequences for the mother and fetus, and few treatments are currently available for their prevention or treatment.

Although the etiology of placental insufficiency is not fully understood, an imbalance of pro- and anti-angiogenic and inflammatory factors may contribute to it [1,2]. The development of the placenta requires extensive angiogenesis and vasculogenesis, and the maternal uterine spiral arteries must be invaded and remodeled by extravillous trophoblasts to allow for increased blood flow to the fetus [3]. This process requires adequate expression of angiogenic and remodeling genes including the vascular endothelial growth factor (VEGF) family. Inadequate trophoblast invasion is a characteristic of many placental pathologies. When this process is incomplete, blood flow to the placenta is compromised, and oxygen supply may be sporadic, leading to placental injury from hypoxia/reoxygenation. Oxidative stress, excessive apoptosis, and inflammation result, compromising trophoblast function and preventing efficient transfer of nutrients [4]. Anti-angiogenic factors in the maternal circulation, including soluble fms-like tyrosine kinase-1 (sFlt-1) and soluble endoglin (sEng), may contribute to the pathogenesis of preeclampsia symptoms including hypertension and proteinuria, and can be used as biomarkers or predictors of risk when measured in early gestation [5,6]. Together, these dysregulated processes interact to contribute to the pathogenesis of placental disorders such as preeclampsia and IUGR.

The essential nutrient choline is required for the synthesis of the neurotransmitter acetylcholine, the membrane phospholipid phosphatidylcholine, and the methyl donor and osmolyte betaine [7]. These biomolecules have crucial roles in supporting pregnancy via their effects on cell growth, DNA methylation, and signaling processes [8]. Choline has previously been shown to reduce levels of sFlt-1 in a randomized dietary intervention trial of maternal choline supplementation during the third trimester of pregnancy in healthy women [9]. Further, choline deficiency has been shown to increase inflammation and apoptotic processes in a cell culture model of human placental trophoblasts [10]; meanwhile, supplementing the maternal diet with additional choline decreases biomarkers of both processes in wildtype mouse placenta [11]. We, thus, hypothesized that choline supplementation would be beneficial for pregnancies complicated by placental insufficiency.

Dlx3 (distal-less homeobox 3) haploinsufficiency in mice has been shown to result in restricted fetal growth and placental defects [12]. This homeodomain-containing transcription factor is required for the development of the maternal–fetal interface [13]. Placentas lacking one copy of this gene display inadequate vascularization and abnormal development of the placental labyrinth [12], which is the area of nutrient exchange between the mother and fetus. Heterozygous embryos are viable but their placentas display abnormalities including impaired remodeling of maternal spiral arteries as well as increased placental oxidative stress and apoptosis [12]. In mice that are homozygous null for *Dlx3*, placental failure occurs between embryonic days 9.5–12.5 resulting in extremely restricted fetal growth and subsequently death [13]. Notably, we have previously shown that maternal choline supplementation (4X versus 1X choline) in *Dlx3*+/− dams increases fetal weights during mid-gestation in wildtype, heterozygous, and null embryos [14]. Most important to this body of work is the evidence supporting a role of DLX3 in human placental insufficiency (reviewed in Reference [15]).

In the present study, we sought to use the *Dlx3*+/− mouse model of placental insufficiency to investigate the effects of maternal choline supplementation on biomarkers of placental function and development across gestation. To accomplish these aims, we used tissue samples that were previously collected from *Dlx3*+/− pregnant dams randomized to consume one of three levels of choline intake [14].

2. Materials and Methods

2.1. Mice and Diets

All animal protocols and procedures used in this study were approved by the Institutional Animal Care and Use Committees at Cornell University, and were conducted in accordance with the Guide for the Care and Use of Laboratory Animals. *Dlx3*+/− mice were genotyped using tail DNA with three-primer duplex PCR (Table S1). Primers were designed to amplify a wildtype band, a knockout band, or both (indicating a heterozygote). Mice were housed in microisolator cages (Ancare, Bellmore, NY, USA) in an environmentally-controlled room (22–25 °C and 70% humidity) with a 12-hour light–dark cycle. During breeding, mice were given ad libitum access to commercial rodent chow (Teklad, Madison, WI, USA) and water. *Dlx3*+/− females were mated with *Dlx3*+/− males in a pair-wise manner, and their offspring were genotyped at time of weaning (3 weeks of age). Heterozygous pups were given ad libitum access to the 1X choline control diet containing 1.4 g choline chloride/kg (Dyets #103345). *Dlx3+/−* female mice were then randomized five days before mating with *Dlx3+/−* male mice and received either the 1X choline control diet, the 2X choline diet containing 2.8 g choline chloride/kg (Dyets #103346), or the 4X choline diet containing 5.6 g choline chloride/kg (Dyets #103347); all provided ad libitum. Embryonic (E) day 0.5 was designated via the presence of a vaginal plug. Pregnant mice were euthanized via carbon dioxide asphyxiation at four different gestational time points: E10.5, E12.5, E15.5, and E18.5.

2.2. Tissue Collection and Processing

After pregnant dams were sacrificed, embryos and placentas were carefully dissected with minimal decidual contamination and weighed. For approximately 1/3 of the litter, the implantation site was fixed in 10% formalin for histological analyses after removal of the embryo for genotyping. For the remaining placentas, at gestational time points E12.5, E15.5, and E18.5, placentas were bisected across the chorionic plate; one half was stabilized in RNAlater for mRNA analysis, while the remaining half was immediately frozen in liquid nitrogen and stored at −80 °C for metabolite analysis. Due to the smaller tissue size, E10.5 placentas were designated for mRNA analysis or metabolite analysis, alternately. Fetal DNA was extracted for *Dlx3* genotyping and sex determination using a commercial kit (Qiagen Inc., Germantown, MD, USA). Sex genotyping was performed using PCR for the *Sry* gene with a commercial kit (Qiagen Inc., Germantown, MD, USA). Primers are listed in Table S1.

2.3. Quantitative Real-Time RT-PCR

RNA was extracted from placentas maintained in RNAlater using TRIzol reagent (Invitrogen, Waltham, MA, USA). Two to three *Dlx3* heterozygous placentas per dam were randomly selected for extraction. RNA concentration and quality were assessed with a NanoDrop ND-1000 instrument (Thermo Fisher Scientific, Waltham, MA, USA), and samples with an A260/A280 ratio above 1.8 were used for quantification. Reverse transcription was performed using the ImProm-II Reverse Transcription System (Promega, Madison, WI, USA). Quantitative PCR was performed using SYBR® Green in a Roche LightCycler480 (Roche, IN, USA). All primers for the targeted genes (*Vegfa, Pgf, Eng, Mmp14, Tnfα, NfκB, Il1b*) were designed using NCBI Primer-BLAST (Table S1). Reaction conditions were as follows: 95 °C for 5 min, followed by 40 cycles for 15 s at 95 °C, 30 s annealing (see Table S1 for annealing temperatures), and 30 s at 72 °C. PCR product specificity was monitored using melting curve analysis at the end of the amplification cycles. Fold changes were calculated using the ΔCt method [16] normalized to the expression level of the housekeeping gene *Tbp* (TATA box binding protein), which has previously been shown to be stable in placental tissue [17], and in response to varying choline supply [18]. At E10.5, both wildtype and heterozygous placentas were used due to limited tissue availability, and *Dlx3* genotype was included in the statistical model. All qPCR analyses were performed in triplicate.

2.4. LC-MS/MS

Concentrations of acetylcholine were measured in the placenta using LC-MS/MS according to the method of Holm et al. [19] with modifications based on our equipment [20].

2.5. Placental Morphometry

Placental tissues fixed in 10% formalin were paraffin embedded and sectioned at 10 μm. Immunohistochemistry was performed on formalin-fixed sections as described previously [21]. For the analysis of maternal spiral artery areas, placental sections were incubated with smooth muscle actin (SMA) antibody (1:50, DakoCytomatin, Glostrup, Denmark), followed by a secondary antibody. Slides were imaged using an Aperio Scanscope (Vista, CA, USA). Maternal spiral arteries were manually defined based on the staining location and the presence of non-nucleated red blood cells. Aperio ImageScope software, version 102.0.7.5, was used to quantify the area. Data are presented as the ratio of artery luminal area to total arterial area. For the analysis of the placental labyrinth area, placental sections were incubated with biotinylated GSL 1-isolectin B4 (1:100, Vector Laboratories, Burlingame, CA, USA) and 3-amino-9-ethylcarbazole (AEC; Invitrogen, Carlsbad, CA, USA), and counterstained with hematoxylin. Isolectin is a marker of endothelial cells and has been used previously to stain vasculature in other mouse tissues. The placental labyrinth compartment was defined manually based on staining location, and area was calculated using Aperio ImageScope software (Vista, CA, USA). Data are expressed as mm^2 of cross-sectional labyrinth area.

2.6. Placental Apoptosis

Placental apoptosis was assessed using the terminal deoxynucleotidyl transferase dUTP nick end labeling (TUNEL) assay. A commercial kit (Millipore, Billerica, MA, USA) was used according to the manufacturer's instructions. Sections were imaged using an Aperio ScanScope and the number of TUNEL-positive cells was determined in the decidua and labyrinth by the average number of TUNEL-positive cells in several randomly selected fields. Field sizes were as follows: for E10.5, five fields of 250×250 μm^2; for E12.5, five fields of 350×350 μm^2; and for E15.5 and E18.5, ten fields of 500×500 μm^2.

2.7. Statistical Analysis

For all outcome variables, data were analyzed separately for each gestational day using a linear mixed model. All statistical models included choline treatment as a fixed effect, and a maternal identifier (ID) as a random effect. Litter size, fetal genotype (except for the gene expression outcomes at E12.5, E15.5, and E18.5, which only included heterozygous pups), and fetal sex (except when the data were stratified by fetal sex) were controlled for in the models as fixed effects. Normality of the data was assessed by evaluating the distribution of residuals. Due to the hypothesis-driven nature of the study and the relatively small sample sizes, corrections for multiple analyses were not performed and statistical interactions were not assessed. Data are presented as means $\pm$ SEM. $p \leq 0.05$ was considered statistically significant and $0.05 < p < 0.10$ was considered to indicate trends. All analyses were performed using SPSS software, Version 23 (IBM, Chicago, IL, USA).

3. Results

We previously reported that maternal choline supplementation increased placental and fetal weights at E10.5 in offspring of *Dlx3+/−* dams regardless of fetal genotype [14]. These data can also be found in Table S2 which depicts embryo weight, placental weight, crown rump length, placental efficiency, and litter size in *Dlx3+/−* dams in response to maternal choline intakes (1X control, 2X, and 4X) at E10.5, E12.5, E15.5, and E18.5.

3.1. Placental Morphometry

Because the *Dlx3* model is associated with labyrinth abnormalities, we sought to determine whether choline treatment increased placental weight by increasing the size of the labyrinth. At E10.5, 4X choline placentas had 73% larger labyrinth area versus 2X choline ($p = 0.014$), and tended to be ~46% larger than 1X control placentas ($p = 0.092$, Figure 1A and 1B). At E12.5 and E15.5, there were no significant differences in labyrinth size by choline treatment. At E18.5, 2X placental labyrinths were ~25% smaller compared to 1X controls ($p = 0.037$) and tended to be ~20% smaller than 4X choline placentas ($p = 0.081$, Figure 1A).

3.2. Placental Apoptosis

We performed the terminal deoxynucleotidyl transferase dUTP nick end labeling assay (TUNEL) to assess placental levels of apoptosis at all four gestational time points. At E10.5, choline treatment tended to result in ~49% lower TUNEL scores (average # TUNEL-positive cells per field) in the 4X choline placentas ($p = 0.053$ versus 1X controls) (Figure 2A). At E12.5, 4X choline placentas had ~58%

lower TUNEL scores (p = 0.048 versus 1X controls) (Figure 2A,B). No differences in TUNEL score were detected between choline treatment groups at E15.5 and E18.5 (Figure 2A).

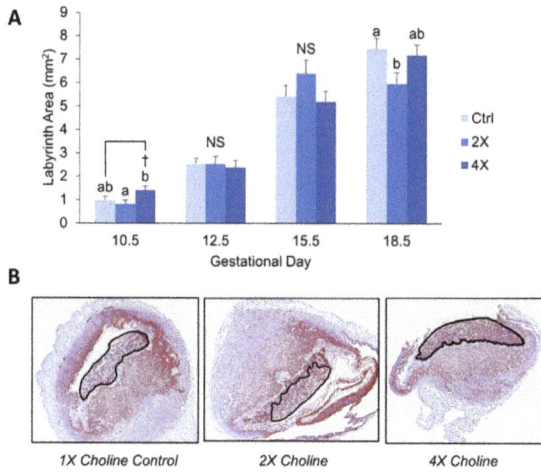

Figure 1. Placental labyrinth area at E10.5, E12.5, E15.5, and E18.5 by choline treatment (**A**). Representative images of placental labyrinths at E10.5 are shown in (**B**). Data were analyzed using mixed linear models with choline treatment as a fixed effect and maternal ID as a random effect. Litter size, fetal genotype, and fetal sex were controlled for in the models as fixed effects. Values are presented as mean ± SEM. Different letters denote significant differences between means of the treatments at $p \leq 0.05$. † denotes $p < 0.1$. n = 7–12 placentas per treatment per time point. NS, nonsignificant.

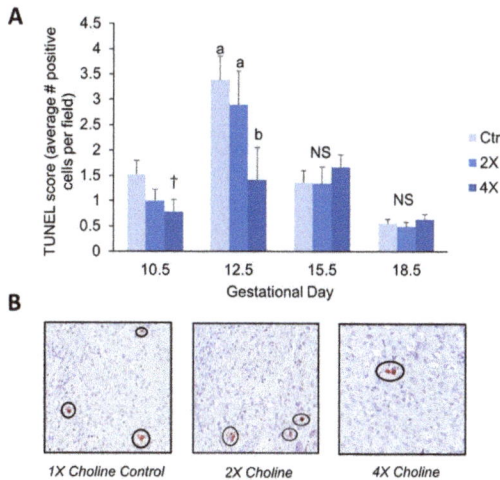

Figure 2. TUNEL score (calculated as the average number of TUNEL-positive cells per field) at E10.5, E12.5, E15.5, and E18.5 by maternal choline treatment (**A**). Representative images of TUNEL staining at E12.5 are shown in (**B**). Data were analyzed using mixed linear models with choline treatment as a fixed effect and maternal ID as a random effect. Litter size, fetal genotype, and fetal sex were controlled for in the models as fixed effects. Values are presented as mean ± SEM. Different letters denote significant differences between means of the treatments at $p \leq 0.05$. † denotes $p < 0.1$ versus 1X choline controls. n = 7–15 placentas per treatment per time point. NS, nonsignificant.

3.3. Placental Artery Remodeling

Because we had previously found an effect of maternal choline supplementation on spiral artery remodeling in wildtype mice [11], we investigated whether it would have a similar function in a model of placental insufficiency. We assessed the luminal ratio of maternal spiral arteries, defined as (luminal area)/total arterial area. Luminal ratio did not differ by choline treatment or *Dlx3* genotype at any gestational time point.

3.4. Placental Expression of Angiogenic Genes

Because altered levels of pro-angiogenic factors have been implicated in the development of preeclampsia and other pregnancy disorders, we measured mRNA expression of several key modulators of placental angiogenesis throughout pregnancy in *Dlx3*+/− placentas (Figure 3A–D). For this outcome, we stratified by fetal sex due to our previous findings showing effects of fetal sex on angiogenic gene expression [11].

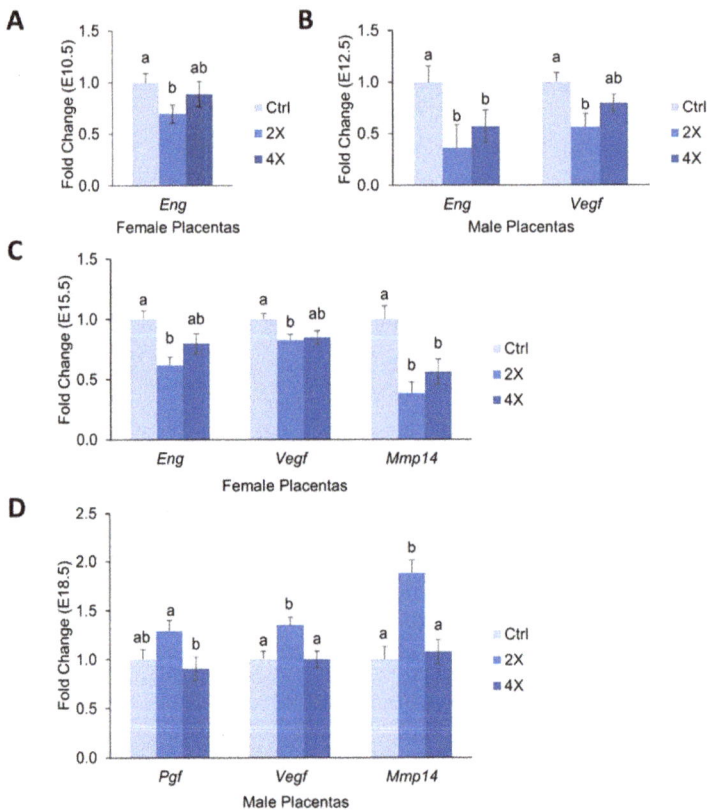

Figure 3. Placental mRNA abundance of angiogenic genes at (**A**) E10.5, (**B**) E12.5, (**C**) E15.5, and (**D**) E18.5 by maternal choline treatment. Data are expressed as the fold-change relative to the housekeeping gene *Tbp*. Data were analyzed using mixed linear models with choline treatment as a fixed effect and maternal ID as a random effect. Litter size and fetal genotype (for E10.5; heterozygous pups were used for E12.5, E15.5, and E18.5) were controlled for in the models as fixed effects. Values are presented as mean ± SEM. Different letters denote significant differences between means of the treatments at $p \leq 0.05$. $n = 20$ placentas per treatment per time point.

At E10.5, expression of *Eng* was ~31% lower in the female 2X choline placentas versus 1X controls ($p = 0.029$) (Figure 3A). No effects of choline treatment on *Eng* expression were detected for the male placentas, nor did choline treatment alter *Vegfa*, *Pgf*, or *Mmp14* expression at E10.5 in either sex.

At E12.5, 2X and 4X choline males had lower expression of *Eng* vs. 1X controls (~64% and ~43%, respectively, $p = 0.005, 0.013$) (Figure 3B). Similarly, male 2X choline placentas had ~44% lower expression of *Vegfa* ($p = 0.026$ versus 1X) (Figure 3B). No significant effects of choline treatment on these angiogenic factors were detected in females; nor did choline treatment influence *Pgf* or *Mmp14* expression at E12.5.

At E15.5, expression of *Eng* in female placentas was ~38% lower in the 2X choline group ($p = 0.002$ vs. 1X). Similarly, 2X choline female placentas had ~17% lower expression of *Vegfa* vs. 1X controls ($p = 0.031$) (Figure 3C). Expression of *Mmp14* was ~42% lower in female 2X choline placentas ($p = 0.019$, vs. 1X) and ~41% lower in 4X choline placentas ($p = 0.015$, vs. 1X) (Figure 3C). No effects of choline treatment on these angiogenic factors were detected in males; nor did choline treatment influence *Pgf* expression in either fetal sex at E15.5.

At E18.5, male placentas in the 2X choline group had ~35% higher expression of *Vegfa* versus 1X controls and 4X choline groups ($p = 0.011$ and 0.01, respectively). Similarly, expression of *Pgf* tended to be ~29% higher in 2X choline males versus 1X control males ($p = 0.091$) and was ~42% higher versus 4X choline ($p = 0.091$). Male 2X choline placentas also had ~62% higher expression of *Mmp14* versus 1X placentas ($p = 0.006$) (Figure 3D). No effects of choline treatment on these angiogenic factors were detected in females; nor did *Eng* expression differ by choline treatment at E18.5 in either fetal sex.

3.5. Placental Expression of Inflammatory Genes

Abnormal regulation of inflammation has been shown in various placental pathologies; therefore, we also measured mRNA expression of several major inflammatory regulators in the *Dlx3+/−* placentas (Figure 4A–C). Again, data were stratified by fetal sex due to our previous work showing the strong effects of fetal sex on inflammatory processes [11].

At E10.5, there were no significant differences in *Tnfα*, *Nfκb*, or *Il1b* expression among choline treatment groups. At E12.5, 2X choline male placentas had a lower expression of Tnfα (~57% versus 1X) and tended to have lower expression of *Nfκb* (~50%, $p = 0.096$ versus 1X) (Figure 4A). No effects of choline treatment on these inflammatory genes were detected in females; nor did expression of *Il1b* differ by treatment.

At E15.5, female 2X choline placentas had ~33% lower expression of *Nfκb* versus 1X controls ($p = 0.020$). Expression of *Il1b* was ~36% lower in 2X choline placentas of both sexes versus 1X controls ($p = 0.034$, Figure 4B), and also in males alone ($p = 0.031$).

At E18.5, expression of *Il1b* was ~32% lower in 4X choline pups of male and female placentas combined ($p = 0.02$) (Figure 4C), a finding that did not reach statistically significant levels in either sex alone. Female 4X choline placentas tended to have ~39% lower expression of *Nfκb* versus 1X control females ($p = 0.058$) (Figure 4C). No differences in Tnfα expression were seen among choline groups at E15.5 or E18.5.

3.6. Placental Acetylcholine

Because acetylcholine has been linked to angiogenic and inflammatory signaling in the placenta [22,23], we measured concentrations of placental acetylcholine throughout gestation. At E12.5, 2X choline placentas had ~136% higher concentrations of acetylcholine versus 1X controls ($p = 0.011$), and ~107% higher concentrations versus 4X choline placentas ($p = 0.020$). At E10.5, E15.5, and E18.5, acetylcholine concentrations did not differ by choline treatment (Figure 5).

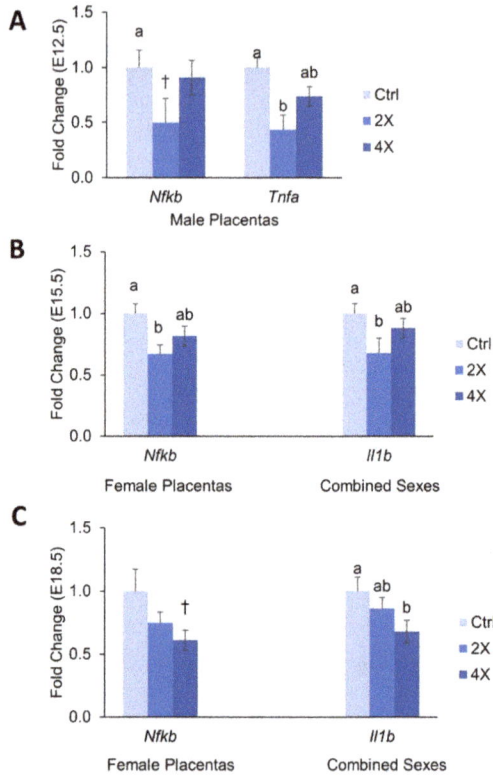

Figure 4. Placental mRNA abundance of inflammatory genes at (**A**) E12.5, (**B**) E15.5, and (**C**) E18.5 by maternal choline treatment. Data are expressed as the fold-change relative to the housekeeping gene *Tbp*. Data were analyzed using mixed linear models with choline treatment as a fixed effect and maternal ID as a random effect. Litter size and fetal genotype (for E10.5; heterozygous pups were used for E12.5, E15.5, and E18.5) were controlled for in the models as fixed effects. Values are presented as mean ± SEM. Different letters denote significant differences between means of the treatments at $p \leq 0.05$. † denotes $p < 0.1$ versus 1X choline controls. $n = 20$ placentas per treatment per time point.

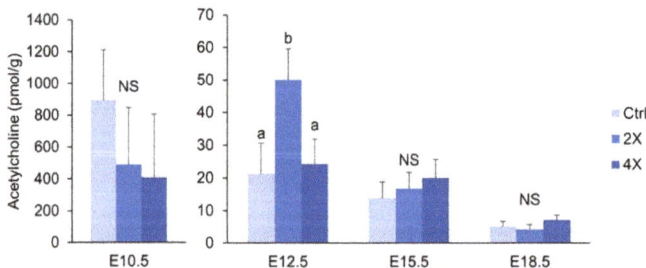

Figure 5. Placental acetylcholine concentrations (pmol/gram tissue) at E10.5, E12.5, 15.5, and 18.5 by maternal choline treatment (1X, 2X, and 4X choline). Data were analyzed using mixed linear models with choline treatment as a fixed effect and maternal ID as a random effect. Litter size, fetal genotype, and fetal sex were controlled for in the models as fixed effects. Values are presented as mean ± SEM. Different letters denote significant differences between means of the treatments at $p \leq 0.05$. $n = 20$ placentas per treatment per time point. NS, nonsignificant.

4. Discussion

4.1. Maternal Choline Supplementation in the Dlx3+/− Pregnant Dam Increases Placental Labyrinth Size and Decreases Placental Apoptosis in Mid-Gestation

Because we had previously reported a higher placental weight at E10.5 with maternal choline supplementation in *Dlx3+/−* dams [14], we sought to determine whether this effect could be explained by alterations in the size of the placental labyrinth or apoptosis levels. Development of the labyrinth region, which facilitates nutrient transfer between mother and fetus, is defective in *Dlx3−/−* animals [13]. At E10.5, a high dose of choline (4X the recommended intake) yielded a larger labyrinth size compared to the 2X choline dose, and tended to yield a larger labyrinth size compared to the 1X choline dose. Thus, an increase in surface area for nutrient transfer may have contributed to the larger embryo weights we previously reported in offspring (both +/− and +/+) of *Dlx3+/−* mothers whom received 4X choline supplementation [14].

An additional explanation for the larger placental weights could be through reductions in apoptosis. For example, 4X (versus 1X) choline placentas had ~58% lower TUNEL scores at E12.5, and a tendency for lower scores (49% lower) at E10.5. These findings concur with previous results showing reductions in apoptosis with choline supplementation in human trophoblast cells [10] and in placentas of wildtype mice [11]. Although apoptosis is required for normal placental development, elevated levels of apoptosis have been reported in preeclamptic and IUGR placentas [24–26]. Notably, the elevated levels of apoptosis in *Dlx3+/−* placentas had previously been rescued using a strong antioxidant, TEMPOL [12]. Therefore, a reduction in placental apoptosis in mid-gestation via maternal choline supplementation may have beneficial effects in reducing the risk of developing placental complications later in gestation.

In a preliminary histological examination of spiral artery remodeling, we did not find evidence that maternal choline supplementation altered arterial luminal area percentage in the *Dlx3+/−* mouse. This is in contrast to our previous findings in wildtype dams, where 4X choline significantly increased luminal area percentage at E10.5, E12.5, E15.5, and E18.5 [11]. It is possible that the pathological phenotype of spiral artery remodeling in the *Dlx3+/−* dam was too severe to be ameliorated by choline supplementation. However, due to the small size of our histology cohort, this finding should be confirmed in a larger study.

Although prior work has shown that *Dlx3* is required for normal placental morphogenesis (13) and reduced *Dlx3* gene dose results in elevated placental cell oxidative stress and apoptosis coincident with altered vascular remodeling (12), we did not detect any differences in labyrinth size, apoptosis levels, or spiral artery remodeling between *Dlx3+/+* and *Dlx3+/−* placentas. We previously found that *Dlx3+/−* fetuses had comparable weights, but a higher expression of growth factor genes versus their *Dlx3+/+* littermates when their mothers consumed a high-quality pregnancy diet [14], suggesting that the *Dlx3+/−* placenta may activate compensatory mechanisms that lead to results similar to wildtype placentas for certain outcomes.

4.2. Effects of Maternal Choline Supplementation on Placental Inflammatory and Angiogenic Gene Expression Vary by Gestational Time Point and Fetal Sex

Inflammation and angiogenesis have been shown to be dysregulated in pregnancy complications including preeclampsia, IUGR, and spontaneous abortion [1,27,28]. Because of this, we measured placental mRNA expression of major modulators of these processes to determine whether choline can influence their placental expression in the *Dlx3+/−* mouse.

Overall patterns seen included the tendency for pro-inflammatory and pro-angiogenic markers to be downregulated in response to choline supplementation, with the 2X dose frequently having a larger effect than that of 4X. For example, compared to 1X choline, 2X choline significantly reduced the expression of the proinflammatory factors *Tnfα*, *Nfκb*, and *Il1b* at various gestational time points of pregnancy; a finding that was not consistently observed with 4X choline. Previous studies have shown that choline deficiency increases the expression of pro-inflammatory cytokines in a human placental trophoblast cell culture model [10], and that maternal choline supplementation reduces inflammatory response in pregnant rats challenged with lipopolysaccharide [29]. The results seen in the current study with a 2X choline dose provide additional support for a role of choline in mitigating inflammation, and suggest that efforts to increase maternal choline intake may be a nutritional strategy to reduce placental inflammation and improve pregnancy outcomes especially since less than ten percent of U.S. pregnant women meet choline intake recommendations [30].

The weakening of the choline-induced anti-inflammatory effects with the 4X treatment may suggest variability whereby maternal choline supplementation has an anti-inflammatory effect up to a certain concentration, beyond which its effects are attenuated. Alternatively, a strong growth-promoting effect of 4X maternal choline supplementation was detected in these mice at E10.5 [14], which was followed by a gradual slowing of growth such that only minor differences were detected in fetal weights in late gestation (E18.5). Thus, the effects of 4X choline on inflammatory (and angiogenic) processes in the placenta may have been weakened by compensatory mechanisms engaged to prevent exaggerated fetal growth.

We also observed downregulation of placental expression of the proangiogenic factor endoglin with maternal choline supplementation at E10.5 and E15.5 in female placentas and at E12.5 in males. These effects were mirrored by similar downregulation of proangiogenic *Vegfa*, which has been shown to be elevated or decreased in preeclamptic patients depending on the study [31–33]. It is possible that the larger labyrinth observed at E10.5 in the current study, combined with the superior placenta efficiency observed previously in these mice [14], resulted in a decreased need for placental angiogenesis, leading to a downregulation of pro-angiogenic factors.

Endoglin also serves as the precursor to soluble VEGF receptor endoglin (sEng), an anti-angiogenic factor that prevents VEGF from acting on target tissues [5], and contributes to the development of placental dysfunction. In the current study, expression of *Mmp14*, the matrix metalloproteinase that cleaves endoglin into its pathogenic soluble form [34], was significantly lower at E15.5 in females with choline supplementation, which is suggestive of decreased generation of sENG. In males, however, placental expression of *Mmp14* was higher at E18.5 with 2X choline supplementation, suggesting greater generation of sENG. This putative increase in sENG in late gestation could have a beneficial role in preventing preterm birth by blunting the parturition promoting effects of VEGF signaling through PGF and VEGF [31,32], both of which also were upregulated at this time point.

The effects of maternal choline supplementation on placental gene expression were sex specific, as previously reported in wildtype mouse pregnancy [11]. Differential expression of angiogenic factors according to fetal sex has been reported in both normal [33] and preeclamptic [35] human pregnancies. Although the mechanisms remain unclear, sex-specific differences in epigenetic regulation and hormonal environment have been suggested to be contributing factors [36,37]. Our findings add to the body of evidence demonstrating that fetal sex should be accounted for when examining placental and fetal outcomes during pregnancy.

4.3. Placental Concentrations of Acetylcholine are Minimally Affected by Maternal Choline Supplementation

Because acetylcholine has been reported to play a role in angiogenic [23] and inflammatory [22] signaling in the placenta, we hypothesized that choline may be modulating gene expression by altering acetylcholine levels. Surprisingly, we did not detect an increase in placental acetylcholine concentrations in response to maternal choline supplementation at E10.5, E15.5, or E18.5. At E12.5, acetylcholine levels were higher in the 2X, but not 4X, choline group. The overall lack of effect of maternal choline supplementation on placental acetylcholine concentrations could reflect rapid uptake of the acetylcholine molecule by the developing fetus as we previously reported that 4X choline increased acetylcholine concentrations in the fetal brain of wildtype mice [38].

4.4. Strengths and Limitations

The study strengths include: (i) the use of a standardized diet and three choline intake levels; (ii) the inclusion of four gestational time points, which allows for a dynamic view of the changes that occur in the placenta throughout gestation; and (iii) the use of an animal model with a hemochorial structure similar to the primate placenta. Nonetheless, several limitations should be noted. The small sample size combined with the relatively high degree of variability for most of the outcome data precluded our ability to assess the interactive effects of fetal genotype and fetal sex with choline treatment. An additional limitation of the current study was the analyses of mRNA abundance without concurrent analyses of proteins. Finally, our histological analyses were included as a hypothesis-generating examination of choline's effects in compromised pregnancies, and should be confirmed in larger cohorts.

5. Conclusions

In conclusion, maternal choline supplementation modulated placental development and function in a mouse model of placental insufficiency, providing some evidence that choline may be a useful therapy during pregnancy to prevent or overcome development of placental disorders that impact fetal and maternal health. Decreases in pro-inflammatory gene expression and placental apoptosis are especially encouraging and align with previous results showing similar effects of choline in different experimental models. Since many pregnant women do not currently meet the recommended intake levels of choline [30], further research is warranted to investigate the effects of increased maternal choline intake on human placental function.

Supplementary Materials: The following are available online at http://www.mdpi.com/2072-6643/11/2/374/s1. Table S1: Primers for genotyping and RT-qPCR. Table S2: Embryo weight, placental weight, crown rump length, and placental efficiency and litter size in *Dlx3+/−* dams in response to three different maternal choline treatments (control, 2X and 4X) at E10.5, E12.5, E15.5, and E18.5.

Author Contributions: The author contributions were as follows: conceptualization, J.H.K., X.J., M.S.R. and M.A.C.; investigation, J.H.K, S.T.K. and J.Y.; data curation, J.H.K, V.G.F., S.P.L. and E.W.; formal analysis, J.H.K.; writing—original draft preparation, J.H.K.; writing—review and editing, M.S.R. and M.A.C.; supervision, M.S.R. and M.A.C.; funding acquisition, X.J., M.S.R. and M.A.C.

Funding: This research was funded by USDA grant NIFA 2012-67017-30176.

Conflicts of Interest: The authors declare no conflict of interest. The funders had no role in the design of the study; in the collection, analyses, or interpretation of data; in the writing of the manuscript, or in the decision to publish the results.

References

1. Chaddha, V.; Viero, S.; Huppertz, B.; Kingdom, J. Developmental biology of the placenta and the origins of placental insufficiency. *Semin. Fetal Neonatal Med.* **2004**, *9*, 357–369. [CrossRef] [PubMed]
2. Azizieh, F.; Raghupathy, R.; Makhseed, M. Maternal Cytokine Production Patterns in Women with Pre-eclampsia. *Am. J. Reprod. Immunol.* **2005**, *54*, 30–37. [CrossRef] [PubMed]
3. Cartwright, J.E.; Whitley, G.S.J. Trophoblast-mediated spiral artery remodelling: A role for apoptosis. *J. Anat.* **2009**, *215*, 21–26.
4. Cheng, M.-H.; Wang, P.-H. Placentation abnormalities in the pathophysiology of preeclampsia. *Expert Rev. Mol. Diagn.* **2009**, *9*, 37–49. [CrossRef] [PubMed]
5. Venkatesha, S.; Toporsian, M.; Lam, C.; Hanai, J.-I.; Mammoto, T.; Kim, Y.M.; Bdolah, Y.; Lim, K.-H.; Yuan, H.-T.; Libermann, T.A.; et al. Soluble endoglin contributes to the pathogenesis of preeclampsia. *Nat. Med.* **2006**, *12*, 642–649. [CrossRef] [PubMed]
6. Boij, R.; Svensson-Arvelund, J.; Nilsson-Ekdahl, K.; Sandholm, K.; Lindahl, T.L.; Pálonek, E.; Garle, M.; Berg, G.; Ernerudh, J.; Jenmalm, M.; et al. Biomarkers of Coagulation, Inflammation, and Angiogenesis are Independently Associated with Preeclampsia. *Am. J. Reprod. Immunol.* **2012**, *68*, 258–270. [CrossRef] [PubMed]

7.   Jiang, X.; West, A.A.; Caudill, M.A. Maternal choline supplementation: A nutritional approach for improving offspring health? *Trends Endocrinol. Metab.* **2014**, *25*, 263–273. [CrossRef] [PubMed]

8.   Caudill, M.A. Pre- and Postnatal Health: Evidence of Increased Choline Needs. *J. Am. Diet. Assoc.* **2010**, *110*, 1198–1206. [CrossRef]

9.   Jiang, X.; Bar, H.Y.; Yan, J.; Jones, S.; Brannon, P.M.; West, A.A.; Perry, C.A.; Ganti, A.; Pressman, E.; Devapatla, S.; et al. A higher maternal choline intake among third-trimester pregnant women lowers placental and circulating concentrations of the antiangiogenic factor fms-like tyrosine kinase-1 (sFLT1). *FASEB J.* **2013**, *27*, 1245–1253. [CrossRef]

10. Jiang, X.; Jones, S.; Andrew, B.Y.; Ganti, A.; Malysheva, O.V.; Giallourou, N.; Brannon, P.M.; Roberson, M.S.; Caudill, M.A. Choline Inadequacy Impairs Trophoblast Function and Vascularization in Cultured Human Placental Trophoblasts. *J. Cell. Physiol.* **2014**, *229*, 1016–1027. [CrossRef]

11. Kwan, S.T. (Cecilia); King, J.H.; Yan, J.; Jiang, X.; Wei, E.; Fomin, V.G.; Roberson, M.S.; Caudill, M.A. Maternal choline supplementation during murine pregnancy modulates placental markers of inflammation, apoptosis and vascularization in a fetal sex-dependent manner. *Placenta* **2017**, *53*, 57–65. [PubMed]

12. Clark, P.; Brown, J.; Li, S.; Woods, A.; Han, L.; Sones, J.; Preston, R.; Southard, T.; Davisson, R.; Roberson, M.; et al. Distal-less 3 haploinsufficiency results in elevated placental oxidative stress and altered fetal growth kinetics in the mouse. *Placenta* **2012**, *33*, 830–838. [CrossRef]

13. Morasso, M.I.; Grinberg, A.; Robinson, G.; Sargent, T.D.; Mahon, K.A. Placental failure in mice lacking the homeobox gene Dlx3. *Proc. Natl. Acad. Sci. USA* **1999**, *96*, 162–167. [CrossRef] [PubMed]

14. King, J.H.; Kwan, S.T.C.; Yan, J.; Klatt, K.C.; Roberson, M.S.; Caudill, M.A. Maternal Choline Supplementation Alters Fetal Growth Patterns in a Mouse Model of Placental Insufficiency. *Nutrients* **2017**, *9*, 765. [CrossRef] [PubMed]

15. Murthi, P.; Kalionis, B.; Rajaraman, G.; Keogh, R.J.; Costa, F.D.S. The Role of Homeobox Genes in the Development of Placental Insufficiency. *Fetal Diagn. Ther.* **2012**, *32*, 225–230. [CrossRef] [PubMed]

16. Schmittgen, T.D.; Livak, K.J. Analyzing real-time PCR data by the comparative CT method. *Nat. Protoc.* **2008**, *3*, 1101–1108. [CrossRef] [PubMed]

17. Meller, M.; Vadachkoria, S.; Luthy, D.; Williams, M. Evaluation of housekeeping genes in placental comparative expression studies. *Placenta* **2005**, *26*, 601–607. [CrossRef] [PubMed]

18. Mehedint, M.G.; Craciunescu, C.N.; Zeisel, S.H. Maternal dietary choline deficiency alters angiogenesis in fetal mouse hippocampus. *Proc. Natl. Acad. Sci. USA* **2010**, *107*, 12834–12839. [CrossRef]

19. Holm, P.I.; Ueland, P.M.; Kvalheim, G.; Lien, E.A. Determination of Choline, Betaine, and Dimethylglycine in Plasma by a High-Throughput Method Based on Normal-Phase Chromatography-Tandem Mass Spectrometry. *Clin. Chem.* **2003**, *49*, 286–294. [CrossRef]

20. Yan, J.; Wang, W.; Gregory, J.F., III; Malysheva, O.; Brenna, J.T.; Stabler, S.P.; Allen, R.H.; Caudill, M.A. MTHFR C677T genotype influences the isotopic enrichment of one-carbon metabolites in folate-compromised men consuming d9-choline. *Am. J. Clin. Nutr.* **2011**, *93*, 348–355. [CrossRef]

21. Berghorn, K.A.; Clark, P.A.; Encarnacion, B.; DeRegis, C.J.; Folger, J.K.; I Morasso, M.; Soares, M.J.; Wolfe, M.W.; Roberson, M.S. Developmental expression of the homeobox protein Distal-less 3 and its relationship to progesterone production in mouse placenta. *J. Endocrinol.* **2005**, *186*, 315–323. [CrossRef] [PubMed]

22. Jonge, W.J.; Ulloa, L. The alpha7 nicotinic acetylcholine receptor as a pharmacological target for inflammation. *Br. J. Pharmacol.* **2009**, *151*, 915–929. [CrossRef] [PubMed]

23. Arias, H.R.; Richards, V.E.; Ng, D.; Ghafoori, M.E.; Le, V.; Mousa, S.A. Role of non-neuronal nicotinic acetylcholine receptors in angiogenesis. *Int. J. Biochem. Cell Biol.* **2009**, *41*, 1441–1451. [CrossRef] [PubMed]

24. DiFederico, E.; Genbacev, O.; Fisher, S.J. Preeclampsia Is Associated with Widespread Apoptosis of Placental Cytotrophoblasts within the Uterine Wall. *Am. J. Pathol.* **1999**, *155*, 293–301. [CrossRef]

25. Allaire, A. Placental apoptosis in preeclampsia. *Obstet. Gynecol.* **2000**, *96*, 271–276. [PubMed]

26. Ishihara, N.; Matsuo, H.; Murakoshi, H.; Laoag-Fernandez, J.B.; Samoto, T.; Maruo, T. Increased apoptosis in the syncytiotrophoblast in human term placentas complicated by either preeclampsia or intrauterine growth retardation. *Am. J. Obstet. Gynecol.* **2002**, *186*, 158–166. [CrossRef] [PubMed]

27. Mestan, K.; Yu, Y.; Matoba, N.; Cerda, S.; Demmin, B.; Pearson, C.; Ortiz, K.; Wang, X. Placental Inflammatory Response Is Associated with Poor Neonatal Growth: Preterm Birth Cohort Study. *Pediatrics* **2010**, *125*, 891–898. [CrossRef] [PubMed]

28. Christiansen, O.B.; Nielsen, H.S.; Kolte, A.M. Inflammation and miscarriage. *Semin. Fetal Neonatal Med.* **2006**, *11*, 302–308. [CrossRef]
29. Zhang, M.; Han, X.; Bao, J.; Yang, J.; Shi, S.-Q.; Garfield, R.E.; Liu, H. Choline Supplementation During Pregnancy Protects Against Gestational Lipopolysaccharide-Induced Inflammatory Responses. *Reprod. Sci.* **2017**, *25*, 74–85. [CrossRef]
30. Wallace, T.C.; Fulgoni, V.L. Usual Choline Intakes Are Associated with Egg and Protein Food Consumption in the United States. *Nutrients* **2017**, *9*, 839. [CrossRef]
31. Wada, Y.; Ozaki, H.; Abe, N.; Mori, A.; Sakamoto, K.; Nagamitsu, T.; Nakahara, T.; Ishii, K. Role of Vascular Endothelial Growth Factor in Maintenance of Pregnancy in Mice. *Endocrinology* **2013**, *154*, 900–910. [CrossRef] [PubMed]
32. Lappas, M. Nuclear factor- B mediates placental growth factor induced pro-labour mediators in human placenta. *Mol. Hum. Reprod.* **2012**, *18*, 354–361. [CrossRef] [PubMed]
33. Scott, N.M.; Hodyl, N.A.; Murphy, V.E.; Osei-Kumah, A.; Wyper, H.; Hodgson, D.M.; Smith, R.; Clifton, V.L. Placental Cytokine Expression Covaries with Maternal Asthma Severity and Fetal Sex. *J. Immunol.* **2009**, *182*, 1411–1420. [CrossRef] [PubMed]
34. Kaitu'U-Lino, T.J.; Palmer, K.R.; Whitehead, C.L.; Williams, E.; Lappas, M.; Tong, S. MMP-14 Is Expressed in Preeclamptic Placentas and Mediates Release of Soluble Endoglin. *Am. J. Pathol.* **2012**, *180*, 888–894. [CrossRef] [PubMed]
35. Muralimanoharan, S.; Maloyan, A.; Myatt, L. Evidence of sexual dimorphism in the placental function with severe preeclampsia. *Placenta* **2013**, *34*, 1183–1189. [CrossRef] [PubMed]
36. Martin, E.; Smeester, L.; Bommarito, P.A.; Grace, M.R.; Boggess, K.; Kuban, K.; Karagas, M.R.; Marsit, C.J.; O'Shea, T.M.; Fry, R.C.; et al. Sexual epigenetic dimorphism in the human placenta: Implications for susceptibility during the prenatal period. *Epigenomics* **2017**, *9*, 267–278. [CrossRef] [PubMed]
37. Yang, X.; Schadt, E.E.; Wang, S.; Wang, H.; Arnold, A.P.; Ingram-Drake, L.; Drake, T.A.; Lusis, A.J. Tissue-specific expression and regulation of sexually dimorphic genes in mice. *Genome Res.* **2006**, *16*, 995–1004. [CrossRef]
38. Kwan, S.T. (Cecilia); King, J.H.; Yan, J.; Wang, Z.; Jiang, X.; Hutzler, J.S.; Klein, H.R.; Brenna, J.T.; Roberson, M.S.; Caudill, M.A.; et al. Maternal Choline Supplementation Modulates Placental Nutrient Transport and Metabolism in Late Gestation of Mouse Pregnancy. *J. Nutr.* **2017**, *147*, 2083–2092.

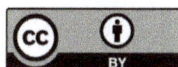

nutrients

MDPI

Article

Blind Analysis of Food-Related IgG Identifies Five Possible Nutritional Clusters for the Italian Population: Future Implications for Pregnancy and Lactation

Gabriele Piuri [1], Enrico Ferrazzi [1,2] and Attilio Francesco Speciani [1,*]

[1] Inflammation Society, 18 Woodlands Park, Bexley DA52EL, UK; gabriele.piuri@me.com (G.P.); enrico.ferrazzi@unimi.it (E.F.)
[2] Fondazione IRCCS Cà Granda, Ospedale Maggiore Policlinico, Department of Clinical Sciences and Community Health, University of Milan, 20122 Milan, Italy
* Correspondence: attilio.speciani@me.com

Received: 1 April 2019; Accepted: 15 May 2019; Published: 17 May 2019

Abstract: Background: The influence of diet in pregnant women on the immune tolerance process is intricate. Food-specific immunoglobulin G (IgG) was associated with exposure to particular food antigens. The IgG antibodies can cross the placental barrier and enter into the colostrum, and maternal IgG is amply present in breast milk. This justifies studying the immunological connection between food-specific IgG antibodies and the mother–fetus relationship. This study was designed to analyze food-specific IgG concentrations and possible food-specific IgG concentration clusters in a large cohort of subjects with a common food culture. Methods: Food-specific IgG antibody concentrations were detected in 18,012 Caucasian or Southern European subjects over 18 years of age. We used an unsupervised hierarchical clustering algorithm to explore varying degrees of similarity among food-specific IgG antibodies. Results: We identified five food groups by the evaluation of food-specific IgG values: one includes foods with a high nickel content, the second cluster is associated with gluten, the third cluster includes dairy products, the fourth one is connected to fermented foods, and the last group is correlated with cooked oils. Discussion: The knowledge derived from studying a large sample allows us to determine food-specific IgG values from a single pregnant woman, compare it to an epidemic standard, and establish modifications required in her lifestyle to modulate her nutritional habits.

Keywords: pregnancy; lactation; weaning; food-related IgG; food clusters; non-IgE-mediated food reactions

1. Introduction

Recently published reviews support the biological association of food-specific immunoglobulin G (IgG) with exposure to particular food antigens [1,2]. IgG antibodies, especially IgG4, are highly related to the immune tolerance of food antigens, and IgG can be responsible for the attenuation of the immunological response. These protective antibodies might regulate the immune response by avoiding the binding of the antigen to the IgE already present on the surface, or by inhibiting the maturation of the dendritic cells, preventing the activation of possible allergic pathways [3]. IgG4 antibodies have diverse anti-inflammatory actions compared to other IgG subclasses. One of these differences is the reduced capacity to induce complement activation due to a low affinity for the C1q and Fc receptors. Due to their ability to bind different antigens in diverse sites, these antibodies do not precipitate antigens [4].

The relationship between IgE-mediated anaphylaxis and more subtle hyper-immune responses associated with high IgG titer is being increasingly studied and has now been precisely defined. Antigens can cause systemic anaphylaxis through the classical pathway by cross-linking IgE bound to mast cell FcεRI or through the alternative path by forming complexes with IgG. New studies have shown an IgG-dependent mechanism of anaphylaxis that involves IgG, FcγRs on macrophages, basophils and neutrophils, complement-derived peptides C3a and C5a, B-cell activating factor (BAFF), and platelet-activating factor (PAF) [5]. According to Finkelman [6–8] and Muñoz-Cano et al. [9], IgG, macrophages, basophils, and neutrophils may even be involved in human anaphylaxis. This delicate blinding of food antigens can be dysregulated by an excess of these specific food antigens related to IgG and activate inflammatory processes [8].

This fine-tuned immune equilibrium permits alien food antigens to land safely on the gut mucosa as they are processed and allowed to pass through the mucosal surface and become nutritional elements for the microbiota, becoming accepted as "legal aliens". This complex recognition occurs on the most notable large external surface in the human body, which is 200 times wider than skin. The repetitive and continuous consumption of a particular food that corresponds to a higher production of specific antibodies can fracture the equilibrium, increase inflammatory mediators [8], and damage the delicate gap junctions in the gut mucosa [10].

High concentrations of food-specific IgG antibodies have been successfully identified as foes in non-IgE-mediated food reactions. Bentz et al. reported significantly higher food-specific IgG antibodies in patients with Crohn's disease in contrast with healthy controls [11]. The same patients showed significant clinical improvement in inflammatory bowel disease (IBD) symptoms when the foods associated with highly specific IgG were removed from the diet [11]. In agreement with these findings, Cai et al. observed high levels of IgG antibodies to specific food antigens in patients affected by IBD [12]. Alpay et al. evaluated the effect of a personalized nutritional approach based on food-specific IgG in sequences of migraine attacks in a randomized, double-blind, cross-over, headache-diary-based trial on patients diagnosed with migraines without auras [13]. A similar double-blind, placebo-controlled, dietary re-challenge trial was performed by Biesiekierski [14] to prove that the symptoms of irritable bowel syndrome (IBS) could be reduced in patients without proven celiac disease and with clinical sensitivity to gluten. A similar study demonstrated that clinical symptoms of IBS were significantly reduced in patients affected by Sjogren's syndrome who underwent a diet characterized by high concentrations of food-specific IgG [15]. IBS is a less-defined pathological condition, yet increased gastrointestinal permeability and gut inflammation were observed by Shulman in children [16]. Similar patterns of food-specific IgG and IgG4 were observed in eosinophilic esophagitis [17], and such deposits of IgG4 may even distinguish patients with gastro-esophageal reflux disease versus eosinophilic esophagitis.

The Western diet is prone to causing this imbalance [18] and is characterized by a lack of variety and seasonality that could elicit excessive antibody production against food antigen clusters. In parallel, the lack of fiber in a diet produces a poor prebiotic environment, directly affecting the gut microbiota. These conditions might convert the role of the microbiota from an anti-inflammatory partner of dendritic cells in the intestinal mucosa into an aggressive collection of pro-inflammatory bacteria.

We hypothesized that high food-specific IgG concentrations in subjects suffering from organ or systemic inflammation might be critical in a pro-inflammatory scenario. This study was designed to analyze food-specific IgG concentrations and possible food-specific IgG concentration clusters in a large cohort of subjects with a common food culture and affected by gastroenteric inflammatory symptoms and/or other tissue or systemic inflammations.

2. Materials and Methods

2.1. Subjects

All of 18,012 patients suspected a relationship between food intake and symptoms such as bloating, constipation, diarrhea, heartburn, gastritis, or other signs and symptoms of possible gastroenteric inflammation. They were all Caucasian or Southern European subjects over 18 years of age. Written consent to this observational study was obtained by all participants who self-enrolled in the study, according to privacy regulations. Sample collection was performed by finger pricks using a nylon swab for the storage of dried blood (Copan Diagnostics, Inc., Murrieta, CA, USA). Blood samples were delivered to a laboratory (Diagnostica Spire S.r.l. Reggio Emilia, Italy) and analyzed within less than seven days from sample collection to ensure the data accuracy. Food-specific IgG antibody concentrations were detected by employing ELISA plates produced by Immunolab GmbH (Kassel, Germany) customized for 44 common Italian food antigens. Lower and upper detection limits for IgG antibodies were 0.0 U/mL and 100 U/mL, respectively.

2.2. Statistical Methods

The frequency distribution of food-specific IgG concentrations in this population was determined for each food antigen tested. Non-parametric descriptive statistics (median and interquartile range) were adopted for non-normal (D'Agostino and Pearson normality test) or bimodal distributions.

We used an unsupervised hierarchical clustering algorithm to explore varying degrees of similarity among food-specific IgG, adapting the statistical methods used by Eisen et al. [19]. The object of using this algorithm was to compute a dendrogram that assembled all food-specific IgG into a single tree. For any food-specific IgG, an upper-diagonal similarity matrix containing similarity scores for all pairs of food-specific IgG was calculated. The matrix was scanned to identify the highest value, representing the most similar pair of food-specific IgG. A node was created joining these two foods, and a new food-specific IgG level was computed for the node by averaging observations for the joined elements. The similarity matrix was then updated with this new node, replacing the two joined elements, and the process was repeated (n − 1) times until only a single element remained. The algorithm initially had 44 food-specific IgG antibodies (one for each antigen), which were gradually grouped together into higher-degree clusters according to their similarities. The algorithm stopped when all food-specific IgG antibodies were grouped into the same cluster. The bar on the left side of the dendrogram indicates the dissimilarity (1 − Correlation) for every node. A lower dissimilarity suggests a higher correlation between the foods, or the clusters of foods, linked together by a node and can be useful to better understand the relationship between the different foods.

3. Results

Food-specific IgG values were measured in 18,012 Italian patients (74.1% women, mean age 44.5 ± 15.5 years). Table 1 shows the IgG concentration for each of the 44 food antigens tested in alphabetical order and the type of distribution observed. Most IgG distributions were asymmetrical. For food-specific IgG with a bimodal distribution, we indicate medians with an interquartile range of both modes. Due to exposure to different food antigens, the IgG concentrations were very low for foods that showed levels of IgG <1 U/mL, such as olives, peaches, tea, honey, red grapes, and zucchini. High levels were found for foods that showed concentrations of IgG >20 U/mL, such as processed cheese, cow milk, and common wheat. Notably, the IgG values with a bimodal distribution were higher compared with IgG values with an asymmetrical distribution.

Table 1. List of tested foods, median and interquartile range of corresponding immunoglobulin G (IgG) values, and type of frequency distribution. For food-related IgG with a bimodal distribution, the interquartile range of both modes is indicated.

Food–Antigen	IgG Levels U/mL	Distribution
Almonds	8.35 (4.55–14.25)	Asymmetrical
Aspergillus fumigatus	3.95 (1.63–10.75)	Asymmetrical
Barley	9.16 (5.06–15.36)	Asymmetrical
Barley malt	1.17 (0.55–2.54)	Asymmetrical
Buckwheat	6.99 (3.43–12.49)	Asymmetrical
Candida albicans	2.48 (0.97–7.00)	Asymmetrical
Canned tuna	3.24 (1.42–6.21)	Asymmetrical
Champignon mushrooms	4.05 (1.38–9.60)	Asymmetrical
Chicken	0.78 (0.29–1.60)	Asymmetrical
Corn	1.32 (0.67–2.51)	Asymmetrical
Eggs	8.63 (3.01–21.58)	Asymmetrical
Goat milk	8.18 (3.92–17.39)	Asymmetrical
Hazelnuts	5.19 (2.46–9.5)	Asymmetrical
Honey	0.07 (0.00–0.41)	Asymmetrical
Kamut	6.47 (3.87–11.27)	Asymmetrical
Kiwis	3.16 (1.55–6.72)	Asymmetrical
Lentils	0.65 (0.25–1.51)	Asymmetrical
Mozzarella cheese	8.71 (4.7–15.56)	Asymmetrical
Oats	1.97 (0.99–4.28)	Asymmetrical
Olives	0.01 (0.00–0.16)	Asymmetrical
Onion	0.71 (0.32–1.40)	Asymmetrical
Oranges	0.19 (0.02–0.79)	Asymmetrical
Parmesan cheese	8.77 (3.45–18.72)	Asymmetrical
Peaches	0.01 (0.00–0.16)	Asymmetrical
Peanuts	7.83 (4.28–13.71)	Asymmetrical
Porcini mushrooms	2.83 (1.1–7.08)	Asymmetrical
Potato	3.34 (1.56–6.30)	Asymmetrical
Red grapes	0.08 (0.00–0.50)	Asymmetrical
Rice	0.52 (0.10–1.48)	Asymmetrical
Ricotta cheese	13.71 (7.32–28.15)	Asymmetrical
Rye	1.28 (0.61–2.65)	Asymmetrical
Soy	0.97 (0.45–2.05)	Asymmetrical
Spinach	0.20 (0.01–0.97)	Asymmetrical
Tea	0.02 (0.00–0.19)	Asymmetrical
Tomato	3.94 (1.20–9.10)	Asymmetrical
Walnuts	0.41 (0.07–1.19)	Asymmetrical
Zucchini	0.08 (0.00–0.60)	Asymmetrical
Beer yeast	3.80 (1.87–6.81) 17.92 (9.01–30.36)	Bimodal
Common wheat	11.07 (7.95–14.61) 32.53 (24.83–41.21)	Bimodal
Cow milk	8.54 (4.68–13.10) 37.55 (27.60–49.70)	Bimodal
Durum wheat	12.04 (7.86–16.47) 34.64 (28.39–42.74)	Bimodal
Pork	1.17 (0.53–2.75) 10.74 (6.05–18.16)	Bimodal
Processed cheese	14.72 (8.86–21.90) 47.19 (38.76–58.96)	Bimodal
Spelt	6.42 (3.71–9.89) 23.46 (18.01–30.26)	Bimodal

Figure 1 shows four models with both asymmetrical and bimodal frequency distribution. We provide diagrams of food-specific IgG values of all 44 foods tested in the Supplementary Materials (Figure S1). Figure 2 shows the dendrogram produced from the results of the clustering algorithm, which identifies five food groups by the evaluation of food-specific IgG values (for every node $p < 0.001$). The first group includes foods with a high nickel content, such as tomato, kiwi fruit, peanuts, almonds, and buckwheat. Inside this group, a second cluster can be identified that includes wheat and associated grains such as Kamut, spelt, and barley. The third cluster includes dairy products (such as cow's and goat's milk as well as Parmesan, mozzarella, and ricotta cheese). The fourth one includes yeasts such as *Candida albicans* and *Saccharomyces cerevisiae* and porcini and champignon mushrooms. This cluster is likely connected to fermented foods. The last group contains roasted nuts (peanuts and almonds) and is probably correlated with heated and cooked oils.

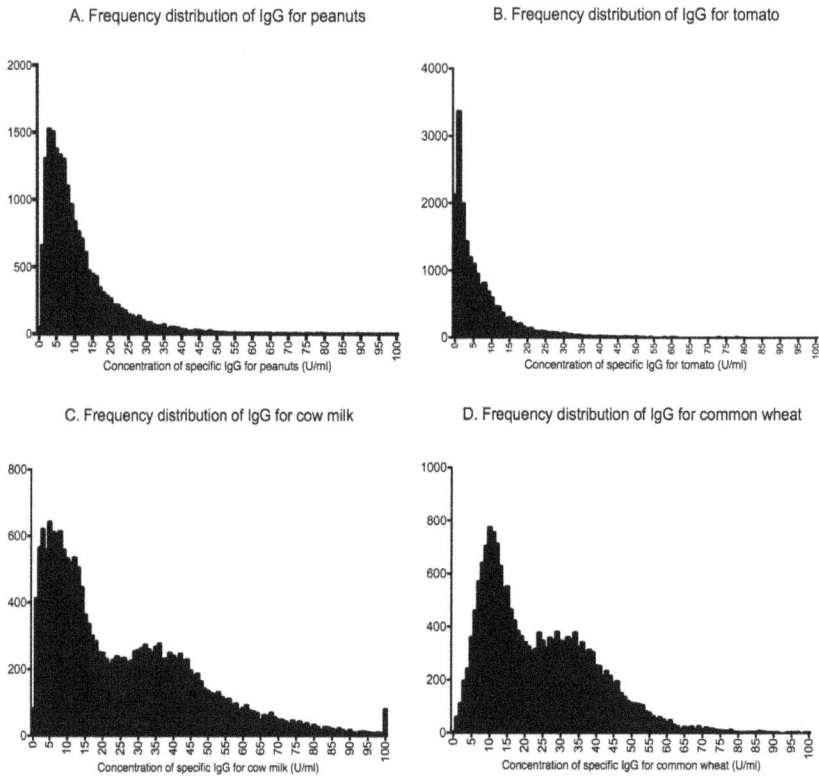

Figure 1. Examples of asymmetrical and bimodal distribution of frequencies for food-specific IgG. (**A,B**) Graphs showing two examples (for peanuts and tomato, respectively) of asymmetrical distribution of IgG. (**C,D**) Graphs showing two examples (for cow's milk and common wheat, respectively) of bimodal distribution of IgG.

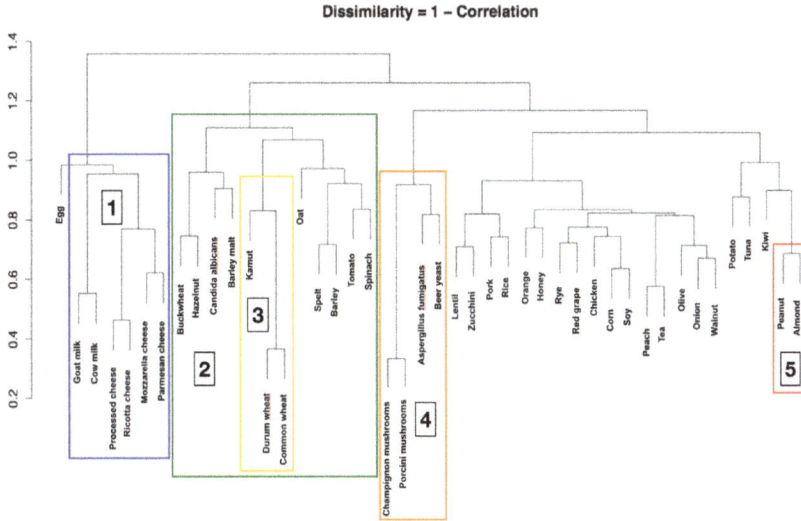

Figure 2. Dendrogram resulting from the clustering algorithm. It is possible to identify five large food clusters: (1) milk and dairy products, (2) foods with high content of nickel, (3) wheat-related grains, (4) fermented foods, and (5) roasted nuts and cooked oils (for every node *p* < 0.001). The bar on the left side of the dendrogram indicates the dissimilarity (1 – Correlation) for every node.

4. Discussion

4.1. Main Findings and Interpretation

The dendrogram obtained by the blind post-hoc matrix, correlated by similarity, allowed us to observe significant correlations between food-specific IgG antibodies that seem to correspond to typical Italian food habits [20–22]. Goat's and cow's milk, processed cheese, and mozzarella and Parmesan cheese were strongly correlated. The first node between processed cheese and ricotta cheese had the highest similarity. The second highest similarities were found via the dendrogram algorithm and were between mozzarella and Parmesan cheese and between goat's and cow's milk. These strict statistical similarities between IgG concentrations were found within dairy products. Such strict correlations, apparently biologically based, were also observed in yeasts (yeast and mushrooms) and in cereals containing gluten. The latter group is probably part of a larger cluster of foods containing nickel. The dendrogram algorithm also segregated a larger group of less strict correlations ranging at a dissimilarity level of 0.8 instead of the 0.3–0.5 dissimilarity level of the previously described clusters. A possible common denominator of these food-specific IgG could be represented by roasted nuts (peanuts and almonds), which are correlated with cooked oils.

The second relevant finding of this large cohort is represented by the distribution of the 44 food-specific IgG levels measured. As expected, the vast majority showed a modal distribution with a marked skewness toward lower concentrations. In eight of the food-specific IgG antibodies, the distribution was bimodal. These latter IgG levels showed significantly higher concentrations compared with IgG concentrations with mono-modal asymmetrical distribution. IgG levels for milk in this Italian population were among these bimodal distributions. The first Gaussian likely represents occasional consumers of milk and dairy products, whereas the second Gaussian reflects daily consumers. Although the use of dairy products is widespread in Italy, a large part of the adult Italian population does not consume milk regularly due to actual or suspected lactase non-persistence [23]. In contrast, the low concentration of specific IgG antibodies for peanuts reflects the nutritional habits of Italians, the vast majority of whom eat peanuts only occasionally.

The differences between IgG levels for different foods could be explained either by eating behaviors connected with increased or reduced intake or by the immunogenicity of the specific food antigen [1,2]. According to these tenets, the difference in the absolute values of IgG for consumers of large amounts of wheat (median concentration 18.22 U/mL) and for consumers of large amounts of honey (median concentration 0.07 U/mL) could be explained by intrinsic antigenic properties.

The production of food-specific IgG antibodies is directly related to the recurrent or prevalent intake of specific foods and can cause an immune reaction inducing, under specific conditions, an increase in inflammatory mediators [8]. The immune system does not specifically recognize foods by IgG, as in the case of IgE, but rather with an approach of similarity, identifying food antigen clusters that reflect the eating habits within different populations. According to this knowledge, the evaluation of the different distribution curves of IgG levels in the Italian population allows us to better understand the possible role of IgG production and how these antibodies can highlight a specific nutritional excess of a food cluster, suggesting a different dietary approach to inflammatory diseases. In agreement with Finkelman [6–8], the increased amount of contact with antigenic foods leads to the production of food-specific IgG for a large number of different foods, thus avoiding an absolute prevalence of a single specific antibody to a specific food group. With this information, the activation of a reasonable inflammatory response can be possibly prevented or modulated.

4.2. Speculations and Further Hypothesis for Future Implications in Pregnancy and Lactation

The influence of diet in pregnant women on the immune tolerance process is intricate. Thus, diet must be analyzed, not only from a compositional standpoint but also from an evolutionary point of view. Pregnancy symptoms, such as nausea and vomiting in the first trimester, might protect both the pregnant woman and the embryo from potentially harmful substances present in food [24], while, in the last trimester, cravings for food expose the fetus to a higher number of antigens and increase immune contact with the outside environment, yielding an immune imprinting. The fetus' immune knowledge of the outer world is guaranteed by the IgG produced by the mother. The IgG antibodies can cross the placental barrier and enter into the colostrum, and maternal IgG is amply present in breast milk. This justifies studying the immunological connection between food-specific IgG antibodies and the mother–fetus relationship [5]. This intrauterine information has allowed mammals to regard specific foods as sources of energy. The body knows if the food is sufficient for intimate contact with the organism and uses it as a nutrient.

4.3. Strength and Limitations

To the best of our knowledge, this is the first study of food-specific IgG involving thousands of subjects who have the same macro-ethnicity—Caucasians of Southern European ancestry—and who self-enrolled based on common gastro-enteric symptoms. Data on over 18,000 subjects were blindly analyzed by an independent third party that was unaware of the meaning of the codes attributed to each food-specific IgG. A major limitation of the statistical evidence observed is represented by the heterogeneity of the population recruited and by the fact that a direct correlation with different signs and symptoms was not available post hoc. However, the coherence of the distribution of IgG concentrations and the coherence of the clusters identified by the dendrogram algorithm with respect to the Italian food consumption profile allowed us to consider our findings genuine in the ongoing debate on food antigens and gastro-enteric IgG production, immune tolerance, and inflammation.

5. Conclusions

The dendrogram algorithm appeared to operate in a process resembling the immune system recognition of food antigens and similar related antigens. This finding allowed us to observe, confirm, and better specify the existence of five large clusters of different foods that appear to react in the same way to IgG antibodies.

Nutrients **2019**, *11*, 1096

Supplementary Materials: The following are available online at http://www.mdpi.com/2072-6643/11/5/1096/s1, Figure S1: Graphs showing the frequency distribution of food-specific IgG concentration for each of the 44 food antigens tested.

Author Contributions: Conceptualization, G.P., E.F. and A.F.S.; Methodology, G.P. and A.F.S.; Software, G.P.; Validation, G.P., E.F. and A.F.S.; Formal Analysis, G.P.; Investigation, G.P., E.F. and A.F.S.; Resources, G.P.; Data Curation, G.P.; Writing—Original Draft Preparation, G.P. and A.F.S.; Writing—Review & Editing, G.P., E.F. and A.F.S.; Visualization, G.P.; Supervision, A.F.S.; Project Administration, G.P.; Funding Acquisition, A.F.S.

Funding: This research received no external funding.

Conflicts of Interest: The authors declare no conflict of interest.

References

1. Ligaarden, S.C.; Lydersen, S.; Farup, P.G. IgG and IgG4 Antibodies in Subjects with Irritable Bowel Syndrome: A Case Control Study in the General Population. *BMC Gastroenterol.* **2012**, *12*, 166. [CrossRef]
2. Speciani, A.F.; Piuri, G.; Ferrazzi, E. IgG Levels to Food Correlate with Nutritional Exposure to Food Antigens but a Methodological Weakness of this Research Prevents the Recognition of Yeast-Related Foods as a Possible Cause of Irritable Bowel Syndrome (IBS). Comment to IgG and IgG4 Antibodies in Subjects with Irritable Bowel Syndrome: A Case Control Study in the General Population Solveig C Ligaarden*, Stian Lydersen and Per G Farup BMC Gastroenterology 2012, 12:166. *BMC Gastroenterol.* **2012**, *12*, 166.
3. Wisniewski, J.; Agrawal, R.; Woodfolk, J.A. Mechanisms of Tolerance Induction in Allergic Disease: Integrating Current and Emerging Concepts. *Clin. Exp. Allergy* **2013**, *43*, 164–176. [CrossRef]
4. Kolfschoten, M.V.D.N.; Schuurman, J.; Losen, M.; Bleeker, W.K.; Martinez, P.M.; Vermeulen, E.; Bleker, T.H.D.; Wiegman, L.; Vink, T.; Aarden, L.A.; et al. Anti-Inflammatory Activity of Human IgG4 Antibodies by Dynamic Fab Arm Exchange. *Science* **2007**, *317*, 1554–1557. [CrossRef] [PubMed]
5. Piuri, G. Individual Food Clusters Excess and Low-Grade Inflammation in Pregnancy. In *Metabolic Syndrome and Complications of Pregnancy*, 1st ed.; Ferrazzi, E., Sears, B., Eds.; Springer Science Publisher: New York, NY, USA; Heidelberg, Germany, 2015; pp. 23–33.
6. Finkelman, F.D. Anaphylaxis: Lessons from Mouse Models. *J. Allergy Clin. Immunol.* **2007**, *120*, 506–515. [CrossRef]
7. Khodoun, M.V.; Strait, R.; Armstrong, L.; Yanase, N.; Finkelman, F.D. Identification of Markers that Distinguish IgE-From IgG-Mediated Anaphylaxis. *Proc. Natl. Acad. Sci. USA* **2011**, *108*, 12413–12418. [CrossRef]
8. Finkelman, F.D.; Khodoun, M.V.; Strait, R. Human IgE-Independent Systemic Anaphylaxis. *J. Allergy Clin. Immunol.* **2016**, *137*, 1674–1680. [CrossRef] [PubMed]
9. Muñoz-Cano, R.; Picado, C.; Valero, A.; Bartra, J. Mechanisms of Anaphylaxis Beyond IgE. *J. Investig. Allergol. Clin. Immunol.* **2016**, *26*, 73–82. [CrossRef]
10. Fritscher-Ravens, A.; Schuppan, D.; Ellrichmann, M.; Schoch, S.; Röcken, C.; Brasch, J.; Bethge, J.; Böttner, M.; Klose, J.; Milla, P.J. Confocal Endomicroscopy Shows Food-Associated Changes in the Intestinal Mucosa of Patients with Irritable Bowel Syndrome. *Gastroenterology* **2014**, *147*, 1012–1020.e4. [CrossRef]
11. Bentz, S.; Hausmann, M.; Piberger, H.; Kellermeier, S.; Paul, S.; Held, L.; Falk, W.; Obermeier, F.; Fried, M.; Schölmerich, J.; et al. Clinical Relevance of IgG Antibodies against Food Antigens in Crohn's Disease: A Double-Blind Cross-Over Diet Intervention Study. *Digestion* **2010**, *81*, 252–264. [CrossRef]
12. Cai, C.; Shen, J.; Zhao, D.; Qiao, Y.; Xu, A.; Jin, S.; Ran, Z.; Zheng, Q. Serological Investigation of Food Specific Immunoglobulin G Antibodies in Patients with Inflammatory Bowel Diseases. *PLoS ONE* **2014**, *9*, e112154. [CrossRef] [PubMed]
13. Alpay, K.; Ertaş, M.; Orhan, E.K.; Üstay, D.K.; Lieners, C.; Baykan, B. Diet Restriction in Migraine, Based on IgG against Foods: A Clinical Double-Blind, Randomised, Cross-Over Trial. *Cephalalgia* **2010**, *30*, 829–837. [CrossRef]
14. Biesiekierski, J.R.; Newnham, E.D.; Irving, P.M.; Barrett, J.S.; Haines, M.; Doecke, J.D.; Shepherd, S.J.; Muir, J.G.; Gibson, P.R. Gluten Causes Gastrointestinal Symptoms in Subjects without Celiac Disease: A Double-Blind Randomized Placebo-Controlled Trial. *Am. J. Gastroenterol.* **2011**, *106*, 508–514. [CrossRef]
15. Kim-Lee, C.; Suresh, L.; Ambrus, J.L. Gastrointestinal Disease in Sjogren's Syndrome: Related to Food Hypersensitivities. *Springerplus* **2015**, *4*, 766. [CrossRef]

16. Shulman, R.J.; Eakin, M.N.; Czyzewski, D.I.; Jarrett, M.; Ou, C.-N. Increased Gastrointestinal Permeability and Gut Inflammation in Children with Functional Abdominal Pain and Irritable Bowel Syndrome. *J. Pediatr.* **2008**, *153*, 646–650. [CrossRef]

17. Clayton, F.; Fang, J.C.; Gleich, G.J.; Lucendo, A.J.; Olalla, J.M.; Vinson, L.A.; Lowichik, A.; Chen, X.; Emerson, L.; Cox, K.; et al. Eosinophilic Esophagitis in Adults is Associated with IgG4 and not Mediated by IgE. *Gastroenterology* **2014**, *147*, 602–609. [CrossRef] [PubMed]

18. Thorburn, A.N.; Macia, L.; Mackay, C.R. Diet, Metabolites, and "Western-Lifestyle" Inflammatory Diseases. *Immunity* **2014**, *40*, 833–842. [CrossRef]

19. Eisen, M.B.; Spellman, P.T.; Brown, P.O.; Botstein, D. Cluster Analysis and Display of Genome-Wide Expression Patterns. *Proc. Natl. Acad. Sci. USA* **1998**, *95*, 14863–14868. [CrossRef] [PubMed]

20. Fatati, G. [Italian eating behavior: Survey 2011]. *Recenti Prog. Med.* **2012**, *103*, 225–233.

21. Pala, V.; Sieri, S.; Palli, D.; Salvini, S.; Berrino, F.; Bellegotti, M.; Frasca, G.; Tumino, R.; Sacerdote, C.; Fiorini, L.; et al. Diet in the Italian EPIC Cohorts: Presentation of Data and Methodological Issues. *Tumori J.* **2003**, *89*, 594–607. [CrossRef]

22. Riccioni, G.; Menna, V.; Di Ilio, C.; D'Orazio, N. Food-Intake and Nutrients Pattern in Italian Adult Male Subjects. *Clin. Ther.* **2004**, *155*, 283–286.

23. Hjartåker, A.; Lagiou, A.; Slimani, N.; Lund, E.; Chirlaque, M.D.; Vasilopoulou, E.; Zavitsanos, X.; Berrino, F.; Sacerdote, C.; Ocké, M.C.; et al. Consumption of Dairy Products in the European Prospective Investigation into Cancer and Nutrition (EPIC) Cohort: Data from 35 955 24-h Dietary Recalls in 10 European countries. *Public Health Nutr.* **2002**, *5*, 1259–1271. [CrossRef] [PubMed]

24. Sherman, P.W.; Flaxman, S.M. Nausea and Vomiting of Pregnancy in an Evolutionary Perspective. *Am. J. Obstet. Gynecol.* **2002**, *186*, S190–S197. [CrossRef] [PubMed]

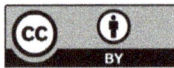

Article

Exposure to Vitamin D Fortification Policy in Prenatal Life and the Risk of Childhood Asthma: Results from the D-Tect Study

Fanney Thorsteinsdottir [1,*], Ekaterina Maslova [2,3], Ramune Jacobsen [1,4], Peder Frederiksen [1], Amélie Keller [1], Vibeke Backer [5] and Berit Lilienthal Heitmann [1,6,7]

[1] Fanney Thorsteinsdottir, Research Unit for Dietary Studies, The Parker Institute, Bisbebjerg og Frederiksberg Hospital, Nordre Fasanvej 57, 2000 Frederiksberg, Denmark; ramune.jacobsen@sund.ku.dk (R.J.); peder.frederiksen@regionh.dk (P.F.); amelie.cleo.keller@regionh.dk (A.K.); berit.lilienthal.heitmann@egionh.dk (B.L.H.)
[2] Department of Primary Care and Public Health, Imperial College London, London W6 8RP, UK; ekaterina.maslova14@imperial.ac.uk
[3] Centre for Fetal Programming, Department of Epidemiology Research, Statens Serum Institut, 2300 Copenhagen, Denmark
[4] Department of Pharmacy, University of Copenhagen, 2100 Copenhagen, Denmark
[5] Department of Respiratory Medicine, Bispebjerg University Hospital, 2400 Copenhagen, Denmark; backer@dadlnet.dk
[6] The Boden Institute of Obesity, Nutrition, Exercise & Eating Disorders, University of Sydney, Sydney, NSW 2006, Australia
[7] The Department of Public Health, Section for General Practice, University of Copenhagen, 2100 Copenhagen, Denmark
*   Correspondence: fanney.thorsteinsdottir@regionh.dk; Tel.: +45-3816-3103

Received: 4 March 2019; Accepted: 18 April 2019; Published: 24 April 2019

Abstract: Prenatal vitamin D insufficiency may be associated with an increased risk of developing childhood asthma. Results from epidemiological studies are conflicting and limited by short follow-up and small sample sizes. The objective of this study was to examine if children born to women exposed to the margarine fortification policy with a small dose of extra vitamin D during pregnancy had a reduced risk of developing asthma until age 9 years, compared to children born to unexposed women. The termination of a Danish mandatory vitamin D fortification policy constituted the basis for the study design. We compared the risk of inpatient asthma diagnoses in all Danish children born two years before (n = 106,347, exposed) and two years after (n = 115,900, unexposed) the termination of the policy. The children were followed in the register from 0–9 years of age. Data were analyzed using Cox proportional hazards regression. The Hazard Ratio for the first inpatient asthma admission among exposed versus unexposed children was 0.96 (95%CI: 0.90–1.04). When stratifying by sex and age, 0–3 years old boys exposed to vitamin D fortification showed a lower asthma risk compared to unexposed boys (HR 0.78, 95%CI: 0.67–0.92). Prenatal exposure to margarine fortification policy with extra vitamin D did not affect the overall risk of developing asthma among children aged 0–9 years but seemed to reduce the risk among 0–3 years old boys. Taking aside study design limitations, this could be explained by different sensitivity to vitamin D from different sex-related asthma phenotypes in children with early onset, and sex differences in lung development or immune responses.

Keywords: asthma; fortification; vitamin D; social experiment

---

1. Introduction

Asthma is one of the most common chronic conditions among children [1]. It is a complex heterogeneous disease that affects both the respiratory and the immune system [2]. It manifests by many phenotypes that vary by sex, age at onset, presence of obesity, as well as the severity of atopy, allergic sensitization, bronchial obstruction, and hyperresponsiveness. Although genetic factors and childhood exposure to environmental triggers, such as tobacco smoke, air pollution, viral infections or aeroallergens play a major role in the development of childhood asthma [3], it has been suggested that environmental exposures during gestation may also be important [4]. Asthma is more prevalent among boys until puberty when a shift towards higher prevalence among girls and women is observed [5,6]. In children, this is thought to be due to sex differences in lung development and inflammatory profile [7].

Vitamin D is a fat-soluble vitamin and a secosteroid hormone playing an important role in both skeletal and non-skeletal functions [8]. It readily crosses the placenta and the fetal supply is totally dependent on the supplies of the mother [9]. Results from animal and human studies have shown that prenatal vitamin D insufficiency may influence both the intrauterine immune system [10] and lung development [11,12], causing permanent changes to these systems. Such changes constitute a plausible biological basis to suggest that vitamin D insufficiency during gestation may have a programming effect contributing to the risk of childhood asthma. This is especially relevant given the high prevalence of vitamin D insufficiency in pregnant women [13]. The research on the association between prenatal vitamin D status and childhood asthma risk in the offspring is quite extensive. Results from several systematic reviews and meta-analyses of observational studies, however, have been inconsistent [14–18]. Two randomized clinical trials (RCT) have recently been conducted; both found non-significant 20% reduced risk of asthma/recurrent wheeze among 0–3 year old children whose mothers were supplemented with vitamin D during pregnancy [19,20], while a combined analysis of the two trials showed a significant reduction in offspring's asthma/recurrent wheeze risk after vitamin D supplementation in pregnancy [21]. Despite sex differences in asthma prevalence and possible sex difference in the effect of vitamin D on asthma development, few observational studies and none of the RCTs have run analyses differentiated by sex. Furthermore, most of the previous studies had limited numbers of participants and short follow-up periods [14–18,21].

In Denmark, between 1937 and 1985, it was mandatory to fortify margarine with 1.25 µg vitamin D per 100 g [22]. The fortification accounted for on average 13% (3–29%) of total vitamin D intake from food in the Danish population [22]. Despite that, the mandatory margarine fortification policy was canceled in June 1985. This study utilized the design of this societal experiment grounded on the distinct in time termination of the Danish margarine vitamin D fortification policy. The objective of the present study was to examine if children born to women exposed to the margarine fortification policy with a small dose of extra vitamin D during pregnancy had a reduced risk of developing asthma until age 9 years compared to children whose mothers were unexposed to the fortification policy during pregnancy. Furthermore, this study examined whether the association between exposure and asthma risk varied by age, sex, and month of birth.

2. Methods

2.1. Study Design

This study is a part of the D-tect project and a detailed study design description has been published elsewhere [23]. Briefly, all individuals born in Denmark during the two years before the termination of the vitamin D policy in 1985 were considered as exposed to vitamin D fortification during prenatal life, and all individuals born during the two years after the termination (excluding a wash-out period), were considered unexposed to vitamin D fortification. The washout period consisted of 9 months for the duration of a full-term pregnancy and an additional 6 months to allow for fortified products to be commercially replaced by non-fortified products (Figure 1).

Termination of margarine fortification: 1. June 1985

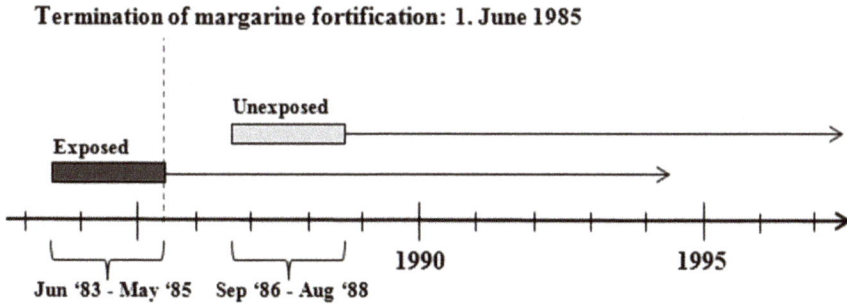

Figure 1. Study design and study population.

All children born alive in Denmark from June 1983–May 1985 and from September 1986–August 1988 were identified using the Danish Civil Registration System (CRS) and included in this study. The CRS was established in 1968 and includes information on all individuals alive and with permanent residence in Denmark at that time, and those who were born in or immigrated to Denmark afterwards [24]. All individuals in Denmark are assigned a unique identification number (CPR number) that can be used to identify the individual in all national registers and databases. From the CRS we retrieved information on the date of birth, date of death (if any), date of emigration or lost to follow up (residence unknown to Danish authorities).

Individuals from our study population were followed in the Danish National Patient Register (DNPR) to identify childhood asthma diagnoses. The DNPR is a national administrative register established in 1977 that contains information on all hospital admissions, including discharge diagnoses, according to the international classification of diseases (ICD) system [25]. Outpatient admissions in DNPR were systematically registered from 1995, and to ensure comparable exposure groups with complete follow-up among both exposed and unexposed individuals we only analyzed inpatient asthma admissions in this study.

According to Danish law, ethical approval is not required for register-based studies. Permission to access data was granted by Forskerservice, Statens Serum Institut (J.no. FSEID-00001369). The Danish Data Protection Agency provided permission to process data (J.no. 2012-41-1156). The study is registered at ClinicalTrials.gov (NCT03330301).

2.2. Definition of Outcome

Childhood asthma was defined as asthma diagnoses from birth to the age of 9 years. We considered puberty as a cut-off for distinguishing childhood asthma from adult asthma, as puberty is the period when there is a sex-based shift in the prevalence of asthma from male predominance to female predominance. In a previous study conducted among Danish children aged 6.0–19.9 years, the mean age for the pre-pubertal stage was 10.88 (SD ± 8.66–13.11) years for girls and 11.83 (SD ± 9.92–13.75) for boys [26], defining the age of 9 as a certain cut-off for pre-pubertal stage.

Asthma was defined based on ICD-8 codes 493.00, 493.01, 493.08 and 493.09; and from 1994 onwards on ICD-10 codes DJ45, DJ45.0, DJ45.1, DJ45.8, DJ45.9, DJ46.0, and DJ46.9. The registry diagnoses of asthma have been previously validated against medical records [27].

2.3. Statistical Analysis

We conducted a time-to-event analysis focusing on the time of first inpatient asthma diagnosis. If asthma was not diagnosed at the age of 9, or if the child became inactive in the CRS (emigrated, lost to follow up or dead) before the age of 9, censoring took place. We used a Cox proportional hazard model with age as the underlying time scale to assess the hazard ratios of first inpatient asthma diagnosis in the group that was exposed to extra vitamin D from fortification during gestation compared to the group that was unexposed to extra vitamin D from fortification. The assumption of proportional hazard was examined using Schoenfeld residuals [28]. Data were presented as the time at risk, incident rate, and hazard ratio (95% confidence interval). Descriptive statistics were presented in frequencies (N) and percentages (%). In multivariable analysis, we adjusted for sex and month of birth. As we included entire birth cohorts of all individuals born in Denmark in adjacent years around the fortification termination, other potential confounders were considered to be equally distributed in both exposure groups, thus adjustment for other confounders was not deemed necessary.

To test our hypothesis that the greatest risk reduction would be observed among those who had most of their prenatal period during the darkest months, we examined if the effect of vitamin D fortification on asthma risk was modified by month of birth by the likelihood ratio test; the statistical tests were two-sided at a 5% significance level. In addition, as decided a priory, we conducted analyses stratified by sex and age at the time of asthma diagnosis hypothesizing potential effect modification by sex and age, since the prevalence of asthma is higher among boys especially in the first few years of life, and both sex and age are important characteristics of different asthma phenotypes [29].

All data management and descriptive statistics were performed using Stata 13 (StataCorp. 2013. Stata Statistical Software: Release 13. College Station, TX, USA, www.stata.com), whereas all statistical analyses were performed using R version 3.3.3 (R Foundation for Statistical Computing, Vienna, Austria, www.R-project.org).

3. Results

Out of 222,247 children included in the study, 106,347 were born to mothers exposed to the margarine fortification policy with extra vitamin D during pregnancy; 115,900 were born to unexposed mothers. Among the exposed children, 1427 (64% boys) had inpatient asthma admission before the age of 9 years; and among unexposed children, 1613 (65% boys) had inpatient asthma admission before the age of 9 years (Figure 2 and Supplementary Table S1).

We did not observe a difference in inpatient asthma admission risk between children exposed and unexposed to the margarine fortification policy with extra vitamin D during the prenatal period (HR 0.96, 95% CI: 0.90–1.03). Furthermore, there was no effect modification by month of birth ($p = 0.28$). The Schoenfeld residuals indicated violation of the proportional hazards assumption with respect to exposure status, and when stratified by age at first diagnoses, we found that among the 0–3 years old, those exposed to extra vitamin D from fortification were less likely to have an inpatient asthma admission (HR 0.86, 95% CI: 0.75–0.98) compared to unexposed ones. Further stratification by sex revealed that reduced risk was confined to the 0–3-year-old boys. Boys of 0–3 years exposed to the margarine fortification policy with extra vitamin D were less likely to have an inpatient asthma admission (HR 0.78, 95% CI: 0.67–0.92) compared to unexposed ones. Adjusting for sex and month of birth gave similar results (Table 1 and Figure 3).

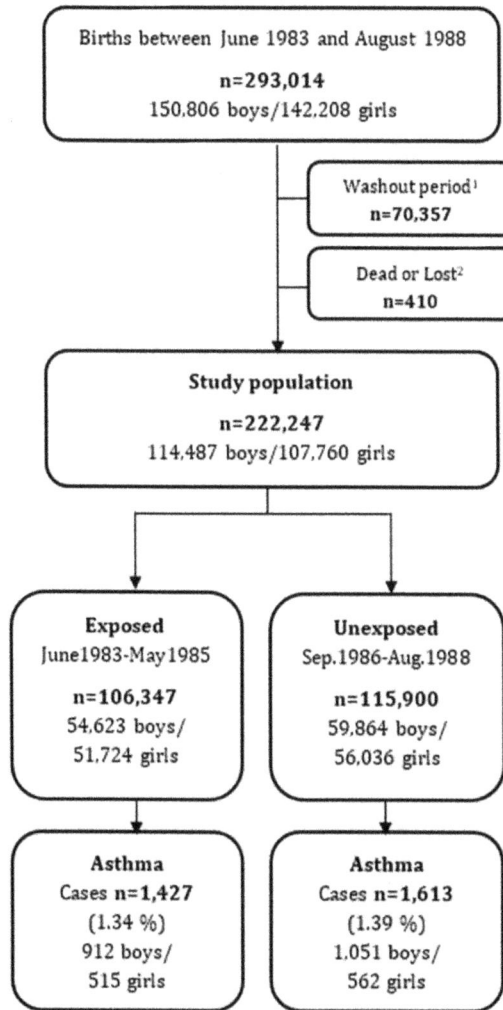

Figure 2. Flowchart of the study population.

Births between June 1983 and August 1988
n=293,014
150,806 boys/142,208 girls

Washout period[1]
n=70,357

Dead or Lost[2]
n=410

Study population
n=222,247
114,487 boys/107,760 girls

Exposed
June 1983-May 1985
n=106,347
54,623 boys/
51,724 girls

Unexposed
Sep. 1986-Aug. 1988
n=115,900
59,864 boys/
56,036 girls

Asthma
Cases **n=1,427**
(1.34 %)
912 boys/
515 girls

Asthma
Cases **n=1,613**
(1.39 %)
1,051 boys/
562 girls

[1] 6 months for fortified products to be commercially replaced, and full 9 month pregnancy after termination of mandatory margarine fortification.
[2] Dead or lost to follow up before birth or on the day of birth.

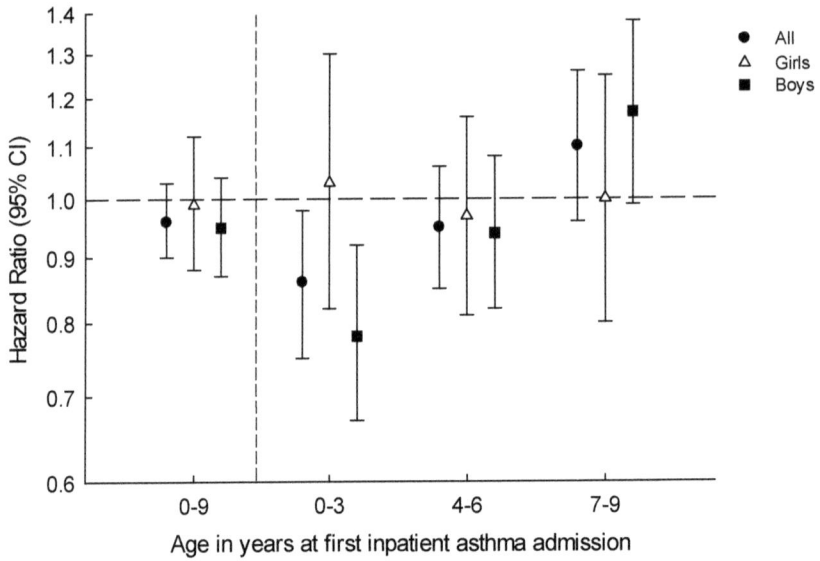

Figure 3. Hazard ratio of childhood asthma among those prenatally exposed to the margarine fortification with vitamin D policy, compared to those unexposed.

Table 1. Incidence, years at risk, rate, and hazard ratio (HR) of childhood asthma among those prenatally exposed to the margarine fortification with vitamin D policy, compared to those unexposed.

| | Exposed | | | Unexposed | | | | | Adjusted † | | p for Interaction |
	Admissions	Time at Risk (Years)	Rate per 100,000 Years at Risk	Admissions	Time at Risk (Years)	Rate per 100,000 Years at Risk	HR	(95% CI)	HR	(95% CI)	with Month of Birth
All	1427	938,797	152.0	1613	1,022,110	157.8	0.96	(0.90–1.03)	0.96	(0.90–1.04)	0.28
0–3 years	393	315,879	124.4	498	343,928	144.8	0.86	(0.75–0.98)	0.86	(0.75–0.98)	0.63
4–6 years	596	312,640	190.6	682	340,339	200.4	0.95	(0.85–1.06)	0.95	(0.85–1.06)	0.02
7–9 years	438	310,278	141.2	433	337,843	128.2	1.10	(0.96–1.26)	1.10	(0.96–1.26)	0.78
Girls	515	457,866	112.5	562	496,107	113.3	0.99	(0.88–1.12)	0.99	(0.88–1.12)	0.30
0–3 years	146	153,849	94.9	153	166,624	91.8	1.03	(0.82–1.30)	1.03	(0.82–1.30)	0.98
4–6 years	221	152,494	144.9	248	165,223	150.1	0.97	(0.81–1.16)	0.97	(0.81–1.16)	0.14
7–9 years	148	151,523	97.7	161	164,259	98.0	1.00	(0.80–1.25)	1.00	(0.80–1.24)	0.41
Boys	912	480,931	189.6	1,051	526,003	199.8	0.95	(0.87–1.04)	0.95	(0.87–1.04)	0.50
0–3 years	247	177,304	194.6	345	162,030	152.4	0.78	(0.67–0.92)	0.78	(0.67–0.92)	0.24
4–6 years	375	175,116	247.8	434	160,146	234.2	0.94	(0.82–1.08)	0.95	(0.82–1.09)	0.10
7–9 years	290	173,583	156.7	272	158,755	182.7	1.17	(0.99–1.38)	1.16	(0.99–1.37)	0.71

† = adjusted for sex and month of birth, except girls and boys are only adjusted for month of birth.

4. Discussion

Overall, we did not see a difference in the risk of asthma between children of both sexes age 0–9 years born to mothers exposed to the margarine fortification policy with a small extra dose of vitamin D during their entire pregnancy compared to those who were born to mothers who were unexposed. However, our analysis indicated that young children (0–3 years old), and in particular boys born to exposed mothers, had more than 20% lower hazards for developing asthma compared to boys born to unexposed mothers.

Several observational studies have examined the association between prenatal vitamin D and the development of asthma in the offspring, however, the results have been mixed. There are several potential reasons for this inconsistency. The observational studies have differed in study design, number of participants, adjustment for covariates, the time at exposure assessment, the source material for biomarker analysis, the concentration of maternal or cord blood 25(OH)D, and the assay method. Early observational studies looking at vitamin D intake during pregnancy, usually assessed by food frequency questionnaire (FFQ), and later development of asthma and wheezing, tended to find inverse associations [30–32]. Vitamin D may have served as a marker of a healthier diet in general and other dietary-related factors such as differences in the maternal microbiome [33]. The cohort studies examining maternal or cord blood 25(OH)D tended to find no association between 25(OH)D level in pregnancy and offspring asthma [34–36]. This was true across different timing of exposure and outcome assessment as well as geographical settings. Total 25(OH)D level may not be a sufficient indicator of the biologically available vitamin D, as other factors such as level of vitamin D binding protein could influence the metabolism and bioavailability [37,38]. These studies also did not look at the difference in asthma risk between different sex nor stratify according to pre-pregnancy vitamin D status which may be more important for reducing asthma risk than vitamin D status in pregnancy. In two recent randomized trials where mothers were supplemented with daily dose of 60 and 100 µg vitamin D respectively during pregnancy [19–21], inverse associations between 25(OH)D level and asthma/recurrent wheeze were strongest among women with a high 25(OH)D status at baseline (≥75 nmol/L). This could indicate that the programming effect already takes place in early pregnancy or even prior to pregnancy, and therefore, having optimal vitamin D status already at conception might be important for reducing the risk of childhood asthma. This may be supported by the results from observational studies assessing vitamin D intake as women with higher vitamin D intake during pregnancy are likely to have had the same dietary pattern prior to pregnancy and thus have higher vitamin D status at conception. In our study, the mothers were exposed to extra vitamin D from fortification both during a long period prior to pregnancy and during the entire pregnancy. Thus, it is expected that the exposed mothers had a higher vitamin D status pre-pregnancy than unexposed mothers. It is important to stress that the vitamin D dose administered to the subjects in the two trials was substantially higher than what women were exposed to from fortification in our study. We have previously calculated, based on the fortification dose (1.25 µg/100g) and margarine intake statistics, that an average additional 0.4–0.6 µg of vitamin D per day could be provided by the fortified margarine [39]. Compared to vitamin D supplementation in the two trials (i.e. 60 and 100 µg), and in light of the recommended total intake of 10 µg vitamin D per day for skeletal actions [40], the Danish margarine fortification policy provided a very low extra vitamin D dose. However, the optimal vitamin D dose for the prenatal development of the immune system and/or lung development is unknown. Much higher supplementation doses provided in the two previously mentioned trials seemed to be inadequate to reach a level of sufficiency among women during their pregnancy to prevent asthma development in the offspring. In our study, a constant intake of a very low extra dose of vitamin D via fortified foods consumption over entire pregnancy (and before pregnancy), might have been sufficient to reduce the risk in the offspring with the highest risk of developing asthma, the youngest boys [7,41]. Methodological advantages and disadvantages of our societal experiment design study, if compared to clinical trials, are discussed below under strengths and limitations.

Asthma phenotypes are defined based on age at debut, the presence of atopy, allergic sanitization, lung function, responsiveness to steroids, obesity, sex, and inflammatory profile. Many of these different phenotypes vary according to age, making age an important parameter in identifying asthma phenotypes [42]. Therefore, to try to isolate specific phenotypes, we stratified the analysis by age at onset. Our results of a slight reduction in the risk of inpatient asthma admission among 0–3 years old boys born to mothers who were exposed to the margarine fortification policy with extra vitamin D during pregnancy are in accordance with the results from the combined analysis of the two recently published RCTs showing a 26% reduction in the risk of asthma/recurrent wheeze at age 0–3 years among those born to mothers who took vitamin D supplementation during pregnancy [21]. This could indicate that vitamin D has an effect on asthma phenotypes that are prevalent in the youngest children, especially boys, or that the programming effect is relatively weaker than the effect of the risk factors accumulating during childhood. On the other hand, among children younger than 6 years, and particularly those younger than 3 years, the asthma diagnosis is based on symptoms (wheezing, cough, and breathlessness), clinical history of these symptoms, or family history of asthma or atopy, whereas among older children and adults asthma is diagnosed based on symptoms and confirmed with objective measures (spirometry, beta2 agonist reversibility test, bronchial provocation test, and peak flow measurements) [3]. Wheezing is the most common clinical manifestation of asthma onset. As very young children who experience severe and persistent wheezing are more likely to also have asthma in childhood or adulthood [43,44], persistent wheezing in very young children usually is considered to be an asthma indication. At the same time, many young children often experience wheezing due to viral respiratory tract infections (RTI) without having or later developing asthma [44]. Notably, a recent review on the association between maternal vitamin D status and RTI in offspring showed an inverse association between exposure to vitamin D and RTIs (highest vs. lowest 25(OH)D level: OR 0.64, 95% CI: 0.47–0.87), but no association with asthma or wheezing [18]. Hence, it cannot be ruled out that the protective effect observed among the 0–3-year-olds in our study was driven by a proportion of children misdiagnosed with asthma because of wheezing due to viral RTI.

In regard to the sex differences, there are anatomic differences in lung size, maturity, and function between the sexes with boys having larger lungs than girls, however, girls have higher forced expiratory flow rates [7]. The lungs of newborn boys are also less mature than the lungs of newborn girls [45] and thus are more vulnerable to respiratory infection, and consequently, asthma. Moreover, severe allergic asthma, or asthma with multiple sensitizations to allergens, characterized by early onset, high eosinophil count, and a low response to corticosteroid, is more prevalent among boys [29]. Children included in our study were children with asthma diagnosed during hospitalization, thus our outcome measure captured the more severe cases of asthma. It is therefore possible that the protective association observed among the youngest boys in our study was driven by the effects on an allergic type of asthma. Interestingly, despite sex differences in the prevalence of asthma, and different asthma phenotypes in boys and girls [44], very few studies have examined whether the effect of prenatal vitamin D exposure on the development of asthma is sex-specific. We identified only one other study that conducted sex-stratified analyses, and similarly to the results of the present study, the authors found an inverse association between maternal vitamin D and asthma risk at 6 years among boys only [46]. Consequently, vitamin D status in fetal life may contribute differently to the regulation of the immunologic responses in boys and girls.

Based on the present study, we cannot conclude that exposure to the margarine fortification policy with extra vitamin D during the prenatal period influences the risk of offspring asthma. However, our results and those of prior studies may indicate that vitamin D intake, even in small amounts, early in pregnancy or even before conception could influence the risk of asthma development, especially among more vulnerable groups such as very young male children. Future studies of the association between prenatal vitamin D and offspring asthma risk should assess vitamin D status or intervene with vitamin D supplements periconceptually or prior to pregnancy. Furthermore, they should focus on different phenotypes of asthma, using biomarkers shown to have a good prognostic value, and assessment of possible sex differences.

Strengths and Limitations

In this study we utilized a societal experiment of an abrupt abolishment of an obligatory vitamin D fortification, that exposed all individuals living in Denmark to extra vitamin D from fortified margarine during a distinct period of time when the fortification policy was implemented, and not thereafter. A semi-ecological study design has both strengths and limitations.

The strength is that we could include all individuals born in Denmark from entire birth cohorts from the Danish population, capturing all inpatient asthma admissions, which makes our results generalizable for the entire Danish population. This was possible due to the excellent Danish administrative and health registers, extensively used in Danish epidemiological research [47,48]. Additionally, asthma diagnoses in DNPR have been previously validated [27]. Another strength of the design was that potential confounding (i.e., from differences in socioeconomic status, obesity, maternal lifestyle and diet during pregnancy) can be considered to be equally distributed in both the exposed and the unexposed groups as they included all individuals born in adjacent birth cohorts around the time of the policy change. Nevertheless, secular trends in potential confounders during this short period of time between 1983–1988 could have introduced residual confounding. Intake of margarine was remarkably stable during the years around the policy change, and we were not able to identify changes in national recommendations for intake and/or supplementation of vitamin D or in fortification practice. However, a study from Denmark shows that smoking among women, a risk factor for offspring asthma, decreased slightly during this period [49]. This would have attenuated our findings and therefore speaks in favor of a true association between exposure to the margarine fortification policy with extra vitamin D and the development of asthma. Furthermore, we know that overweight and obesity, a risk factor for asthma, has been increasing among women [50], and from 1987–1988 there were changes in fiscal policy in Denmark that caused economic challenges for many households [51,52]. It can be speculated that this economic crisis influenced overall diet quality, such as decreased the intake of fish or fish oil, which is also shown to have a protective effect on asthma development among offspring.

The limitation of this semi-ecological study design is that information on our exposure represents ecological data; we do not have any information on actual vitamin D intake, neither from the fortified margarine nor from other dietary sources and hence cannot make actual intake recommendations. A further limitation of the study is that we only included in-patient discharge diagnoses and not outpatients diagnoses and diagnoses by general practitioners, as the DNPR does not collect this information. Consequently, we have a subgroup of asthmatic children, most likely those with severe or uncontrolled asthma, and can generalize our results only to this group. Another study limitation related to the nature of register data, which does not specify different phenotypes of asthma, nor clinical parameters. To approximate this information, we conducted analyses stratified by age and sex; however, even though the phenotypes differ by age and sex, there are other parameters that are equally important, such as sensitization to allergens, responsiveness to steroids, and inflammatory profile that would also be interesting to examine.

5. Conclusions

Our study, based on the societal experiment concerning margarine fortification with vitamin D in Denmark, suggests that prenatal exposure to a small dose of extra vitamin D from fortification may be associated with a lower risk of childhood asthma among boys aged 0–3 years, but not among older children or the youngest girls. Asthma phenotypes with very early onset that have different vitamin D sensitivity and/or sex differences in lung development or immune responses may explain our findings. However, residual confounding effects due to the semi-ecological design of the study cannot be ruled out.

Supplementary Materials: The following are available online at http://www.mdpi.com/2072-6643/11/4/924/s1, Table S1: Characteristics of the study population in numbers and percentages.

Author Contributions: B.L.H. designed the study. F.T., B.L.H., E.M. and R.J. formulated the research question. P.F. performed the statistical analysis. F.T. drafted the manuscript. All authors interpreted the results, critically reviewed the manuscript, approved the final version and agreed on the submission of the manuscript.

Funding: This research was funded by the Danish Agency for Science, Technology and Innovation, the Ministry of Science, Higher Education (grant 0603-00453B).

Acknowledgments: This study was a part of the D-tect study funded by the Danish Agency for Science, Technology and Innovation, the Ministry of Science, Higher Education, under the instrument "Strategic Research Projects" (grant 0603-00453B). The funders had no role in study design, data collection and analysis, decision to publish, or preparation of the manuscript.

Conflicts of Interest: The authors declare no conflict of interest.

References

1. Masoli, M.; Fabian, D.; Holt, S.; Beasley, R. The global burden of asthma: Executive summary of the GINA Dissemination Committee Report. *Allergy* **2004**, *59*, 469–478. [CrossRef] [PubMed]
2. Bush, S.; Kleinert, S.; Pavord, I.D. The asthmas in 2015 and beyond: A Lancet Commission. *Lancet* **2015**, *385*, 1273–1275. [CrossRef]
3. Pedersen, S.E.; Hurd, S.S.; Lemanske, R.F.; Becker, A.; Zar, H.J.; Sly, P.D.; Soto-Quiroz, M.; Wong, G.; Bateman, E.D. Global strategy for the diagnosis and management of asthma in children 5 years and younger. *Pediatr. Pulmonol.* **2011**, *46*, 1–17. [CrossRef] [PubMed]
4. De Luca, G.; Olivieri, F.; Melotti, G.; Aiello, G.; Lubrano, L.; Boner, A.L. Fetal and early postnatal life roots of asthma. *J. Matern. Fetal. Neonatal. Med.* **2010**, *23*, 80–83. [CrossRef] [PubMed]
5. Postma, D.S. Gender Differences in Asthma Development and Progression. *Gend. Med.* **2007**, *4* (Suppl. B), S133–S146. [CrossRef]
6. Almqvist, C.; Worm, M.; Leynaert, B. Impact of gender on asthma in childhood and adolescence: A GA2LEN review. *Allergy* **2008**, *63*, 47–57. [CrossRef]
7. Pignataro, F.S.; Bonini, M.; Forgione, A.; Melandri, S.; Usmani, O.S. Asthma and gender: The female lung. *Pharmacol. Res.* **2017**, *119*, 384–390. [CrossRef]
8. Wimalawansa, S.J. Non-musculoskeletal benefits of vitamin D. *J. Steroid. Biochem. Mol. Biol.* **2018**, *175*, 60–81. [CrossRef]
9. Larque, E.; Morales, E.; Leis, R.; Blanco-Carnerdo, J.E. Maternal and Foetal Health Implications of Vitamin D Status during Pregnancy. *Ann. Nutr. Metab.* **2018**, *72*, 179–192. [CrossRef] [PubMed]
10. Chi, A.; Wildfire, J.; McLoughlin, R.; Wood, R.A.; Bloomberg, G.R.; Kattan, M.; Gregen, P.; Gold, D.R.; Witter, F.; Chen, T.; et al. Umbilical cord plasma 25-hydroxyvitamin D concentration and immune function at birth: The Urban Environment and Childhood Asthma study. *Clin. Exp. Allergy* **2011**, *41*, 842–850. [CrossRef] [PubMed]
11. Chen, L.; Wilson, R.; Bennet, E.; Zosky, R. Identification of vitamin D sensitive pathways during lung development. *Respir Res.* **2016**, *17*, 47. [CrossRef] [PubMed]
12. Kho, A.T.; Sharma, S.; Qiu, W.; Gaedigk, R.; Klanderman, B.; Niu, S.; Anderson, C.; Leeder, J.S.; Weiss, S.T.; Tantisira, K.G. Vitamin D related genes in lung development and asthma pathogenesis. *BMC Med. Genom.* **2013**, *6*, 47. [CrossRef]
13. Hollis, B.; Wagner, C. Nutritional vitamin D status during pregnancy: Reason for concern. *CMAJ* **2006**, *174*, 1287–1290. [CrossRef]
14. Nurmatov, U.; Devereux, G.; Sheikh, A. Nutrients and foods for the primary prevention of asthma and allergy: Systematic review and meta-analysis. *J. Allergy Clin. Immunol.* **2011**, *127*, 724–733. [CrossRef] [PubMed]
15. Beckhaus, A.A.; Garcia-Marcos, L.; Forno, E.; Pacheco-Gonzalez, R.M.; Celedón, J.C.; Castro-Rodriguez, J.A. Maternal nutrition during pregnancy and risk of asthma, wheeze, and atopic diseases during childhood: A systematic review and meta-analysis. *Allergy* **2015**, *70*, 1588–1604. [CrossRef] [PubMed]
16. Feng, H.; Xun, P.; Pike, K.; Wills, A.K.; Chawes, B.L.; Bisgaard, H.; Cai, W.; Wan, Y.; He, K. In utero exposure to 25-hydroxyvitamin D and risk of childhood asthma, wheeze, and respiratory tract infections: A meta-analysis of birth cohort studies. *J. Allergy Clin. Immunol.* **2017**, *139*, 1508–1517. [CrossRef]

17. Song, H.; Yang, L.; Jia, C. Maternal vitamin D status during pregnancy and risk of childhood asthma: A meta-analysis of prospective studies. *Mol. Nutr. Food Res.* **2017**, *61*, 1600657. [CrossRef] [PubMed]
18. Pacheco-Gonzalez, R.M.; Garcia-Marcos, L.; Morales, E. Prenatal vitamin D status and respiratory and allergic outcomes in childhood: A meta-analysis of observational studies. *Pediatr. Allergy Immunol.* **2018**, *29*, 243–253. [CrossRef]
19. Chawes, B.L.; Bønnelykke, K.; Stokholm, J.; Vissing, N.H.; Bjarnadóttir, E.; Schoos, A.M.; Wolsk, H.M.; Pedersen, T.M.; Vinding, R.K.; Thorsteinsdóttir, S.; et al. Effect of vitamin d3 supplementation during pregnancy on risk of persistent wheeze in the offspring: A randomized clinical trial. *JAMA* **2016**, *315*, 353–361. [CrossRef]
20. Litonjua, A.A.; Carey, V.J.; Laranjo, N.; Harshfield, B.J.; McElrath, T.F.; O'Connor, G.T.; Sandel, M.; Iverson, R.E.; Lee-Paritz, A.; Strunk, R.C.; et al. Effect of prenatal supplementation with vitamin d on asthma or recurrent wheezing in offspring by age 3 years: The vdaart randomized clinical trial. *JAMA* **2016**, *315*, 362–370. [CrossRef]
21. Wolsk, H.M.; Chawes, B.L.; Litonjua, A.A.; Hollis, B.W.; Waage, J.; Stokholm, J.; Bønnelykke, K.; Bisgaard, H.; Weiss, S.T. Prenatal vitamin D supplementation reduces risk of asthma/recurrent wheeze in early childhood: A combined analysis of two randomized controlled trials. *PLoS ONE* **2017**, *12*, e0186657. [CrossRef]
22. Nordic Council of Ministers. The fortification of foods with vitamins and minerals. In *Tilsætning af Vitaminer og Mineraler til Levnedsmidler*; Nordic Council of Ministers: Copenhagen, Denmark, 1989.
23. Jacobsen, R.; Abrahamsen, B.; Bauerek, M.; Holst, C.; Jensen, C.B.; Knop, J.; Raymond, K.; Rasmussen, L.B.; Stougaard, M.; Sørensen, T.I.A.; et al. The influence of early exposure to vitamin D for development of diseases later in life. *Bmc Public Health* **2013**, *13*, 515. [CrossRef]
24. Pedersen, C.B. The Danish Civil Registration System. *Scand. J. Public Health* **2011**, *39* (Suppl. 7), 22–25. [CrossRef] [PubMed]
25. Lynge, E.; Sandegaard, J.L.; Rebolj, M. The Danish National Patient Register. *Scand. J. Public Health* **2011**, *39* (Suppl. 7), 30–33. [CrossRef] [PubMed]
26. Juul, A.; Teilmann, G.; Scheike, T.; Hertel, N.T.; Holm, K.; Laursen, E.M.; Main, K.M.; Skakkebæk, N.E. Pubertal development in Danish children: Comparison of recent European and US data. *Int. J. Androl.* **2006**, *29*, 247–255. [CrossRef] [PubMed]
27. Moth, G.; Vedsted, P.; Schiøtz, P.O. National registry diagnoses agree with medical records on hospitalized asthmatic children. *Acta Pædiatr.* **2007**, *96*, 1470–1473. [CrossRef] [PubMed]
28. Therneau, T.M.; Grambsch, P.M. *Modeling Survival Data: Extending the Cox Model*; Statistics for Biology and Health; Springer: New York, NY, USA, 2000; Volume XIV, p. 350.
29. Just, J.; Saint Pierre, P.; Amat, F.; Gouvis-Echraghi, R.; Lambert-Guillemot, N.; Guiddir, T.; Annesi Maesano, I. What lessons can be learned about asthma phenotypes in children from cohort studies? *Pediatric Allergy Immunol.* **2015**, *26*, 300–305. [CrossRef] [PubMed]
30. Erkkola, M.; Kaila, M.; Nwaru, B.I.; Kronberg-Kippilä, C.; Ahonen, S.; Nevalainen, J.; Veijola, R.; Pekkanen, J.; Ilonen, J.; Simell, O.; et al. Maternal vitamin D intake during pregnancy is inversely associated with asthma and allergic rhinitis in 5-year-old children. *Clin. Exp. Allergy* **2009**, *39*, 875–882. [CrossRef] [PubMed]
31. Camargo, C.A.; Rifas-Shiman, S.L.; Litonjua, A.A.; Rich-Edwards, J.W.; Weiss, S.T.; Gold, D.R.; Kleinman, K.; Gillman, M.W. Maternal intake of vitamin D during pregnancy and risk of recurrent wheeze in children at 3 y of age. *Am. J. Clin. Nutr.* **2007**, *85*, 788–795. [CrossRef] [PubMed]
32. Devereux, G.; Litonjua, A.A.; Turner, S.W.; Craig, L.C.; McNeill, G.; Martindale, S.; Helms, P.J.; Seaton, A.; Weiss, S.T. Maternal vitamin D intake during pregnancy and early childhood wheezing. *Am. J. Clin. Nutr.* **2007**, *85*, 853–859. [CrossRef] [PubMed]
33. Vuillermin, P.J.; Macia, L.; Nanan, R.; Tang, M.L.; Collier, F.; Brix, S. The maternal microbiome during pregnancy and allergic disease in the offspring. *Semin Immunopathol.* **2017**, *39*, 669–675. [CrossRef]
34. Camargo, C.A.; Ingham, T.; Wickens, K.; Thadhani, R.; Silvers, K.M.; Epton, M.J.; Town, G.I.; Pattemore, P.K.; Espinola, J.A.; Crane, J. Cord-blood 25-hydroxyvitamin D levels and risk of respiratory infection, wheezing, and asthma. *Pediatrics* **2011**, *127*, e180–e187. [CrossRef] [PubMed]
35. Chawes, B.L.; Bonnelykke, K.; Jensen, P.F.; Schoos, A.M.; Heickendorff, L.; Bisgaard, H. Cord blood 25(OH)-vitamin D deficiency and childhood asthma, allergy and eczema: The COPSAC2000 birth cohort study. *PLoS ONE* **2014**, *9*, e99856. [CrossRef]

36. Gazibara, T.; den Dekker, H.T.; de Jongste, J.C.; McGrath, J.J.; Eyles, D.W.; Burne, T.H.; Reiss, I.K.; Franco, O.H.; Tiemeier, H.; Jaddoe, V.W.; et al. Associations of maternal and fetal 25-hydroxyvitamin D levels with childhood lung function and asthma: The Generation R Study. *Clin. Exp. Allergy* **2016**, *46*, 337–346. [CrossRef] [PubMed]

37. Gopal-Kothandapani, J.S.; Evans, L.F.; Walsh, J.S.; Gossiel, F.; Rigby, A.S.; Eastell, R.; Bishop, N.J. Effect of vitamin D supplementation on free and total vitamin D: A comparison of Asians and Caucasians. *Clin. Endocrinol.* **2019**, *90*, 222–231. [CrossRef]

38. Bikle, D.D.; Malmstroem, S.; Schwartz, J. Current Controversies: Are Free Vitamin Metabolite Levels a More Accurate Assessment of Vitamin D Status than Total Levels? *Endocrinol. Metab. Clin. North Am.* **2017**, *46*, 901–918. [CrossRef]

39. Jacobsen, R.; Hypponen, E.; Sorensen, T.I.; Vaag, A.A.; Heitmann, B.L. Gestational and Early Infancy Exposure to Margarine Fortified with Vitamin D through a National Danish Programme and the Risk of Type 1 Diabetes: The D-Tect Study. *PloS ONE* **2015**, *10*, e0128631. [CrossRef]

40. *Nordic Nutrition Recommendations 2012*; Nordic Council of Ministers: Copenhagen, Denmark, 2004; Volume 5.

41. Stevenson, D.K.; Verter, J.; Fanaroff, A.A.; Oh, W.; Ehrenkranz, R.A.; Shankaran, S.; Donovan, E.F.; Wright, L.L.; Lemons, J.A.; Tyson, J.E. Sex differences in outcomes of very low birthweight infants: The newborn male disadvantage. *Arch. Dis. Child. Fetal Neonatal Ed.* **2000**, *83*, F182–F185. [CrossRef]

42. Just, J.; Bourgoin-Heck, M.; Amat, F. Clinical phenotypes in asthma during childhood. *Clin. Exp. Allergy* **2017**, *47*, 848–855. [CrossRef]

43. Guilbert, T.W.; Mauger, D.T.; Lemanske, R.F. Childhood asthma-predictive phenotype. *J. Allergy Clin. Immunol. Pract.* **2014**, *2*, 664–670. [CrossRef]

44. Martinez, F.D.; Wright, A.L.; Taussig, L.M.; Holberg, C.J.; Halonen, M.; Morgan, W.J. Asthma and wheezing in the first six years of life. The Group Health Medical Associates. *N. Engl. J. Med.* **1995**, *332*, 133–138. [CrossRef]

45. Torday, J.S.; Nielsen, H.C.; Fencl Mde, M.; Avery, M.E. Sex differences in fetal lung maturation. *Am. Rev. Respir. Dis.* **1981**, *123*, 205–208.

46. Zosky, G.R.; Hart, P.H.; Whitehouse, A.J.; Kusel, M.M.; Ang, W.; Foong, R.E.; Chen, L.; Holt, P.G.; Sly, P.D.; Hall, G.L. Vitamin D deficiency at 16 to 20 weeks' gestation is associated with impaired lung function and asthma at 6 years of age. *Ann. Am. Thorac. Soc.* **2014**, *11*, 571–577. [CrossRef]

47. Pedersen, C.B.; Gotzsche, H.; Moller, J.O.; Mortensen, P.B. The Danish Civil Registration System. A cohort of eight million persons. *Dan Med. Bull.* **2006**, *53*, 441–449.

48. Schmidt, M.; Schmidt, S.A.; Sandegaard, J.L.; Ehrenstein, V.; Pedersen, L.; Sorensen, H.T. The Danish National Patient Registry: A review of content, data quality, and research potential. *Clin. Epidemiol.* **2015**, *7*, 449–490. [CrossRef] [PubMed]

49. Olsen, J.; Frische, G.; Poulsen, A.O.; Kirchheiner, H. Changing smoking, drinking, and eating behaviour among pregnant women in Denmark. Evaluation of a health campaign in a local region. *Scand. J. Soc. Med.* **1989**, *17*, 277–280. [CrossRef] [PubMed]

50. Bendixen, H.; Holst, C.; Sorensen, T.I.; Raben, A.; Bartels, E.M.; Astrup, A. Major increase in prevalence of overweight and obesity between 1987 and 2001 among Danish adults. *Obes. Res.* **2004**, *12*, 1464–1472. [CrossRef] [PubMed]

51. Ministry of Treasury. *Tre Reformer af Personskatterne 1987–2002*; Ministry of Treasury: Copenhagen, Denmark, 2001.

52. Jensen, A. Kuren der rystede Danmark. Available online: https://www.berlingske.dk/samfund/kuren-der-rystede-danmark (accessed on 23 April 2019).

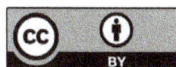

Article

Priming of Hypothalamic Ghrelin Signaling and Microglia Activation Exacerbate Feeding in Rats' Offspring Following Maternal Overnutrition

Roger Maldonado-Ruiz [1,2], Marcela Cárdenas-Tueme [3], Larisa Montalvo-Martínez [1,2], Roman Vidaltamayo [4], Lourdes Garza-Ocañas [5], Diana Reséndez-Perez [3] and Alberto Camacho [1,2,*]

[1] Department of Biochemistry, College of Medicine, Universidad Autónoma de Nuevo León, Monterrey, C.P. 64460, México; rogalmalruiz@gmail.com (R.M.-R.); lj_montalvo.mtz@hotmail.com (L.M.-M.)
[2] Neurometabolism Unit. Center for Research and Development in Health Sciences, Universidad Autónoma de Nuevo León, Monterrey, C.P. 64460, México
[3] Department of Cell Biology and Genetics, College of Biological Sciences, Universidad Autónoma de Nuevo León, Monterrey, C.P. 64460, México; marcela.cdns@gmail.com (M.C.-T.); diaresendez@gmail.com (D.R.-P.)
[4] Department of Basic Science, School of Health Sciences, Universidad de Monterrey, San Pedro Garza, N.L. 66238, México; roman.vidaltamayo@udem.edu
[5] Departamento de Farmacologia y Toxicología, College of Medicine, Universidad Autonoma de Nuevo Leon, Monterrey, C.P. 64460, México; logarza@live.com.mx
* Correspondence: acm590@hotmail.com; Tel.: +01-52(81)8329-4050

Received: 30 March 2019; Accepted: 29 May 2019; Published: 31 May 2019

Abstract: Maternal overnutrition during pregnancy leads to metabolic alterations, including obesity, hyperphagia, and inflammation in the offspring. Nutritional priming of central inflammation and its role in ghrelin sensitivity during fed and fasted states have not been analyzed. The current study aims to identify the effect of maternal programming on microglia activation and ghrelin-induced activation of hypothalamic neurons leading to food intake response. We employed a nutritional programming model exposing female Wistar rats to a cafeteria diet (CAF) from pre-pregnancy to weaning. Food intake in male offspring was determined daily after fasting and subcutaneous injection of ghrelin. Hypothalamic ghrelin sensitivity and microglia activation was evaluated using immunodetection for Iba-1 and c-Fos markers, and Western blot for TBK1 signaling. Release of TNF-alpha, IL-6, and IL-1β after stimulation with palmitic, oleic, linoleic acid, or C6 ceramide in primary microglia culture were quantified using ELISA. We found that programmed offspring by CAF diet exhibits overfeeding after fasting and peripheral ghrelin administration, which correlates with an increase in the hypothalamic Iba-1 microglia marker and c-Fos cell activation. Additionally, in contrast to oleic, linoleic, or C6 ceramide stimulation in primary microglia culture, stimulation with palmitic acid for 24 h promotes TNF-alpha, IL-6, and IL-1β release and TBK1 activation. Notably, intracerebroventricular (i.c.v.) palmitic acid or LPS inoculation for five days promotes daily increase in food intake and food consumption after ghrelin administration. Finally, we found that i.c.v. palmitic acid substantially activates hypothalamic Iba-1 microglia marker and c-Fos. Together, our results suggest that maternal nutritional programing primes ghrelin sensitivity and microglia activation, which potentially might mirror hypothalamic administration of the saturated palmitic acid.

Keywords: ghrelin; hypothalamic inflammation; microglia; nutritional programing

1. Introduction

Maternal obesity or maternal overnutrition during pregnancy and lactation programs an adverse uterine milieu leading to defects in organ function and metabolism in offspring [1,2]. Programing involves a new setting of peripheral and central pathways including energy expenditure and appetite regulation, which potentially increase the susceptibility for obesity and metabolic-related pathologies in adult offspring [2]. Maternal nutritional programming by cafeteria diet (CAF) in murine models sets metabolic alterations including impaired insulin sensitivity, hypertension, endothelial dysfunction, increased adiposity [3–5], and altered appetite regulation (hyperphagia) [2,6].

Food intake is actively regulated by ghrelin, which is the only known appetite-inducing peptide produced by endocrine cells of the gastric mucosa [7,8]. Ghrelin induces a powerful orexigenic signal by activating the secretagogue receptors of growth hormone (GHSR) expressed in the hypothalamic POMC of the arcuate nucleus (ARC) and the NPY/AgRP neurons of the paraventricular nucleus (PVH) [7,8]. Maternal programming by overnutrition increases plasma ghrelin levels in both dams and their offspring [9]; Additionally, neonatal overfeeding disrupts ghrelin signaling [10] and induces overweight into adulthood in both males and females [11,12]. Maternal nutritional programming by overnutrition also stimulates proliferation of neuroepithelial and neuronal precursor cells in the hypothalamus during the embryonic period, leading to differentiation and proliferation of orexigenic peptide-producing neurons [13]. Furthermore, a recent clinical study demonstrated that the maternal prenatal lipid profile was associated with the offspring's eating behavior and energy intake [14]. This evidence proposes that maternal nutritional programming might set an orexigenic phenotype in the offspring by increasing plasma ghrelin levels and orexigenic neuronal expression in the hypothalamic nucleus.

Maternal obesity or maternal overnutrition is also associated with a positive inflammatory profile, known as metabolic inflammation. For instance, free fatty acids accumulation in plasma during maternal programming promote a central and peripheral inflammatory response through toll-like receptor 4 (TLR-4) activation [15–17]. In addition, clinical evidence showed substantial increased expression of TLR-4, IL-6, and IL-8 in the placenta of obese women [18], and TLR-4 ablation in the ARC nucleus of murine models prevents obesity [19].

In the brain, hypothalamic microglia actively responds to accumulation of saturated fatty acids following caloric exposure in murine models [11,12]. We have reported that the saturated lipid palmitic acid leads to the activation of the TLR-4-TBK1 pathway in the hypothalamus of obese murine models, which correlates with insulin resistance [20]. Of note, initial reports identified that chronic microglia activation following caloric exposure correlates with ghrelin resistance in the hypothalamus [21]. Conversely, genetic ablation of microglia leads to anorexia and weight loss [22]. Of importance, seminal studies have identified that plasma lipid profile selectively regulates ghrelin sensitivity. For instance, lipid infusions in humans suppresses the GHSR effects of ghrelin [23]. Additionally, in vitro studies identified that prolonged exposure to unsaturated fatty acids activates ghrelin sensitivity, potentially due to an increase in the GHSR in lipid rafts [24]. This evidence suggests that unsaturated or saturated plasma lipid profiles promote microglia activation, leading to positive or negative ghrelin sensitivity, respectively. It is unknown whether overnutrition during maternal programming primes hypothalamic ghrelin signaling in offspring, promoting increased food intake in adulthood. The current study was designed to identify the effect of maternal nutritional programming by caloric exposure on ghrelin-induced activation of hypothalamic neurons and food intake regulation in the offspring.

2. Materials and Methods

2.1. Reagents and Antibodies

Reagents and antibodies used in our experimental design are showed in Tables 1 and 2, respectively.

Table 1. List of reagents

Reagent	Catalog	Application (conc.)	Manufacturer
Ghrelin		i.c.v	Sigma-Aldrich, St. Louis, MO, USA
Dulbecco's Modified Eagle's Medium high glucose	G8903 D5648	PC	Sigma-Aldrich, St. Louis, MO, USA
L-15 Medium (Leibovitz)	L4386	PC	Sigma-Aldrich, St. Louis, MO, USA
Palmitic acid	P0500	i.c.v. and PC	Sigma-Aldrich, St. Louis, MO, USA
Palmitoleic acid	P9417	PC	Sigma-Aldrich, St. Louis, MO, USA
Linoleic acid	L1376	PC	Sigma-Aldrich, St. Louis, MO, USA
Stearic acid	S47S1	PC	Sigma-Aldrich, St. Louis, MO, USA
N-hexanoyl-D-esfingosin	H6524	PC	Sigma-Aldrich, St. Louis, MO, USA
lipopolysaccharide (LPS) *Escherichia coli* 0111: B4	L2630	i.c.v. and PC	Sigma-Aldrich, St. Louis, MO, USA
Rat TNF-α ELISA Ready-SET-Go!	88-7340	ELISA	eBioscience, San Diego, CA, USA
Rat IL-6 ELISA kit	RAB0311	ELISA	Sigma-Aldrich, St. Louis, MO, USA
Rat IL-1β ELISA kit	RAB0277	ELISA	Sigma-Aldrich, St. Louis, MO, USA

PC: primary microglia cell culture; i.c.v: intracerebroventricular injection.

Table 2. List of antibodies

Antibody	Catalog	Application (conc.)	Host	Manufacturer
Anti-NAK	ab40676	WB (1:1000)	Rabbit	abcam, Cambridge, MA, USA
Anti-p-NAK S172	ab109272	WB (1:1000)	Rabbit	abcam, Cambridge, MA, USA
Anti-p-NF-κB p65 S536	3033S	WB (1:1000)	Rabbit	Cell Signaling, Beverly, MA, USA
Anti-p- NF-κB p65	8242S	WB (1:1000)	Rabbit	Cell Signaling, Beverly, MA, USA
Anti- β-Actin	8457P	WB (1:5000)	Rabbit	Cell Signaling, Beverly, MA, USA
Anti-rabbit IgG-HRP	sc-2370	WB (1:1000)	Cow	Santa Cruz Biotech., Dallas, TX, USA
Alexa fluor 488 anti-rabbit	A-11034	IF (1:1000)	Goat	Thermo Fisher Scientific, Waltham, MA, USA
Alexa fluor 546 anti-rabbit	A-11035	IF (1:1000)	Goat	Thermo Fisher Scientific, Waltham, MA, USA
Anti-c-fos	ab190289	IF (1:1000)	Rabbit	abcam, Cambridge, MA, USA
Anti-Iba-1	ab178847	IF (1:200)	Rabbit	abcam, Cambridge, MA, USA

WB: western blot; IF: Immunofluorescence.

2.2. Animals and Housing

All the experiments were performed using two-month-old wild-type female Wistar rats (initial body weight 200–250 g). Animals were handled according to the NIH guide for the care and use of laboratory animals (NIH Publications No. 80–23, revised in 1996). We followed the Basel Declaration to implement the ethical principles of Replacement, Reduction and Refinement of experimental animal models. Our study was approved by the local Animal Care Committee (BI0002). Rats were housed individually in Plexiglas-style cages, maintained at 20–23 °C in a temperature-controlled room with a 12-h light/dark cycle. Water was available ad libitum in the home cage. Food availability is described below.

2.3. Diets

The standard chow diet formula contained 57% carbohydrates, 13% lipids, and 30% proteins, caloric density = 3.35 kcal/g (LabDiet, St. Louis, MO 63144, 5001, Cat. D12450B). Cafeteria (CAF) diet was made of liquid chocolate, biscuits, bacon, fries potatoes, standard diet, and pork paté based on a 1:1:1:1:1:1:2 ratio, respectively; total calories 3.72 kcal/g in 39% carbohydrates, 49% lipids, 12% proteins, and 513.53 mg of sodium, caloric density = 3.72 kcal/g, as we reported before [5]. It is important to note that the CAF diet simulates the feeding habits of human populations in North America [25].

2.4. Maternal Nutritional Programming Model

Programing and mating experiments were performed using 12-week-old male and 10-weel-old virgin female Wistar rats. Animals were acclimated to the animal facility seven days prior to the nutritional programming protocol in standard conditions with ad libitum access to food and water. Female rats ($n = 6$) were randomized into two batches of three animals each, one for the control chow diet and the second for the CAF diet, as we reported [5]. After randomization, female rats were exposed ad libitum to specific formula diets three weeks before mating. Rats were mated with age-matched Wistar males for two days and males were removed from the home cage. Pregnancy diagnosis was performed in females after mating by vaginal plug. Female rats lacking copulation plugs were returned to the home cage for a second mating. Pregnant rats were kept on the same diet until birth and lactation. Male offspring from mothers exposed to Chow or CAF diets were weaned at post-natal day 21, grouped into 10–12 subjects per group and exposed to control Chow diet (Control Chow and CAF programmed groups) for nine weeks. During the experiment, body weight and food intake were measured weekly (Figure 1a).

2.5. Analysis of Ghrelin Signaling for Chow and CAF Exposure in Offspring

The offspring from mothers exposed to Chow ($n = 10$–12) or CAF ($n = 10$–12) diet were fasted for 16 h by removing their food at 18:00 PM. To measure total food intake, Chow and CAF diets were weighed and placed inside the cages, where they were left for 4 h, after which food was removed and weighed. Additionally, after removing the food, Chow or CAF programmed offspring were injected intradermically with 0.2 micrograms/kg of ghrelin ($n = 10$–12) or saline ($n = 10$–12), and food was placed in their cages for 2 h (see Table 1 for reagents). Rats were allowed to eat ad libitum, and then food was removed and weighed.

This procedure allowed each subject to be its own control for the ghrelin effect. Next, rats were intracardially perfused and processed for immunohistochemistry against c-Fos for neuronal and Iba-1 for microglia activation (see Table 2 for antibodies), as described below.

2.6. Intracardiac Perfusion

After 2 h of ghrelin administration, the offspring was anesthetized by 1 mL pentobarbital (PiSA Agropecuaria) i.p. overdose. A dermal dissection was performed from the abdominal region to the upper part of the thoracic cage, exposing the heart. Then, the left ventricle of the heart was perforated following its apex and a cut was made in the right atrium in order to open the circulatory system. Rats were intracardially perfused with 250 mL 0.1 M phosphate-buffered saline (PBS) + 10 U/mL heparin followed by 250 mL paraformaldehyde 4% in PBS 0.1M (PFA) using an infusion pump (Fisher Scientific GP1000) at a flow rate of 15 mL/min. The brains were collected, and samples were stored in 4% PFA + PBS 0.1 M at 4 °C for 24 hours and changed to 10%, 20%, and 30% sucrose before cutting. We obtained 40-μm coronal sections in the rostral-caudal direction between bregma −1.58 and −1.94 mm for the ARC, and between bregma −0.70 and −0.94 mm for the PVN using a cryostat; the sections were processed for immunohistochemistry as described below. Anatomical limits of each brain region were identified using the Paxinos and Watson Atlas [26].

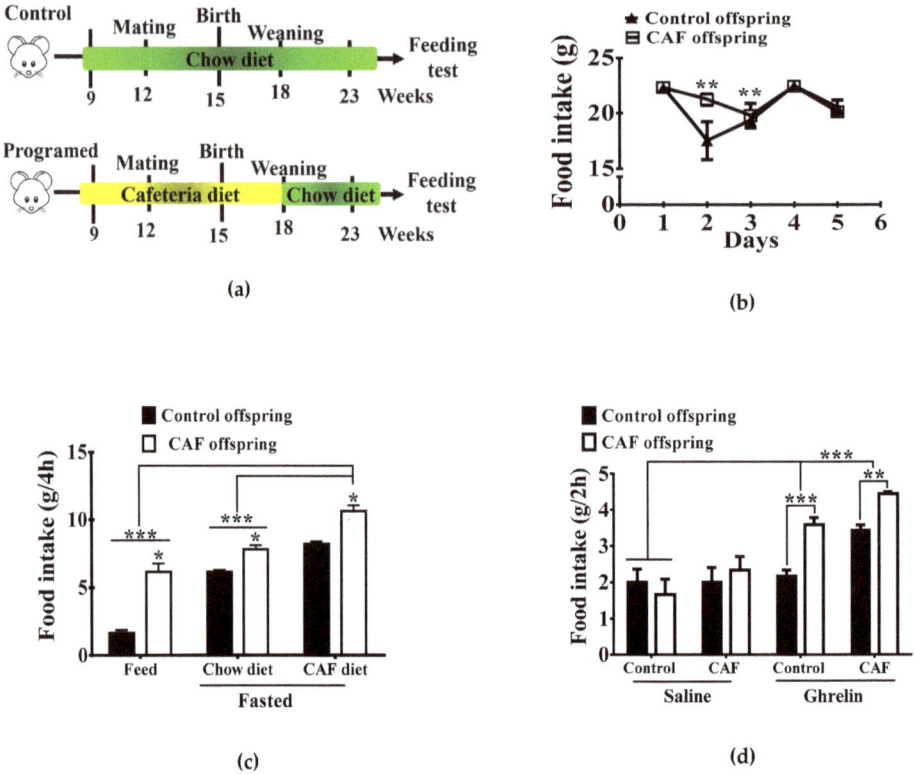

(a)

(b)

(c)

(d)

Figure 1. Effect of maternal nutritional programming on food intake in male offspring. (**a**) Maternal programing was performed by exposing Chow or CAF diet for nine weeks including pre-pregnancy, pregnancy and lactation. After weaning the offspring of both (CAF and Chow diets) was exposed to Chow diet for 5 weeks, by two months of age (week 23) we performed the feeding test. (**b**) Daily food intake by both Chow offspring and CAF diet offspring. (**c**) Chow and CAF diet consumption during 4 h in offspring after fasting for 16 h and refeeding. (**d**) Food intake for 2 h after administration with ghrelin 0.2 μg/Kg SC. (control diet group $n = 10$–12; cafeteria diet (CAF) group $n = 10$–12; the graphs show normalized data of the mean ± S.E.M. Two-way ANOVA followed by Tukey multiple comparation test; * $p < 0.05$, ** $p < 0.01$, *** $p < 0.001$).

2.7. Tissue Sample Collection

The second batch of offspring ($n = 10$–12 each) were sacrificed by decapitation at nine weeks of age. Blood samples were collected in 500-μL tubes (Beckton Dickinson) and plasma fraction was isolated by centrifugation at 4 °C and frozen at −80 °C. ARC and PVN-DMN of hypothalamus were dissected and frozen immediately at 80 °C for Western blot analysis.

2.8. Stereotaxic Surgery and I.C.V. Ghrelin Administration

A third batch of rats was selected for stereotaxic brain surgeries to selectively stimulate the hypothalamic region. In brief, all surgeries were carried out using aseptic techniques and animals were injected with ketamine (100 mg/kg, i.p.) + xylazine (10 mg/kg, i.p.) to induce anesthesia and analgesia, respectively. By eight weeks of age, male rats ($n = 36$) were implanted with a cannula in the third ventricle following the stereotaxic coordinates, AP: −2.56, mL: 0, DV: −9.4 according to the rat brain atlas [26]. The animals were allowed to recover for seven days and placed into three experimental groups ($n = 8$/group) for five days i.c.v administration of: 1) artificial cerebrospinal fluid (ACSF)

(Control), 2) 40 µg/µL palmitic acid (PAL), and 3) 2 µg/µL lipopolysaccharide (LPS) (*Escherichia coli* 0111: B4). We performed a single i.c.v administration of ACSF, PAL or LPS using an infusion pump at 2 µL flux rate. We quantified total food intake per day as well as glucose and insulin following the i.c.v administration of 1µg/µL ghrelin.

2.9. Glucose and Insulin Tolerance Test (GTT, ITT) and Ghrelin Sensitivity Assessments

Following i.c.v administration, males were fasted for 8 or 12 h and were intraperitoneally injected with 1 U of insulin/100 g or 40% glucose/kg body weight, respectively. Blood glucose levels were quantified at 0, 15, 30, 45, 60, 90, and 120 min, as described previously [5]. A week after GTT and ITT assessments, rats were i.c.v. injected with ghrelin (1 µg/µL) and we quantified total food intake for two hours. Subjects were transcardially perfused as described and processed for immunohistochemistry analysis as described below.

2.10. Microglia Primary Culture and Treatments

Cerebral cortices from the postnatal day 2 (P2) Wistar rat pups were surgically dissected, harvested, the meninges and blood vessels were removed, and the parenchyma minced and triturated in Leibovitz's L-15 Medium (Thermo Fisher Scientific, Waltham, Massachusetts) + 0.1% bovine serum albumin (BSA) with 4.5 g/L glucose, 100 U/mL penicillin, and 0.1 mg/mL streptomycin. Suspended cells were filtered (70 mm) and plated on T-75 Flasks containing 10 mL of Dulbecco's Modified Eagle's medium (DMEM) (SIGMA, San Luis, MO, USA); media were replenished every two days, resulting in mixed glial monolayers. Two weeks later, the flasks were shaken (200 rpm) for two hours (37 °C) to specifically release microglia.

Microglia culture were 70–80% confluent and stimulated for 24h with one of each fatty acids as follow: 100 µM palmitic acid, 100 µM palmitoleic acid, 100 µM stearic acid and 100 µM linoleic acid (Sigma-Aldrich, San Luis, MO, USA), 25 µM N-hexanoyl-D-sphingosine (C6) or 0.1 µg/mL LPS. Culture medium was recovered to perform the IL-6, IL-1β, and TNF-alpha ELISA tests. All fatty acids were first solubilized in DMEM media containing 10% of free fatty acid BSA, then administered in each well. Microglia were harvested and total protein was extracted using lysis buffer for Western blot analysis as described below.

2.11. Cytokine Measurements

Levels of IL-6, IL-1β, and TNF- alpha in culture medium of microglia following fatty acids or LPS stimulation were measured by ELISA (Sigma-Aldrich, St. Louis, MO, USA), following the manufacturer's instructions.

2.12. Immunohistochemistry Analysis by Confocal Imaging

Frozen brain sections were air dried at room temperature (RT) for one hour to prevent sections from falling off the slides during antibody incubations. Afterwards, the slices were washed three times for 5 min with 1X PBS + 0.1% TritonX-100 (PBST) and the slices were blocked in PBST + 10% goat serum for an hour. Subsequently, brain sections were incubated with PBST + 5% goat serum with the primary antibody anti-Iba-1 (1:200) or anti-c-Fos (1:1000) at 4 °C overnight. Subsequently, the slices were washed in PBST three times and then incubated for three hours with the secondary antibodies Alexa Fluor 488 Rabbit Goat Anti-Rabbit (IgG) for C-Fos or Alexa Fluor 546 Goat Anti-Rabbit (IgG) for Iba-1, each diluted in PBST + 5% goat serum (1:1000). Afterwards, brain sections were washed three times with PBST and air-dried at RT. Finally, brain sections were mounted using Vectashield with DAPI (Vector Laboratories, Burlingame, CA, USA) on coverslips.

2.13. Western Blot Analysis

Microglia culture samples and ARC and PVN-DMN hypothalamic biopsies were incubated in lysis buffer solution (150 mM NaCl, 25 mM Tris–HCl pH 7.5, containing 50 mM NaF, 10 mM NaP2O7, 1 mM Sodium orthovanadate, complete protease inhibitor cocktail (Roche, Mannheim, Germany) 0.5% Triton X-100) followed by sonication (for 5 s at 1500 Hz on ice). Samples were centrifuged for 10 min at 1500× g and protein concentration were determined by the bicinchoninic acid (BCA) assay at a concentration of 40 µg/µL. Samples were mixed with Laemmli buffer and then heated t 90 °C for 5 min and subjected to SDS–PAGE. Proteins were electrophoretically transferred to nitrocellulose membranes. The membrane was then blocked for 2 h at RT in TBS-T buffer (10mM Tris, 0.9% NaCl, 0.1% Tween 20, pH 7.5) containing 5% BSA. Membranes were incubated overnight with primary antibodies at 4 °C: TBK1 (1:1000), TBK1-pSer172, anti-NF-κB (1:1000), NF-κB-pSer536 (1:1000), anti-actin (1:2000). Membranes were washed (4 times/5 min) in TBS-T and incubated for 1 h with horseradish peroxidase (HRP)-conjugated secondary antibody. Proteins were detected by ECL, which were read employing the ChemiDoc™ XRS+ System (BIO-RAD) and quantified densitometrically with the 1.31V ImageJ software (Wayne Rasband, National Institutes of Health, Bethesda, MD, USA).

2.14. Statistical Analysis

Statistical analyses were conducted using the Prism 7 GraphPad software. Western blot data were analyzed using the unpaired Student's *t*-test. We used two-way ANOVA followed by Tukey for multiple comparations. Data are presented as mean ± SD. The significance levels displayed on figures are as follows: * $p < 0.05$, ** $p < 0.01$, *** $p < 0.001$.

3. Results

3.1. Maternal Nutritional Programming Exacerbates Ghrelin Sensitivity in Offspring, Leading to an Increase in Food Intake

First, we aimed to identify the effect of maternal nutritional programming by caloric exposure on basal and ghrelin-induced food intake regulation in the offspring. We found that offspring showed a significant transient increase of food intake by day two during the five days schedule, with no changes on total basal food intake (Figure 1b). Additionally, offspring programmed by the CAF diet exhibited an increase in Chow and CAF food intake after 14 h fasting when compared with offspring exposed to Chow diet during programming (Figure 1c). Of note, incentive food intake behavior in the programmed offspring was sensitive to ghrelin administration. We found that subcutaneous ghrelin injection significantly increased Chow and CAF diet intake in offspring programmed by maternal CAF compared with Chow programmed offspring (Figure 1d). These results suggest that maternal programming by CAF diet actively promotes food intake by potentially priming ghrelin sensitivity in offspring.

3.2. Maternal Programming by CAF Exposure Sets Activation of Hypothalamic Ghrelin-Sensitive C-Fos Neurons in Offspring

Next, we sought to identify if ghrelin sensitivity correlated with neuronal response and microglia activation in the hypothalamic ARC nucleus. We used a 120-min time-frame schedule following systemic ghrelin administration to identify central neuronal c-fos activation in the ARC nucleus leading to food intake response, as reported [27]. We found that offspring programmed by a maternal CAF diet exposure showed substantial microglia activation evidenced by an increase in the Iba-1 marker (Figure 2a). Additionally, CAF diet exposure promoted a higher neuronal c-fos expression in ARC when compared with matched controls (Figure 2b). Together, these results confirm that maternal programming is able to sensitize central neuronal activation in the hypothalamus of offspring following systemic ghrelin administration, which correlates with central microglia activation.

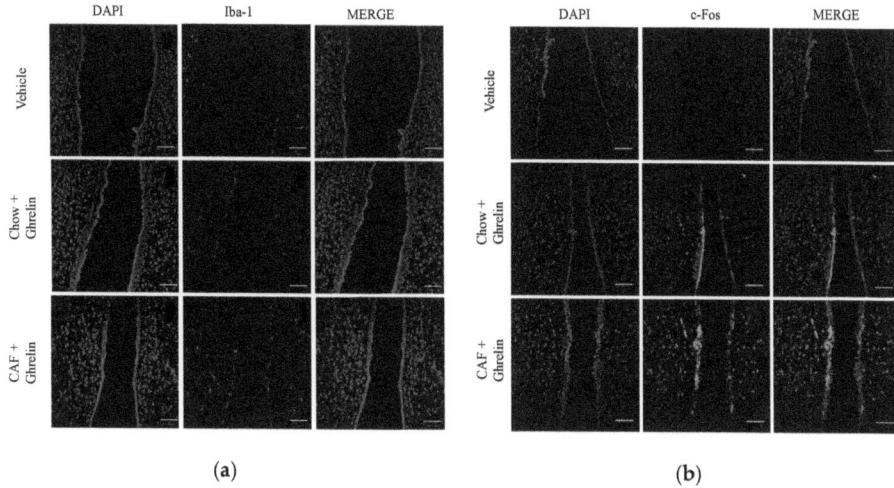

(a)   (b)

Figure 2. Maternal programming leads to microglia activation and c-Fos response in hypothalamus. Offspring was programmed by CAF diet exposure as previously described, and 0.2 micrograms/kg ghrelin was intradermically administered, and subjects were intracardially perfused with 0.1M PBS + heparin followed by PBS + 4% PFA. Hypothalamic sections were obtained using a cryostat, according to the Paxinos and Watson Atlas. Immunofluorescence to identify microglia activation was performed using the Iba-1 antibody (1:200) following by the secondary antibody Alexa Fluor 546 Goat Anti-Rabbit (IgG) (1:1000) (a). c-Fos activation was identified by anti c-Fos (1:1000) and Alexa Fluor 488 Rabbit Goat Anti-Rabbit (1:1000) (b). Brain sections were mounted using Vectashield with DAPI (Vector Laboratories) on coverslips. (*n* = 3). PBS, phosphate-buffered saline, PFA, paraformaldehyde.

3.3. Saturated Lipids Activate a Pro-Inflammatory Stage in Microglia

To identify whether positive energy balance in offspring after programming selectively displayed microglia activation and ghrelin sensitivity, we initially characterized potential lipid species showing a pro-inflammatory profile using a microglia in vitro system. We performed saturated or unsaturated fatty acids stimulation for 24 h and quantified TNF-alpha, IL-6, and IL-1β release, as described. We found that the C16:0-saturated palmitic acid incubation efficiently promotes TNF-alpha, IL-6 and IL-1β release when compared with control, whereas the C18:0 long-chain stearic acid promotes TNF-alpha release with no changes in IL-6 and IL-1β (Figure 3a–c). Additionally, palmitoleic acid (C16:1), the monounsaturated form of palmitic acid promoted the production of IL-6, whereas the C6 ceramide (C18:1/6:0) decreased it (Figure 3b). Finally, the polyunsaturated linoleic acid (C18:2) incubation did not show changes in the pro-inflammatory profile of microglia (Figure 3a–c).

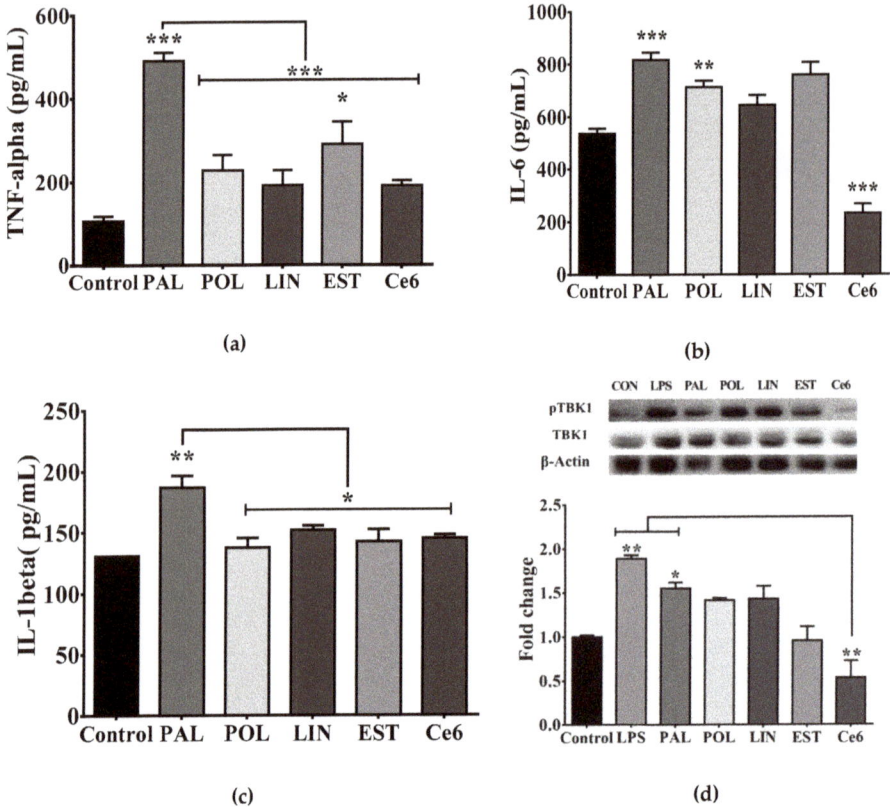

Figure 3. Palmitic acid incubation leads to cytokine production and TBK1 pathway activation in primary microglia. (**a**) TNF-alpha secretion, (**b**) IL-6 secretion or (**c**) IL-1β secretion by primary microglia culture following 1% BSA-FFA (Control); 100 μM palmitic acid, palmitoleic acid, linoleic acid or stearic acid or 25 μM C6 ceramide incubation for 24h. TNF-alpha, IL-6 and IL-1β secretion were quantified by ELISA following the manufacturer's instructions ($n = 4$). (**d**) TBK1 phosphorylation following saturated and unsaturated fatty acids stimulation was identified using western blot analysis. The graphs show normalized data of the mean ± S.E.M. Two-way ANOVA followed by Tukey multiple comparation test; * $p < 0.05$, ** $p < 0.01$, *** $p < 0.001$). TBK1, TANK-binding kinase 1, BSA-FFA, Bovine serum albumin-free fatty acids (FFA).

We previously reported that palmitic acid leads to the TLR4-TBK1 pathway activation in the hypothalamus of obese murine models, which correlates with systemic insulin resistance [20]. We identified whether stimulation with saturated and unsaturated fatty acids lead to TBK1 activation in microglia cultures. Our results show that both the positive inflammatory reagent, LPS, and palmitic acid elicit a significant activation of the TBK1 pathway in microglia cells (Figure 3d). Of importance, the C6 ceramide blocks the TBK1 pathway activation (Figure 3d), which correlates with no changes in TNF-alpha and IL-1β release (Figure 3a,b) with a decrease in the IL-6 release (Figure 3c). Our results confirmed the saturated palmitic acid as a reliable lipid species leading to pro-inflammatory state in microglia cells.

3.4. Hypothalamic Palmitic Acid Inoculation Promotes Increase in Total Food Intake

We determined whether central administration of the pro-inflammatory modulator palmitic acid disrupted plasma glucose homeostasis and/or food intake response. We found that i.c.v administration of palmitic acid for 5 days partially increased plasma glucose levels following insulin administration, however, it did not change total glucose homeostasis evidenced by area under the curve (AUC) quantification (Figure 4a,b). Additionally, we found no changes in glucose homeostasis addressing by the GTT (Figure 4c,d).

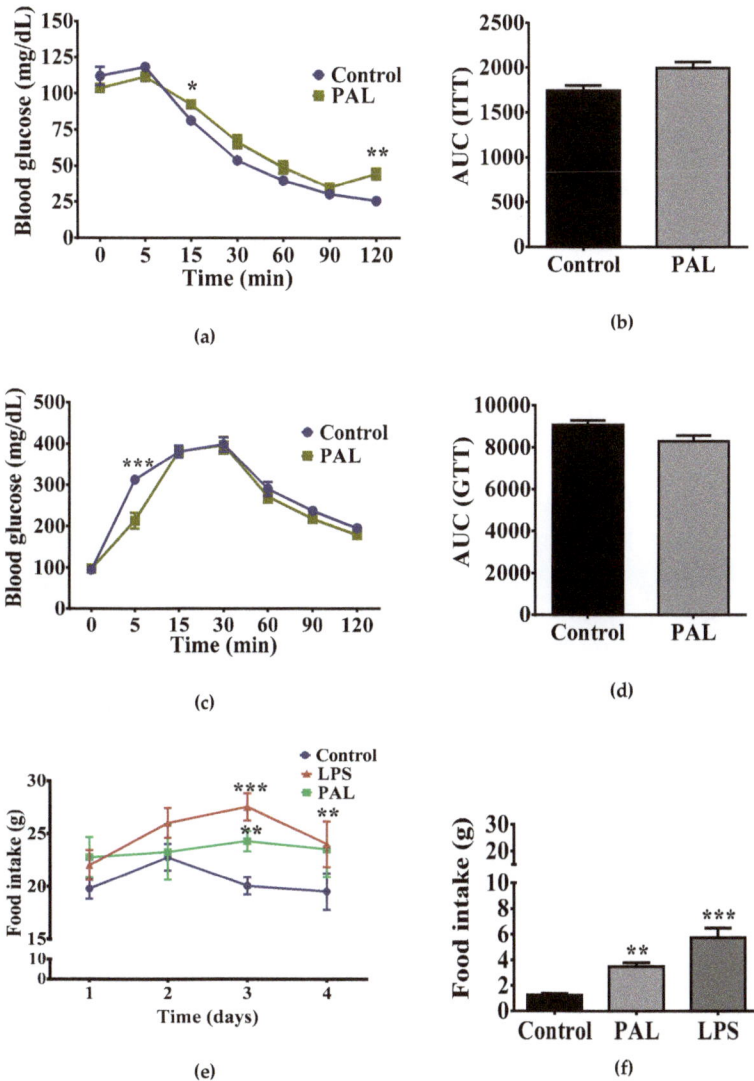

Figure 4. Chronic i.c.v. palmitic acid administration sensitizes ghrelin signaling leading to food intake increase. ITT and area under the curve (AUC) (**a–b**) and GTT and AUC (**c–d**) were analyzed following i.c.v of 2 µg/mL LPS or 40 µg/µL palmitic acid administration for five days. Daily food intake quantification following palmitic acid, LPS or ACSF administration (**e**). Ghrelin-sensitive food intake was analyzed by day 5 after 2 h, 1 µg/µL ghrelin i.c.v. administration (**f**). The graphs show normalized data of the mean ± S.E.M., Student's *t*-test, * $p < 0.05$). ($n = 4$, the results are shown as the mean ± S.E.M. Two-way ANOVA followed by Tukey multiple comparation test; * $p < 0.05$, ** $p < 0.01$, *** $p < 0.001$). LPS, Lipopolysaccharides, ACSF, artificial cerebrospinal fluid.

Next, we hypothesized that the pro-inflammatory modulator palmitic acid might reproduce the increase in food intake found in the offspring of mothers exposed to CAF diet. We administered LPS, palmitic acid or vehicle via i.c.v for five days and we quantified basal food intake and food intake following i.c.v administration of ghrelin (1 μg/μL). We found a time-dependent increase of daily total food intake during LPS or palmitic acid schedule when compared with ACSF administration (Figure 4e). Additionally, we identified that five days of palmitic acid administration results in a 3.5-fold increase of food intake following i.c.v. administration of ghrelin when compared with the control group (Figure 4f). Of note, i.c.v. administration of the pro-inflammatory reagent LPS reproduces the total food intake induced by ghrelin administration (Figure 4f). These results support the hypothesis that saturated lipids sensitize hypothalamic ghrelin signaling, leading to exacerbation of food intake.

3.5. Hypothalamic Saturated Lipids Stimulation Activates Microglia and Ghrelin-Sensitive Neurons

At this final stage, we integrated the in vivo and in vitro results identified in Figures 1–4, supporting the effect of saturated palmitic acid on microglia activation and increased food intake in programmed offspring. We determined that palmitic acid promoted hypothalamic microglia activation and that it correlated with ghrelin-sensitive neuronal activation. We found that i.c.v. palmitic acid administration for five days following by ghrelin stimulation promoted a significant increase of microglia activation in the ARC of the hypothalamus, evidenced by immunofluorescence stain of the IBA1 marker when compared with the vehicle (Figure 5a). We also confirmed that palmitic acid promoted an increase in the c-fos immunosignal, confirming neuronal activation in the ARC nucleus (Figure 5b).

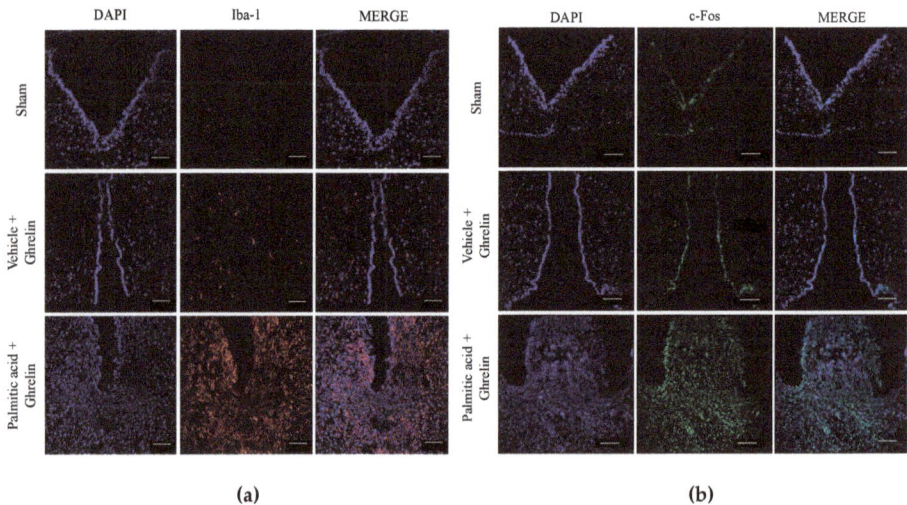

Figure 5. *Cont.*

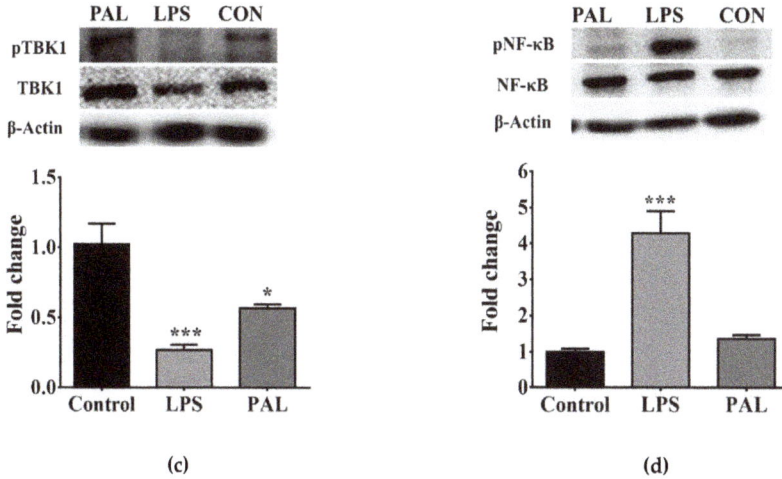

(c)   (d)

Figure 5. Palmitic acid promotes microglia activation and c-fos response in hypothalamus. Rats were i.c.v. administered with, ACSF, 2 μg/μL LPS or 40μg/μL palmitic acid for 5 days and vehicle or ghrelin was injected into the third ventricle by day 5. Immunofluorescence against Iba-1 marker (microglia activation) (**a**) or c-fos activation were performed as described in Figure 4 (**b**). (**c** and **d**) Changes in TBK1 and NF-κB phosphorylation in the ARC of hypothalamus were identified using western blot analysis following i.c.v. ACSF, LPS or palmitic acid administration for five days (*n* = 4 per group). The graphs show normalized data of the mean ± S.E.M. Two-way ANOVA followed by Tukey multiple comparation test; * *p* < 0.05, *** *p* < 0.001). TBK1, TANK-binding kinase 1, BSA-FFA, Bovine serum albumin-free fatty acids, ACSF, cerebrospinal fluid, PAL, palmitic acid, LPS, lipopolysaccharide.

Finally, microglia activation in the ARC nucleus of the hypothalamus after palmitic acid administration was also evaluated by analyzing the TLR4-TBK1 pathway. Western blot analysis showed a decrease of the nuclear factor kappa B (NF-κB) phosphorylation following palmitic acid stimulation, which is also promoted by LPS (Figure 5c). As expected, LPS administration promoted a four-fold increase of NF-κB phosphorylation in the ARC of the hypothalamus and no changes were found after stimulation with palmitic acid (Figure 5d).

4. Discussion

Extensive evidence has confirmed that maternal obesity or maternal overnutrition during pregnancy and lactation negatively modulate peripheral and central pathways disturbing basal energy homeostasis and appetite regulation in the offspring [1,2]. We, and others, have identified that maternal nutritional programming by CAF diet exposure in murine models sets metabolic alterations [3–5] and defective behaviors, including addiction-like behavior [6,28], which potentially contributes to hyperphagia [2]. Here, by using in vitro and in vivo experimental approaches we suitably identified the lipotoxic effect of the saturated lipid species palmitic acid as a potential trigger to promote hypothalamic microglia activation and actively sensitize the central effects of ghrelin on food intake. Notably, we also discovered that maternal programming by CAF diet exposure also reproduces the effect of palmitic acid in the hypothalamus by priming the central ghrelin response for feeding in the offspring. Based on our results, we propose that palmitic acid might be considered a lipid species capable of dynamically priming hypothalamic ghrelin sensitivity to food intake in the offspring of mothers programmed by caloric diets.

A key contribution of our study is that nutritional programming by CAF exposure increases basal feeding response and ghrelin-sensitivity in the offspring. Initially, daily food intake was not increased on CAF diet –programmed groups, however, we did observe hyperphagia following plasma increase of ghrelin levels by fasting or SC ghrelin injection. As already proposed, maternal programming by caloric exposure increases ghrelin levels in the offspring [9], which may contribute to the hyperphagic phenotype during fasting in our model. On this context, in a parallel scenario we identified that maternal programming primes hypothalamic neuronal activation in the offspring, evidenced by an increase in c-fos expression in the ARC nucleus, which is also exacerbated by i.c.v. or subcutaneous ghrelin administration. This suggests that priming of central ghrelin signaling exacerbates feeding in the context of fasting or pharmacologic plasma ghrelin increase. Our data agree with the effects of maternal nutritional programming by caloric diets in murine models, which stimulates the proliferation of orexigenic peptide–producing neurons [13] and leads to hyperphagia in the offspring [2]. Notably, the effect of plasma lipidomic profile leading to food intake in humans suggests that the higher prenatal triglycerides plasma concentrations in humans were associated with higher food responsiveness in offspring at 5 years old [14]. These results are also in line with murine models showing that increased perinatal triglyceride concentrations correlate with hyperphagia in the offspring [29]. Together, these results propose that nutritional programing by CAF diet primes the ghrelin response for Chow and CAF feeding in the offspring.

Maternal obesity or maternal overnutrition promotes free fatty acid accumulation in plasma, which is associated with central and peripheral inflammatory response, potentially throughout the TLR-4 pathway [13–15]. In fact, TLR-4, IL-6, and IL-8 expression have been identified in the placenta of obese women when compared with lean women [16]. In murine models, plasma accumulation of saturated fatty acids in diet-induced obesity activates hypothalamic microglia [18,19]. In fact, there is an interactive crosstalk integrating central and peripheral immunity regulating hypothalamic nodes for metabolic and feeding homeostasis [16]. For instance, we have reported that the saturated lipid palmitic acid leads to the TLR-4-TBK1 pathway activation in the hypothalamus of obese murine models, which correlates with insulin resistance [19]. Here we hypothesized that maternal programming by CAF exposure sets a plasma lipotoxic profile in the offspring, leading to central microglia activation. Our experimental in vitro data allowed us to propose that, in contrast to the unsaturated lipid species such as the palmitoleic acid, linoleic acid or even, the C6 ceramide, the saturated lipid species palmitic acid, is an effective pro-inflammatory mediator in microglia activating the IL-6, IL-1β and TNF-alpha cytokines release. Additionally, LPS stimulation in microglia cells closely reproduces the pro-inflammatory profile found during palmitic acid stimulation, supporting the negative effect of palmitic acid.

One of the most outstanding results in our study is the major effect of hypothalamic palmitic acid inoculation on sensitizing ghrelin response for food intake. Ghrelin has been reported as a molecule that prevents the lipotoxic effects of palmitic acid stimulation in diverse cell types, including hepatocytes, pancreatic β-cells, and myoblasts [30–32]. In fact, ghrelin also exerts immunomodulatory effects on macrophages, T lymphocytes and microglia, guiding these cells towards an anti-inflammatory phenotype during obesity-induced inflammation [16,33]. In addition, ghrelin regulates by antagonizing TNF-α/NF-κB and TLR-4 signaling pathways [16,34] associated whit metabolic inflammation on the brain [35]. In any case, does hypothalamic microglia activation by palmitic acid explains the priming ghrelin response in the offspring programmed by CAF diet exposure? Programming the offspring with CAF diet exposure closely replicates microglia activation in the ARC nucleus of the hypothalamus, evidenced by an increase in the Iba-1 marker staining. Our results agree with previous data showing that systemic LPS inoculation activates central microglia [11,12,36]. In the beginning, clinical evidence, reported that the microglial inhibitor minocycline induced weight loss as a major side-effect [37]. Experimental basic evidence confirms that transient pharmacologic microglia depletion in murine models leaded to food intake decrease and weight loss [22]. Supporting our findings, neonatal overfed rats show hypothalamic microglia activation positive for Iba-1 and IL-6 and NF-κB expression, which correlates with accelerated weight gain [38]. However, additional experimental evidence does not support this scenario by showing that LPS, certain cytokines (e.g., IL-1β and TNF-α) and dietary lipids sets, in fact, a pathological state known as sickness-associated anorexia [16,39], which actively induces

IL-1β and TNF-α mRNA expression in the ARC nucleus of the hypothalamus [40]. Additionally, weight loss and anorexia in mice do not show a peripheral or central pro-inflammatory phenotype [22], and pharmacologic microglia ablation does not promote changes in mice body weight [41].

We suggest that an explanation to this discrepancy might be associated with a time-dependent pro-inflammatory profile including LPS, palmitic acid and dietary lipids in our model, and potential hormone and metabolic profiles modulating central and peripheral immune activation. For instance, inflammation and gliosis are detected in rat and mouse ARC nucleus within the first few days following high-fat diet exposure, before obesity develops [42], suggesting that a positive inflammatory profile promotes central leptin and insulin resistance [16], which potentially leads to an increase in plasma leptin levels favoring weight gain [43]. Additionally, hypothalamic microglia activation by lipid over supply might prime ghrelin sensitivity, potentially due to an increase in the GHSR into lipid rafts [24]. In any case, based on these data we propose that during the maternal CAF diet programming, palmitic acid might be one lipid species capable of promoting central microglia activation in the offspring.

Our study still lacks evidence if maternal programming by a CAF diet leads to plasma and brain increases of palmitic acid to support its effect on microglia activation and ghrelin sensitivity. Reports have shown that mice exposed to a western-style high fat diet for 16 weeks experienced a C16:0 saturated lipid increase in plasma and brain [44], including hippocampus [45]. In fact, an increase in plasma palmitic acid has been identified in healthy overweight subjects showing upper tertiles (T3) according to L4 visceral fat area [46]. Importantly, the direct effect of palmitic acid intake on brain function and its correlation with positive inflammatory immune profile in humans, was recently identified, showing that three-week high palmitic acid diet intake promotes an increase in the basal ganglia activation which correlates with IL-6, IL-18, and IL-1β plasma accumulation [47]. Finally, experimental evidence has also confirmed that the integrity of the blood brain barrier is compromised following western diet exposure in mice [48], which tentatively suggests that selective fatty acids incorporation into the brain might be favored during blood-brain barrier disruption and contribute to palmitic acid flux to the hypothalamus, a region lacking a blood-brain barrier.

5. Conclusions

Our results support the hypothesis that maternal programming by CAF diet exposure primes a hypothalamic ghrelin response leading to food intake exacerbation in male offspring. Of note, caloric programing also replicates the central microglia activation and ghrelin sensitivity found during intraventricular palmitic acid administration. We propose that palmitic acid might be considered a lipid species involved in priming of hypothalamic ghrelin sensitivity to food intake in the offspring during CAF diet exposure.

Author Contributions: Conceptualization: R.M.-R., M.C.-T., and A.C.; investigation: R.M.-R., M.C.-T., L.M.-M., R.V., D.R.-P., and A.C.; methodology: R.M.-R., M.C.-T., L.M.-M., R.V., and A.C.; supervision: R.V., D.R.-P., L.G.-O and A.C.; visualization: R.V., D.R.-P., L.G.-O and A.C.; writing—review and editing: R.M.-R., M.C.-T., L.G.-O and A.C.

Funding: This work was funded by National Council of Science and Technology in Mexico (CONACYT) (CB-2015-255317 to Alberto Camacho and CB-2013-220342 to Roman Vidaltamayo), 582196 CONACYT for Larisa Montalvo-Martínez, 573686 CONACYT for Roger Maldonado-Ruiz, 650620 CONACYT for Marcela Cárdenas-Tueme and División de Extensión, Consultoría e Investigación, Universidad de Monterrey grants (Plan de Investigación 2018 and 2019) to R. Vidaltamayo.

Acknowledgments: The authors thank M.S. Alejandra Arreola-Triana for her support on editing this manuscript.

Conflicts of Interest: The authors declare no conflict of interest.

References

1. Alfaradhi, M.Z.; Kusinski, L.C.; Fernandez-Twinn, D.S.; Pantaleão, L.C.; Carr, S.K.; Ferland-McCollough, D.; Yeo, G.S.H.; Bushell, M.; Ozanne, E.S. Maternal Obesity in Pregnancy Developmentally Programs Adipose Tissue Inflammation in Young, Lean Male Mice Offspring. *Endocrinology* **2016**, *157*, 4246–4256. [CrossRef] [PubMed]

2. Reynolds, C.M.; Segovia, S.A.; Vickers, M.H. Experimental models of maternal obesity and neuroendocrine programming of metabolic disorders in offspring. *Front. Endocrinol. (Lausanne)* **2017**, *8*, 1–11. [CrossRef]

3. Frihauf, J.B.; Fekete, É.M.; Nagy, T.R.; Levin, B.E.; Zorrilla, E.P. Maternal Western diet increases adiposity even in male offspring of obesity-resistant rat dams: Early endocrine risk markers. *Am. J. Physiol. Integr. Comp. Physiol.* **2016**, *311*, R1045–R1059. [CrossRef] [PubMed]

4. Taylor, P.D.; Samuelsson, A.-M.; Poston, L. Maternal obesity and the developmental programming of hypertension: A role for leptin. *Acta Physiol.* **2014**, *210*, 508–523. [CrossRef] [PubMed]

5. Cardenas-Perez, R.E.; Fuentes-Mera, L.; de la Garza, A.L.; Torre-Villalvazo, I.; Reyes-Castro, L.A.; Rodriguez-Rocha, H.; Garcia-Garcia, A.; Corona-Castillo, J.C.; Tovar, A.R.; Zambrano, E.; et al. Maternal overnutrition by hypercaloric diets programs hypothalamic mitochondrial fusion and metabolic dysfunction in rat male offspring. *Nutr. Metab. (London)* **2018**, *15*, 38. [CrossRef] [PubMed]

6. Camacho, A.; Montalvo-Martinez, L.; Cardenas-Perez, R.E.; Fuentes-Mera, L.; Garza-Ocañas, L. Obesogenic diet intake during pregnancy programs aberrant synaptic plasticity and addiction-like behavior to a palatable food in offspring. *Behav. Brain Res.* **2017**, *330*, 46–55. [CrossRef]

7. Nakazato, M.; Murakami, N.; Date, Y.; Kojima, M.; Matsuo, H.; Kangawa, K.; Matsukura, S. A role for ghrelin in the central regulation of feeding. *Nature* **2001**, *409*, 194–198. [CrossRef]

8. Perelló, M.; Zigman, J.M. The Role of Ghrelin in Reward-Based Eating. *Biol. Psychiatry* **2012**, *72*, 347–353. [CrossRef] [PubMed]

9. Słupecka, M.; Romanowicz, K.; Woliński, J. Maternal high-fat diet during pregnancy and lactation influences obestatin and ghrelin concentrations in milk and plasma of Wistar rat dams and their offspring. *Int. J. Endocrinol.* **2016**, *2016*, 1–9. [CrossRef] [PubMed]

10. Sominsky, L.; Ziko, I.; Spencer, S.J. Neonatal overfeeding disrupts pituitary ghrelin signalling in female rats long-term; Implications for the stress response. *PLoS ONE* **2017**, *12*, e0173498. [CrossRef] [PubMed]

11. Valdearcos, M.; Douglass, J.D.; Robblee, M.M.; Dorfman, M.D.; Stifler, D.R.; Bennett, M.L.; Gerritse, I.; Fasnacht, R.; Barres, B.A.; Thaler, J.P.; et al. microglial inflammatory signaling orchestrates the hypothalamic immune response to dietary excess and mediates obesity susceptibility. *Cell Metab.* **2017**, *26*, 185–197. [CrossRef] [PubMed]

12. Valdearcos, M.; Robblee, M.M.; Benjamin, D.I.; Nomura, D.K.; Xu, A.W.; Koliwad, S.K. microglia dictate the impact of saturated fat consumption on hypothalamic inflammation and neuronal function. *Cell Rep.* **2014**, *9*, 2124–2139. [CrossRef]

13. Chang, G.-Q.; Gaysinskaya, V.; Karatayev, O.; Leibowitz, S.F. Maternal high-fat diet and fetal programming: Increased proliferation of hypothalamic peptide-producing neurons that increase risk for overeating and obesity. *J. Neurosci.* **2008**, *28*, 12107–12119. [CrossRef] [PubMed]

14. Dieberger, A.; de Rooij, S.; Korosi, A.; Vrijkotte, T. Maternal lipid concentrations during early pregnancy and eating behaviour and energy intake in the offspring. *Nutrients* **2018**, *10*, 1026. [CrossRef] [PubMed]

15. Rogero, M.; Calder, P. Obesity, inflammation, toll-like receptor 4 and fatty acids. *Nutrients* **2018**, *10*, 432. [CrossRef]

16. Maldonado-Ruiz, R.; Fuentes-Mera, L.; Camacho, A. Central modulation of neuroinflammation by neuropeptides and energy-sensing hormones during obesity. *Biomed Res. Int.* **2017**, *2017*, 1–12. [CrossRef] [PubMed]

17. Milanski, M.; Degasperi, G.; Coope, A.; Morari, J.; Denis, R.; Cintra, D.E.; Tsukumo, D.M.L.; Anhe, G.; Amaral, M.E.; Takahashi, H.K.; et al. Saturated fatty acids produce an inflammatory response predominantly through the activation of TLR4 signaling in hypothalamus: Implications for the pathogenesis of obesity. *J. Neurosci.* **2009**, *29*, 359–370. [CrossRef] [PubMed]

18. Yang, X.; Li, M.; Haghiac, M.; Catalano, P.M.; O'Tierney-Ginn, P.; Mouzon, S.H. Causal relationship between obesity-related traits and TLR4-driven responses at the maternal–fetal interface. *Diabetologia* **2016**, *59*, 2459–2466. [CrossRef]

19. Zhao, Y.; Li, G.; Li, Y.; Wang, Y.; Liu, Z. Knockdown of Tlr4 in the arcuate nucleus improves obesity related metabolic disorders. *Sci. Rep.* **2017**, *7*, 7441. [CrossRef]
20. Delint-Ramirez, I.; Ruiz, R.M.; Torre-Villalvazo, I.; Fuentes-Mera, L.; Ocañas, L.G.; Tovar, A.; Camacho, A. Genetic obesity alters recruitment of TANK-binding kinase 1 and AKT into hypothalamic lipid rafts domains. *Neurochem. Int.* **2015**, *80*, 23–32. [CrossRef]
21. Naznin, F.; Toshinai, K.; Waise, T.M.Z.; NamKoong, C.; Moin, A.S.M.; Sakoda, H.; Nakazato, M. Diet-induced obesity causes peripheral and central ghrelin resistance by promoting inflammation. *J. Endocrinol.* **2015**, *226*, 81–92. [CrossRef]
22. De Luca, S.N.; Sominsky, L.; Soch, A.; Wang, H.; Ziko, I.; Rank, M.M.; Spencer, S.J. Conditional microglial depletion in rats leads to reversible anorexia and weight loss by disrupting gustatory circuitry. *Brain Behav. Immun.* **2019**, *77*, 77–91. [CrossRef] [PubMed]
23. Broglio, F.; Gottero, C.; Benso, A.; Prodam, F.; Destefanis, S.; Gauna, C.; Maccario, M.; Deghenghi, R.; van der Lely, A.J.; Ghigo, E. Effects of ghrelin on the insulin and glycemic responses to glucose, arginine, or free fatty acids load in humans. *J. Clin. Endocrinol. Metab.* **2003**, *88*, 4268–4272. [CrossRef] [PubMed]
24. Delhanty, P.J.D.; van Kerkwijk, A.; Huisman, M.; van de Zande, B.; Verhoef-Post, M.; Gauna, C.; Hofland, L.; Themmen, A.P.N.; van der Lely, A.J. Unsaturated fatty acids prevent desensitization of the human growth hormone secretagogue receptor by blocking its internalization. *AJP Endocrinol. Metab.* **2010**, *299*, E497–E505. [CrossRef] [PubMed]
25. Sampey, B.P.; Vanhoose, A.M.; Winfield, H.M.; Freemerman, A.J.; Muehlbauer, M.J.; Fueger, P.T.; Newgard, C.B.; Makowski, L. Cafeteria diet is a robust model of human metabolic syndrome with liver and adipose inflammation: comparison to high-fat diet. *Obesity* **2011**, *19*, 1109–1117. [CrossRef]
26. Paxinos, G.; Watson, C. *The Rat Brain in Stereotaxic Coordinates*, 6th ed.; Academic Press: San Diego, CA, USA, 2007; 456p.
27. Cabral, A.; Valdivia, S.; Fernandez, G.; Reynaldo, M.; Perello, M. divergent neuronal circuitries underlying acute orexigenic effects of peripheral or central ghrelin: Critical role of brain accessibility. *J. Neuroendocrinol.* **2014**, *26*, 542–554. [CrossRef]
28. De la Garza, A.; Garza-Cuellar, M.; Silva-Hernandez, I.; Cardenas-Perez, R.; Reyes-Castro, L.; Zambrano, E.; Gonzalez-Hernandez, B.; Garza-Ocañas, L.; Fuentes-Mera, L.; Camacho, A. Maternal flavonoids intake reverts depression-like behaviour in rat female offspring. *Nutrients* **2019**, *11*, 572. [CrossRef]
29. Sullivan, E.L.; Smith, M.S.; Grove, K.L. perinatal exposure to high-fat diet programs energy balance, metabolism and behavior in adulthood. *Neuroendocrinology* **2011**, *93*, 1–8. [CrossRef]
30. Wang, W.; Zhang, D.; Zhao, H.; Chen, Y.; Liu, Y.; Cao, C.; Han, L.; Liu, G. Ghrelin inhibits cell apoptosis induced by lipotoxicity in pancreatic β-cell line. *Regul. Pept.* **2010**, *161*, 43–50. [CrossRef]
31. Zhang, S.; Mao, Y.; Fan, X. Inhibition of ghrelin o-acyltransferase attenuated lipotoxicity by inducing autophagy via AMPK–mTOR pathway. *Drug Des. Devel. Ther.* **2018**, *12*, 873–885. [CrossRef]
32. Mosa, R.M.H.; Zhang, Z.; Shao, R.; Deng, C.; Chen, J.; Chen, C. Implications of ghrelin and hexarelin in diabetes and diabetes-associated heart diseases. *Endocrine* **2015**, *49*, 307–323. [CrossRef] [PubMed]
33. Harvey, R.E.; Howard, V.G.; Lemus, M.B.; Jois, T.; Andrews, Z.B.; Sleeman, M.W. The Ghrelin/GOAT system regulates obesity-induced inflammation in male mice. *Endocrinology* **2017**, *158*, 2179–2189. [CrossRef] [PubMed]
34. Qu, R.; Chen, X.; Hu, J.; Fu, Y.; Peng, J.; Li, Y.; Chen, J.; Li, P.; Liu, L.; Cao, J.; et al. Ghrelin protects against contact dermatitis and psoriasiform skin inflammation by antagonizing TNF-α/NF-κB signaling pathways. *Sci. Rep.* **2019**, *9*, 1348. [CrossRef]
35. Maldonado-Ruiz, R.; Montalvo-Martínez, L.; Fuentes-Mera, L.; Camacho, A. Microglia activation due to obesity programs metabolic failure leading to type two diabetes. *Nutr. Diabetes* **2017**, *7*, e254. [CrossRef]
36. Muhammad, T.; Ikram, M.; Ullah, R.; Rehman, S.; Kim, M. Hesperetin, a Citrus flavonoid, attenuates lps-induced neuroinflammation, apoptosis and memory impairments by modulating TLR4/NF-κB signaling. *Nutrients* **2019**, *11*, 648. [CrossRef] [PubMed]
37. Levkovitz, Y.; Mendlovich, S.; Riwkes, S.; Braw, Y.; Levkovitch-Verbin, H.; Gal, G.; Fennig, S.; Treves, I.; Kron, S. A Double-blind, randomized study of minocycline for the treatment of negative and cognitive symptoms in early-phase schizophrenia. *J. Clin. Psychiatry* **2010**, *71*, 138–149. [CrossRef]

38. Ziko, I.; de Luca, S.; Dinan, T.; Barwood, J.M.; Sominsky, L.; Cai, G.; Kenny, R.; Stokes, L.; Jenkins, T.A.; Spencer, S.J. Neonatal overfeeding alters hypothalamic microglial profiles and central responses to immune challenge long-term. *Brain. Behav. Immun.* **2014**, *41*, 32–43. [CrossRef]

39. Van Niekerk, G.; Isaacs, A.W.; Nell, T.; Engelbrecht, A.-M. Sickness-Associated Anorexia: Mother Nature's Idea of Immunonutrition? *Mediators Inflamm.* **2016**, *2016*, 1–12. [CrossRef] [PubMed]

40. Wisse, B.E.; Ogimoto, K.; Tang, J.; Harris, M.K.; Raines, E.W.; Schwartz, M.W. Evidence that lipopolysaccharide-induced anorexia depends upon central, rather than peripheral, inflammatory signals. *Endocrinology* **2007**, *148*, 5230–5237. [CrossRef]

41. Djogo, T.; Robins, S.C.; Schneider, S.; Kryzskaya, D.; Liu, X.; Mingay, A.; Gillon, C.J.; Kim, J.H.; Storch, K.-F.; Boehm, U.; et al. Adult NG2-glia are required for median eminence-mediated leptin sensing and body weight control. *Cell Metab.* **2016**, *23*, 797–810. [CrossRef]

42. Thaler, J.; Yi, C.; Schur, E.; Guyenet, S.; Hwang, B.; Dietrich, M.; Zhao, X.; Sarruf, D.; Izgur, V.; Maravilla, K.; et al. Obesity is associated with hypothalamic injury in rodents and humans. *J. Clin. Investig.* **2011**, *122*, 153. [CrossRef]

43. Morton, G.J.; Meek, T.H.; Schwartz, M.W. Neurobiology of food intake in health and disease. *Nat. Rev. Neurosci.* **2014**, *15*, 367–378. [CrossRef] [PubMed]

44. Rodriguez-Navas, C.; Morselli, E.; Clegg, D.J. Sexually dimorphic brain fatty acid composition in low and high fat diet-fed mice. *Mol. Metab.* **2016**, *5*, 680–689. [CrossRef] [PubMed]

45. Spinelli, M.; Fusco, S.; Mainardi, M.; Scala, F.; Natale, F.; Lapenta, R.; Mattera, A.; Rinaudo, M.; Puma, D.D.L.; Ripoli, C.; et al. Brain insulin resistance impairs hippocampal synaptic plasticity and memory by increasing GluA1 palmitoylation through FoxO3a. *Nat. Commun.* **2017**, *8*, 2009. [CrossRef]

46. Kang, M.; Lee, A.; Yoo, H.J.; Kim, M.; Kim, M.; Shin, D.Y.; Lee, J.H. Association between increased visceral fat area and alterations in plasma fatty acid profile in overweight subjects: a cross-sectional study. *Lipids Health Dis.* **2017**, *16*, 248. [CrossRef]

47. Dumas, J.A.; Bunn, J.Y.; Nickerson, J.; Crain, K.I.; Ebenstein, D.B.; Tarleton, E.K.; Makarewicz, J.; Poynter, M.E.; Kien, C.L. Dietary saturated fat and monounsaturated fat have reversible effects on brain function and the secretion of pro-inflammatory cytokines in young women. *Metabolism* **2016**, *65*, 1582–1588. [CrossRef]

48. Hsu, T.M.; Kanoski, S.E. Blood-brain barrier disruption: Mechanistic links between Western diet consumption and dementia. *Front. Aging Neurosci.* **2014**, *6*, 6. [CrossRef]

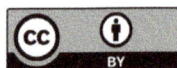

nutrients

MDPI

Article

SIRT1 Attenuates Kidney Disorders in Male Offspring Due to Maternal High-Fat Diet

Long T. Nguyen [1,*], Crystal H. Mak [2], Hui Chen [1,2], Amgad A. Zaky [1], Muh G. Wong [1], Carol A. Pollock [1] and Sonia Saad [1,2]

[1] Renal medicine, Kolling Institute, Royal North Shore Hospital, University of Sydney, Sydney, New South Wales 2065, Australia; hui.chen-1@uts.edu.au (H.C.); amgadadolf@hotmail.com (A.A.Z.); muhgeot.wong@sydney.edu.au (M.G.W.); carol.pollock@sydney.edu.au (C.A.P.); sonia.saad@sydney.edu.au (S.S.)

[2] School of Life Sciences, Faculty of Science, University of Technology Sydney, Sydney, New South Wales 2007, Australia; Crystal.H.Mak@student.uts.edu.au

[*] Correspondence: long.t.nguyen@sydney.edu.au; Tel.: +61-299-264-788

Received: 22 November 2018; Accepted: 8 January 2019; Published: 11 January 2019

Abstract: Maternal obesity has been associated with kidney disorders in male offspring. Our previous studies have demonstrated that Sirtuin (SIRT)1, an essential regulator of metabolic stress responses, is suppressed in the offspring as the result of maternal high-fat diet (HFD) consumption, which is likely to underpin the adverse metabolic and renal outcomes. To examine if SIRT1 overexpression or activation early in life can protect the offspring kidney, wild-type (WT) and transgenic (Tg) offspring were born to the same diet-induced obese female C57BL/6 mice through breeding with hemizygous SIRT1-transgenic (Tg) male mice and examined for renal pathological changes. In separate experiments, SIRT1 activator SRT1720 (25 mg/kg/2 days i.p) was administrated in WT offspring over 6 weeks of postnatal high-fat diet exposure. The results show that offspring born to obese dams have increased kidney weight, higher levels of renal triglycerides, and increased expression of oxidative stress, inflammatory, and fibrotic markers, as well as increased albuminuria compared to offspring of control dams. Both SIRT1 overexpression and SRT1720 treatment attenuated renal lipid contents and expression of lipogenesis, oxidative stress, and inflammatory markers; however, fibrosis was modestly reduced and albuminuria was not affected. The findings suggest that SIRT1 therapy can ameliorate some pathological mechanisms of kidney programming due to maternal obesity but may not be sufficient to prevent the resulting chronic kidney injury.

Keywords: Obesity; chronic kidney disease; foetal programming; sirtuin

---

1. Introduction

Obesity is a global health concern due to its prevalence and impact on the development of various diseases such as type 2 diabetes and hypertension, as well as secondary comorbidities including chronic kidney diseases (CKD). In obese people, the levels of circulating lipid and fatty acids are much higher than in non-obese individuals and can thus accumulate into non-adipose tissues such as heart, liver, pancreas, and kidney. Renal lipid accumulation or 'lipotoxicity' has been suggested to be the direct cause of structural and functional changes in mesangial cells, podocytes, and tubular cells [1,2], leading to obesity-related nephropathy [3]. Additionally, obesity-mediated diabetes and hypertension also contribute to the development of CKD.

Recent evidence suggests that the effects of obesity on CKD can also be intergenerational due to intrauterine foetal programming. Maternal obesity and high-fat diet consumption during pregnancy have been found to not only result in metabolic disorders such as glucose intolerance, insulin resistance, hyperlipidaemia, and hepatic steatosis [4–7], but also disrupt renal lipid metabolism and induce oxidative stress [8], albuminuria, glomerulosclerosis, and tubulointerstitial fibrosis in the offspring [9]. The molecular mechanisms and mediating factors of such intergenerational effects are still poorly understood.

Our recent studies suggest that Sirtuin (SIRT)1, an essential regulator of metabolism and stress responses [10,11], may play an important role in maternal obesity-induced foetal programming [12], particularly metabolic disorders such as insulin resistance and hepatic steatosis [8,13]. In kidney, we have shown in a rat model that SIRT1 expression is suppressed in male offspring born to obese dams in association with increased renal lipid accumulation [8]. SIRT1 is known to promote lipid catabolism in muscle and liver by activating peroxisome proliferator-activated receptor gamma coactivator 1 alpha (PGC-1α) [14,15], an essential regulator of mitochondria biosynthesis and fatty acid oxidation, while suppressing de novo lipogenesis through sterol regulatory element-binding protein (SREBP)-1c, carbohydrate-responsive element-binding protein (ChREBP), and peroxisome proliferator-activated receptor gamma (PPARγ) [16,17], leading to attenuated lipotoxicity. SIRT1-deficient mice have elevated kidney inflammation [18] and urinary albumin excretion [19]. SIRT1 activation by SRT1720 increases the expression of antioxidant enzymes including superoxide dismutase (SOD), glutathione peroxidase (GPx-1), and glutathione, leading to attenuated levels of fibrotic injury due to unilateral ureteral obstruction (UUO) [20]. With regard to CKD, SIRT1 activation by resveratrol increases (SOD)2 expression and reduces the levels of oxidative stress markers 8-OHdg and nitrotyrosine in a mouse model of type 2 diabetes [21]. Likewise, SIRT1 transgenic mice demonstrate ameliorated diabetic nephropathy [19].

As such, we hypothesised that upregulation of SIRT1 signalling at early postnatal ages will improve the male offspring's renal outcomes. In this study, using two different models, we confirm the protective roles of SIRT1 in foetal kidney programming due to maternal obesity.

2. Methods

2.1. Animals

The study was approved by the Animal Care and Ethics Committee of the University of Sydney (RESP/15/22). All methods were performed in accordance with the relevant guidelines and regulations in the Australian Code of Practice for the Care and Use of Animals for Scientific Purposes. Female C57BL/6 mice (8 weeks) or SIRT1 transgenic (SIRT1-Tg) mice were fed a high-fat diet (HFD, 20 kJ/g, 43.5% calorie as fat, Specialty Feed, Glen Forrest, WA, Australia) or standard rodent chow (11 kJ/g, 14% calorie as fat, Gordon's Speciality Stockfeeds, Yanderra, NSW, Australia) for 6 weeks before mating and throughout gestation and lactation [6]. As our previous showed sex-specific regulation of SIRT1 by maternal HFD, all female mice were culled on postnatal day (P) 1 and male mice were adjusted to 4-6 pups/ litter.

In the first experiments, wild-type (WT) female mice were mated with Tg male mice to produce both WT and Tg offspring without maternal genotypic modification (Figure 1A). Three main groups were studied: WT offspring born to control dams (MC, $n = 20$), WT offspring born to HFD-fed dams (MHF, $n = 26$), and Tg offspring born to HFD-fed dams (MHFS, $n = 11$). The original Tg colony was a generous gift from Dr. Lindsay Wu (University of New South Wales, Australia). Mice were genotyped in accordance to the Jackson Laboratory genotyping protocol for the B6.Cg-Col1a1[tm1(CAG-Sirt1)Dsin]/Mmjax strain using crude DNA extracted with DirectPCR Lysis Reagent (Mouse Tail) (Viagen Biotech, California, USA) and culled at weaning (P20) for kidney studies. In the second experiments, male offspring from chow or HFD-fed WT breeders (MC and MHF, respectively) were fed chow or HFD from P20 to week 9 (OC and OHF, respectively). Animals born to HFD-fed dams and/or fed on HFD themselves were administered a low dose of SIRT1 activator SRT1720 (S, 25 mg/kg/2 days i.p, Selleckchem, Houston, TX, USA) or vehicle control (Figure 1B). The experimental design resulted in five groups: MC/OC ($n = 9$), MC/OHF ($n = 17$), MHF/OHF ($n = 15$), MC/OHF/S ($n = 9$), and MHF/OHF/S ($n = 9$). These offspring were culled at week 9.

All pups were deeply anaesthetised with 3% isoflurane and euthanised upon cardiac puncture for blood collection after 5h fasting. Phosphate-buffered saline (PBS, 1%) was used for whole body perfusion. Tissues were snapped frozen and stored at −80 °C or fixed in neutral buffered formalin (10%) for approximately 36 h for later analyses.

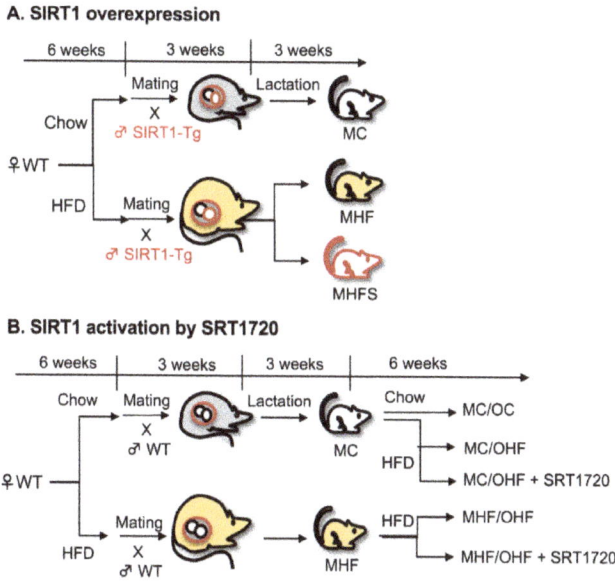

Figure 1. Animal models of SIRT1 overexpression (**A**) and activation (**B**) in offspring. SIRT: sirtuin; MC: offspring of chow-fed dams; MHF: offspring of HFD-fed dams; MHFS: MHF offspring with SIRT1 overexpression. OC: chow-fed offspring; OHF: HFD-fed offspring; WT: wild-type; Tg: transgenic, HFD: high-fat diet.

2.2. Urine Collection and Urinary Albumin Creatinine Ratio Analysis

The urine of P20 offspring was collected directly from the bladder during culling, while that of week 9 offspring was collected after a 24-h stay in metabolic cages. The urine was stored in −80 °C and examined for creatinine (Cayman, MI, USA) and albumin (Abcam, VIC, Australia) according to the manufacturers' instructions. Urinary albumin creatinine ratio (UACR) was used to account for potential differences in hydration in the animal cohort.

2.3. Protein and Lipid Extraction from Tissues

The tissues were homogenized in Triton X-100 lysis buffer (pH 7.4, 150 mM NaOH, 50 mM Tris-HCl, 1% Triton X-100, Roche protease inhibitor) using TissueRuptor (Qiagen, Hilden, Germany). Lipid and protein were extracted and the concentration was measured according to our previously published protocols [8] using Roche triglyceride reagent GPO-PAP (Roche Life Science, NSW, Australia) and Pierce BCA Protein Assay Kit (Thermo Scientific, VIC, Australia) according to the manufacturer's instructions. Lipid concentrations were normalised to the weight of tissue homogenized. Protein concentrations were standardised to 5 µg/µL.

2.4. Quantitative RT-PCR

Total RNA of renal tissues was isolated using RNeasy Plus Mini Kit (Qiagen Pty Ltd., CA, USA) according to the manufacturer's instructions, while fat tissues and hypothalamus's RNA were extracted using Trizol Reagent (Sigma-Aldrich). The purified total RNA was used as a template to generate first-strand cDNA using the First Strand cDNA Synthesis Kit (Roche Life Science, NSW, Australia). The amplicons of target genes were amplified with SYBR Green probes (iTaq Universal SYBR Green Supermix, Bio-Rad, NSW, Australia) using an ABI Prism 7900 HT Sequence Detection System (Applied Biosystems, CA, USA). Primers were as per our previous publications [8,13]. Gene expression was standardized to β-actin mRNA and log-transformed.

2.5. Immunoblotting

The proteins were electrophoresed and electroblotted onto the Hybond nitrocellulose membrane (Amersham Pharmacia Biotech, Amersham, UK), which were then incubated with a primary antibody at 4 °C overnight. The primary antibodies used for immunoblotting included manganese superoxide dismutase (MnSOD, rabbit, dilution 1:2000, EMD Millipore, North Ryde, NSW, Australia) and GPx-1 (goat, dilution 1:500, R&D System, Minneapolis, MN, USA). β-actin (goat, dilution 1:3000, Santa Cruz, TX, USA) was used as the housekeeping protein. Subsequently, the membrane were incubated with a horseradish peroxidase-conjugated secondary antibodies (1:5000, Cell Signalling, MA, USA). The immunoblots were developed by adding the Luminata Western HRP Substrates (Millipore, MA, USA) to the membrane and exposed for an appropriate duration using ImageQuant LAS 4000 (Fujifilm, Tokyo, Japan). ImageJ (National Institutes of Health, USA) was used for densitometric analyses.

2.6. SIRT1 Activity Assay

Nuclear protein was extracted according to the protocol 'Nuclear protein extraction without the use of detergent (Sigma-Aldrich, Dublin, Ireland) using a hypotonic lysis buffer (10 mM 4-(2-hydroxyethyl)-1-piperazineethanesulfonic acid (HEPES), pH 7.9, with 1.5 mM MgCl2 and 10 mM KCl, 1 mM Dithiothreitol), followed by centrifuge to separate nuclear and cytoplasmic fractions. The nuclear proteins were extracted using extraction buffer (20 mM HEPES, pH 7.9, with 1.5 mM MgCl2, 0.42 M NaCl, 0.2 mM EDTA, 25% (v/v) glycerol, 1 mM Dithiothreitol). No protease inhibitor was used in the extraction to avoid interference with SIRT1 activity measurement. SIRT1 activity was then measured using the SIRT1 activity assay kit (Abcam, Cambridge, UK) as per manufacturer's instruction.

2.7. Immunohistochemistry

Immunohistochemistry (IHC) staining was performed as previously described [8]. Briefly, tissues were fixed in 10% formalin for 36-h and embedded in paraffin or frozen-embedded in OCT solution (Tissue-Tek). Paraffin sections were prepared at a 4-µm thickness and mounted on microscope slides (Trajan Scientific and Medical, VIC, Australia). Antigen retrieval was performed at 99 °C for 20 min in 0.01 M, pH 6.0 citric buffer. Endogenous peroxidase was deactivated with 3% H2O2 (Sigma-Aldrich, Dublin, Ireland). The slides were then blocked by Protein Block Serum-Free (Dako, Glostrup, Denmark), and incubated with one of the primary antibodies, which included Fibronectin, Collagen type I (dilution 1:750, Abcam, Cambridge, UK), and 8-hydroxy-2′ -deoxyguanosine (8-OHdg, dilution 1:200, Cell Signalling Technology, MA, USA). After overnight incubation at 4 °C, biotinylated secondary anti-rabbit IgG antibodies (Dako) were incubated for 30 mins and finally horseradish peroxidase (HRP)-conjugated streptavidin (Dako) for 10 mins. Using a light microscope (Leica DM750 photomicroscope with ICC50W digital camera), six consecutive non-overlapping fields from each kidney section were photographed at 20× magnification. Image J (National Institutes of Health, USA) was used to quantitate the staining area percentage.

2.8. Statistical Analysis

Data are expressed as column (mean ± SEM) or box plots (25th to 75th percentiles, whisker extends from the minimum to the maximum value). One-way ANOVA followed by Bonferroni post-hoc tests were used.

3. Results

3.1. SIRT1 Overexpression Suppresses Renal Lipid Accumulation in MHF Offspring

As can be seen from Figure 2A,B, WT offspring born to dams fed a HFD showed increased kidney weight ($p < 0.001$) and triglyceride levels ($p < 0.01$), which were reversed by SIRT1 overexpression in the MHFS mice ($p < 0.01$ and $p < 0.05$, respectively). No changes in the percentages of kidney weight per body weight were found. The mRNA and protein expression, as well as activity of SIRT1 in the offspring kidney in this study was significantly reduced by MHF ($p < 0.05$, Figure 2B). Consistently, the mRNA expression of PGC-1α was downregulated ($p < 0.05$) and that of ChREBP and SREBP-1c was upregulated ($p < 0.05$, Figure 2C). Increased expression of SIRT1 was confirmed in MHFS mice by both qRT-PCR and immunoblot ($p < 0.001$ and $p < 0.05$, respectively). SIRT1 activity were significantly increased in MHFS offspring ($p < 0.05$, Figure 2B). SIRT1 overexpression in MHFS offspring significantly increased PGC-1α expression and suppressed ChREBP ($p < 0.01$) but had no effect on SREBP-1c.

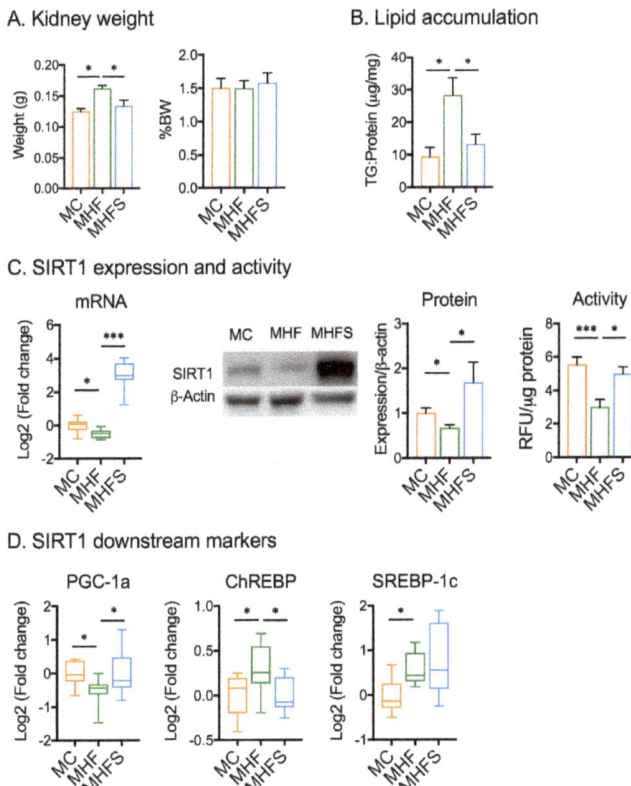

Figure 2. SIRT1 overexpression reduces kidney weight and lipid accumulation in offspring born to obese dams. (**A**) Kidney weight ($n = 11$–26). (**B**) Kidney triglyceride level ($n = 6$). (**C**) SIRT1 expression and activity ($n = 6$). (**D**) The expression of downstream markers of SIRT1 ($n = 6$). Data are expressed by mean ± SEM or box plot (min to max, the central lines indicate the median). SIRT: sirtuin; PGC-1α: peroxisome proliferator-activated receptor gamma coactivator 1 alpha; SREBP-1c: sterol regulatory element-binding protein, ChREBP: carbohydrate-responsive element-binding protein; MC: offspring of chow-fed dams; MHF: offspring of HFD-fed dams; MHFS: MHF offspring with SIRT1 overexpression. * $p < 0.05$, *** $p < 0.001$.

3.2. SIRT1 Overexpression Suppresses Renal Oxidative Stress and Inflammation Markers in MHF Offspring

WT offspring born to HFD-fed dams showed increased renal expression of inducible nitric oxide synthase (iNOS, $p < 0.05$) and prostaglandin-endoperoxide synthase (COX2, $p < 0.05$, Figure 3A), indicating increased production of reactive nitrogen and oxygen species (RNS and ROS, respectively). Concomitantly, the protein expression of antioxidant enzymes MnSOD but not GPx-1 was suppressed ($p < 0.05$, Figure 3B). 8-OHdG, which indicates oxidative damage of the DNA, was significantly increased due to MHF ($p < 0.01$, Figure 3C). SIRT1 overexpression in MHFS offspring normalised MnSOD protein expression ($p < 0.05$), and suppressed 8-OHdG accumulation ($p < 0.05$), suggesting reduced oxidative stress.

A. ROS and RNS production

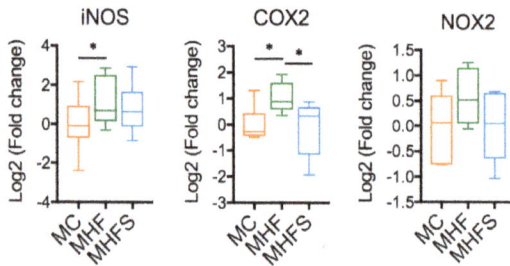

B. Antioxidant defence

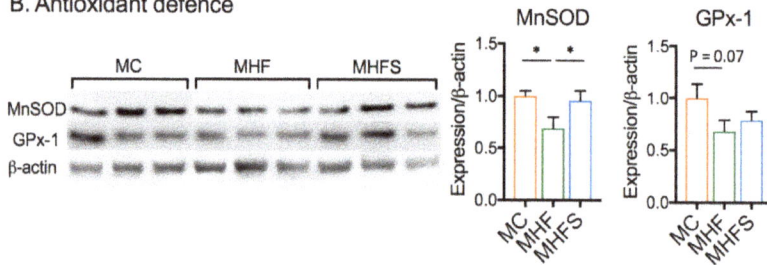

C. DNA oxidative damage

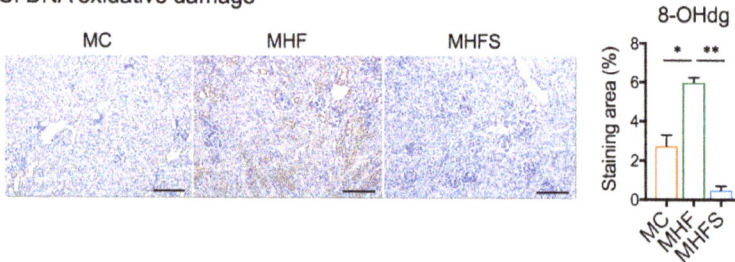

Figure 3. SIRT1 overexpression attenuates renal oxidative stress in offspring born to obese dams. (**A**) mRNA expression of oxidative stress markers ($n = 6$). (**B**) Protein expression of antioxidant enzymes. (**C**) Immunohistochemistry (IHC) staining and quantification of 8-hydroxy-2′-deoxyguanosine (8-OHdG) ($n = 6$). Data are presented as mean ± SEM or box plot (min to max, the central lines indicate the median). SIRT: sirtuin; iNOS inducible nitric oxide synthase; COX2: prostaglandin-endoperoxide synthase; NOX: NADPH oxidase; MnSOD: manganese superoxide dismutase; GPx: Glutathione peroxidase; MC: Offspring of chow-fed dams; MHF: offspring of HFD-fed dams; MHFS: MHF offspring with SIRT1 overexpression. * $p < 0.05$, ** $p < 0.01$.

3.3. SIRT1 Overexpression Attenuates Renal Inflammation but not Albuminuria in MHF Offspring

The mRNA expression of inflammation markers including Macrophage chemotactic protein (MCP)-1 and Tumour necrosis factor alpha (TNF)α were upregulated in MHF offspring ($p < 0.05$, Figure 4A). The expression of F4/80, a macrophage marker, was also significantly elevated ($p < 0.05$, Figure 4A). SIRT1 overexpression significantly suppressed the expression of F4/80 ($p < 0.05$) but not MCP-1 and TNFα.

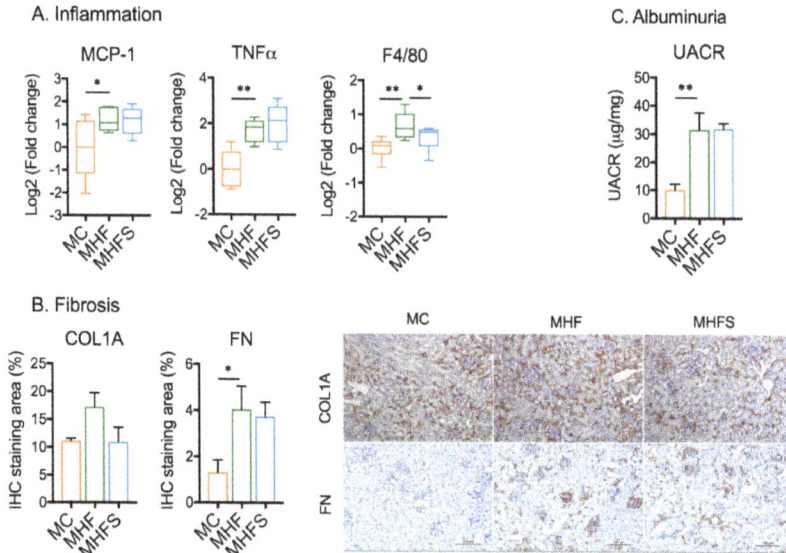

Figure 4. SIRT1 overexpression reduces markers of macrophage but not fibrosis and albuminuria in offspring born to obese dams. (**A**) mRNA expression of inflammation. (**B**) IHC staining quantification of fibrotic markers ($n = 6$). (**C**) Urinary albumin creatinine ratio UACR ($n = 6$). Data are presented as mean ± SEM or box plot (min to max, the central lines indicate the median). MCP: Macrophage chemotactic protein; TNFα: Tumour necrosis factor alpha; COL: collagen; FN: fibronectin. MC: offspring of chow-fed dams; MHF: offspring of HFD-fed dams; MHFS: MHF offspring with SIRT1 overexpression. * $p < 0.05$, ** $p < 0.01$.

The protein expression of COL1A was not significantly changed despite a trend to increase at this early age (Figure 4B). In contrast, fibronectin FN deposition particularly in glomeruli was increased by MHF ($p < 0.05$), suggesting increased fibrogenesis. As a likely result, UACR was significantly elevated ($p < 0.01$, Figure 4C), reflecting albuminuria. Despite attenuation of oxidative and inflammatory markers, SIRT1 overexpression had no significant effects on the expression of both markers, as well as UACR.

3.4. SRT1720 Attenuates Renal Lipogenesis in Offspring Due to Maternal and Postnatal HFD Consumption

At postnatal week 9, offspring fed a HFD for 6 weeks (OHF) had increased kidney net weight ($p < 0.01$) in comparison to chow-fed offspring (Figure 5A). Maternal HFD consumption exacerbated this effect ($p < 0.01$). Kidney weight/body weight ratio and kidney triglyceride levels were only increased in offspring exposed to both maternal and postnatal HFD ($p < 0.05$, Figure 5B), suggesting the significant contribution of maternal HFD consumption to offspring's kidney lipid metabolism. SIRT1's mRNA expression, protein expression, and activity were significantly decreased due to OHF ($p < 0.05$, Figure 5C). There was no further reduction in MHF/OHF offspring. In contrast to our expectation, PGC-1 α expression was increased by OHF ($p < 0.05$, Figure 5D). ChREBP mRNA expression was significantly increased in MC/OHF offspring ($p < 0.05$). SREBP-1c levels were unchanged. There was no additive effects from MHF on the regulation of these markers.

A. Kidney weight
B. Lipid accumulation

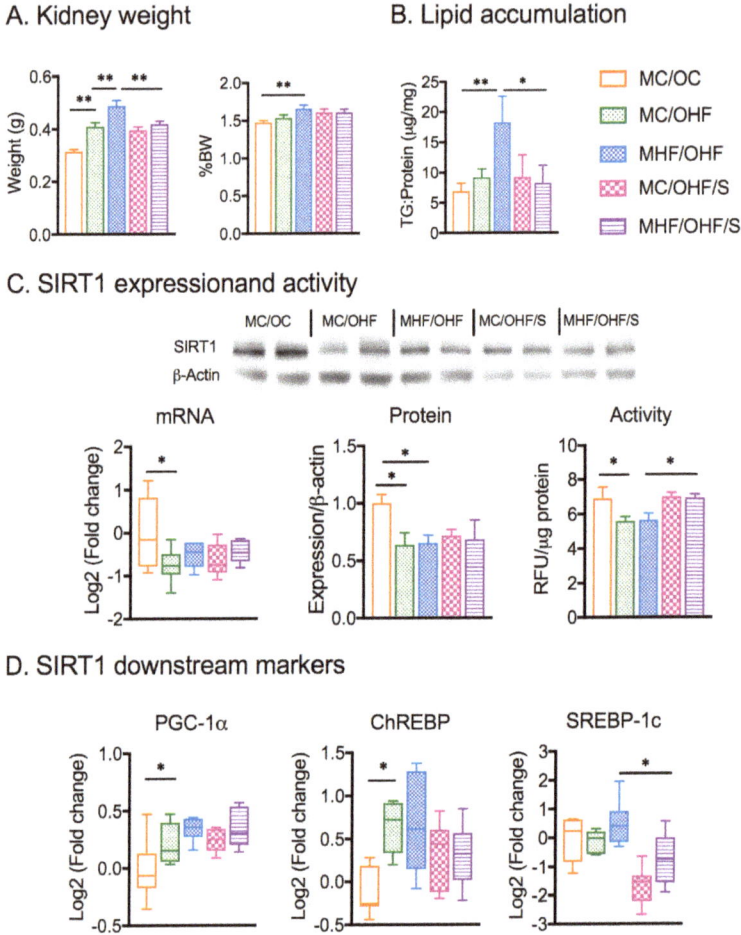

C. SIRT1 expressionand activity

D. SIRT1 downstream markers

Figure 5. SRT1720 suppresses renal lipid accumulation in offspring due to maternal and postnatal HFD consumption. (**A**). Kidney weight ($n = 9$–17). (**B**) Kidney triglyceride level ($n = 8$). (**C**) SIRT1 expression and activity. (**D**) mRNA expression of SIRT1 downstream markers ($n = 8$). Data are expressed by mean ± SEM or box plot (min to max, the central lines indicate the median). SIRT: sirtuin; PGC-1α: peroxisome proliferator-activated receptor gamma coactivator 1 alpha; SREBP-1c: sterol regulatory element-binding protein, ChREBP: carbohydrate-responsive element-binding protein; MC: offspring of chow-fed dams; OC: chow-fed offspring; MHF: offspring of HFD-fed dams; OHF: HFD-fed offspring; S: SRT1720. * $p < 0.05$, ** $p < 0.01$.

SRT1720 administration significantly reduced kidney net weight ($p < 0.01$, Figure 5A) and renal level of triglycerides ($p < 0.05$, Figure 5B) in MHF/OHF/S offspring. As expected, the agonist did not increase mRNA or protein expression of SIRT1 but normalised its activity in these offspring ($p < 0.05$ Figure 5C). Such increase was associated with reduced mRNA expression of SREBP-1c ($p < 0.05$, Figure 5D). However, no significant changes were found in the expression of the other two downstream markers.

3.5. SRT1720 Suppresses Renal Oxidative Stress and Inflammation Markers in Offspring Due to Maternal and Postnatal HFD Consumption

In contrast to P20, no changes in mRNA expression of iNOS and COX2 in the offspring kidney were found in the offspring born to obese dams and/or fed a postnatal HFD in comparison to the control MC/OC (Figure 6A). However, the expression of NADPH oxidase (NOX)2 was significantly increased ($p < 0.01$). On the other hand, MnSOD and GPx-1 protein expression was not significantly changed, demonstrating a trend to adaptation of antioxidant defence in the offspring in adolescent following postnatal HFD exposure (Figure 6B). 8-OHdG accumulation was significantly higher in the offspring from HFD-fed dams compared to the control group ($p < 0.01$, Figure 6C), reflecting increased DNA oxidative damage despite normal antioxidant levels. SRT1720 treatment significantly suppressed renal expression of NOX2 in MHF/OHF/S offspring ($p < 0.05$). In line with NOX2 expression, the levels of 8-OHdG were significantly suppressed by SRT1720 treatment ($p < 0.05$, Figure 6B), suggesting ameliorated oxidative stress.

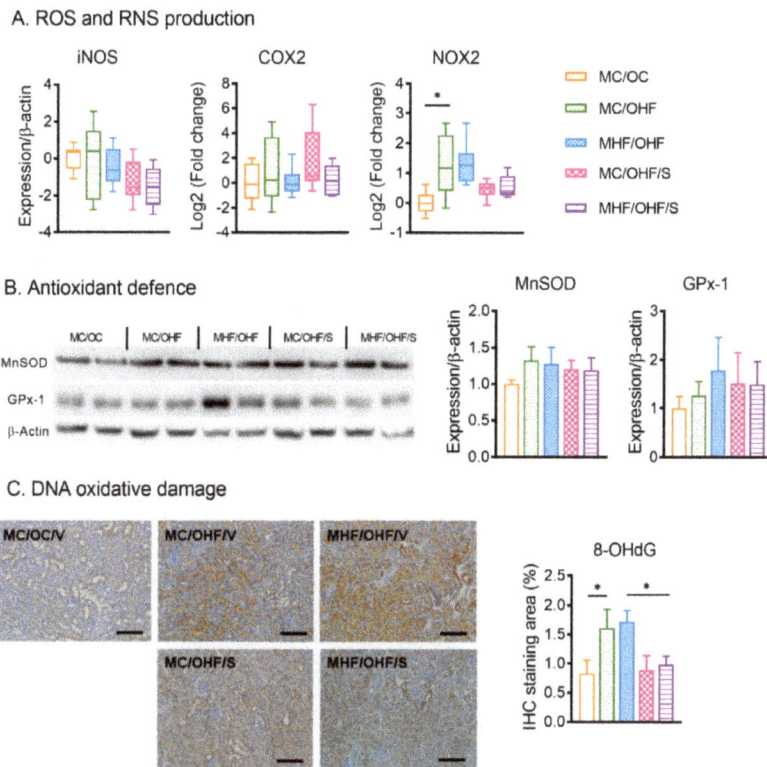

Figure 6. SRT1720 attenuates renal oxidative stress in offspring due to maternal and postnatal HFD consumption. (**A**) mRNA expression of oxidative stress markers ($n = 8$). (**B**) Protein expression of antioxidant enzymes ($n = 8$). (**C**) IHC staining and quantification of 8-hydroxy-2'-deoxyguanosine (8-OHdG) ($n = 8$). Data are presented as mean ± SEM or box plot (min to max, the central lines indicate the median). iNOS inducible nitric oxide synthase; COX2: prostaglandin-endoperoxide synthase; NOX: NADPH oxidase; MnSOD: manganese superoxide dismutase; GPx: Glutathione peroxidase; MC: offspring of chow-fed dams; OC: chow-fed offspring; MHF: offspring of HFD-fed dams; OHF: HFD-fed offspring; V or VEH: vehicle control; S or SRT: SRT1720. * $p < 0.05$.

3.6. SRT1720 Attenuates Renal Fibrogenesis but not Albuminuria in Offspring Due to Maternal and Postnatal HFD Consumption

Maternal HFD consumption significantly increased the expression of inflammation marker MCP-1 (vs MC/OHF, $p < 0.05$) and macrophage marker F4/80 (vs MC/OC, $p < 0.05$) in the offspring (Figure 7A). SRT1720 significantly suppressed MCP-1 ($p < 0.05$), TNFα ($p < 0.01$), and F4/80 ($p < 0.05$) mRNA levels. Consistent with the results at weaning, maternal HFD consumption significantly exacerbated renal extracellular matrix (ECM) deposition of COL1A ($p < 0.05$) and FN ($p < 0.05$) in offspring in adolescence (Figure 7B). Such an effect was not evident in animals exposed to postnatal HFD only. SRT1720 administration suppressed the expression of COL1A ($p < 0.05$) but not FN ($p < 0.05$) in MHF/OHF offspring. In line with the changes of fibrotic markers, UACR was significantly elevated by postnatal HFD with and without maternal HFD pre-exposure ($p < 0.01$, Figure 7C). The increase was modulated by SRT1720 treatment only in MC/OHF/S offspring ($p < 0.05$).

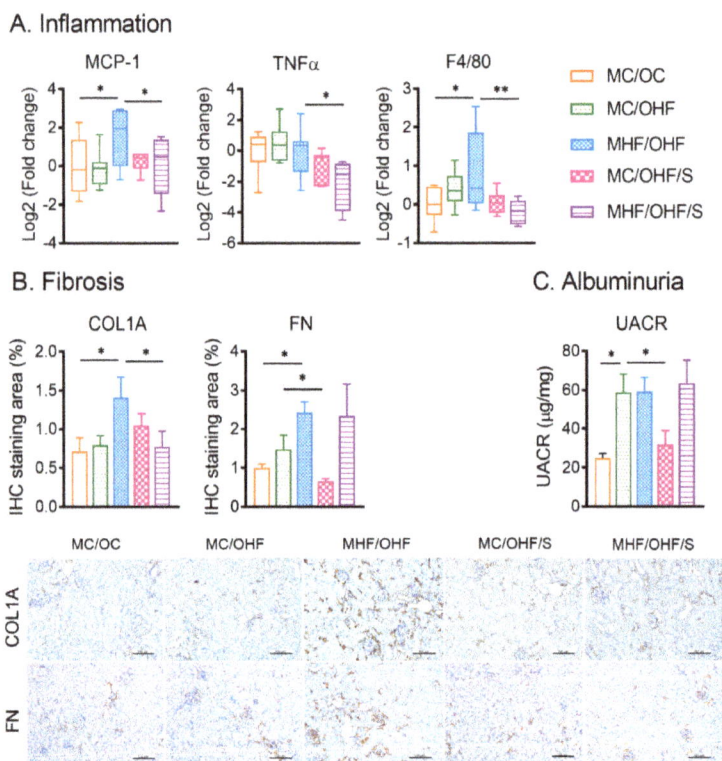

Figure 7. SRT1720 attenuates renal inflammation and fibrosis but not the urinary albumin creatinine ratio in offspring due to maternal and postnatal HFD consumption. (**A**) mRNA expression of inflammatory markers. (**B**) Immunohistochemistry quantification of fibrotic markers ($n = 8$). (**C**) Urinary albumin creatinine ratio UACR ($n = 8$). Data are presented as mean ± SEM. MCP: Macrophage chemotactic protein; TNFα: Tumour necrosis factor alpha; COL: collagen; FN: fibronectin. MC: offspring of chow-fed dams; OC: chow-fed offspring; MHF: offspring of HFD-fed dams; OHF: HFD-fed offspring; S: SRT1720. * $p < 0.05$, ** $p < 0.01$.

4. Discussion

Maternal obesity is a risk factor of metabolic disorders such as diabetes and hyperlipidaemia in the offspring, which in turn can contribute to the early development and progression of CKD. In the present study, we confirm that maternal high-fat consumption-induced obesity can lead to increased lipid accumulation, oxidative stress, inflammation, and fibrosis in the offspring at weaning and adolescence. Importantly, these pathological changes are associated with reduced SIRT1 expression and activity. The upregulation of SIRT1 signalling by means of genetic modification or administration of SIRT1 agonist SRT1720 is found to attenuate renal lipid deposition, oxidative stress, and inflammation but not fibrosis and albuminuria due to maternal obesity.

It is noteworthy that we have also examined metabolic disorders in the same model and showed that offspring born to obese dams had increased body weight, hyperlipidaemia and hyperglycaemia at weaning [13] and adolescence [22], which were significantly reversed by SIRT1 overexpression/activation. As these metabolic disorders are important risk factors of CKD, the improvements in systemic glucose and lipid metabolism by SIRT1 may also contribute to the attenuated kidney disorders due to maternal HFD in the offspring. A future study using kidney-specific SIRT1 overexpression mice is required to clarify its direct and indirect effects.

In kidney, SIRT1 overexpression in MHFS offspring led to the recovered expression of PGC-1α, as well as the suppression of ChREBP. On the other hand, SRT1720 administration suppressed SREBP1 expression. PGC-1α is involved in mitochondrial biosynthesis and fatty acid oxidation [23,24]. Defective expression of fatty acid oxidation genes including PGC-1α in renal tubular epithelial cells has been implicated in the development of kidney fibrosis [25,26]. ChREBP and SREBP1 have been shown to be up-regulated in the kidney of diabetic mice [27–29]. The ablation of either protein was able to prevent lipotoxicity, oxidative stress, inflammation, fibrosis, and albuminuria. The results provide corroborative evidence as to the significance of SIRT1 signalling in the regulation of renal lipotoxicity and nephropathy due to maternal obesity.

Oxidative stress is induced by the imbalance between the production of reactive oxygen/nitrogen species (ROS/RNS) and antioxidant capacity. Elevated oxidative stress has been suggested to be the major instigator of diabetic nephropathy [30], leading to glomerular inflammation and tubulointerstitial fibrosis. In this study, in concert with increased lipid accumulation, MHF offspring have elevated renal oxidative stress, as reflected by the increased levels of iNOS, COX2, and 8-OHdG, as well as reduction of MnSOD at weaning. In adolescence, NOX2 and 8-OHdG were elevated. The increases in iNOS and 8-OHdG are consistent with our previous studies [8,31]. Particularly, iNOS has been characterised as one of the earliest effects of diabetes on kidney [32]. iNOS is a major source of nitric oxide (NO), while NO tends to be deficient in the advanced stages of CKD [33], which may explain the unchanged expression of iNOS at week 9. MnSOD levels were recovered at week 9, likely due to a compensatory effect to prolonged oxidative stress. The result is in line with a previous study by Ruggerio et al. [34], in which they fed C57BL/6 mice a HFD for 12 or 16 weeks and found an adaptation of mitochondrial biogenesis, antioxidant and respiratory machinery in the kidney despite the evident of oxidative stress. Indeed, PGC-1α, the pivotal regulator of mitochondrial biogenesis, was also increased in the offspring following postnatal HFD exposure in our study. No additive effects were induced by maternal HFD consumption with regard to oxidative stress markers, suggesting the parts of the maternal effects have been overwhelmed by postnatal HFD. Such phenomenon has been demonstrated in our previous studies [35].

SIRT1 overexpression suppressed COX2 levels at weaning, which is in line with the study by Jung et al. showing a downregulation of COX2 in aged rat kidney following short-term caloric restriction [36]. In addition, SIRT1 overexpression/activation also normalised MnSOD expression and 8-OHdG accumulation at weaning, and suppressed NOX2 and 8-OHdG levels at week 9, thus confirming the protective effects of SIRT1 therapy against maternal obesity-induced kidney oxidative damage at different developmental stages. SIRT1 overexpression and activation had no effects on iNOS expression, which may suggest a less potent role of SIRT1 in modulation of nitrosative stress. The results also imply differences between SIRT1 overexpression and SRT1720 in their mechanisms to regulate oxidative stress.

Apart from oxidative stress, the study also showed significant increases in inflammatory markers including MCP-1 and F4/80. The elevated levels of renal fibrosis markers including COL1A and

Nutrients **2019**, *11*, 146

FN and albuminuria in offspring of HFD-fed dams at both weaning and week 9 are consistent with our previous reports, clearly confirming that maternal obesity contributes to the risk of CKD in offspring [8,31]. SIRT1 overexpression significantly suppressed F4/80, and SRT1720 treatment reduced MCP-1, TNFα, and F4/80 in the offspring exposed to maternal HFD, suggesting the anti-inflammatory effects of SIRT1 against maternal obesity-induced kidney inflammation. Although SIRT1 activation suppresses COL1A deposition in MHF/OHF/S offspring kidney in adolescence, FN levels were not affected. Similarly, although albuminuria by SRT1720 was reduced in the offspring on postnatal HFD, which is consistent with a previous study in diabetic animals [19], it persisted in those pre-exposed to maternal high-fat diet, suggesting that offspring affected by maternal obesity are likely to resist SIRT1 therapy regarding albuminuria. A combination with gestational weight control and other therapies may be necessary to increase the effectiveness. Besides, natural SIRT1 activators such as resveratrol, or NAD+precursors can be tested on humans to further investigate the clinical relevance of the therapy [37].

Collectively, the study demonstrates that SIRT1 plays essential roles in kidney programming, upregulation of which can partially suppresses renal lipid accumulation, oxidative stress, inflammation, and fibrogenesis in the offspring born to obese mothers. However, further studies are required to address persistent albuminuria.

Author Contributions: L.T.N. designed and conducted all main experiments, performed data analysis, prepared figures and wrote the manuscript. C.H.M. performed experiments and data analysis. A.A.Z. assisted with tissue processing for histology. M.G.W. assisted with renal pathology analysis. H.C, C.A.P., and S.S. coordinated the execution of the project and was involved in the experiment design. H.C, C.A.P., and S.S reviewed data analysis and the manuscript.

Funding: L.N. was supported by Sydney Medical School's ECR PhD Scholarship and Amgen research scholarship.

Acknowledgments: We acknowledge Lindsay Wu from The University of New South Wales, Australia for kindly sharing the SIRT1-transgenic colony.

Conflicts of Interest: The authors declare no conflict of interest.

Abbreviations

8-OHdg	8-hydroxy-2′-deoxyguanosine
ACEC	Animal Care and Ethics Committee
ChREBP	Carbohydrate response-element-binding protein
COL	Collagen
COX	Prostaglandin-endoperoxide synthase
ECM	Extracellular matrix
F4/80	Marker of macrophage
FN	Fibronectin
iNOS	Inducible nitric oxide synthase
HFD	High-fat diet
MCP-1	Macrophage chemotactic protein 1
MHF	Maternal high-fat diet consumption
NOX	NADPH oxidase
OHF	High-fat feeding in offspring
PGC-1α	Peroxisome proliferator-activated receptor gamma coactivator 1-α
PPAR	Peroxisome proliferator-activated receptors
ROS	Reactive oxygen species
SIRT	Silent information regulator
S	SRT1720
SREBP	Acetylated sterol regulatory element binding proteins
TNFα	Tumour necrosis factor α
UACR	Urine albumin/creatinine ratio
V	Vehicle control

MDPI

St. Alban-Anlage 66

4052 Basel

Switzerland

Tel. +41 61 683 77 34

Fax +41 61 302 89 18

www.mdpi.com

Nutrients Editorial Office

E-mail: nutrients@mdpi.com

www.mdpi.com/journal/nutrients